D1766952

The Library
Hadlow College
Hadlow
Tonbridge
Kent TN11 0AL
Tel: 01732 853245

Hadlow
college

Date of Return	Date of Return	Date of Return
ONE WEEK LOAN		
3 0 OCT 2012	ONE WEEK LOAN	
0 7 NOV 2012 ONE WEEK LOAN		
ONE WEEK LOAN		
1 6 OCT 2013		
2 2 JAN 2014		
ONE WEEK LOAN		
ONE OCT 2014 LOAN		
2 1 OCT 2014		
ONE WEEK LOAN		
5 OCT 2015		

This is a 7 day loan book
higher fines will be charged

Please note that fines will be charged if this book is returned late

EQUINE WOUND MANAGEMENT

Second Edition

EQUINE WOUND MANAGEMENT

Second Edition

Ted S. Stashak, DVM, MS, Diplomate ACVS, Professor Emeritus Equine Surgery
Department of Clinical Sciences
College of Veterinary Medicine and Biomedical Sciences
Colorado State University
Fort Collins, Colorado

Christine Theoret, DMV, PhD, Diplomate ACVS
Director, Comparative Tissue Healing Laboratory
Associate Professor
Département de biomédecine vétérinaire
Faculté de médecine vétérinaire
Université de Montréal
Saint-Hyacinthe, Québec

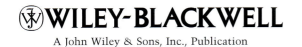

WILEY-BLACKWELL

A John Wiley & Sons, Inc., Publication

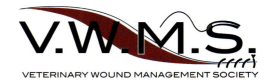

VETERINARY WOUND MANAGEMENT SOCIETY

First edition first published 1991
Second edition first published 2008
© 1991 Lea & Febiger
© 2008 Wiley-Blackwell

Blackwell Publishing was acquired by John Wiley & Sons in February 2007. Blackwell's publishing program has been merged with Wiley's global Scientific, Technical, and Medical business to form Wiley-Blackwell.

Editorial Office
2121 State Avenue, Ames, Iowa 50014-8300, USA

For details of our global editorial offices, for customer services, and for information about how to apply for permission to reuse the copyright material in this book, please see our website at www.wiley.com/wiley-blackwell.

Library of Congress Cataloguing-in-Publication Data

Equine wound management / [edited by] Ted S. Stashak, Christine Theoret. – 2nd ed.
    p. ; cm.
  Rev. ed. of: Equine wound management / Ted S. Stashak. 1991.
  Includes bibliographical references and index.
  ISBN-13: 978-0-8138-1223-6 (alk. paper)
  ISBN-10: 0-8138-1223-2 (alk. paper)
  1. Horses–Wounds and injuries–Treatment. 2. Horses–Surgery. I. Stashak, Ted S. II. Theoret, Christine.
III. Stashak, Ted S. Equine wound management.
  [DNLM: 1. Horses–injuries. 2. Horses–surgery. 3. Wounds and Injuries–therapy.
4. Wounds and Injuries–veterinary. SF 951 E647 2008]
  SF951.S77 2008
  636.1'08971–dc22

                                2008016810

A catalogue record for this book is available from the U.S. Library of Congress.

Set in 10 on 12 pt Palatino by SNP Best-set Typesetter Ltd., Hong Kong
Printed in Singapore by Markono Print Media Pte Ltd

Disclaimer

2 2010

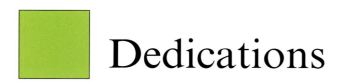

Dedications

To my wife, Gloria, and my children, Angela, Stephanie, and Ryan, for their love and untiring support.
To my parents, Theodore and Ann, for emphasizing the value of an education.

Ted S. Stashak

To my parents, Susan and André, for encouraging excellence.
Pour Alain qui me procure cet équilibre ô si bénéfique et pour Mozelle, Marek et Francesca qui me comble de leur allégresse!
Gràcies, en especial, a la Pilar i en Jordi per la seva visió positiva i generosa contribució en aquest llibre.

Christine Theoret

Table of Contents

Preface

The second edition of this textbook was long overdue. Indeed, since the first edition appeared in 1991, a number of ground-breaking studies have modernized the art of wound management in both human and veterinary patients. New topical medications, interactive dressings, and surgical procedures are now available, enabling veterinarians to treat serious injuries once deemed incurable. Moreover, research has shown, unequivocally, that many aspects of the horse's healing response are unique, such that a textbook dedicated to the art and science of wound management in this species would be a most valuable tool for equine practitioners. Subsequent to the recent publication of two journal volumes on this topic (*Clinical Techniques in Equine Practice*, June 2004, TS Stashak, guest editor; *Veterinary Clinics of North America*, April 2005, CL Theoret, guest editor), it seemed most opportune to provide readers with a single, comprehensive source of theoretical and practical information, enhanced by an abundance of helpful tables, line drawings, and color figures. Thus, the purpose of this book is to provide an authoritative, state-of-the-art text on equine wounds and their management.

The first chapter provides an update on the physiology of cutaneous wound healing, with a special focus on the newly discovered mediators that govern the mechanisms underlying repair. Horses have a distinctive response to trauma; therefore, the second section of the chapter endeavors to describe the major differences from the relatively normal healing profile of ponies. The chapter concludes with an enlightening discussion of innovative solutions to the specific problems encountered when dealing with a traumatic wound in a horse.

Chapter 2 addresses selected factors that can exert a negative impact on the physiologic mechanisms that contribute to repair. This is followed by a review of wound management practices that influence infection and healing. The chapter emphasizes the importance of thoroughly assessing the wound and the patient as well as various measures such as hemostasis, cleansing, debriding, and disinfecting the wound in the first few hours following injury. The subject is approached in the order in which a case involving a wound would be evaluated and managed clinically. Because infection is a major cause of delayed healing, this chapter emphasizes management practices that reduce its incidence.

The third chapter is devoted to topical wound treatments. It includes an updated list of dressings and wound-care products. The authors have prepared a number of valuable tables in an effort to guide the practitioner through the maze of commercially available products; they outline indications and suggest the best use for each. This chapter is enhanced by a new and separate section focusing on the use of biologic scaffolds engineered from the extracellular matrix as a potential therapeutic option for treating soft tissue injuries in veterinary medicine.

The fourth chapter leads the reader through the decision-making process preceding the closure of a traumatic wound. Factors which may preclude this approach are considered, as are the selection of suture materials and patterns as well as the use of drains and alternative, innovative approaches to wound closure in the event that this method is deemed appropriate.

Chapter 5 begins with a review of the physical and biomechanical properties of skin which will help the practitioner develop an appropriate surgical plan. That is followed by a detailed description of practical reconstructive techniques that can be used in conjunction with primary or delayed wound closure.

The next series of chapters (6, 7, and 8) is devoted to the management of wounds in various regions of the body: the head, the neck and body, and the distal extremities, with a focus on how to treat degloving injuries and how to prevent or manage the species-specific problem of exuberant granulation tissue.

Chapters 9 and 10 focus on the fact that a fair proportion of traumatic wounds in horses compromise deep, underlying structures. They present detailed anatomical reviews that should enable the practitioner to identify involvement of synovial structures or tendons/ligaments and promptly instigate the recommended therapy to improve the overall prognosis.

Chapter 11 addresses skin grafting, which should be considered for a wound that cannot heal by epithelialization and contraction or be closed using conventional or reconstructive suturing techniques. This chapter describes the principles and various techniques of free skin grafting, the advantages and disadvantages of each technique, and the effects of grafts on the wound.

Chapters 12 through 14 focus on the management of wounds suffering from serious debilitating conditions: severe infection, burn injury, and tumor development. Chapter 12 emphasizes the proper selection of antibiotic agents and reviews methods for optimizing their delivery and efficacy at the site of infection. Chapter 13 reviews the pathophysiology of burn injury and associated pulmonary damage and advises the reader on the appropriate treatment for immediate disorders as well as long-term wound care. While burns are uncommon in horses, management of such injuries can be expensive and time consuming. Moreover, cardiovascular involvement, smoke inhalation, and corneal ulceration can compromise the outcome. Finally, Chapter 14 addresses the transformation of a wound into a sarcoid tumor, which suspends the healing process, often indefinitely. It provides the reader with tips on recognizing and solving this unusual problem.

Chapter 15, which addresses laser surgery, was added to this edition of the textbook in response to the wider usage of this modality in veterinary medicine following the introduction in the 1990s of a more affordable waveguide-delivered CO_2 laser. The author discusses various clinical applications of laser surgery pertaining to wound management: debridement, removal of exuberant granulation tissue, graft bed preparation.

Chapter 16 is a well-illustrated chapter intended to guide the practitioner in the art of applying bandages, splints, and casts to support wound healing in different regions of the body.

We thank the contributing authors for their willingness to bring all of their valuable experience to this textbook. We are indebted to these people who generously contributed their clinical insight and current research data.

Acknowledgments

First, I wish to thank Ray Kersey, veterinary consulting editor for Wiley-Blackwell, for his persistence in approaching me regarding a long overdue revision of the first edition of *Equine Wound Management*. I also want to recognize Erin Gardner, commissioning editor, for her attention to detail and follow-up on the plans discussed at our initial meeting that finally led to a contract being signed. Antonia Seymour, publishing director, professional; Nancy Simmerman, editorial assistant; and all of the editorial staff at Wiley-Blackwell have been most patient and helpful with the delays in this revision; for this I am most thankful.

Once committed to the revision, and after realizing the magnitude of the family commitments facing me following my retirement from Colorado State University, I realized that I needed to identify a co-editor. Subsequent to my experience as guest editor for a wound management journal issue, the choice became clear, and I am so pleased that Dr. Christine Theoret agreed to join me in this endeavor. I am also very grateful to her for her willingness to take the lead during times when I was faced with family medical issues that had to take precedence over my editorial responsibilities.

I thank Jenger Smith, a professional photographer who has been involved with several of my textbooks, for continuing to provide the best possible color images for this publication. I am also grateful to Dave Carlson, the medical illustrator for the first edition, for agreeing to provide many new excellent illustrations. I am deeply indebted to Dennis Sylvain, librarian at the Veterinary Teaching Hospital at Colorado State University, for his willingness to do the numerous literature searches required to present the most current information. Truly, without his help it would have been most difficult for me to complete this revision.

I am most grateful to our colleagues and referring practitioners for allowing us the courtesy of using some of their case material as examples. I also acknowledge our residents, barn nurses, and students for the care and treatment of many of the cases presented in the text.

Finally, I would like to acknowledge our clients whose interest in providing the best care for their horses allowed us the opportunity to explore new avenues of treatment which we have shared with the readers of this textbook.

Ted S. Stashak with Christine Theoret

Contributors

Ted S. Stashak, DVM, MS, Diplomate ACVS
Professor Emeritus, Equine Surgery
Colorado State University
Santa Rosa, CA 95409
Tel.: (707) 539-1941
Fax: (240) 559-1941, then enter PIN number 8576
Email: tstashak@sbcglobal.net

Christine L. Theoret, DMV, PhD, Diplomate ACVS
Director, Comparative Tissue Healing Laboratory
Associate Professor, Equine Surgical Anatomy
Faculté de médecine vétérinaire
Université de Montréal
C.P. 5000 St-Hyacinthe
Québec, Canada
J2S 7C6
Tel: (450) 773-8521, extension 8517
Fax: (450) 778-8109
Email: christine.theoret@umontreal.ca

Stephen F. Badylak, PhD, DVM, MD
McGowan Institute for Regenerative Medicine
100 Technology Drive, Suite 200
University of Pittsburgh
Pittsburgh, PA 15219
Tel.: (412) 235-5144
Fax: (412) 235-5224
Email: badylaks@upmc.edu

Cooper Williams, DVM
720 Houcksville Road
Hampstead, MD 21074
Tel.: (410) 239-2323
Email: cooperwilliamsvmd@comcast.net

Julie Myers-Irvin, PhD
University of Pittsburgh
Office of Research, Health Sciences
401 Scaife Hall
Pittsburgh, PA 15261
Tel.: (412) 383-5213
Email: jmyers_irvin@hs.pitt.edu

Spencer Barber, DVM, Diplomate ACVS
Professor, Equine Surgery
Western College of Veterinary Medicine
University of Saskatchewan
52 Campus Dr.
Saskatoon, SK
Canada S7N 5B4
Tel.: (306) 966-7063
Fax: (306) 966-7159
Email: spence.barber@usask.ca

Gary M. Baxter, VMD, MS, Diplomate ACVS
Professor, Equine Surgery
Colorado State University
300 West Drake
Ft. Collins, CO 80523
Tel: (970) 297-4471 or 297-0382
Fax: (970) 297-1275
Email: gary.baxter@colostate.edu

Christophe Céleste, DrVet, MS, Diplomate ACVS
and ECVS
Clinician, Equine Emergency and Surgery
Faculté de médecine vétérinaire
Université de Montréal
C.P. 5000 St-Hyacinthe
Québec, Canada
J2S 7C6
Tel: (450) 778-8100
Email: christophe.celeste@umontreal.ca

Ellis Farstvedt, DVM, MS, Diplomate ACVS
CSR Equine, Copper Spring Ranch
1373 South Pine Butte Road
Bozeman, MT 59718
Tel.: (406) 522-4044 or (602) 531-7588 (cell)
Email: ellis@csrequine.com

Jorge Gomez, DVM, MS, Diplomate ACVS
Hagyard Equine Medical Institute
4250 Ironworks Pike
Lexington, KY 40511
Tel.: (859) 233-0026
Email: jgomez@hagyard.com

R. Reid Hanson, DVM, Diplomate ACVS and
  ACVECC
Professor, Equine Surgery
College of Veterinary Medicine
J.T. Vaughan Hall
1500 Wire Road
Auburn University
Auburn, Alabama 36849
Tel.: (334) 844-4490
Fax: (334) 844-4368
Email: hansorr@auburn.edu

Henry Jann, DVM, MS, Diplomate ACVS
Associate Professor, Equine Surgery
College of Veterinary Medicine
Oklahoma State University
Stillwater, OK 74078-2042
Tel: (405) 744-8596
Fax: (405) 744-6262
Email: jann@okstate.edu

Derek C. Knottenbelt, OBE, BVM&S, DVMS,
  Diplomate ECEIM, MRCVS
Professor, Equine Internal Medicine
University of Liverpool
Neston
Wirral, UK
CH64 7TE
Email: knotty@liv.ac.uk

James A. Orsini, DVM, Diplomate ACVS
Associate Professor, Equine Surgery
Director, International Laminitis Institute at PennVet
  New Bolton Center
School of Veterinary Medicine
University of Pennsylvania
Kennett Square, PA 19348
Tel: (610) 925-6402
Fax: (610) 925-8120
Email: orsini@vet.upenn.edu

Yvonne A. Elce, DVM, Diplomate ACVS
Clinical Assistant Professor, Equine Surgery
College of Veterinary Medicine
The Ohio State University
601 Vernon L. Tharp Street
Columbus OH 43210
Tel: (614) 292-9683
Email: elce.1@osu.edu

Beth M. Ross, DVM, Diplomate ACVS
126 Montana Dr.
Chadds Ford, PA 19317
Tel: (484) 770-8135
Email: bmrossdvm@hotmail.com

Jim Schumacher, DVM, MS, Diplomate ACVS,
  MRCVS
Professor, Equine Surgery
College of Veterinary Medicine
University of Tennessee
Knoxville, TN 37901-1071
Tel: (865) 755-8239
Fax: (865) 974-5773
Email: jschumac@utk.edu

Kenneth E. Sullins, DVM, MS, Diplomate ACVS
Professor, Equine Surgery
Va-Md Regional College of Veterinary Medicine
Leesburg, VA 20177
Tel: (703) 771-6827
Fax: (703) 771-6877 or 771-6810
Email: sullins@vt.edu

Jacintha M. Wilmink, DVM, PhD, Diplomate RNVA
Woumarec (wound management and reconstruction
  in horses)
Hamsterlaan 4
6705 CT Wageningen
The Netherlands
Tel: **31 (0)317 414462
Fax: **31 (0)317 414462
Email: jwilmink@tiscali.nl

David A. Wilson, DVM, MS, Diplomate ACVS
Professor, Equine Surgery
Section Head, Equine Medicine and Surgery
Acting Hospital Director
Department of Veterinary Medicine and Surgery
University of Missouri
900 E Campus Dr.
Columbia, MO 65211
Tel: (573) 882-3513
Fax: (573) 884-0173
Email: wilsonda@missouri.edu

EQUINE WOUND MANAGEMENT

Second Edition

1 Wound Healing

1.1 Physiology of Wound Healing

Christine L. Theoret, DMV, PhD, Diplomate ACVS

Introduction

A vital trait of living organisms, continually subjected to insults from the environment, is their capacity for self repair. Whether the injury is surgical or accidental, it will generate an attempt by the host to restore tissue continuity. Two processes are involved in healing: regeneration and repair. Regeneration entails the replacement of damaged tissue with normal cells of the type lost and is only possible in tissues with a sustained population of cells capable of mitosis, such as epithelium, bone, and liver. Repair is a "stop-gap" reaction designed to re-establish the continuity of interrupted tissues with undifferentiated scar tissue (see Figure 4.12 in Chapter 4). Repair is therefore the "second best" method of healing, producing a result which is less biologically useful than the tissue it replaced and possibly adversely affecting adjacent normal tissues.

Traumatic wounds occur commonly in horses. The objective of repair is re-establishment of an epithelial cover and recovery of tissue integrity, strength, and function. Partial-thickness cutaneous wounds, e.g., abrasions and erosions, heal primarily by migration and proliferation of epidermal cells from the remaining underlying epithelium as well as the adnexal structures (hair follicles, sweat and sebaceous glands), with little participation of inflammatory or mesenchymal cells. In contrast, repair of full-thickness cutaneous wounds hinges principally on three coordinated phases: acute inflammation, cellular proliferation, and finally, matrix synthesis and remodeling with scar formation (Figure 1.1). These processes rely on the complex interaction between cells, their surrounding matrix, and the mediators that govern their numerous activities.

Veterinarians can positively influence wound repair by understanding its mechanisms, which will ensure selection of appropriate wound management techniques. Hippocrates once said, "Healing is a matter of time, but it is sometimes a matter of opportunity."

Over the past decade, research aimed at unveiling and possibly augmenting the reparative mechanisms of the body has yielded advances in the field of cytokines and the ability to readily synthesize most molecules associated with wound repair.[2] This chapter aims to provide an update on the physiological, cellular, biochemical, and molecular aspects of wound repair.

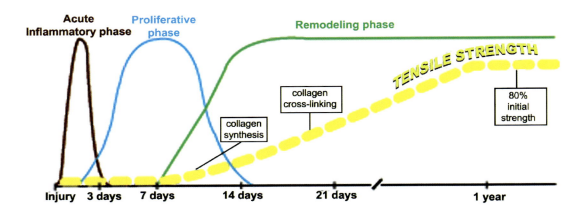

Figure 1.1. Temporal profile of various processes and gain in tensile strength occurring during normal cutaneous wound repair. Reprinted from *Clinical Techniques in Equine Practice*, 3, Theoret CL, Update on wound repair, pp. 110–122, Copyright (2004), with permission from Elsevier.

Phases of Wound Repair

Acute Inflammation

Inflammation prepares the wound for the subsequent reparative phases. It purges the body of alien substances and disposes of dead tissue, while the participating cellular populations liberate mediators to amplify and sustain the events to follow. Inflammation encompasses vascular and cellular responses whose intensity is strongly correlated to the severity of trauma.

Vascular Responses

The injured endothelial cell membrane releases phospholipids that are transformed into arachidonic acid and its metabolites, which mediate vascular tone and permeability as well as platelet aggregation. The first response of the damaged blood vessel is vasoconstriction, lasting 5–10 minutes, after which vasodilation, primarily of the small venules, ensues and facilitates diapedesis of cells, fluids, and proteins across the vessel wall into the extravascular space. Coagulated blood and aggregated platelets together form a clot (provisional matrix) within the wound that, despite providing limited strength, seals off the defect and prevents further bleeding. The clot also functions as a scaffold through the presence of a large number of binding sites on blood proteins that are recognized by special surface receptors (integrins) found on migrating inflammatory and mesenchymal cells.

Activated platelets are among the earliest promoters of inflammation, via the release of potent chemoattractants and mitogens from their storage granules. These serve as signals to initiate and amplify the reparative phases of healing and are detailed later in this chapter. Over time, the surface clot desiccates to form a scab that protects the wound from infection. This scab is in turn lysed by plasmin, a serine proteinase, and sloughs along with dead inflammatory cells and bacteria as healing proceeds underneath. The provisional extracellular matrix (ECM) will be replaced by granulation tissue in the next phase of repair.

Cellular Responses

Leukocytes are recruited from the circulating blood pool to the site of injury by the numerous vasoactive mediators and chemoattractants supplied by the coagulation and activated complement pathways, by platelets, by mast cells, and by injured or activated mesenchymal cells.[3] These signals initiate the processes of rolling, activation, tight adhesion, and finally transmigration of inflammatory cells through the microvascular endothelium. Chemoattractants additionally stimulate the release of enzymes by the activated neutrophils, which facilitate their penetration through vascular basement membranes upon migration. Neutrophil diapedesis is further facilitated by increased capillary permeability following the release of a spectrum of vasodilatory agents. Cellular influx begins within minutes and neutrophil numbers progressively increase to reach a peak 1 to 2 days after injury. Neutrophils act as a first line of defense in contaminated wounds by destroying debris and bacteria through phagocytosis and subsequent enzymatic and oxygen-radical mechanisms. The principal degradative proteinases released by the neutrophils to rid the site of denatured ECM components are neutrophil-specific interstitial collagenase, neutrophil elastase, and cathepsin G. Neutrophil migration and phagocytosis cease when contaminating particles are cleared from the site of injury. Most cells then become entrapped within the clot, which is sloughed during later phases of repair. The neutrophils remaining within viable tissue die in a few days and are phagocytosed by the tissue macrophages or modified wound fibroblasts. This marks the termination of the early inflammatory phase of repair. Although the neutrophils help create a favorable wound environment and serve as a source of pro-inflammatory cytokines, they are not essential to repair in uninfected wounds.[4]

The rapid increase in macrophage numbers under inflammatory conditions is predominantly caused by the emigration of monocytes from the vasculature, followed by differentiation into macrophages to assist resident tissue macrophages at the wound site for a period of days to weeks. In this manner, the responsive and adaptable pluripotent monocytes can morph into macrophages whose functional properties are determined by the conditions they encounter at the site of mobilization. Similar to neutrophils, the macrophages are phagocytes and thus carry out debridement and microbial killing. Unlike neutrophils, wound macrophages play a key role in the reparative phases of healing. Indeed, adherence to the ECM (which consists of a cross-linked supporting framework of collagen fibrils and elastin fibers, saturated with proteoglycans and other glycoproteins) stimulates monocytes to transform into a phenotype with the ability to continually synthesize and express the various cytokines necessary for their survival as well as for the initiation and propagation of new tissue formation in wounds (Figure 1.2).

A classic series of experiments in the 1970s determined that wounds depleted of both circulating blood monocytes and tissue macrophages exhibit not only severe retardation of tissue debridement but also a marked delay in fibroblast proliferation and subsequent wound fibrosis.[5] Although it has long been considered that the inflammatory response is instrumental in supplying mediators that orchestrate the cell and tissue movements

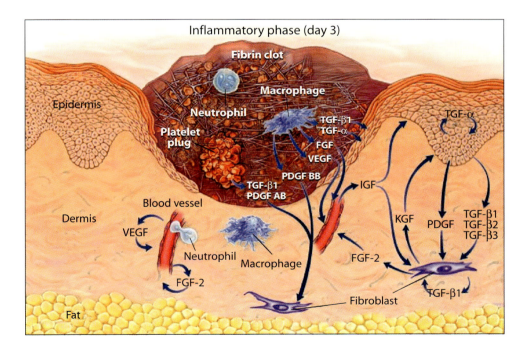

Figure 1.2. Illustration of a full thickness cutaneous wound showing the cellular and molecular components present 3 days after injury. FGF = basic fibroblast growth factor; IGF = insulin-like growth factor; KGF = keratinocyte growth factor; PDGF = platelet-derived growth factor; TGF = transforming growth factor; VEGF = vascular endothelial growth factor. Modified from Singer and Clark.[3]

necessary for repair, it was recently shown that mice genetically lacking macrophages and functioning neutrophils are able to repair skin wounds within a similar time frame to wild-type siblings, and that repair appears scar free, possibly in response to an altered local cytokine and growth factor profile.[6] Conversely, clues from the liver suggest that, although macrophages direct fibrosis, they might also be the best equipped cells to resolve it.[7]

Upon arrival at the site of inflammation, macrophages participate in bacterial killing via mechanisms that parallel those of the neutrophil. Three inducible secreted neutral proteinases have been identified in macrophages: elastase, collagenase and plasminogen activator (PA). These proteinases aid in degradation of damaged tissue and debris, which must be cleared before repair can proceed. Despite the new data gleaned from the study on macrophageless mice, acute inflammation is still considered crucial to the normal outcome of wound repair, particularly in horses where wounds are frequently exposed to infective agents.

Macrophages are regarded as the major inflammatory cell not only responsible for debridement, but also for recruitment of other inflammatory and mesenchymal cells, and subsequent induction of angiogenesis, fibroplasia and epithelialization. Paradoxically, prolonged inflammation will retard healing and encourage the development of chronic proliferation of fibroblastic granulation. This is thought to contribute to the pathogenesis of a number of diseases characterized by disproportionate scarring, such as pulmonary fibrosis, hepatic cirrhosis, glomerulonephritis, and dermal keloids in humans. Extensive scarring or fibrosis of any organ may cause catastrophic loss of function of that organ. In the horse, a comparable condition is the development of exuberant granulation tissue in full-thickness cutaneous wounds (see Treatment of Exuberant Granulation Tissue in Chapter 8).

Inflammation is a sequence of events: production of mediators; rolling, tethering, and adhesion of neutrophils to vascular endothelium with subsequent migration through endothelium and basement membranes; altered vascular permeability with passage of fluid into tissues; neutrophil phagocytosis of invading organisms, and release of biologically active materials; emigration of monocytes from the local vasculature; and maturation of monocytes into inflammatory macrophages with subsequent removal of the components of inflammation. Resolution of inflammation should therefore address each one of these events and halt or potentially reverse it. However, despite the importance of the processes by which inflammation normally resolves, little research has been done in this area.

Apoptosis, or programmed cell death, is the universal pathway for the elimination of unneeded cells and tissues in a phagocytic process that does not elicit additional inflammation.[8] This mechanism prevails during all phases of wound repair because each relies on rapid increases in specific cell populations that either prepare the wound for repair (inflammatory cells) or deposit new matrices and mature the wound (mesenchymal cells), but then must be eliminated prior to progression to the next phase. Indeed, a mature wound is typically acellular.

In conclusion, it appears that the termination of inflammation is a complex and closely regulated sequence of events. There are several steps at which the resolution process could go astray, leading to suppuration, chronic inflammation (Figure 1.3), and/or excessive fibrosis.

Cellular Proliferation

Fibroplasia

The proliferative phase of repair comes about as inflammation subsides, and is characterized by the appearance of red, fleshy granulation tissue, which ultimately fills the defect. Although the earliest part of this phase is very active on a cellular basis, this does not immediately translate into a gain in wound strength. Indeed, during the first 3 to 5 days following injury, mesenchymal cells such as fibroblasts, endothelial, and epithelial cells are rapidly invading the wound in preparation for matrix synthesis and maturation or for coverage; however, these latter reinforcing mechanisms lag somewhat. Granulation tissue is formed by three elements that move into the wound space simultaneously: macrophages debride and produce cytokines and growth factors, which stimulate angiogenesis and fibroplasia; fibroblasts proliferate and synthesize new ECM components; and new blood vessels carry oxygen and nutrients necessary for the metabolism and growth of mesenchymal cells, and confer to the granulation tissue its characteristic red, granular appearance (Figure 1.4).[3]

This stroma, rich in fibronectin and hyaluronan, replaces the fibrin-containing clot to provide a physical barrier to infection, and importantly, it provides a surface across which mesenchymal cells can migrate. A number

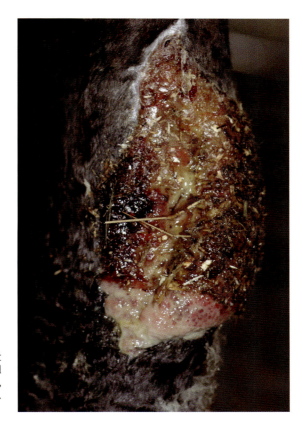

Figure 1.3. This metatarsal wound failed to heal for 7 months as a result of chronic low-grade inflammation due to exposure as well as superficial and deep infection. The wound in fact became larger rather than smaller, illustrating suspension of the healing process. Courtesy of Dr. D. Knottenbelt.

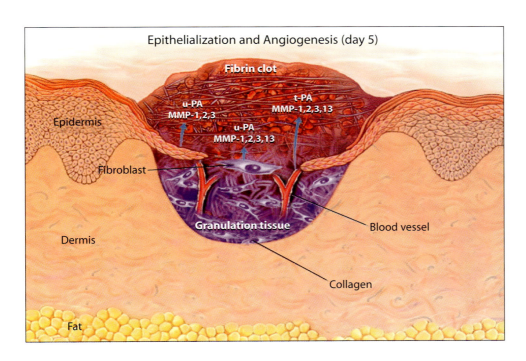

Figure 1.4. Illustration of a full-thickness cutaneous wound 5 days after injury showing angiogenesis, fibroplasia, and epithelialization. uPA = urokinase-type plasminogen activator; tPA = tissue-type plasminogen activator; MMP = matrix metalloproteinase. Modified from Singer and Clark.[3]

of matrix molecules as well as chemoattractants, cytokines, and growth factors released by inflammatory cells are believed to stimulate fibroblasts from adjacent uninjured dermis and subcutaneous tissue to proliferate and express integrin receptors to assist migration into the wound space. Integrins are transmembrane proteins that act as the major cell-surface receptors for ECM molecules and thus mediate interactions and transduction of signals between cells and their environment. They are particularly critical to the migratory movements exhibited by wound healing cells such as epithelial and endothelial cells, as well as fibroblasts. Migration immediately precedes advancing capillary endothelial buds but follows macrophages, which have cleared a path by phagocytozing debris. Fibroblasts themselves also possess an active proteolytic system to aid migration into the cross-linked fibrin blood clot: proteinases include PA, various collagenases, gelatinase, and stromelysin.[9]

Once fibroblasts have arrived within the wound space, they proliferate and then switch their function to protein synthesis and commence the gradual replacement of provisional matrix by a collagen-rich one, probably under the influence of various cytokines and growth factors. As the wound matures, there is a marked increase in the ratio of type I (mature) to type III (immature) collagen; proteoglycans also become abundant within the mature matrix. The greatest rate of connective tissue accumulation within the wound occurs 7 to 14 days after injury, which translates into the period of most rapid gain in tensile strength (Figure 1.1).

Thereafter, collagen content levels off as fibroblasts down-regulate their synthetic mechanisms; this corresponds to a much slower gain in wound strength, which occurs as the wound remodels. The fibroblast-rich granulation tissue is subsequently replaced by a relatively avascular and acellular scar as the capillary content regresses and fibroblasts either undergo apoptosis[10] or acquire smooth-muscle characteristics and transform into myofibroblasts that participate in wound contraction. The latter phenomena are regulated by the physiological needs and/or the microenvironmental stimuli present at the wound site. It appears that if the signal to down-regulate fibroblast activity is delayed beyond a specific time point, apoptosis is permanently impaired, which ultimately leads to an imbalance between collagen synthesis and degradation[11] and the formation of excessive scar tissue.

Angiogenesis

Besides initiating the inflammatory response through interaction with leukocytes, microvascular endothelial cells play a key role in the proliferative phase of repair. The formation of new capillary blood vessels from pre-existing ones (angiogenesis) is necessary to sustain the granulation tissue newly formed within the wound bed. Angiogenesis, in response to tissue injury and hypoxia, is a complex and dynamic process mediated by diverse soluble factors from both serum and the surrounding ECM environment, in particular angiogenic inducers including growth factors, chemokines and angiogenic enzymes, endothelial-specific receptors, and adhesion molecules such as integrins,[12] many of which are released during the inflammatory phase of repair.

Construction of a vascular network requires sequential steps that include augmented microvascular permeability, the release of proteinases from activated endothelial cells with subsequent local degradation of the basement membrane surrounding the existing vessel, migration and sprouting of endothelial cells into the interstitial space, endothelial cell proliferation and formation of granulation tissue and differentiation into mature blood vessels, eventually followed by regression and involution of the newly formed vasculature as tissue remodels.[13] Angiogenesis is dependent not only on the cells and cytokines present, but also on the production and organization of ECM components which act as both scaffold support through which endothelial cells may migrate and as reservoir and modulator for growth factors. Thus, endothelial cells at the tip of capillaries begin their migration into the wound in response to angiogenic stimuli and absence of neighboring cells on the second day following injury.

Cytoplasmic pseudopodia extend through fragmented basement membranes; subsequently, the entire endothelial cell migrates into the perivascular space. Cells remaining in the parent vessel near the tip of the angiogenic sprouts begin to proliferate, providing a continuous source of microvascular endothelial cells for angiogenesis. When a new capillary sprout first develops it is solid; after it fuses with a neighboring sprout to form an arcade, it becomes canalized and erythrocytes pass into and through it.

Lumen formation probably involves the joining of plasma membranes of individual and/or adjacent cells, as well as extensive intracellular vacuolization followed by fusion of the vacuoles to form "ring cells," which ultimately fuse to form seamless capillaries. Capillaries then become stable as endothelial cells interact with the new basement membrane within 24 hours of new vessel formation. Once the reconstitution of stroma is complete, there is no longer the need for a rich vascular supply. Angiogenic stimuli are down-regulated or the local concentration of inhibitors increases and most of the recently formed capillary network quickly involutes through the activity of matrix metalloproteinases (MMPs),[14] in particular MMP-1 and MMP-10,[15] and apoptosis of endothelial cells. The wound color becomes paler as the rich capillary bed disappears from the granulation tissue.

Epithelialization

All body surfaces are covered by epithelium, which acts as a discriminating barrier to the environment. As such, epithelium provides the primary defense against hostile surroundings and is a major factor in maintaining internal homeostasis by limiting fluid and electrolyte loss. The outer multilayered stratified squamous epithelium (the epidermis) interfaces with the musculoskeletal framework by means of a connective tissue layer (the dermis) and a fibro-fatty layer (the subcutis). Epidermis is attached to the dermis at the level of the basement membrane, a thin, glycoprotein-rich layer composed primarily of laminin and type IV collagen. This attachment is mediated by hemidesmosomes, which physically attach the basal cells of the epidermis to the underlying dermis, as well as by vertically oriented type VII collagen anchoring fibrils, which bind the cytoskeleton.[16]

It is critical to survival that an extensive full-thickness wound be covered without delay. In addition to the aforementioned hemostatic activities, which establish a temporary barrier, centripetal movement of the residual epithelium below the clot participates in wound closure. Although epithelial migration commences 24 to 48 hours following wounding, the characteristic pink rim of new epithelium (Figure 1.5) is not macroscopically visible until 4 to 6 days later, although this is variable since the rate of wound closure depends on the animal species as well as the wound site, substrate, and size.

For example, epithelialization is accelerated in a partial-thickness wound because migrating cells will arise not only from the residual epithelium at the wound periphery but also from remaining epidermal appendages. Furthermore, the basement membrane is intact in this type of injury, precluding a lengthy regeneration. On the other hand, during second intention healing of a full-thickness wound, epithelialization must await the formation of a bed of granulation tissue to proceed. Wounds in the flank region of a horse epithelialize at a rate of 0.2 mm/day, compared with a rate as slow as 0.09 mm/day for wounds in the distal region of limbs.[17]

In preparation for migration, basal epidermal cells at the wound margin undergo phenotypic alterations that favor mobility and phagocytic activity. Additionally, various degradative enzymes necessary for the proteolysis of ECM components are up-regulated within cells at the leading edge, facilitating ingestion of the clot and debris found along the migratory route. The migratory route is determined by the array of integrin receptors expressed on the surface of migrating epithelial cells, for various ECM proteins. Indeed, a fundamental reason why migrating epidermis dissects the fibrin eschar from wounds is that they cannot interact with the fibrinogen and its derivatives found within the clot since they lack the appropriate integrin.[18] Once the wound surface is covered by epithelial cells that contact one another, further migration is inhibited by the expression within the ECM of laminin, a major cell adhesion factor for epithelial cells, from the margin of the wound inward.

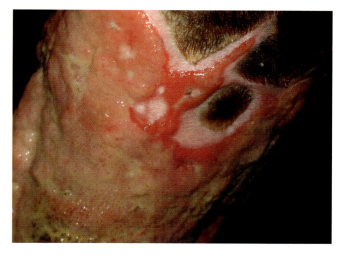

Figure 1.5. Large full-thickness metatarsal wound that healed partially by second intention and was subsequently grafted successfully. The wound showed excellent epithelialization from the healing margin of the wound. Note the island of epithelium corresponding to a graft. The healthy epithelial tissue is characterized by an area of hyperemia adjacent to it. Courtesy of Dr. D. Knottenbelt.

Although initial cell migration does not require an increase in cellular multiplication, epidermal cells at the wound margin do begin to proliferate 1 to 2 days after injury to replenish the migratory front. This corresponds histologically to epithelial hyperplasia (Figure 1.6), as cellular mitosis increases 17-fold within 48 to 72 hours. The new cells leapfrog over those at the wound margin and adhere to the substratum, only to be replaced in turn by other cells coming from above and behind. The newly adherent monolayer subsequently restratifies to restore the original multilayered epidermis.

In full-thickness wounds healing by second intention, such as those commonly managed in equine practice, provisional matrix is eventually replaced by a mature basement membrane zone. Repairing epidermis reassembles its constituents from the margin toward the center of the wound.[3] Epidermal cells then revert to a quiescent phenotype and become attached to this new basement membrane through hemidesmosomes and to the underlying neodermis through type VII collagen fibrils. This particular aspect of epithelialization is time-consuming, occurring long after total wound coverage is apparent, which may explain the continued fragility of neoepidermis for extended periods following macroscopically complete repair. This is particularly evident in large wounds of the limb, where epidermis at the center is often thin and easily traumatized (Figures 1.7a and 1.7b).

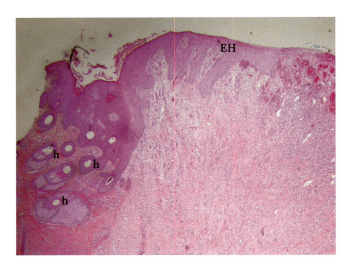

Figure 1.6. Photomicrograph of wound edge biopsy. Normal unwounded skin to the left demonstrating epidermal appendages (h = hair follicles); new hyperplastic epithelium (EH) to the right, overlying granulation tissue bed. Reprinted from *Clinical Techniques in Equine Practice*, 3, Theoret CL, Update on wound repair, pp. 110–122, Copyright (2004), with permission from Elsevier.

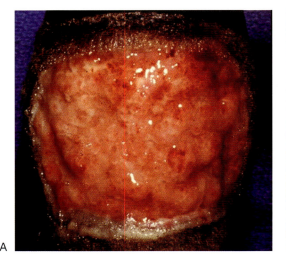

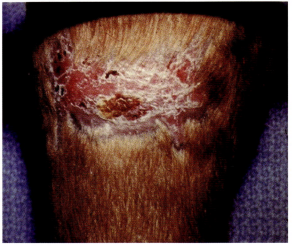

A

B

Figure 1.7. (a) A 5-day-old, full-thickness, experimentally created wound over the dorsal fetlock. Granulation tissue is beginning to fill the wound bed. (b) The same wound, 75 days following creation. Neoepidermis is thin, dry, and hairless, and could be easily traumatized. Courtesy of Dr. T. Stashak.

Matrix Synthesis and Remodeling

In addition to epithelialization, contraction contributes to the successful closure of full-thickness wounds. Contraction is defined as a process whereby both dermis and epidermis bordering a full-thickness skin deficit are drawn from all sides centripetally over the exposed wound bed.[19] This usually occurs during the second week following injury. Wound contraction not only accelerates closure, but also enhances the cosmetic appearance and strength of the scar because proportionally less wound area must be covered by newly formed inferior quality epithelium, which is fragile and lacks normal nervous, glandular, follicular, and vascular components (see Figures 4.12 and 1.7b). For this reason, a high degree of contraction is a desired feature of wound repair, at least in the horse.

A number of theories have been proposed to explain wound contraction; however, most authorities agree that it involves a finely orchestrated interaction of ECM, cytokines/growth factors, and cells, in particular a specialized fibroblast phenotype: the myofibroblast. These are the most abundant cellular elements of healthy granulation tissue and are aligned within the wound along the lines of contraction. The most striking feature of the myofibroblasts is a well-developed alpha smooth muscle actin (α-SMA) microfilamentous system, arranged parallel to the cell's long axis and in continuity with ECM components via various integrins. In addition to these cell-substratum links, intercellular connections such as gap junctions and hemidesmosomes ensure that neighboring cells exert tension on one another. Factors producing and regulating contraction are presently unknown, but appear to include various cytokines/growth factors.

Wound contraction is divided into three phases. An initial lag phase (wherein skin edges retract and the wound area increases temporarily for 5 to 10 days) occurs prior to significant fibroblastic invasion into the wound, which is a prerequisite for contraction. Subsequently a period of rapid contraction is followed by one of slow contraction as the wound approaches complete closure. The number of myofibroblasts found in a wound appears proportional to the need for contraction; thus, as repair progresses and the rate of contraction slows, this number decreases accordingly.

During wound contraction, the surrounding skin stretches by intussusceptive growth and the wound takes on a stellate appearance. Contraction ceases in response to one of three events: the wound edges meet and contact inhibition halts both the processes of epithelialization and contraction; tension in the surrounding skin becomes equal to or greater than the contractile force generated by the α-SMA of the myofibroblasts; or, in the case of chronic wounds, a low myofibroblast count in the granulation tissue may result in failure of wound contraction despite laxity in the surrounding skin. In the latter case, the granulation tissue is pale and consists primarily of collagen and ground substance. Wound contraction is greater in regions of the body with loose skin than in regions where skin is under tension, such as the distal aspect of horse limbs. Although it is speculated that the shape of the wound may influence the process of contraction, this does not appear relevant in wounds at the distal extremities of horse limbs where skin is tightly stretched and not easily moved.[20]

As contraction concludes, myofibroblasts disappear, either by reverting to a quiescent fibroblast phenotype or by apoptosis,[10] primarily in response to reduced tension within the ECM.[21] The myofibroblast persists in fibrotic lesions where it may be involved in further ECM accumulation and pathologic contracture, a condition leading to significant morbidity, particularly when it involves joints or body orifices, but is rarely encountered in the horse.

The conversion of ECM from granulation to scar tissue constitutes the final phase of wound repair and consists of connective tissue synthesis, lysis, and remodeling, also referred to as maturation. Proteoglycans replace hyaluronan during the second week of repair, support the deposition and aggregation of collagen fibers, and provide the mature matrix with better resilience. Collagen macromolecules provide the wound tensile strength as their deposition peaks within the first week in primary wound repair and between 7 and 14 days in second intention healing. Although this corresponds to the period of most rapid gain in strength, only 20% of the final strength of the wound is achieved in the first 3 weeks of repair. At this time, collagen synthesis is balanced by collagen lysis, which normally prevents accumulation of excessive amounts of collagen and formation of pathologic scars.

The balance between synthesis and degradation determines the overall strength of a healing wound at a particular time. The first newly deposited collagen tends to be oriented randomly and therefore provides little tensile strength, whereas during remodeling the fibers reform along lines of stress and therefore resist dehiscence more effectively. Cross-linking in the later formed collagen is also more effective, although never to the same extent as in the original tissue. The new collagen weaves into that which preexisted and also appears to bond to the ends of old collagen fibers. These welds are points of weakness, which may rupture under stress.

Collagen degradation within a wound depends on the presence of various proteolytic enzymes released from inflammatory and mesenchymal cells. Most are of the MMP family of zinc-dependent endopeptidases that are collectively capable of degrading virtually all ECM components. Although MMPs are not constitutively expressed in skin, up-regulation occurs whenever proteolysis is required, such as during cell migration and matrix remodeling. Inactive precursors of the MMPs are cleaved in the extracellular space by proteinases such as plasmin and trypsin, leftover from the inflammatory and proliferative phases, but also by other MMPs.

To date, more than 20 different MMPs, all distinct gene products, have been characterized (Table 1.1)[9] and are generally divided into four major groups. The best-known subgroup of MMPs are the collagenases (MMP-1, -8, and -13), which possess the unique ability to cleave the triple helix of native types I, II, and III collagens, the rate-limiting step of collagen degradation. The fragments generated are thermally unstable and denature into their constitutive polypeptide chains, forming gelatin peptides. Basal epithelial cells at the migratory front of epithelialization are the predominant source of collagenase during active wound repair,[9] while the resolution of granulation tissue also depends on the activity of collagenase, in this case expressed by dermal fibroblasts.

Table 1.1. Major matrix metalloproteinases (MMPs) involved in wound repair.

MMP name	MMP #	Substrates	Source
Collagenases			
Interstitial collagenase	MMP-1	Collagen (I, II, III, VII, IX)	Epithelial cell, fibroblast
Neutrophil collagenase	MMP-8	Collagen (I, II, III)	PMN
Collagenase 3	MMP-13	Collagen (I, II, III, IV)	Endothelial cell, fibroblast
Stromelysins			
Stromelysin-1	MMP-3	PGs, laminin, fibronectin,	Epithelial cell
Stromelysin-2	MMP-10	Collagen (III, IV, IX, X)	Epithelial cell, fibroblast
Stromelysin-3	MMP-11	Collagen IV, fibronectin, gelatin, laminin	Fibroblast
Gelatinases			
Gelatinase A (72 kDa)	MMP-2	Gelatin, collagen (I, IV), elastin	Most cells
Gelatinase B (92 kDa)	MMP-9	Gelatin, collagen (IV, V), elastin	Inflammatory cell, epithelial cell, fibroblast
Matrilysin	MMP-7	PGs, elastin, fibronectin, laminin, gelatin, collagen IV	Epithelial cell
Membrane-type MMPs			
MT1-MMP	MMP-14	Collagen (I, III), fibronectin	
MT2-MMP	MMP-15	Vitronectin, pro-MMPs	
MT3-MMP	MMP-16	Collagen (III), fibronectin	
MT4-MMP	MMP-17	Gelatin, pro-gelatinase A	
MT5-MMP	MMP-20	Collagen (V), aggrecan, COMP	Tooth enamel

PMN = polymorphonuclear granulocyte
PG = proteoglycan
COMP = cartilage oligomeric matrix protein

The stromelysins, members of another subgroup of MMPs, possess broad substrate specificity. Stromelysin-1 and -2 are strong proteoglycanases and can also degrade basement membranes, laminin, and fibronectin, while stromelysin-3 is only weakly proteolytic. Although stromelysin-2 expression is strictly confined to the epidermis, stromelysin-1 is also abundantly expressed by dermal fibroblasts in the granulation tissue associated with wounds. Because of its broad substrate specificity, it may be important in remodeling the matrix, in particular the newly formed basement membrane, during repair.[9]

There are two metallogelatinases: the 72 kilodalton (kDa) gelatinase (gelatinase A) which, unlike other MMPs, is produced constitutively by most cells types, and the 92 kDa gelatinase (gelatinase B), produced by most inflammatory cells as well as by epithelial cells. Both types efficiently degrade denatured collagens (gelatins) and also attack basement membranes, fibronectin, and insoluble elastin. Matrilysin is the smallest MMP (28 kDa) but is a stronger proteoglycanase than stromelysin and also degrades basement membranes, insoluble elastin, laminin, fibronectin, and gelatin.

Homeostasis between collagen synthesis and degradation during the remodeling phase depends on the simultaneous presence of MMPs and non-specific inhibitors such as α2-macroglobulin and α1-antiprotease, as well as natural specific inhibitors, the tissue inhibitors of metalloproteinases (TIMPs). TIMPs are a gene family of four structurally related members, TIMP-1 through -4, that inhibit conversion of MMPs from a zymogen to an activated state and that irreversibly bind to the catalytic site of active MMPs. The role of TIMPs in wound repair is not limited to remodeling, since they also promote growth in a wide range of cell types and are thought to stabilize the basement membrane of regenerating epidermis, as well as inhibit angiogenesis and induce apoptosis.

Inhibition of MMP activity during the acute inflammatory phase enhances the strength of the wound reached during the repair phase despite accompanying decreases in the inflammatory response and new collagen synthesis. This is thought to result from decreased collagen turnover or increased collagen maturation and cross-linking, or both.[22] However, under most circumstances, an imbalance between MMPs and TIMPs will lead to abnormal resolution and delayed repair. Indeed, although the presence of MMPs is essential for normal wound maturation, it may also be responsible for the inability of chronic wounds to heal. For example, chronic wound fluid is characterized by elevated levels of proteinases, particularly MMP-9 and serine proteinases, which lead to excessive protein degradation and the inactivation of critical growth factors. Chronic wounds also contain reduced levels of TIMPs, in particular TIMP-1.[23] It is interesting to note that as epithelialization progresses, production of MMPs by epithelial cells is turned off, allowing the formation of hemidesmosomal adhesions between cells and the basement membrane.

Wound remodeling continues for up to 2 years. During that time there is no net increase in collagen content, but rather a rearrangement of collagen fibers into a more organized lattice structure, under the influence of local mechanical factors, progressively increasing the tensile strength of scar tissue. The majority of type III collagen fibers laid down early in the healing process are replaced by collagen type I, fibers become increasingly cross-linked, and the normal skin ratio of 4:1 type I to type III collagen is re-established. Glycosaminoglycans are steadily degraded until they reach concentrations found in normal dermis. The duration of the maturation phase depends on a variety of factors including the patient's genetic makeup, age, location of the wound on the body, type of injury, and duration of inflammation. At maximum strength, cutaneous wounds remain 15–20% weaker than the normal surrounding tissue, although this varies markedly among species (Figure 1.1).[24]

Mediators of Wound Repair

Wound repair relies on a complex amalgamation of interactive processes involving formed elements of blood (e.g., erythrocytes, platelets, leukocytes), ECM, and mesenchymal cells. Although histological and morphometric observations have permitted a detailed description of the kinetics of cellular and macromolecular components involved in repair, much remains to be learned about the regulation of such activities. Restoration of structural integrity and partial functional properties appears to rely on soluble mediators synthesized by cells present in the wound or in the surrounding tissue which coordinate migration, proliferation, and protein synthesis by the various cell populations involved in the repair process.

Cytokines, defined as 4–60 kDa signaling glycoproteins released by most nucleated cells, are among the most important soluble mediators regulating wound repair. They act in concentrations of 10^9–10^{12} M in an autocrine (same cell), paracrine (adjacent cell), or endocrine (distant cell) fashion. For cytokines to exert an effect, the target cell must express a surface receptor to the specific mediator. Receptors are proteins with an extracellular site to bind the cytokine and a transmembranous site to transmit the signal to the intracellular site where it must reach nuclear DNA for a specific response to occur. Cells may have different numbers of receptors for different factors; the concentration of factors in the area and the number of receptors that are bound determine the response generated. Growth factors are cytokines, which exert primarily mitogenic influences. The cytokines that play a significant role in wound repair are summarized in Table 1.2.

Table 1.2. Cytokines involved in wound repair.

Name	Abbreviation	Source	Major function
Colony stimulating factor	CSF	Macrophage, lymphocyte, fibroblast, endothelial cell	Differentiation and maturation of hematopoietic stem cells
Interferon	IFN	Monocyte and macrophage, lymphocyte, mesenchymal cell	Proinflammatory; release of other cytokines; inhibit fibrosis
Interleukin	IL	All nucleated cells, in particular macrophage and lymphocyte	Proinflammatory; enhance epithelialization, angiogenesis, and remodeling
Tumor necrosis factor	TNF	Macrophage, lymphocyte, mast cell	Proinflammatory; enhance angiogenesis, epithelialization and remodeling
Connective tissue growth factor	CTGF	Fibroblast	Mediator of TGF-β activity (cell proliferation and ECM accumulation)
Epidermal growth factor	EGF	Platelet, saliva	Epithelialization; chemotactic and mitogenic to fibroblast; protein and MMP synthesis (remodeling); angiogenesis (TGF-α)
Transforming growth factor-α	TGF-α	Macrophage, epithelial cell	
Fibroblast growth factor	FGF	Inflammatory cell, fibroblast, endothelial cell	Chemotactic and mitogenic to fibroblast and epithelial cell; protein synthesis; angiogenesis
Insulin-like growth factor	IGF	Liver, platelet	Chemotatic and mitogenic to endothelial cell; migration of epithelial cell; fibroblast proliferation; protein and GAG synthesis
Keratinocyte growth factor	KGF	Fibroblast	Chemotactic and mitogenic to epithelial cell
Platelet-derived growth factor	PDGF	Platelet	Chemotactic to inflammatory cell and fibroblast; mitogenic to mesenchymal cell; protein synthesis; contraction?
Transforming growth factor-β	TGF-β	Platelet, lymphocyte, mast cell, monocyte and macrophage, endothelial cell, epithelial cell, fibroblast	Chemotactic to inflammatory and mesenchymal cell; fibroblast proliferation; protein synthesis; ECM deposition (inhibition of MMP; induction of TIMP); wound contraction
Vascular endothelial growth factor	VEGF	Macrophage; fibroblast; endothelial cell; epithelial cell	Angiogenesis

ECM = extracellular matrix
MMP = matrix metalloproteinase
TIMP = tissue inhibitor of metalloproteinase
GAG = glycosaminoglycan

Cytokines

Colony-Stimulating Factors (CSFs)

Four cytokines classified as colony-stimulating factors (CSFs) have been identified: granulocyte (G) CSF, macrophage (M) CSF, granulocyte-macrophage (GM) CSF, and multilineage (ML) CSF. Many cells involved in repair including macrophages, lymphocytes, fibroblasts, and endothelial cells synthesize CSFs and/or are targets of this cytokine.[25] CSFs influence repair by promoting the differentiation and maturation of hematopoietic stem cells to progenitor cells and, finally, to granulocytes, monocytes, macrophages, and lymphocytes. These mature cells can in turn secrete or produce secondary cytokines with subsequent effects on inflammation, angiogenesis, epithelialization, and fibroplasia. Cloning of equine GM-CSF has recently been achieved.[26]

Interferons (IFNs)

Interferons (IFNs) represent a family of cytokines originally discovered on the basis of their antiviral activity, but which also influence general immunity, activating and modulating lymphocytes, macrophages, natural killer, and dendritic cells. Type I IFNs share the same ubiquitously expressed receptor and include IFN-α, produced by dendritic cells and monocytes/macrophages, and IFN-β, produced by several mesenchymal cell types. Interferon-γ is a type II IFN with its own distinct and more specifically expressed receptor. In horses, IFN-α1, -β and -γ were cloned and sequenced earlier[27]; however, recombinant proteins allowing the analysis of protein, antibodies, and biological activity only became available recently.[28] Interestingly, it was revealed that while recombinant equine IFN-γ does not display substantial antiviral activity, it shows immune modulatory effects on monocytes, at least in vitro. This indicates that IFN-γ may stimulate the inflammatory phase of repair, via release by activated monocytes and macrophages of a plethora of additional cytokines, in particular interleukins (ILs) and growth factors. IFN-γ is thought to prevent excessive fibrosis from occurring in the later stages of repair, which may be of particular significance to wound healing in the horse.[29]

Interleukins (ILs)

Interleukins (ILs) are produced by virtually every nucleated cell (in particular macrophages and lymphocytes) and most cells express IL surface receptors through which the cytokine mediates cell-to-cell and cell-to-matrix interactions. Two different IL-1 peptides exist: IL-1α and IL-1β. There is very close homology between the two and both activate cells and stimulate their proliferation. Interleukin-1 has a wide range of biological activities, many of which are pro-inflammatory, but it also aids in the later phases of repair. Notably, IL-1 is synthesized by epithelial cells in response to injury and favors epithelialization by directly stimulating chemoattraction of epithelial cells, and indirectly enhancing their proliferation by up-regulating keratinocyte growth factor (KGF) production by wound fibroblasts. The autocrine nature of epithelial cell–derived IL-1 is emphasized by the fact that it additionally induces the cell to synthesize IL-1, transforming growth factor (TGF)-α and KGF. Interleukin-1 also influences matrix synthesis and remodeling via stimulation of fibroblast proliferation and enhancement of collagenase production. Equine IL-1α and -β,[30] as well as their natural inhibitor, IL-1 receptor antagonist (IL-1ra's)cDNAs have been cloned, sequenced, and expressed.[31]

Other ILs have also been attributed a role in wound repair. For example, it has been shown, using IL-6–deficient mice, that repair of full-thickness excisional skin wounds requires this particular IL to proceed normally via gene expression of IL-1, chemokines, adhesion molecules, transforming growth factor beta (TGF-β1), and vascular endothelial growth factor (VEGF).[32] Interleukin-8 appears to accelerate maturation of granulation tissue, encouraging the formation of thicker, more mature collagen fibers.[33] Conversely, IL-10 seems inhibitory to ECM remodeling during wound repair, by reducing tumor necrosis factor α (TNFα)–induced fibroblast proliferation, decreasing concentrations of TGF-β1, and inhibiting collagen type I protein synthesis by dermal fibroblasts, at least in vitro.[34]

Tumor Necrosis Factor-α (TNF-α)

Tumor necrosis factor-α (TNF-α) is produced by a variety of cell types including macrophages, T cells, mast cells, and epithelial cells, and exerts principally inflammatory effects. Tumor necrosis factor-α may favor angiogenesis through chemoattraction and proliferation of endothelial cells, and it is also thought to enhance remodeling through fibroblast proliferation and up-regulation of collagenase as well as TIMP-1 levels.[35] Interestingly, loss of TNF-α in tissue macrophages potentiates TGF-β–mediated pathogenic tissue response during wound healing[36], which could favor fibrosis. Finally, TNF-α has been shown to stimulate epithelial cell migration. The gene encoding equine TNF-α has been cloned and characterized.[37]

Growth Factors

Connective Tissue Growth Factor (CTGF)

Connective tissue growth factor (CTGF) secretion by fibroblasts is selectively induced by TGF-β and its biological activities resemble those of platelet-derived growth factor (PDGF).[38] CTGF acts in an autocrine and paracrine fashion upon connective tissue cells, in particular the fibroblast, in which it mediates TGF-β activity, thus indirectly stimulating cell proliferation and ECM accumulation.[39] Connective tissue growth factor expression in blood vessels suggests a potential role in angiogenesis. As such, CTGF is an interesting target for future anti-fibrotic therapies because it is conceivable that inhibition of CTGF may block the pro-fibrotic effects of TGF-β without affecting TGF-β's anti-proliferative and immunosuppressive effects.[40] Although equine CTGF has not been cloned, an antigenic similarity between human and horse CTGF was recently established in a bio-equivalence assay.[41] This same study demonstrated that fibrogenic CTGF is present in horse lacrimal fluid, and derives, at least partly, from the lacrimal gland. This may explain why repair of corneal ulcers in horses is often associated with profound corneal stromal fibrosis and scar formation.

Epidermal Growth Factor (EGF)/Transforming Growth Factor-α (TGF-α)

Although plasma levels of epidermal growth factor (EGF) are undetectable, platelets release substantial amounts upon aggregation. This growth factor is also abundant in saliva, which may represent the physiologic basis for wound licking. As its name implies, EGF enhances epithelialization through various mechanisms: accrued contractility of epithelial cells allows more efficient migration,[42] and both proliferation and differentiation are favored. Furthermore, EGF exerts positive effects on the wound fibroblast, including chemoattraction, mitogenesis, and up-regulation of protein and MMP synthesis, important to the remodeling phase of repair.[18] The coding sequence for equine EGF has been identified, and it shows 60–70% amino acid identity with EGF sequences of other species.[43]

Transforming growth factor-α (TGF-α), which has no amino acid homology with TGF-β, is synthesized by activated macrophages and epithelial cells, and while it is distinct from EGF, it binds to the same cell-surface receptor and exhibits similar biologic activities. Like EGF it is a chemoattractant[44] and mitogenic for epithelial cells and fibroblasts; however, it is considered a more potent inducer of angiogenesis, in particular via initiation of tube formation by microvascular endothelial cells.[45] Interestingly, TGF-α has also been attributed a role in host defense during wound repair, by inducing the expression of antimicrobial peptides in proliferating epithelial cells, which complements the physical barrier against microorganisms formed by new epithelium.[46]

Fibroblast Growth Factor (FGF)

Basic fibroblast growth factor (bFGF), also called heparin-binding growth factor-2, is the most extensively studied member of a growing group of structurally related proteins with high affinity for heparin, and was one of the first angiogenic factors to be characterized.[47] It is synthesized by a number of cell types involved in angiogenesis and wound repair, and is found in the ECM bound to heparin. Although the exact mechanism involved in its cellular release remains unsolved, this is postulated to occur upon damage to the synthesizing cell. Dermal wounding could thus trigger the release of bFGF protein preexisting in cells in the wound area, allowing active bFGF to exert its mitogenic and chemotactic effects on virtually all cells.

Fibroblast growth factors are mitogenic to mesenchymal cells, whereby they influence many of the processes taking place during the proliferative phase of repair. Notably, bFGF promotes endothelial cell migration during granulation tissue formation by induction of cell surface integrins that mediate the binding of endothelial cells to ECM,[13] and is thus considered a potent angiogenic factor, particularly in response to the hypoxic wound environment. Additionally, bFGF can augment epithelialization and may stimulate wound contraction via the enhancement of TGF-β1 activity. Finally, bFGF exerts effects on matrix synthesis and remodeling by reversing the induction of collagen type I production while simultaneously encouraging collagenase production by fibroblasts.[48] A partial coding sequence for equine bFGF has been deduced and deposited in GenBank.[49]

Insulin-Like Growth Factors (IGFs)

The insulin-like growth factors (IGFs) are structurally similar to pro-insulin and have insulin-like activity. There are two forms with separate receptors: IGF-1 and IGF-2. Production of IGF-1 by the liver and other tissues is in part regulated by insulin, estrogen, and growth hormone (GH). Indeed, cell proliferation, tissue differentiation, and protein synthesis engendered by GH are mediated, indirectly, through the production of IGFs.

Unlike other growth factors whose primary source during wound repair is the inflammatory cell, substantial levels of inactive IGF, reversibly bound by high affinity IGF-binding proteins, are present in blood. Once cleaved, the free IGF can exert its autocrine, paracrine, and endocrine actions. Until recently, IGFs were primarily considered mediators of the growth-promoting effects of GH. Lately, it has been shown that IGF-1, released by platelets upon clotting and activated by enzymatic activity, low pH, and decreased oxygen tension present in the wound environment, is a potent chemoattractant and mitogenic for vascular endothelial cells,[50] enhances epithelial cell proliferation in vitro,[51] and stimulates collagen synthesis by fibroblasts.[52] In addition, IGF-1 stimulates epithelial cell membrane protrusion and facilitates cell spreading, which influences the speed of wound epithelialization.[51] Interestingly, IGF-1 induces TGF-β1 mRNA and protein expression,[53] which implies that it may, indirectly, influence even more aspects of repair.

Equine IGF-1 cDNA has been cloned and sequenced.[54]

Keratinocyte Growth Factor (KGF)

Keratinocyte growth factor-1 is a member of the rapidly growing FGF family; it is sometimes referred to as FGF-7 and resembles bFGF (FGF-2). While most FGFs influence proliferation and/or differentiation of numerous cell types, KGF, weakly expressed in skin but 100-fold up-regulated in dermal and granulation tissue fibroblasts after wounding,[55] acts specifically on epithelial cells in a paracrine fashion.[56] It stimulates migration and especially proliferation of these cells, but also affects differentiation of early progenitor cells within dermal appendages in the wound bed and adjacent dermis. Both KGF-1 and -2 were recently found to enhance granulation tissue formation during wound repair by increasing angiogenesis and collagen deposition.[57]

A partial coding sequence for horse KGF-1 (FGF-7) gene is known.[58]

Platelet-Derived Growth Factor (PDGF)

Platelet-derived growth factor (PDGF) is a family of isoforms consisting of homo- or heterodimers of products of two genes, the PDGF A-chain gene and PDGF B-chain gene. Three isoforms of PDGF exist, depending on the bonds formed between the A- and B-chains: AA, AB, and BB.[59] While the predominant isoform in human platelets is PDGF-AB, this is species variable and currently unknown in the horse. However, it was recently determined that the equine PDGF-A gene shares 83.8% sequence and 87.5% predicted peptide homology with human PDGF-A, while the equine PDGF-B gene is similar in length to the human gene, sharing 90.3% and 91.7% nucleotide and peptide identity, respectively.[60]

The platelet, the first cell to invade the site of trauma, is the largest source of PDGF, although a number of connective tissue cell types are also triggered by wounding to express PDGF-like molecules and receptors. Thus, throughout the normal repair process, wound tissues are continuously bathed in PDGF. The patterns of PDGF and PDGF receptor expression suggest a paracrine mechanism of action since the ligands are predominantly expressed in the epidermis whereas the receptors are found in the fibroblast of dermis and granulation tissue.[61]

Platelet-derived growth factor acts initially as a chemoattractant for inflammatory cells and fibroblasts, which it activates in an autocrine fashion. Subsequently it becomes mitogenic for mesenchymal cells through the release of other growth factors, namely TGF-β, from activated macrophages.[62] In this manner, PDGF may participate in angiogenesis and accelerate epithelialization in normal and pathologic wounds, including those of the horse cornea.[63] Furthermore, it stimulates the production of ECM components and increases collagenase activity by the wound fibroblast, in this manner enhancing remodeling. Finally, PDGF's role in contraction remains unclear, although it does not appear to be direct.[64]

Transforming Growth Factor-β (TGF-β)

Transforming growth factor-β (TGF-β) is widely acknowledged as the growth factor with the broadest range of activities in repair, based both on the variety of cell types that produce and/or respond to it and on the spectrum of its cellular responses.[65] In mammals, three isoforms of TGF-β are currently identified (TGF-β 1–3), whose spatial and temporal distributions are specific. TGF-β1 is the most abundant in the majority of tissues, and in platelets it is the only isoform.[65] The cDNA for equine TGF-β1 has been cloned and sequenced; it exhibits 99% identity to mature human TGF-β1.[66]

Transforming growth factor-β can be synthesized and released from virtually all cell types participating in the repair process. A unique feature of this peptide is that it can regulate its own production by monocytes and activated macrophages in an autocrine manner.[65] Autoinduction results in a sustained expression at the wound site and extends the effectiveness of both the initial burst of endogenous TGF-β released upon injury and exogenous TGF-β that may be applied to a wound. Thus, this growth factor is ubiquitous during repair when its major effects are to enhance chemoattraction of inflammatory and mesenchymal cells, in particular fibroblasts, and to modulate the accumulation of ECM.

In the former capacity, TGF-β's effects are exacerbated by its influence on activated macrophages to secrete more TGF-β as well as other angiogenic and fibrogenic mediators. The effects of TGF-β on ECM are more complex and profound than those of any other cytokine and are central to increasing the maturation and strength of wounds. In addition to enhancing fibroblast migration to the site of repair, TGF-β regulates the transcription of a wide variety of ECM proteins.[65] Furthermore, it concurrently inhibits ECM turnover by inducing TIMPs and reducing MMP expression. These particular activities have earned TGF-β the nickname "fibrogenic" cytokine. Indeed, a cause-and-effect relationship was established between TGF-β1/β2 and fibrosis, in various tissues.[67]

Transforming growth factor-β has also been found to promote angiogenesis by stimulating endothelial cell migration, differentiation, and tubule formation, as well as up-regulating their integrin receptors. Transforming growth factor-β's impact on epithelialization has not been completely elucidated; however, it appears to favor epithelial cell migration while inhibiting keratinocyte proliferation; its ability to do both simultaneously relates to its role as a potent stimulator of gene expression, in particular of ECM components, MMPs, and integrins in different target cells.[61]

Finally, TGF-β1 enhances wound contraction by inducing α-SMA expression in granulation tissue myofibroblasts.[68]

Vascular Endothelial Growth Factor (VEGF)

Vascular endothelial growth factor (VEGF), also known as vascular permeability factor, has potent and selective mitogenic, angiogenic, and permeability-enhancing effects on endothelial cells.[69] VEGF is expressed in a range of cells, predominantly macrophages, in response to soluble mediators, cell-bound stimuli, and environmental factors and binds to two endothelial cell-specific receptors. Expression is up-regulated during early wound repair in response to tissue hypoxia, and it correlates with the density of granulation tissue developing within the wound. While VEGF activity is considered essential to optimal wound angiogenesis via stimulation of ECM degradation, and proliferation, migration, and tube formation by endothelial cells,[70] it is not critical to wound healing. A further role recently attributed to VEGF consists of a proliferative stimulus exerted on keratinocytes, which might enhance wound epithelialization.[71] Cloning of equine VEGF cDNA has been achieved.[72]

Other Tissues Involved in Traumatic Wounds

Tendons and Ligaments

The reader is referred to Chapter 10 for detailed information on managing tendon lacerations. Tendons and ligaments are soft connective tissues consisting of closely packed collagen fiber bundles arranged in parallel fashion. The main function of these structures is to transmit tensile loads thereby providing for the motion and stability of joints in the musculoskeletal system.[73] Because the biomechanical properties of the healed tendon or ligament define its functional ability, it is critical to understand specific processes occurring in injured structures.[74]

Tendons and ligaments differ significantly in morphological appearance, biochemical content, and tensile properties. Moreover, it has long been recognized that healing characteristics differ between different ligaments (even within the same joint), making it difficult to describe a "typical healing scenario."[73] Nevertheless, the response to trauma of a ligament with "reasonable healing characteristics" (one located in an extra-articular compartment which is vascular and cellular, and in which stresses are low) is similar to that seen in any connective tissue. As for tendons, they may repair by either intrinsic (via resident tenocytes from the epitendon and endotendon) or extrinsic mechanisms, whereby cells from the surrounding paratendon, or sheath synovium (visceral layer) or subcutis, invade the tissue and support healing.[75] The latter form of repair generally prevails following severe disruption/transection of an equine tendon, which regrettably, compromises the end result via formation of peritendinous adhesions. Though it is true that mature tendons surrounded by a synovial sheath are poorly vascularized and rely principally on synovial fluid diffusion for nutrition,[76] they do have more blood vessels than is commonly accepted, and like any other connective tissue, undergo neovascularization during repair.[75]

While the phases of healing for tendinous/ligamentous tissues resemble those of other connective tissues, tendons and ligaments repair at a slower rate due to their dense, hypocellular composition.[77] Thus, the inflammatory phase may extend into the second week of repair while the proliferative phase with production of amorphous ground substance and aligned collagen occurs from 72 hours until roughly 6 weeks post-injury. In the horse superficial digital flexor tendon, expression of immature collagen (type III) is increased in the first 4 weeks following collagenase-induced injury.[78] Finally, the phase of matrix remodeling and maturation will last up to 1 year or longer following the initial trauma. After approximately 4 months, the collagen bundles having remodeled within an injured equine tendon will appear microscopically, similar to those of a normal, intact tendon.[79] Nevertheless, under the best circumstances, it may take up to twice that time before the repair site attains a strength equivalent to that of adjacent normal tendon.[80]

In many cases, remodeling of repair tissue within tendons and ligaments does not progress to the point of recreating normal tissue such that the scar remains different from the original structure in some important ways.[74] First, it appears that scars contain a number of 'flaws' (e.g., fat cells, inflammatory foci, blood vessels, loose collagen, and disorganized collagen),[81] which, while decreasing in number and size over time, never completely disappear. Second, while changes in the quantities of various key matrix components occur over time, with some of them recovering to within normal ranges, other matrix components do not recover as well. For example, chronic abnormalities in proteoglycan types, collagen types, and collagen fibril size and cross-links have been reported in healing rabbit medial collateral ligament.[82,83]

The repair tissue is weakest between the fifth and seventh day post-wounding. In general, there are improvements in load deformation properties over the first few months of healing; however, as mentioned previously, the properties of a normal uninjured tendon/ligament are likely to never be entirely restored.

New treatment modalities are being explored in an effort to improve the substandard repair of tendon/ligament tissue. An exciting alternative that has also interested veterinary scientists is the local delivery of pluripotent growth factor molecules to the injured tissue. In the horse, expression of both IGF-I and TGF-β was detected in collagenase-damaged superficial digital flexor tendon. Specifically, mRNA levels for TGF-β1 peak early in the wound healing process (1 week). In the first 2 weeks after lesion induction, tissue levels of IGF-I protein decrease approximately 40% compared to normal tendon; however by 4 weeks, these levels exceed those of normal tendon and remain elevated through 8 weeks.[78]

Intralesional injections of recombinant human IGF-I[84] as well as administration of recombinant human PDGF-BB to equine superficial digital flexor tendons in explant culture[85] have recently shown promise (see Chapter 10). Administration of other growth factors such as bFGF, TGF-β, and VEGF, shown to be key molecules implicated in the various phases of tendon/ligament repair in other species[77], has yet to be evaluated in a pure recombinant form in the horse. However, investigators have shown the benefits of culturing equine superficial digital flexor tendon explants in platelet-rich plasma (PRP),[86] an excellent source of growth factors released from platelet α-granules, including PDGF, TGF-β, FGF, VEGF, IGF-I, and EGF.[87] For more information on PRP, see Wound Repair: Problems in the Horse and Innovative Solutions later in this chapter.

Another promising alternative is to make use of mesenchymal stem cells (MSCs) that have the potential to differentiate into a spectrum of specialized tissues including tendon and ligament. Two reports in the horse have documented a positive effect of either adipose-derived adult stem cells[88] or MSCs and bone marrow mononucleated cells[89] on tendon healing. In both cases the pluripotent cells were injected into collagenase-induced lesions within the superficial digital flexor tendon, which caused no adverse effects over 7[88] or 21[89] weeks.

The first study documented that DNA, glycosaminoglycan, and total collagen content were not differentially induced by treatment; however, stem-cell–treated lesions showed improved tendon fiber architecture, reduced inflammatory cell infiltration, and improved tendon fiber density and alignment upon histological examination.[88] The second study documented immunohistochemically an increased expression of type I collagen concomitant with decreased expression of type III collagen protein.[89]

While none of these experimental models fully reproduces the clinical situation of a tendon wound occurring in a horse, valuable information can be gleaned from these studies in regard to the eventual use of innovative modalities to treat a tendon injury.

Nonetheless, despite the promising findings of the aforementioned studies targeting therapies to enhance tendon and ligament repair, no existing approach brings about complete tissue recovery following injury. Many delivery parameters such as amount of recombinant growth factors at the wound site, as well as duration and method of delivery, may prove critical to success. As is true for skin, we must increase our knowledge of both the molecular and cellular mechanisms underlying tendon and ligament repair to better design an effective treatment regimen.

Periosteum

Periosteum, a well-vascularized osteogenic organ, possesses two distinct layers which contribute to wound repair. The outer fibrous layer contains fibroblasts, blood vessels, and fibers of Sharpey (a direct continuation of periosteal collagen fibers around which the bone's cortical lamellae grow) while the inner cambium layer encloses nerves, capillaries, osteoblasts, and MSCs.[90] Periosteal vessels from the outer layer contribute to bone healing because they nourish the outer third of the diaphysis and supplement the epiphysio-metaphyseal vessels and the principal nutrient arteries found within the medullary cavity.[91] The cambium layer serves as a reservoir of undifferentiated pluripotential MSCs[92] and as a source of growth factors playing important roles in the healing and remodeling process taking place at the outer surface of damaged cortical bone.

Many studies have shown that injured periosteum regenerates both cartilage and bone from its progenitor cells;[90] indeed, MSCs from the cambium layer can differentiate into neochondrocytes to produce cartilage tissue that is later replaced by bone and/or can differentiate directly into osteoblasts.[93] One study in horses showed that chondroid tissue displaying morphologic and matrix staining properties similar to those of hyaline cartilage was generated from periosteum obtained from the medial aspect of the proximal tibia and placed intra-articularly.[94] Localized outgrowths of new bone beneath the periosteum are referred to as exostoses. These result from the rapid formation of new or reactive bone following activation and proliferation of osteoblast progenitors in the cambium layer, as may result from avulsion, laceration, or blunt trauma. Trabeculae of woven bone extend from the underlying bone surface at acute angles, and can be readily distinguished histologically from the mature lamellar bone of the cortex. Depending on their size and the inciting cause, exostoses may either persist or gradually be removed by remodeling (Figures 1.8a and 1.8b)[95]. For specific examples of the contribution of periosteum to wound repair, see Chapter 6.

Hoof

The old adage "no hoof, no horse" signals the need to fully understand the mechanisms governing repair of the tissues contained in this specialized anatomic structure. Briefly, the lamellar corium, of dermal origin, overlies the periosteum of the distal (third) phalanx and is tightly interlocked with the epidermal laminae of the hoof. In cases of traumatic avulsion, the stratum germinativum of the epidermal laminae usually remains adhered to the lamellar corium. The living cells thus spared are responsible for the rapid epithelialization and keratinization often seen in the wound bed.[97] The lamellar basement membrane, left intact, is used as a template for proliferating cells.[98]

The hoof wall, or stratum corneum, is of epidermal origin and is usually divided into a stratum externum, which is a thin superficial layer of horn that extends distad from the periople a variable distance; a stratum medium, which is thick and highly keratinized; and a softer stratum internum, which includes the epidermal laminae mentioned previously. The stratum medium is composed of horn tubules which grow from the stratum germinativum of the coronary epidermis that surrounds the coronary papillae. With the coronary corium and

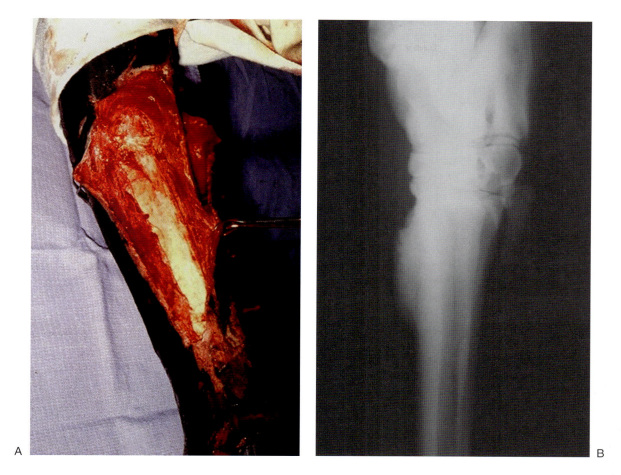

A   B

Figure 1.8. (a) Extensive avulsion injury to the dorsal metatarsal region. This picture was taken at surgery; the periosteum had been stripped from the exposed cortex of the metatarsal bone. Following cleansing and debridement, the edges of the distal half of the wound were apposed with sutures while the proximal half was left open to heal by second intention. A bandage cast splint that extended from the plantar fetlock region to the caudal mid-tibial region was used to immobilize the limb. (b) Lateral radiograph taken following complete healing of the wound. Note the mature (remodeled) exostoses that formed on the dorsal aspect of the metatarsal bone in the region where the wound was allowed to heal by second intention. Courtesy of Dr. T. Stashak.

perioplic corium of dermal origin, the coronary epidermis constitutes the coronary band. Clinically, the underlying modified subcutis, or coronary cushion, is often considered part of the coronary band.

The slow distad growth of the hoof wall (10 mm per month) results from the differences between the primary and secondary epidermal laminae of the stratum internum. Cells of the primary epidermal laminae progressively keratinize while moving distally with the tubules of the stratum medium. The basal cells of the secondary lamellae, on the other hand, adhere to the lamellar corium and do not keratinize. A continuous cycle of breaking and reforming links between the two cell populations is responsible for maintaining a very strong attachment of the hoof wall to the parietal surface of the distal phalanx, while allowing slow distal growth of the horn tubules.[99] Upon reaching the solar surface of the hoof, the keratinized cells of the epidermal laminae form the junction between the hoof wall and the sole. This zone of softer and whiter horn is commonly called the white line (Figure 1.9).

Specific biomechanical properties of the equine foot affect the pattern of injury but also the pattern of repair. Any injury of sufficient force to invade the resistant stratum corneum usually results in a full-thickness wound (Figure 1.10). Full-thickness hoof wounds are rare but when they occur, the rigidity of the stratum corneum usually prevents gaping of the wound margins, encourages fracture as opposed to tear of the hoof capsule, and causes the tissues to completely avulse from the underlying structures rather than just lacerate.[100] Where the hoof wall is thinner and less rigid, at the coronary band and at the heel, lacerations, tears, and partial-thickness wounds are more common. For more information regarding laceration and avulsion injury of the hoof, see Chapter 8.

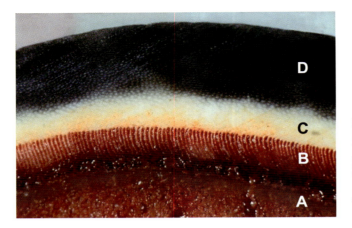

Figure 1.9. Cross-section of the hoof at the level of the white line. A: distal phalanx; B: lamellae; C: white line; D: hoof wall. The keratinized cells of the epidermal laminae usually form a junction between the hoof wall and the sole made of softer and whiter horn and commonly called "white line." Reprinted from *Veterinary Clinics of North America Equine Practice*, 21(1), Céleste C and Szoke M, Management of Equine Hoof Injuries, pp. 167–190, Copyright (2005), with permission from Elsevier.

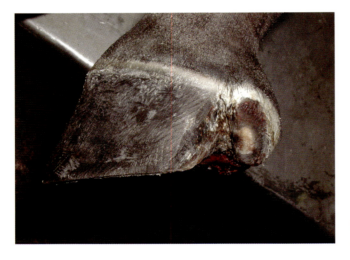

Figure 1.10. Full-thickness hoof wound. Courtesy of Centre Hospitalier Universitaire Vétérinaire de l'Université de Montréal.

Wounds affecting tissues below the coronary band are contained within the rigid stratum corneum such that swelling is impossible during the inflammatory phase. Furthermore, the rigid nature of the hoof may prevent adequate drainage of exudate and spontaneous elimination of foreign bodies and necrotic tissues, leading to sub-solar abscess formation and/or infection of deeper underlying structures. For more information regarding sub-solar abscesses, see Chapter 8. Contraction does not occur in hoof wounds[101] and epithelialization differs. A full-thickness hoof wound involving the frog or sole usually evolves similarly to a full-thickness skin wound, with homogenous epithelial coverage coming from surrounding epithelium and re-establishment of epithelial strata by local epithelial proliferation. In a full-thickness wound involving the hoof wall, epithelium is re-established by progressive hoof wall growth from the coronary band downward rather than by local epithelial proliferation. However, in some hoof wounds and especially those involving the coronary band region, the epithelial margins may be of one or more origins. In these cases, the final appearance and structure of the healed wound will reflect the nature and source of epithelium that filled the defect.[100] Thus, full-thickness wounds involving both skin and the coronary band will often cause the formation of horny spurs or persistent defects in the hoof wall. For more information regarding full-thickness wounds and the formation of horny spurs, see Chapter 8.

Conclusion

The equine practitioner to whom is presented a wounded horse should fully understand the physiologic mechanisms underlying repair to design an appropriate treatment plan. In the following chapters of this book, experienced authors share their opinions on how best to manage specific injuries. The reader will benefit from a thorough knowledge of the different phases of healing as well as the mediators governing them, since these dictate the approach to follow, particularly in complicated wounds such as those afflicted by chronic inflammation and/or an excessive proliferative response.

References

1. Theoret CL: Wound repair and specific reaction to injury. In JA Auer and JA Stick eds. *Equine surgery (3rd edition)*. Philadelphia: W.B. Saunders, 2005, p. 44
2. Kirsner RS, Eaglstein WH: The wound healing process. Dermatol Clin 1993;11:629
3. Singer AJ, Clark RAF: Cutaneous wound healing. New Engl J Med 1999;341:738
4. Simpson DM, Ross R: The neutrophilic leukocyte in wound repair—a study with antineutrophil serum. J Clin Invest 1972;51:2009
5. Leibovich SJ, Ross R: The role of the macrophage in wound repair: a study with hydrocortisone and antimacrophage serum. Am J Pathol 1975;78:71
6. Martin P, D'Souza D, Martin J, et al: Wound healing in the PU.1 null mouse—tissue repair is not dependent on inflammatory cells. Current Biol 2003;13:1122
7. Duffield JS, Forbes SJ, Constandinou CM, et al: Selective depletion of macrophages reveals distinct, opposing roles during liver injury and repair. J Clin Invest 2005;115:56
8. Greenhalgh DG: The role of apoptosis in wound healing. Int J Biochem Cell Biol 1998;30:1019
9. Mignatti P, Rifkin DB, Welgus HG, et al: Proteinases and tissue remodeling. In RAF Clark ed. *The molecular and cellular biology of wound repair (2nd edition)*. New York: Plenum Press, 1996, p. 427
10. Desmoulière A, Redard M, Darby I, et al: Apoptosis mediates the decrease in cellularity during the transition between granulation tissue and scar. Am J Pathol 1995;146:56
11. Luo S, Benathan M, Raffoul W, et al: Abnormal balance between proliferation and apoptotic cell death in fibroblasts derived from keloid lesions. Plast Reconstr Surg 2001;107:87
12. Liekens S, De Clerq E, Neyts J: Angiogenesis: regulators and clinical applications. Biochem Pharmacol 2001;61:253
13. Li J, Zhang Y-P, Kirsner RS: Angiogenesis in wound repair: angiogenic growth factors and the extracellular matrix. Microsc Res Tech 2003;60:107
14. Zhu WH, Guo X, Villaschi S, et al: Regulation of vascular growth and regression by matrix metalloproteinases in the rat aorta model of angiogenesis. Lab Invest 2000;80:545
15. Davis GE, Senger DR: Endothelial extracellular matrix. Biosynthesis, remodeling, and functions during vascular morphogenesis and neovessel stabilization. Circ Res 2005;97:1093
16. Woodley DT: Reepithelialization. In RAF Clark ed. *The molecular and cellular biology of wound repair (2nd edition)*. New York: Plenum Press, 1996, p. 339
17. Stashak TS: Principles of wound healing. In TS Stashak ed. *Equine wound management*. Philadelphia: Lea and Febiger, 1991, p. 11
18. Nanney LB, King LE: Epidermal growth factor and transforming growth factor-β. In RAF Clark ed. *The molecular and cellular biology of wound repair (2nd edition)*. New York: Plenum Press, 1996, p. 171
19. Desmoulière A, Gabbiani G: The role of the myofibroblast in wound healing and fibrocontractive diseases. In RAF Clark ed. *The molecular and cellular biology of wound repair (2nd edition)*. New York: Plenum Press, 1996, p. 391
20. Madison JB, Gronwall RR: Influence of wound shape on wound contraction in horses. Am J Vet Res 1992;53:1575
21. Grinnell F, Zhu M, Carlson MA, et al: Release of mechanical tension triggers apoptosis of human fibroblasts in a model of regressing granulation tissue. Exp Cell Res 1999;248:608
22. Witte MB, Thornton FJ, Kiyama T, et al: Metalloproteinase inhibitors and wound healing: a novel enhancer of wound strength. Surg 1998;124:464
23. Yager DR, Chen SM, Ward SI, et al: Ability of chronic wound fluids to degrade peptide growth factors is associated with increased levels of elastase activity and diminished levels of proteinase inhibitors. Wound Repair Regen 1997;5:23
24. Levenson SM, Geever EF, Crowley LV, et al: The healing of rat skin wounds. Ann Surg 1965;161:293
25. Mann A, Breuhahn K, Schirmacher P, et al: Keratinocyte-derived granulocyte-macrophage colony stimulating factor accelerates wound healing: Stimulation of keratinocyte proliferation, granulation tissue formation, and vascularization. J Invest Dermatol 2001;117:1382
26. Mauel S, Steinbach F, Ludwig H: Monocyte-derived dendritic cells from horses differ from dendritic cells of humans and mice. Immunol 2006;117:463
27. Curran JA, Argyle DJ, Cox P, et al: Nucleotide sequence of the equine interferon gamma cDNA. DNA Seq 1994;4:405
28. Steinbach F, Mauel S, Beier I: Recombinant equine interferons: expression cloning and biological activity. Vet Immunol Immunopathol 2002;84:83

29. Ishida Y, Kondo T, Takayasu T, et al: The essential involvement of cross-talk between IFN-gamma and TGF-beta in the skin wound-healing process. J Immunol 2004;172:1848

30. Howard RD, McIlwraith CW, Trotter GW, et al: Cloning of equine interleukin 1 alpha and equine interleukin 1 beta and determination of their full-length cDNA sequences. Am J Vet Res 1998;59:704

31. Howard RD, McIlwraith CW, Trotter GW, et al: Cloning of equine interleukin 1 receptor antagonist and determination of its full-length cDNA sequence. Am J Vet Res 1998;59:712

32. Lin ZQ, Kondo T, Ishida Y, et al: Essential involvement of IL-6 in the skin wound-healing process as evidenced by delayed wound healing in IL-6–deficient mice. J Leukoc Biol 2003;73:713

33. Moyer KE, Saggers GC, Allison GM, et al: Effects of interleukin-8 on granulation tissue maturation. J Cell Physiol 2002;193:173

34. Moroguchi A, Ishimura K, Okano K, et al: Interleukin-10 suppresses proliferation and remodeling of extracellular matrix of cultured human skin fibroblasts. Eur Surg Res 2004;36:39

35. Mori R, Kondo T, Ohshima T, et al: MMP-1 and TIMP-1 mRNA expression were markedly increased with IL-6 and TNF-alpha treatment and remains unchanged with IL-1beta. Burns 2003;29:527

36. Saika S, Ikeda K, Yamanaka O, et al: Loss of tumor necrosis factor alpha potentiates transforming growth factor beta-mediated pathogenic tissue response during wound healing. Am J Pathol 2006;168:1848

37. Su X, Deem Morris D, McGraw RA: Cloning and characterization of gene TNFα encoding equine tumor necrosis factor alpha. Gene 1991;107:319

38. Igarashi A, Okochi H, Bradham DM, et al: Regulation of connective tissue growth factor gene expression in human skin fibroblasts and during wound repair. Mol Biol Cell 1993;4:637

39. Grotendorst GR: Connective tissue growth factor: A mediator of TGF-β action on fibroblasts. Cytokine Growth Factor Rev 1997;8:171

40. Blom IE, Goldschmeding R, Leask A: Gene regulation of connective tissue growth factor: new targets for antifibrotic therapy? Matrix Biol 2002;21:473

41. Ollivier FJ, Brooks DE, Schultz GS, et al: Connective tissue growth factor in tear film of the horse: detection, identification and origin. Graefes, Arch Clin Exp Ophthalmol 2004;242:165

42. Haase I, Evans R, Pofahl R, et al: Regulation of keratinocyte shape, migration and wound epithelialization by IGF-1- and EGF-dependent signaling pathways. J Cell Sci 2003;116:3227

43. Stewart F, Power CA, Lennard SN, et al: Identification of the horse epidermal growth factor (EGF) coding sequence and its use in monitoring EGF gene expression in the endometrium of the pregnant mare. J Mol Endocrinol 1994;12:341

44. Li Y, Fan J, Chen M, et al: Transforming growth factor-alpha: a major human serum factor that promotes human keratinocyte migration. J Invest Dermatol 2006;126:2096

45. Ono M, Okamuro K, Nakayama Y, et al: Induction of human microvascular endothelial tubular morphogenesis by human keratinocytes: Involvement of transforming growth factor-alpha. Biochem Biophys Res Commun 1992;189:601

46. Sorensen OE, Cowland JB, Theilgaard-Monch K, et al: Wound healing and expression of antimicrobial peptides/polypeptides in human keratinocytes, a consequence of common growth factors. J Immunol 2003;170:5583

47. Abraham JA, Klagsbrun M: Modulation of wound repair by members of the fibroblast growth factor family. In RAF Clark ed. *The molecular and cellular biology of wound repair (2nd edition).* New York: Plenum Press, 1996, p. 195

48. Kuwabara K, Ogawa S, Matsumoto M, et al: Hypoxia-mediated induction of acidic/basic fibroblast growth factor and platelet-derived growth factor in mononuclear phagocytes stimulates growth of hypoxic endothelial cells. Proc Natl Acad Sci USA 1995;92:4606

49. Welter H, Bollwein H, Einspanier R: Direct submission to GenBank (AJ319906) for Equus caballus FGF-2, 2002

50. Taylor WR, Alexander RW: Autocrine control of wound repair by insulin-like growth factor 1 in cultured endothelial cells. Am J Physiol 1993;265:C801

51. Ando H, Jensen PJ: EGF and IGF-1 enhance keratinocyte migration. J Invest Dermatol 1993;100:633

52. Dunaiski V, Belford DA: Contribution of circulating IGF-I to wound repair in GH-treated rats. Growth Horm IGF Res 2002;12:381

53. Ghahary A, Shen Q, Shen YJ, et al: Induction of transforming growth factor beta 1 by insulin-like growth factor-1 in dermal fibroblasts. J Cell Physiol 1998;174:301

54. Otte K, Rozell B, Gessbo A, et al: Cloning and sequencing of an equine insulin-like growth factor I cDNA and its expression in fetal and adult tissues. Gen Comp Endocrinol 1996;102:11

55. Beer HD, Gassmann MG, Munz B, et al: Expression and function of keratinocyte growth factor and activin in skin morphogenesis and cutaneous wound repair. J Investig Dermatol Symp Proc 2000;5:34

56. Werner S: Keratinocyte growth factor: a unique player in epithelial repair processes. Cytokine Growth Factor Rev 1998;9:153

57. Robson MC, Phillips TJ, Falanga V, et al: Randomized trial of topically applied repifermin (recombinant human keratinocyte growth factor-2) to accelerate wound healing in venous ulcers. Wound Repair Regen 2001;9:347

58. Welter H, Bollwein H, Einspanier R: Direct submission to GenBank (AJ439891) for Equus caballus FGF-7, 2002

59. Heldin CH, Westermark B: Role of platelet-derived growth factor *in vivo*. In RAF Clark ed. *The molecular and cellular biology of wound repair (2nd edition)*. New York: Plenum Press, 1996, p. 249

60. Donnelly BP, Nixon AJ, Haupt JL, et al: Nucleotide structure of equine platelet-derived growth factor-A and -B and expression in horses with induced acute tendinitis. Am J Vet Res 2006;67:1218

61. Santoro MM and Gaudino G: Cellular and molecular facets of keratinocyte reepithelialization during wound healing. Exp Cell Res 2005;304:274

62. Pierce GF, Vande Berg J, Rudolph R, et al: Platelet-derived growth factor-BB and transforming growth factor beta 1 selectively modulate glycosaminoglycans, collagen, and myofibroblasts in excisional wounds. Am J Pathol 1991;138:629

63. Haber M, Cao Z, Panjwani N, et al: Effects of growth factors (EGF, PDGF-BB and TGF-beta 1) on cultured equine epithelial cells and keratocytes: implications for wound healing. Vet Ophthalmol 2003;6:211

64. Saba AA, Freedman BM, Gaffield JW, et al: Topical platelet-derived growth factor enhances wound closure in the absence of wound contraction: an experimental and clinical study. Ann Plast Surg 2002;49:62

65. Roberts AB, Sporn MB: Transforming growth factor-β. In RAF Clark ed. *The molecular and cellular biology of wound repair (2nd edition)*. New York: Plenum Press, 1996, p. 275

66. Penha-Goncalves MN, Onions DE, Nicolson L: Cloning and sequencing of equine transforming growth factor–beta-1 (TGF–beta-1) cDNA. DNA Seq 1997;7:375

67. Shah M, Foreman DM, Ferguson MWJ: Neutralization of TGF-β1 and TGF-β2 or exogenous addition of TGF-β3 to cutaneous rat wounds reduces scarring. J Cell Sci 1995;108:985

68. Desmoulière A, Geinoz A, Gabbiani F, et al: Transforming growth factor β1 induces α-smooth muscle actin expression in granulation tissue myofibroblasts in quiescent and growing cultured fibroblasts. J Cell Biol 1993;122:103

69. Dvorak HF, Brown LF, Betmar M, et al: Vascular permeability factor/vascular endothelial growth factor, microvascular hyperpermeability, and angiogenesis. Am J Pathol 1995;146:1029

70. Howdieshell TR, Callaway D, Webb WL, et al: Antibody neutralization of vascular endothelial growth factor inhibits wound granulation tissue formation. J Surg Res 2001;96:173

71. Wilgus TA, Matthies AM, Radek KA, et al: Novel function for vascular endothelial growth factor receptor-1 on epidermal keratinocytes. Am J Pathol 2005;167:1257

72. Miura N, Misumi K, Kawahara K, et al: Cloning of cDNA and high-level expression of equine vascular endothelial growth factor. Direct submission to GenBank (AB053350), 2001

73. Woo SLY, Debski RE, Zeminski J, et al: Injury and repair of ligaments and tendons. Ann Rev Biomed Engin 2000; 2:83

74. Frank CB, Hart DA, Shrive NG: Molecular biology and biomechanics of normal and healing ligaments: a review. Osteoarthr Cartil 1999;7:130

75. Fenwick SA, Hazleman BL, Riley GP: The vasculature and its role in the damaged and healing tendon. Arthritis Res 2002;4:252

76. Gelberman RH: Flexor tendon physiology: tendon nutrition and cellular activity in injury and repair. Instr Course Lect 1985;34:351

77. Tozer S, Duprez D: Tendon and ligament: development, repair and disease. Birth Defects Res C Embryo Today 2005;75:226

78. Dahlgren LA, Mohammed HO, Nixon AJ: Temporal expression of growth factors and matrix molecules in healing tendon lesions. J Orthop Res 2005;23:84

79. Watkins JP, Auer JA, Gay S, et al: Healing of surgically created defects in the equine superficial digital flexor tendon: collagen-type transformation and tissue morphologic reorganization. Am J Vet Res 1985;46:2091

80. Manske PR, Gelberman RH, Vande Berg JS, et al: Intrinsic flexor tendon repair. A morphological study in vitro. J Bone Joint Surg 1984;66:385

81. Shrive N, Chimich D, Marchuk L, et al: Soft tissue "flaws" are associated with the material properties of the healing rabbit medial collateral ligament. J Orthop Res 1995;13:923

82. Frank CB, Shrive NG, McDonald DB, et al: Rabbit medial collateral ligament scar weakness is associated with decreased collagen hydroxypyridinium cross-link density. J Orthop Res 1995;13:157

83. Frank CB, McDonald D, Shrive NG: Collagen fibril diameters in the rabbit medial collateral ligament scar: a longer term assessment. Connect Tissue Res 1997;36:261

84. Dahlgren LA, van der Meulen MC, Bertram JE, et al: Insulin-like growth factor-I improves cellular and molecular aspects of healing in a collagenase-induced model of flexor tendinitis. J Orthop Res 2002;20:910

85. Haupt JL, Donnelly BP, Nixon AJ: Effects of platelet-derived growth factor-BB on the metabolic function and morphologic features of equine tendon in explant culture. Am J Vet Res 2006;67:1595

86. Schnabel LV, Mohammed HO, Miller BJ, et al: Platelet-rich plasma (PRP) enhances anabolic gene expression patterns in flexor digitorum superficialis tendons. J Orthop Res 2007;25:230

87. Pietrzak WS, Eppley BL: Platelet rich plasma: biology and new technology. J Craniofac Surg 2005;16:1043

88. Dahlgren LA, Haupt JL, Yeager AD, et al: Adipose-derived adult stem cells improve aspects of tendon regeneration. Vet Surg 2006;35:E5

89. Crovace A, Lacitignola L, De Siena R, et al: Regeneration of extracellular matrix in collagenase induced tendonitis model in the horse using cultured bone marrow mesenchymal cells and bone marrow mononucleated cells, controlled with placebo: preliminary results. Vet Surg 2006;35:E5

90. Malizos KN, Papatheodorou LK: The healing potential of the periosteum. Injury, Int J Care Injured 2005;36S:13

91. Glowacki J: Angiogenesis in fracture repair. Clin Orthop 1998;355:82

92. Nakahara H, Bruder SP, Goldberg VM, et al: In vivo osteochondrogenetic potential of cultured cells derived from periosteum. Clin Orthop 1990;259:223

93. Scott-Savage P, Hall BK: Differentiative ability of the tibial periosteum for the embryonic chick. Acta Anat (Basel) 1980;106:129

94. Vachon A, McIlwraith CW, Trotter GW, et al: Neochondrogenesis in free intra-articular, periosteal, and perichondrial autografts in horses. Am J Vet Res 1989;50:1787

95. Thompson K: Bones and joints. In MG Maxie ed. *Jubb, kennedy and palmer's pathology of domestic animals (5th edition)*. Philadelphia: Saunders Elsevier, 2007, p. 21

96. Céleste CL, Szoke MO: Management of equine hoof injuries. Vet Clin North Am Equine Pract 2005;21:167

97. Kainer RA: Clinical anatomy of the equine foot. Vet Clin North Am Equine Pract 1989;5:1

98. Pollitt CC, Daradka M: Hoof wall wound repair. Equine Vet J 2004;36:210

99. Leach DH, Oliphant LW: Ultrastructure of the equine hoof wall secondary epidermal lamellae. Am J Vet Res 1983;44:1561

100. Parks AH. Equine foot wounds: general principles of healing and treatment. Proc Am Assoc Equine Pract 1999: 180

101. Fessler JF: Hoof injuries. Vet Clin North Am Equine Pract 1989;5:643

1.2 Differences in Wound Healing between Horses and Ponies

Jacintha M. Wilmink, DVM, PhD, Diplomate RNVA

Horses and Ponies: Same Species, Different Healing Characteristics

Over the course of millions of years the horse evolved from a small forest dweller to a large ungulate which inhabited the vast open plains of the temperate zone. It became a so-called "fright and flight" animal whose instinctive reaction to danger is to run.[1] Evolution took place as a response to various environmental and climatic challenges while selection by mankind resulted in the development of special features. Both evolution and selection led to the large variety of breeds known today.

The equine species can be roughly subdivided into horses and ponies; this is officially a matter of the height at the withers of an adult (ponies are <1.48 meters). Whether ponies are just small horses has been disputed for decades. The discussion of this topic, with respect to wound healing, started in the 1980s, when Bertone, et al. (1985)[2] found in a study on second-intention healing that ponies healed faster without the formation of exuberant granulation tissue (EGT), in contrast to horses. However, other authors reported the development of EGT in ponies,[3,4] and the faster healing of wounds in ponies could not be confirmed.[4] Because a difference in wound healing between horses and ponies might provide information about the basic biology of equine wound healing and about the complications commonly associated with repair in this species, Wilmink, et al. performed a series of experiments to investigate wound healing in both horses and ponies. They proved that ponies heal faster and with fewer complications than do horses[5–7] and demonstrated that these differences were based on the efficiency and capacity of the leukocyte to produce several mediators.[8,9] The details of these studies will be discussed herein.

What remains to be elucidated is the cause of the observed differences in healing between horses and ponies. It may well be that the longer period of domestication of the horse has precluded natural selection against poor healing, since the wounded horse was/is tended to by man. Additionally, the artificial selection of features such as height, athletic capacity, and appearance might have favored the development of some diseases and undesirable characteristics, possibly including the reduced efficiency of leukocytes. Moreover, horses with poorly healed wounds, which limit their athletic ability, are often used for breeding, which may perpetuate the cycle. In contrast, ponies have been domesticated for a much shorter time period, and that suboptimal health status and poor healing capabilities may have been ruled out by natural selection. Moreover, artificial selection within pony breeds has been less intense and many pony breeds maintain subpopulations (and genetic reserves) in the wild. This could explain the better wound healing capacity of ponies compared to horses.

Clinically Apparent Phases during Wound Healing

Wound healing is often divided into general phases of acute inflammation, proliferation, and remodeling. Because these phases overlap and occur simultaneously in all tissue components, it is difficult to distinguish them from one another. Consequently, this division is more theoretical than clinical. In practice it may be more realistic to divide healing into macroscopically apparent events: inflammation, formation of granulation tissue, wound contraction, and epithelialization. Although these events also partially overlap, they largely succeed one another and occur more or less chronologically. Moreover, they are clearly visible to the veterinarian. These events occur as well during primary intention healing, but then they are shorter and not readily visible. Remarkable differences in these phases between horses and ponies and between body and limb wounds determine the speed and efficiency of healing.[5,6] The following simplified review summarizes the main mechanisms of healing.

Inflammatory Phase

During this phase polymorphonuclear (PMN) cells and macrophages migrate to the wound site to clear it of contaminating bacteria and nonviable tissue. This process is referred to as cellular debridement. Macrophages additionally release a plethora of biologically active substances that are essential for the recruitment of more inflammatory and mesenchymal cells and initiate the healing process.[10] For more information see Section 1.1 of this chapter.

Formation of Granulation Tissue

Macrophages, fibroblasts, and endothelial cells move into the wound space as a unit and depend on one another.[11] Macrophages provide a continuing source of cytokines and growth factors necessary for the stimulation of fibroplasia and angiogenesis. Fibroblasts construct new extracellular matrix (ECM) needed to support cell in-growth while blood vessels transport oxygen and nutrients necessary to cell metabolism.[12] Fibroblasts use the fibrin clot as a provisional matrix for migration and rapidly replace it with a new loose ECM consisting of glycoproteins (fibronectin and laminin), proteoglycans (hyaluronic acid), and collagens (initially type III, later type I).[13] The entity of cells and ECM is granulation tissue which fills the gap and is the basis for subsequent wound contraction and epithelial migration.

Wound Contraction

Wound contraction results from the action of differentiated fibroblasts (myofibroblasts) in the granulation tissue, which contain filaments of smooth muscle actin. Contraction of these filaments in the fibroblasts and connection among fibroblasts and with ECM pull the wound margins centripetally (toward the center),[14,15] rapidly reducing the wound surface area by means of intact full-thickness skin. Consequently, wound contraction is a critical determinant of the speed of second intention wound healing as well as the final cosmetic appearance of the scar. Wound contraction is stimulated by certain cytokines but inhibited by chronic inflammation.

Epithelialization

Epithelialization is the slowest phase of the wound healing process and concludes wound closure (1 mm/10 days at the most in limb wounds of horses).[16] Although epithelialization starts a few hours after trauma with the migration of epithelial cells, it becomes macroscopically apparent only about 2 weeks after wounding. Epithelial proliferation occurs after 2 days, triggered by the secretion of cytokines and growth factors by fibroblasts, inflammatory cells, and the keratinocytes themselves.[12,13] Epithelialization is impaired by fibrin remnants of the clot and by chronic inflammation.[17] Newly formed epithelium lacks skin adnexa and is thin and fragile because it is poorly attached to the underlying basement membrane.[18] The part of the wound that has healed by epithelialization remains visible as a superficial scar.

For further details on the physiology of wound repair, see the previous section of this chapter.

First Intention Healing (Primary Wound Closure)

When possible, primary closure of traumatic wounds is preferred because healing is usually faster and the cosmetic results are better than after second intention healing. Unfortunately, primary closure may result in either partial or complete dehiscence of the wound. Whether a wound dehisces or not depends on many factors including those relating to the wound itself, to the animal, to the chosen treatment method, and to the environment.[19,20]

Differences in first intention healing between horses and ponies were evaluated retrospectively in more than 500 equine patients suffering traumatic wounds and admitted to a referral clinic.[7] Patients were identified as horse or pony according to the average adult height at the wither of the breed; ponies measured <1.48 meters, horses measured >1.48 meters. The outcome of primary closure and the occurrence of bone sequestra were recorded. Successful primary closure was defined as complete healing by first intention without any degree of dehiscence (Figures 1.11a and 1.11b). The study revealed that successful primary closure occurs significantly more often in ponies than in horses, while bone sequestra form significantly less often in ponies.

The predominant cause of both wound dehiscence and sequestra formation is wound infection.[7,21–23] Other factors contributing to wound dehiscence are tension on the wound margins, excessive movement of the sutured region, and involvement of certain structures; factors contributing to sequestra formation include exposure of cortical bone and excessive trauma.[24] Factors that may influence the risk of wound infection include the time elapsed since injury, the degree of contamination, the degree of tissue damage, and the thoroughness of wound

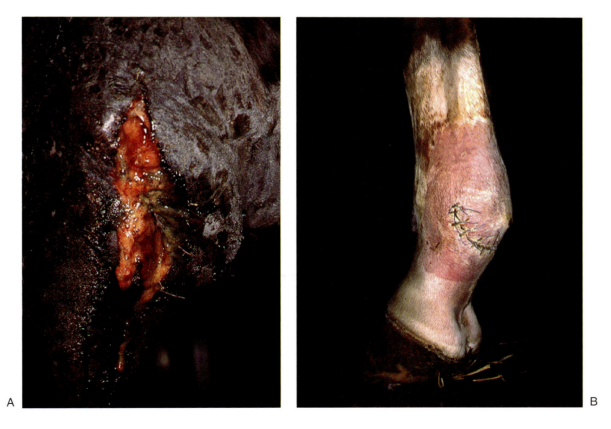

A
B

Figure 1.11. (A) Dehiscence of a wound on the elbow of a horse, sutured 1 week prior, as a result of wound infection. (B) Distal limb wound of a 4-year-old pony with an open fetlock joint and damage to the lateral collateral ligament. The wound was sutured approximately 8 hours after onset and healed successfully, without (partial) dehiscence. Reprinted with permission.[50]

debridement and lavage. The latter is apparently the most important factor that can be modified clinically.[19,20,23] The number of bacteria left in the wound following surgical debridement is critical, in combination with wound factors that facilitate colonization such as dead space, hematoma formation, and devitalized tissue. (For more information on factors involved in the development of infection, see Chapter 2). Although bacterial colonization and development of infection are greatly influenced by the administration of antibiotics, the effectiveness of the patient's own local defense, i.e., its acute inflammatory response, is as least as important to the prevention of infection.[10,11]

In the aforementioned retrospective study, all these factors relating to wound infection were evaluated and compared between horses and ponies.[7] The treated ponies and horses were of similar age and gender. In both groups more than 60% of the wounds were located on the lower limbs (carpus, tarsus, and distal to these sites). The wounds were comparable for location, duration, and degree of contamination; however, the wounds in ponies were generally deeper, with a greater number of ruptured extensor tendons and more cases of damaged periosteum and exposed bone. Primary closure of the wound was attempted in approximately two-thirds of all patients, whether pony or horse. More pony wounds than horse wounds were closed under local anesthesia in the standing animal. Postoperative management differed between horses and ponies: antibiotics and non-steroidal anti-inflammatory drugs (NSAIDs) were given significantly less often to ponies, with no differences in the period of administration and choice of medication. Bandaging techniques and the frequency of application of a rigid cast were comparable for both groups.

The results of the study (i.e., less wound dehiscence and fewer sequestra in ponies) suggest that healing was less compromised by wound infection in ponies despite the unfavorable conditions: ponies had a greater risk of bacterial challenge than horses because of deeper wounds, incomplete debridement achievable in the standing position, and a reduced use of antibiotics. Wound infection occurs when the level of bacterial contamination exceeds the capacity of the local tissue defenses determined by the inflammatory response.[10,11,23] Therefore, the results of this retrospective study imply that the acute inflammatory response in ponies is more effective at reducing bacterial contamination than is that of horses. However, the more frequent use of NSAIDs in horses may have contributed to a reduced effectiveness of the inflammatory response, because of the anti-inflammatory properties of the medication.

Second Intention Healing

Second intention healing of traumatic wounds occurs when closure is not feasible or when a wound dehisces following primary closure, but also in situations where there are economic constraints. Second intention healing was investigated in both horses and ponies by means of standardized deep excisional wounds created on the metatarsi and buttocks.[5,6] All experimental wounds measured 20 by 35 mm and extended to the denuded metatarsal bone or to a depth of 18 mm on the buttocks. During the week following their creation, all wounds increased in size (retracted) (Figure 1.12). Thereafter, the size of buttock wounds of both horses and ponies and of limb wounds of ponies decreased rapidly. In contrast, the limb wounds of horses increased to almost twice their initial dimensions by 2 weeks following their creation, with a subsequent slow decrease to regain their

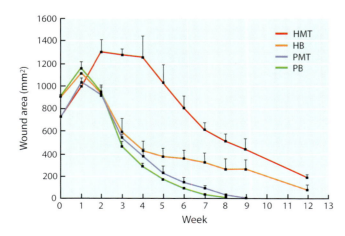

Figure 1.12. Wound area as a function of time (mean + s.e.m.). HMT = metatarsal wounds of horses; HB = body wounds of horses; PMT = metatarsal wounds of ponies; PB = body wounds of ponies. Redrawn with permission.[5]

original size only after 6 weeks. All wounds in ponies healed within 7 to 9 weeks, regardless of their anatomic location, whereas only two of the body wounds in horses healed within the 12-week observation period. The remaining wounds (body and limb) of horses were not closed by the end of the 12-week study. This research revealed that ponies heal significantly faster than do horses (Figure 1.12)[5,6] and that the speed and efficiency of healing seems related to remarkable differences in the phases of the healing process.[5,6] Further studies showed that these differences can be attributed to variations in leukocyte function.[8,9,25]

Inflammatory Phase

The inflammatory response to wounding was more prompt in ponies. The initial leukocytic infiltration of wounds was faster, resulting in a higher number of PMNs during the first 3 weeks of healing, after which the PMNs subsequently disappeared rapidly in these wounds. In contrast, the influx of PMNs was slower in horses and the initial number was smaller, but thereafter the number remained persistently elevated and after 4 weeks it exceeded the number of PMNs counted in pony wounds (Figures 1.13a and 1.13b).[6]

Leukocytes of ponies produced more reactive oxygen species (ROS), such as H_2O_2 or O^- radicals, which are necessary for bacterial killing after phagocytosis.[9] They also produced higher levels of other inflammatory mediators [tumor necrosis factor (TNF)α, interleukin (IL)-1, chemoattractants, transforming growth factor (TGF)-β)],[8,9] essential to the reinforcement of the inflammatory response, to the induction of fibroplasia, and to wound contraction. The superior production of these mediators can thus explain the higher initial influx of leukocytes into wounds of ponies.

The migrated leukocytes in turn release more biologically active substances, thus creating a positive feed-back loop further enhancing the inflammatory response.[10,26] This loop may account for the faster cellular debridement of non-viable tissue and fibrin deposits in ponies leading to the faster development of a healthy granulation bed, whereas in horses the granulation tissue retained an irregular and purulent appearance along with persistent fibrin deposits.[5,6] An enhanced inflammatory response can likewise translate into the more efficient local defense against contaminating bacteria, leading to better prevention of wound infection found in ponies.[7] A stronger acute inflammatory response thus averts the development of chronic, lower grade inflammation and leads to a faster and more thorough preparation of the wound for repair. Indeed, chronic inflammation, such as seen in horses,[6] perpetuates the release of tissue-damaging lysosomal enzymes as well as mediators, such as TGF-β, which over-stimulate fibroplasia leading to the formation of EGT and thus inhibiting contraction.[10,27–29]

In summary, the inflammatory response in ponies is both stronger and more succinct; this pattern appears to be more efficient for the wound healing process. In contrast, the inflammatory response in horses is characterized by a weak onset but persists over time, which may relate to the lower initial production of inflammatory mediators.

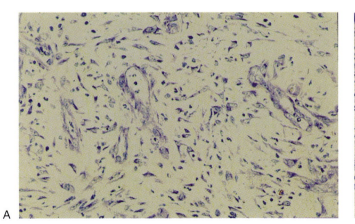 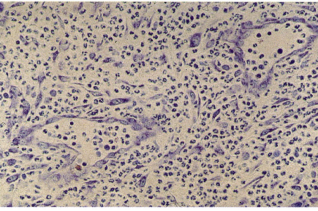

A   B

Figure 1.13. Typical histological appearance (Giemsa stain) of the superficial layer of the granulation tissue of a horse limb wound (A) and a pony buttock wound (B), illustrating the difference in the initial inflammatory response between horses and ponies after 1 week of healing. The initial influx of leukocytes was faster in pony wounds than horse wounds. Reprinted with permission.[6]

Formation of Granulation Tissue

Granulation tissue formed faster in horses than in ponies: the exposed metatarsal bones of horses were completely covered with granulation tissue within 1 week, whereas complete coverage in ponies took nearly 3 weeks (Figures 1.14a and 1.14b).[5] This new and abundant granulation tissue appears to push the wound edges apart, which may explain why limb wounds in horses enlarged so dramatically during the first 2 weeks following their creation (Figure 1.12).

After 2 weeks of healing, all wounds of both horses and ponies were characterized by granulation tissue that protruded somewhat above the level of the surrounding skin (Figures 1.15a, 1.15b, 1.15c, and 1.15d). At week 3, the limb wounds of horses showed EGT at both distal and medial wound margins, whereas in the limb wounds of ponies this was mainly seen distally (Figures 1.16a and 1.16b). The wounds on the buttocks of both horses and ponies had also formed excess granulation tissue which protruded above all wound margins (Figures 1.16c and 1.16d).

After the wounds were left uncovered, EGT disappeared spontaneously during the following week in most wounds, except those on the limbs of horses where the excessive tissue had to be trimmed.[5] The granulation tissue in horses was traversed by grooves and clefts for a much longer period and presented a purulent surface up to week 5 after wound creation, which may relate to the weak and delayed onset and prolongation of the inflammatory phase. In contrast, the granulation tissue of pony wounds was smooth, regular, and of a healthy pink color significantly sooner (Figures 1.17a and 1.17b).[5]

It was apparent microscopically that fibroblasts continued to proliferate in horse wounds even after granulation tissue had filled the wound bed, contrary to fibroblasts of pony origin which ceased proliferating at this time (Figures 1.18a and 1.18b). Additionally, granulation tissue appeared chaotic and subject to persistent inflammation in horses, while it was regularly organized in pony wounds (Figures 1.18a and 1.18b).[6]

As mentioned previously, there may be a causal relationship between persistent inflammation and the continuous proliferation of fibroblasts and synthesis of granulation tissue, via the activity of mediators such as

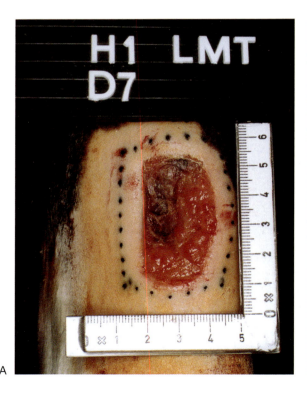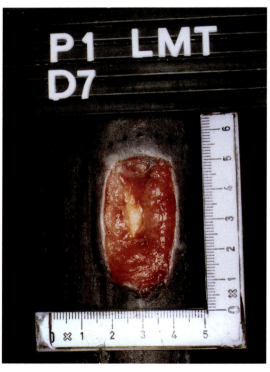

A   B

Figure 1.14. (A) The formation of granulation tissue in horses was fast; the exposed metatarsal bone was completely covered with granulation tissue within 1 week. (B) In contrast, the exposed bone in the ponies was still visible after 1 week and complete coverage with granulation tissue took nearly 3 weeks. Reprinted with permission.[50]

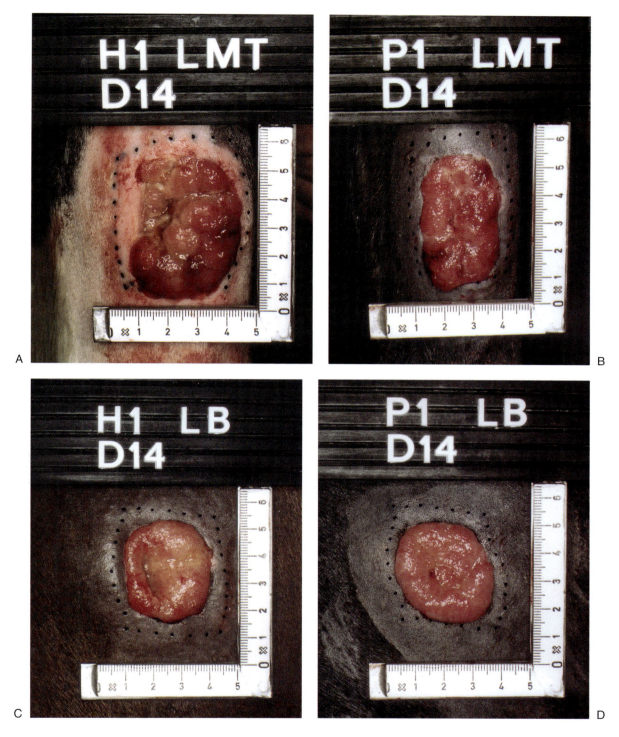

Figure 1.15. After 2 weeks of healing, all limb and buttock wounds of both horses and ponies were characterized by granulation tissue that protruded somewhat above the level of the surrounding skin. (A) Metatarsal wound of a horse, (B) metatarsal wound of a pony, (C) buttock wound of a horse, and (D) buttock wound of a pony. Reprinted with permission.[51]

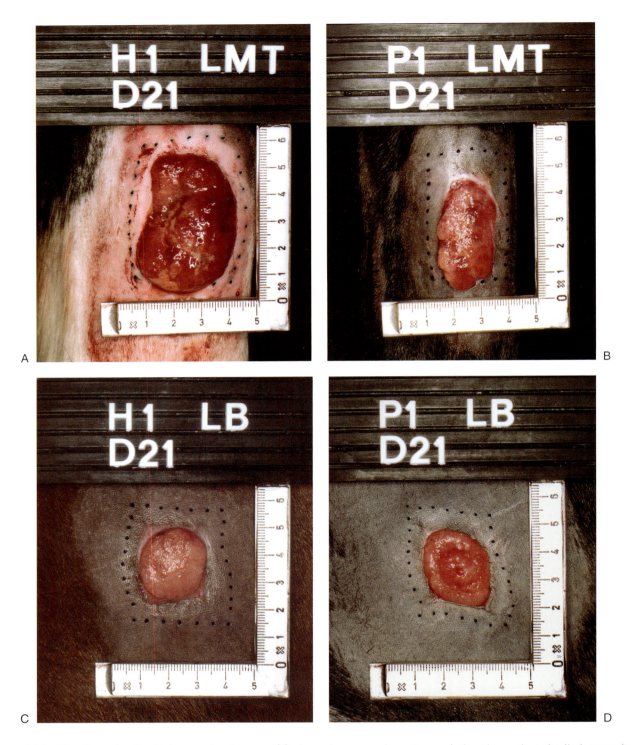

Figure 1.16. After 3 weeks, the limb wounds of horses (A) showed more exuberant granulation tissue than the limb wounds of ponies (B). In the same time frame, the wounds on the buttocks of both horses (C) and ponies (D) had formed some exuberant granulation tissue protruding above all wound margins. Figures 1.16a and 1.16b reprinted with permission.[50]

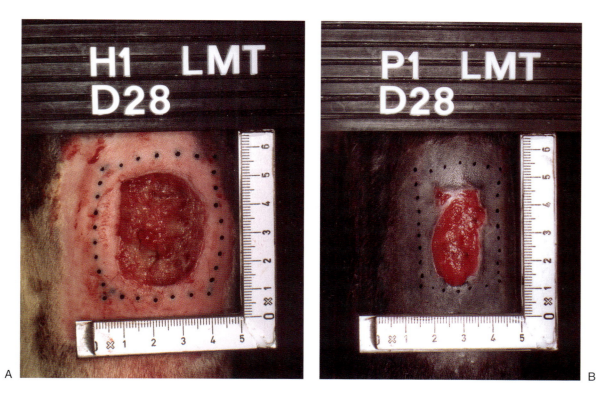

Figure 1.17. (A) The granulation tissue of the limb wounds of horses was traversed by grooves and clefts and presented a purulent surface after 4 weeks, whereas (B) the granulation tissue of pony wounds was smooth, regular, and of a healthy pink color. Reprinted with permission.[50]

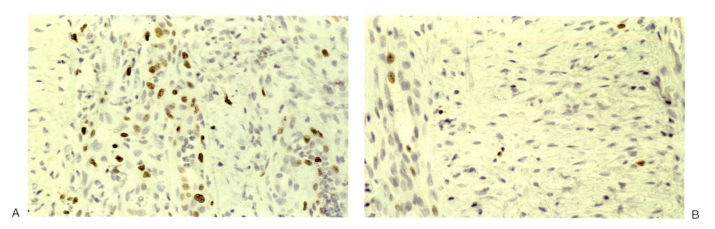

Figure 1.18. Typical histological appearance of the granulation tissue of metatarsal wounds at week 6 (DAP-filter, MIB). (A) In horses, many brown-colored cells, actively synthesizing DNA and preparing for mitosis, were present. Note the irregular arrangement of the fibroblasts in the tissue and the presence of polymorphonuclear granulocytes. (B) In ponies, only a few brown cells are seen in the regularly organized granulation tissue. Reprinted with permission.[6]

TNFα, IL-1, IL-6, platelet derived growth factor (PDGF), TGF-β, and basic fibroblast growth factor (bFGF), which are known to induce fibrosis.[28,30] However, the formation of granulation tissue was less extensive in the wounds of ponies, particularly those located on the limb, despite initially higher levels of TNFα, IL-1, and TGF-β,[5,8,9] which mediate the migration and proliferation of fibroblasts and endothelial cells.[28] Furthermore, fibroblasts from limbs of ponies are known to proliferate faster in vitro than those of horses,[31] contrary to the situation in vivo. Apparently, the balance of mediators, interaction with other factors, and time scale of their presence in vivo is more important than their absolute concentration in determining cellular growth rate, stressing once more the significance of the overall course of the inflammatory response.

The formation of granulation tissue in horses is excessively fast, compared to other species[32] and to what is observed in ponies.[5] The fast formation and the persistent proliferation, related to an unrelenting inflammatory response, clearly contribute to the formation of EGT.[5,6]

Wound Contraction

Wound contraction was faster and significantly more pronounced in ponies than in horses and in body wounds than in limb wounds (Figures 1.19a, 1.19b, 1.19c, and 1.19d).[5] As a result, second-intention wound healing was significantly faster in ponies than in horses and in body wounds than in metatarsal wounds.[5]

Histology showed that the myofibroblasts in newly-formed granulation tissue of ponies were organized into a regular pattern within 2 weeks, in which the cells were oriented perpendicular to the vessels and parallel to the wound surface. This pattern is thought to enhance wound contraction. While the number of fibroblasts and the amounts of smooth muscle actin and collagen did not differ in horse wounds compared to pony wounds, the organization of wound myofibroblasts of horses was delayed (Figures 1.18a and 1.18b).[6]

Wound contraction occurs when the forces exerted by the myofibroblast exceed centrifugal (outward) forces and the local resistance to displacement. Centrifugal forces present in horse and pony skin are similar, as evidenced by the identical enlargement which occurred immediately after creation of experimental wounds (Figure 1.12). Moreover, there is no reason to believe that the local resistance to contraction in horses and ponies should differ. Therefore, variations in wound contraction are most likely related to differences in the contractile force generated by myofibroblasts within the granulation tissue.

Surprisingly, although myofibroblasts are arranged in a more structured pattern in the wounds of ponies,[6] the inherent contraction capacity of fibroblasts from ponies and horses was similar in vitro.[25] This suggests that wound factors, such as the presence of inflammatory mediators, determine the contractile forces exerted by myofibroblasts and hence the extent of wound contraction. Indeed, inflammatory mediators, in particular TGF-β, wield major effects on wound contraction.

Interestingly, it was shown that TGF-β levels are significantly higher in the early granulation tissue of pony wounds.[8] This may explain the faster organization of myofibroblasts and the more extensive wound contraction observed in ponies since TGF-β stimulates the differentiation of fibroblasts into myofibroblasts,[33] induces α-smooth muscle actin, α1β1 and α1β2 integrins, collagen, and fibronectin, all factors necessary to wound contraction,[34] and enhances contractile forces.[35] Furthermore, since other inflammatory mediators such as prostaglandin (PG)E$_1$, PGE$_2$, TNFα, IL-1, IL-6, and interferon (IFN)γ inhibit contractility,[36] the chronic inflammatory response characteristic of horse wounds may exacerbate the deficient contraction noted in these wounds.

In summary, the greater contribution of contraction to wound closure in ponies compared to horses results in a faster second intention wound healing process in ponies (Figures 1.12 and 1.19). The differences in wound contraction are not caused by disparity in the innate contractile capacity of the fibroblasts but by the balance of mediators in the wound environment. The limited contribution of contraction to wound closure in limb wounds of horses can be attributed to the low initial production of TGF-β and the frequent occurrence of chronic inflammation.[5,6,8]

Epithelialization

The mitotic activity of epithelial cells was similar for horses and ponies during the first weeks of healing. It was temporarily reduced in week 3 when EGT was present in all wounds of horses and ponies, limbs and buttocks.[6] After the third week an inverse correlation between the epithelialized area and wound contraction developed such that wounds demonstrating more contraction showed less epithelialization (pony versus horse wounds, buttock versus limb wounds) (Figures 1.19 and 1.20).[5] This likely relates to a decrease in the length of the wound margins furnishing migrating and proliferating epithelial cells. Thus, more epithelialization is seen when limited wound contraction occurs, such as in limb wounds of horses (Figure 1.19).[5] In these wounds epithelialization was significantly faster compared to that occurring in all other wounds, from 6 weeks onward,[5] resulting in the largest area of newly formed inferior quality epithelium and the most pronounced scars (Figures 1.21a and 1.21b).

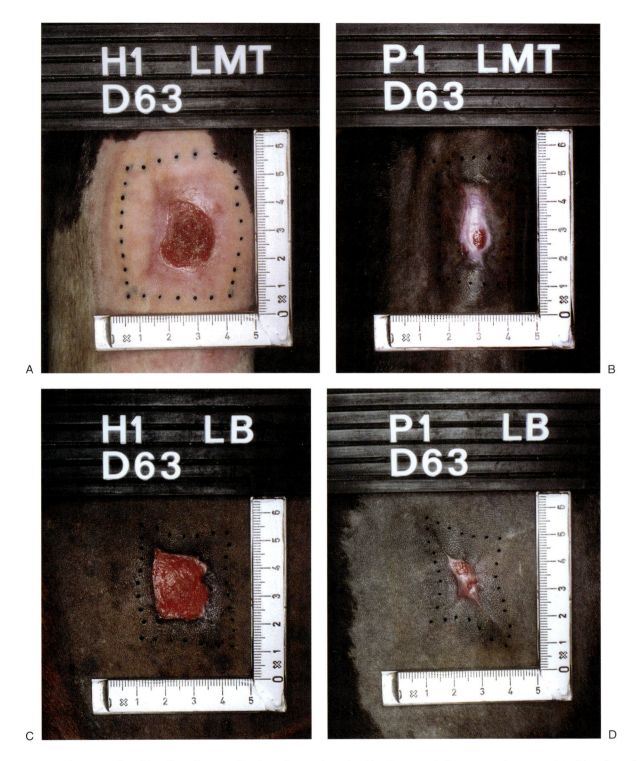

Figure 1.19. After 9 weeks of healing, the contribution of wound contraction to wound closure can be appreciated by observing the tattoo patterns close to the original wound margins. (A) The metatarsal wounds of horses have decreased in size. The tattoos show that only minimal wound contraction occurred, whereas pronounced epithelialization is visible. (B) Wound closure in the metatarsal wounds of ponies was to a large extent the result of wound contraction and some epithelialization. (C) The buttock wounds of horses also showed wound contraction, whereas epithelialization was still limited. (D) The buttock wounds of ponies were closed, mainly by wound contraction and very little epithelialization. The scar of this pony was unfortunately superficially damaged while shaving the hairs around the scar for the photographs. Figures 1.19a and 1.19b reprinted with permission.[50]

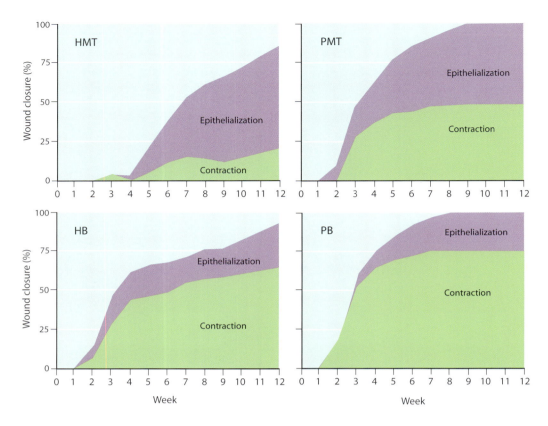

Figure 1.20. Relative contribution of contraction and epithelialization to wound closure. For abbreviations see Figure 1.12. An inverse correlation between the epithelialized area and wound contraction exists, such that wounds demonstrating more contraction show less epithelialization (pony versus horse wounds, body versus limb wounds). Redrawn with permission.[5]

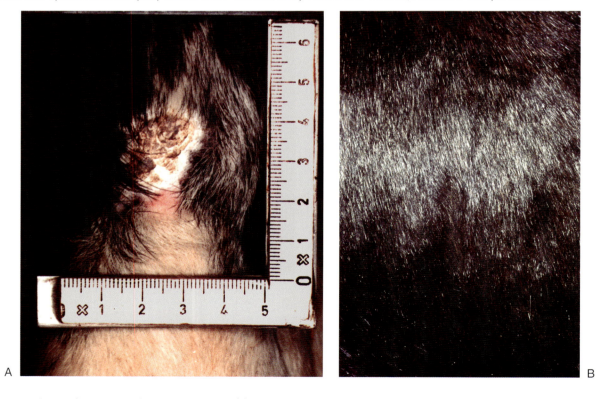

Figure 1.21. Scars of a metatarsal wound of a horse (A) and a buttock wound of a pony (B) 1.5 years after healing. The limb wounds of horses closed mainly by epithelialization, and an unsightly scar was present after complete healing. The buttock wounds of the ponies closed mainly by wound contraction, leaving no visible scar behind. Reprinted with permission.[50]

Epithelialization is also hindered by persistent inflammation which promotes leukocyte release of toxic products and lysosomal enzymes. These not only induce tissue damage but inhibit epithelial mitosis by altering the critical balance of cytokines and growth factors upon which epithelial cells depend.[17] Additionally, epithelial mitosis appears to be negatively influenced by the presence of EGT and/or factors inducing EGT,[37] as suggested by the finding that the mitotic activity of epithelial cells in all wounds was temporarily reduced when EGT was present.[6]

In other words, epithelialization is slower when wound contraction is more rapid, as seen in ponies. The effect of faster epithelialization (as seen in limb wounds of horses) on the speed of wound healing is limited because the process is inherently slow. A more extensive scar is formed when epithelialization is the primary mode of wound closure (Figures 1.21a and 1.21b).

Clinical Implications

Traumatic wounds of ponies heal more favorably than do those of horses. This usually translates into a better prognosis in ponies than in horses as well as reduced costs of treatment. In cases in which a pony owner may be reluctant to invest because of the relatively low economic value of the animal, the better prognosis may justify treatment.

First Intention Healing (Primary Closure)

The results of the study conducted on primary closure illustrate the importance of wound infection as a detrimental factor in the process of healing, and the significant role of the inflammatory response in local defense. As yet, there are no proven ways to stimulate the inflammatory response to improve the local defense mechanisms, implying that prevention of wound infection is of paramount importance, particularly in horses. Therefore, general anesthesia is preferred, especially when treating extensive limb wounds, because thorough irrigation and debridement are more difficult to achieve in the standing patient. Debridement of exposed cortical bone also seems to be essential to protecting it from infection and subsequent formation of bone sequestra.

Infiltration and proliferation of bacteria can be prevented by proper antimicrobial prophylaxis. Broad-spectrum antibiotics should always be given as soon as possible to horses suffering from extensive traumatic wounds, particularly those that expose bone. In case of a referral, the veterinarian who first attends the wounded horse should administer antibiotics. The intravenous route is recommended to ensure immediate and appropriate tissue levels.

The fact that the inflammatory response should initially be stimulated rather than inhibited implies that corticosteroids should not be used; furthermore, the routine use of NSAIDs is disputable. Adverse effects of NSAIDs have been reported on the migration of leukocytes, infection rate, and the healing of wounds.[38–41] NSAIDs may therefore increase the likelihood of wound infection. However, the use of NSAIDs may be inevitable in cases of (expected) severe lameness or abundant swelling that may compromise local circulation. In these selected cases NSAIDs are recommended, but at the lowest possible dose and only for a limited period. Other medications that have a negative influence on the inflammatory response, such as local anesthetics, should not be locally infiltrated into the tissue where regional perineural anesthesia or a line block, performed distant from the wound, can be used.[19]

In conclusion, measures should be taken to reduce contamination and to limit any detrimental effect on the inflammatory response, particularly in horses. In the clinical situation this may translate into a more frequent choice to treat limb wounds of horses, as opposed to ponies, under general anesthesia, especially when there is any doubt about the complexity of a limb wound.

Second Intention Healing

Modulation of the Inflammatory Response

The inflammatory response orchestrates the entire healing process. The acute inflammatory response is a prerequisite for launching healing, whereas chronic inflammation hinders the later phases of wound contraction and epithelialization. In horses the inflammatory response seems too weak initially and fails to resolve in a timely fashion. This implies that inflammation should initially be stimulated and later on be inhibited. In fact, we should aim to model the course of the inflammatory response in a horse wound to a more "pony-like course" (Figure 1.22).

Roughly speaking, this means that inflammation should be encouraged until the wound is filled with granulation tissue, and that it should be inhibited from that point onward to reduce the formation of EGT and facilitate contraction and epithelialization. By modulating the inflammatory response, the successive phases of the healing process will simultaneously be influenced. The initial enhancement of inflammation will also boost the formation of granulation tissue and the initial impetus to wound contraction, whereas the preclusion of chronic inflammation will benefit both wound contraction and epithelialization (for more details see Chapter 8). Therefore, treatment of wounds healing by second intention can be simplified by focusing on the inflammatory phase and can be subdivided in either stimulation or inhibition of the inflammatory response.

Stimulation of the Inflammatory Response

The initial inflammatory response in horses should be encouraged and in no manner be limited. Simultaneously, the formation of granulation tissue will be enhanced, which is desirable until the wound cavity has filled in. First, the need for inflammation and the risk of infection can be reduced by surgical debridement, regardless of whether a wound is to be sutured. Surgical debridement is required when necrosis, exposed cortical bone, or frayed tendons are present in the wound of a horse because cellular debridement, by the inflammatory response, is slow in horses.

Furthermore, it is advisable to bandage the wound with interactive dressings or topical gels that increase inflammation and stimulate healing.[42] Solcoseryl® (Solco Basle Ltd., Birsfelden, Switzerland) was proven experimentally to stimulate inflammation in the wounds of horses.[43] A gel containing activated platelets (Lacerum®, BeluMedX, Little Rock, AK) may also be expected to do this,[44,45] as should alginate dressings, acemannan-

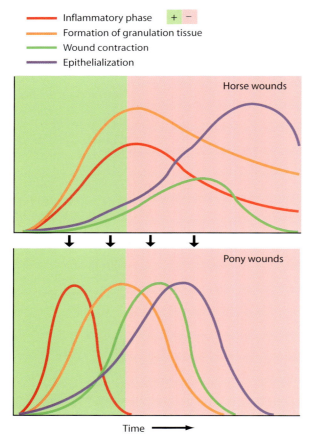

Figure 1.22. Schematic representation of the wound healing phases in horses. Inflammation should initially be stimulated (green shaded area) until the wound is filled with granulation tissue, and thereafter be arrested (pink shaded area) to reduce the formation of exuberant granulation tissue and facilitate contraction and epithelialization. In fact, we should aim to treat horse wounds in such a way that the pattern of healing will resemble that of ponies.

containing hydrogel (Carravet Wound Dressing®, Veterinary Products Laboratories, Phoenix, AZ), Iodosorb® dressings (Smith & Nephew, Hull, UK), honey, and sugar. These products have the potential to activate macrophages but have not specifically been tested in horses.

Bandages themselves favor the inflammatory response by increasing local temperature—which speeds up biological processes in general and angiogenesis in particular—thus supplying leukocytes and lowering pH, which causes a shift of the hemoglobin dissociation curve, increasing availability of oxygen for the leukocytes. Simultaneously, the formation of granulation tissue is enhanced, although the most important stimulus for this is the increase in oxygen-gradient between the granulation tissue and the wound surface and the decrease in tissue pH found under bandages or casts.[3]

Unfortunately, it is not yet possible to stimulate the initial inflammatory response to a greater degree in a more specific way, although this might be beneficial for the progress of wound healing in horses. Interestingly, a product such as Solcoseryl, found to stimulate the acute inflammatory response in horses, did not exert comparable effects in ponies.[43] Apparently, the suboptimal initial inflammatory response in horses can be stimulated more effectively than the already appropriate one in ponies. This suggests that the choice for special dressings and local products enhancing the initial inflammatory response is less critical in ponies.

Inhibition of the early inflammatory response should be avoided. Therefore, the use of corticosteroids is contraindicated and the prolonged administration of moderate to high doses of NSAIDs is questionable. Agents that are toxic to leukocytes, such as insufficiently diluted antiseptics, should be avoided. Additionally, wet bandages and hydrotherapy using cold water can be detrimental because they transiently decrease local tissue temperature and consequently cause vasoconstriction. A decrease in temperature slows biological processes and the ensuing vasoconstriction limits the supply of leukocytes, nutrients, and oxygen to the wound. Therefore, for optimal healing, it is recommended that the wetting agent for a dressing and the fluid used for irrigation be warm (~30°C) to avoid transient vasoconstriction.[46]

Resolution of the Inflammatory Response

As soon as the wound cavity has filled in with granulation tissue, the inflammatory response should no longer be encouraged but inhibited. Chronic inflammation, inherent to limb wounds of horses, enhances the formation of EGT and delays wound contraction through persistently elevated levels of several mediators (see Chapter 8). Possible stimuli causing a chronic inflammatory response should be diagnosed and eliminated.

The wound must be protected from environmental microorganisms and foreign material. This can be achieved by covering the wound surface with inert semi-occlusive dressings. Further, the number of bacteria on the wound surface must be controlled because they are strongly chemoattractive to leukocytes and perpetuate inflammation. Reduction of surface contamination can be achieved by wound excision. Superficial layers of tissue are removed and the number of clefts reduced. This also helps eliminate many leukocytes and mediators that accumulate in the superficial layers of the granulation tissue.

The use of antiseptic wound dressings (e.g., Kerlix® A.M.D. gauze, Covidien Animal Health/Kendall, Dublin, OH), silver chloride–coated dressings (Silverlon®, Argentum, Lakemont, GA) or the local application of antimicrobials for a limited period of 1 or 2 weeks may further decrease surface contamination and chronic inflammation. Systemic antibiotics are less effective because their influence in the most superficial layer of the granulation tissue is limited.

The local use of corticosteroids may be considered if it is necessary to further reduce the chronic inflammatory response. However, corticosteroids should be used infrequently and for short periods (1 or 2 days), because their effect is not limited to the inflammatory response but also impacts the other phases of wound healing. Theoretically, a similar effect could be expected from NSAIDs but the effect of parenteral administration as well as local application on chronic wounds is unknown. On the other hand, high loading doses of oxyphenylbutazone (12 mg/kg for 2 days) and maintenance doses of 6 mg/kg for 5 days administered to a horse with an acute wound significantly reduced inflammation and granulation tissue formation.[38] However, the effect of a local application of corticosteroids is more direct compared to long-term parenterally-administered high doses of NSAIDs.

Treatments that focus on reducing surface contamination and chronic inflammation concomitantly favor wound contraction and epithelialization. First, they limit the number of leukocytes and thus their toxic effects on epithelialization and reduce levels of contraction-inhibiting inflammatory mediators. Second, such treatments reduce the risk of developing EGT along with its detrimental influence on both wound contraction and epithelialization. In fact, such treatments favor contraction and epithelialization indirectly by eradicating detrimental factors; however, specific therapies to directly stimulate these phases are unfortunately not currently available.

That there is a need to specifically target wound contraction, particularly in horses, is clear since the rate of contraction determines the speed of second intention healing and the final cosmetic outcome.[5] Because the differences in wound contraction between horses and ponies appear to be caused by local tissue factors rather than by the innate contractile capacity of fibroblasts, it may indeed be feasible to influence the process.[25] It is known that wound contraction is stimulated by TGF-β[35] but inhibited by many other inflammatory mediators[36] which are abundant during chronic inflammation. In this respect, it is reasonable to expect that the application of TGF-β to wounds in horses would stimulate contraction; however, this was not found in an experimental study,[47] possibly because either the formulation of TGF-β or the application schedule was suboptimal. At this time, efforts to stimulate contraction are aimed at modulating the inflammatory response, as mentioned previously.

Conditions for optimum epithelialization include a smooth, healthy bed of granulation tissue that does not protrude above the level of the adjacent skin, along with a moist wound environment. Therefore, epithelialization will benefit from the measures taken to reduce surface contamination and chronic inflammation because it is inhibited by EGT and by toxic products produced by leukocytes.[10] A moist environment can be provided by semi-occlusive dressings; however, fully-occlusive dressings, with the exception of silicone gel dressings,[48] should be avoided in the management of horse wounds because they prolong healing time and stimulate the production of excess wound exudate and granulation tissue.[49] Foam dressings possess a good absorption capacity which is expected to limit the influence of toxic products released from degenerated leukocytes within exudate. Finally, in large wounds, skin grafting will dramatically enhance epithelialization by increasing the wound margins from which epithelial cells migrate and proliferate.

Because epithelialization is the predominant mechanism of closure of limb wounds in horses, measures to optimize the conditions for epithelialization are more essential in horses than in ponies.

Conclusion

Differences in wound healing between horses and ponies have provided valuable information about the intrinsic process of wound healing and the common complications encountered when managing traumatic wounds in the equine. Ponies heal faster and with fewer complications than do horses. These differences can, to a large extent, be explained by disparity in the local inflammatory response, which in turn relates to differences in the functional capacity of the leukocytes. Research data indicate that in clinical practice a maximal effect of treatment will be obtained if a differential approach is used, optimizing conditions for each successive phase of the wound healing process. In particular, the effect of treatment on the inflammatory response is of paramount importance to the other phases of healing and therefore should always be considered when managing a wound.

References

1. Simpson GG: *Horses: the story of the horse family in the modern world and through sixty million years of history.* New York: Oxford University Press, 1951, p.24
2. Bertone AL, Sullins KE, Stashak TS, et al: Effect of wound location and the use of topical collagen gel on exuberant granulation tissue formation and wound healing in the horse and pony. Am J Vet Res 1985;46:1438
3. Fretz PB, Martin GS, Jacobs KA, et al: Treatment of exuberant granulation tissue in the horse: evaluation of four methods. Vet Surg 1983;12:137
4. Barber SM: Second intention wound healing in the horse: the effect of bandages and topical corticosteroids. Proc Am Assn Equine Practnrs 1990;35:107
5. Wilmink JM, Stolk PWT, van Weeren PR, et al: Differences in second-intention wound healing between horses and ponies: macroscopical aspects. Equine Vet J 1999;31:53
6. Wilmink JM, van Weeren PR, Stolk PWT, et al: Differences in second-intention wound healing between horses and ponies: histological aspects. Equine Vet J 1999;31:61
7. Wilmink JM, van Herten J, van Weeren PR, et al: Study of primary-intention healing and sequester formation in horses compared to ponies. Equine Vet J 2002;34:270
8. Van Den Boom R, Wilmink JM, O'Kane S, et al: Transforming growth factor-β levels during second intention healing are related to the different course of wound contraction in horses and ponies. Wound Rep Regen 2002;10:188

9. Wilmink JM, Veenman JN, van den Boom R, et al: Differences in polymorphonucleocyte function and local inflammatory response between horses and ponies. Equine Vet J 2003;35:561

10. Cotran SC, Kumar V, Robbins SL: Cellular growth and differentiation: normal regulation and adaptations; Inflammation and repair. In Schoen FJ ed. *Robins pathologic basis of disease, vol 1 (5th edition)*. Philadelphia: WB Saunders, 1994, p.35

11. Clark RAF: Cutaneous tissue repair: basic biologic considerations. J Am Acad Dermatol 1985;5:701

12. Clark RAF: Biology of dermal repair. Dermatol Clin 1993;11:647

13. Moulin V: Growth factors in skin wound healing. Eur J Cell Biol 1995;68:1

14. Clark RAF: Basics of cutaneous wound repair. J Dermatol Surg Oncol 1993;19:693

15. Darby I, Skalli O, Gabbiani G: α-Smooth muscle actin is transiently expressed by myofibroblasts during experimental wound healing. Lab Invest 1990;63:21

16. Stashak TS: Principles of wound healing. In Stashak Ted S ed. *Equine wound management*. Philadelphia: Lea and Febiger, 1991, p.1

17. Stadelmann WK, Digenis AG, Tobin GR: Physiology and healing dynamics of chronic cutaneous wounds. Am J Surg 1998;176:26

18. Jacobs KA, Leach DH, Fretz PB, et al: Comparative aspects of the healing of excisional wounds on the leg and body of horses. Vet Surg 1984;13:83

19. Caron JP: Management of superficial wounds. In Auer JA and Stick JA eds. *Equine surgery* (*2nd edition*). Philadelphia: WB Saunders, 1999, p.129

20. Stashak TS: Principles of wound management and selection of approaches to wound closure. In Stashak Ted S ed. *Equine wound management*. Philadelphia: Lea and Febiger, 1991, p.36

21. Moens Y, Verschooten F, De Moor A, et al: Bone sequestration as a consequence of limb wounds in the horse. Vet Radiol 1980;21:40

22. Hanson RR: New concepts in the treatment of large avulsion wounds of the distal extremities. Proc Am Assn Equine Practnrs 2006;52:281

23. Stashak TS: Contributing factors and selected techniques for prevention. Proc Am Assn Equine Practnrs 2006;52:270

24. Hanson RR: Management of avulsion wounds with exposed bone. Clin Tech Equine Pract 2004;3:188

25. Wilmink JM, Nederbragt H, van Weeren PR, et al: Differences in wound contraction between horses and ponies: the in vitro contraction capacity of fibroblasts. Equine Vet J 2001;33:499

26. Rook G, Balkwil F: Cell-mediated immune reactions. In: Crowe L ed. *Immunology* (*5th edition*). London: Mosby International Ltd, 1998, p.121

27. Wahl SM: The role of lymphokines and monokines in fibrosis. Ann N Y Acad Sci 1985;460:224

28. Turck C, Dohlman JG, Goetzl E: Immunological mediators of wound healing and fibrosis. J Cell Physiol 1987;5:89

29. Roberts AB, Sporn MB, Assoian RK, et al: Transforming growth factor type β: rapid induction of fibrosis and angiogenesis in vivo and stimulation of collagen formation in vitro. Proc Nat Acad Sci USA 1986;83:4167

30. Kovacs EJ. Fibrogenic cytokines: the role of immune mediators in the development of scar tissue. Immunol Today 1991;12:17

31. Bacon Miller C, Wilson DA, Keegan KG, et al: Growth characteristics of fibroblasts isolated from the trunk and distal aspect of the limb of horses and ponies. Vet Surg 2000;29:1

32. Chvapil M, Pfister T, Escalada S, et al: Dynamics of the healing of skin wounds in the horse as compared with the rat. Exp Mol Pathol 1979;30:349

33. Desmoulière A, Geinoz A, Gabbiani F, et al: Transforming growth factor-β1 induces α-smooth muscle actin expression in granulation tissue myofibroblasts and in quiescent and growing cultured fibroblasts. J Cell Biol 1993;122:103

34. Ignotz RA, Heino J, Massague J: Regulation of cell adhesion receptors by transforming growth factor-β. J Biol Chem 1989;264:389

35. Montesano R, Orci L: Transforming growth factor β stimulates collagen-matrix contraction by fibroblasts: implications for wound healing. Proc Natl Acad Sci USA 1988;85:4894

36. Ehrlich HP, Wyler DJ: Fibroblast contraction of collagen lattices in vitro: inhibition by chronic inflammatory cell mediators. J Cell Physiol 1983;116:345

37. Van Ruissen F, van Erp PE, de Jongh GJ, et al: Cell kinetic characterization of growth arrest in cultured human keratinocytes. J Cell Sci 1994;107:2219

38. Gorman HA, Wolff WA, Frost WW, et al: The effect of oxyphenylbutazone on surgical wounds of the horse. J Am Vet Med Assoc 1968;152:487

39. Sedgwick AD, Lees P, Dawson J, et al: Cellular aspects of inflammation. Vet Rec 1987;120:529

40. Proper SA, Fenske NA, Burnett SM, et al: Compromised wound repair caused by perioperative use of ibuprofen. J Am Acad Dermatol 1988;18:1173

41. Kahn LH, Styrt BA: Necrotizing soft tissue infections reported with nonsteroidal antiinflammatory drugs. Ann Pharmacother 1997;31:1034

42. Chvapil M, Holubec H, Chvapil T: Inert wound dressing is not desirable. J Surg Res 1991;51:245

43. Wilmink JM, Stolk PTW, van Weeren PR, et al: The effectiveness of the haemodialysate Solcoseryl® for second-intention healing in horses and ponies. J Vet Med 2000;47:311
44. Carter CA, Jolly DG, Worden CE, et al: Platelet-rich plasma gel promotes differentiation and regeneration during equine wound healing. Exp Mol Path 2003;74:244
45. Monteiro S, Lepage OM, Theoret CL: The effects of platelet-rich plasma on the repair of wounds on the distal limb in horses. Am J Vet Res, in press 2008
46. Niemzura RT, DePalma RG: Optimum compress temperature for wound hemostasis. J Surg Res 1979;26:570
47. Steel CM, Robertson ID, Thomas J, et al: Effect of topical rh-TGF-β1 on second intention wound healing in horses. Aust Vet J 1999;77:734
48. Ducharme-Desjarlais M, Lepault E, Celeste C, et al: Determination of the effect of a silicone dressing (CicaCare®) on second intention healing of full-thickness wounds of the distal limb of horses. Am J Vet Res 2005;66:1133
49. Howard RD, Stashak TS, Baxter GM: Evaluation of occlusive dressings for management of full-thickness excisional wounds on the distal portion of the limbs of horses. Am J Vet Res 1993;54:2150
50. Wilmink JM, van Weeren PR: Differences in wound healing between horses and ponies: application of research results to the clinical approach of equine wounds. Clin Techn Equine Pract 2004;3:123
51. Wilmink JM, van Weeren PR: Second intention repair in the horse and pony and management of exuberant granulation tissue. Vet Clin North Am Equine Pract 2005;21:15

Wound Repair: Problems in the Horse and Innovative Solutions

Christine L. Theoret, DMV, PhD, Diplomate ACVS

Introduction

In view of the frequent complications developing during second intention repair of full-thickness wounds in horses, a number of innovative approaches have been proposed to accelerate and improve the quality of repair while abrogating the difficulties that arise as a result of an inefficient but protracted inflammatory response to wounding, an exaggerated fibroblastic activity, and the subsequent retardation of epithelialization and wound contraction. This section reviews some of the more promising treatments recently studied in the equine species in hopes of combating aberrant wound repair. A dynamic, multimodal approach using local and systemic strategies to stimulate repair may hold the key to success. Equine practitioners must thoroughly understand the mechanisms underlying repair to better assess the plethora of novel therapies that flood the market, and consequently better serve their clients and patients.

Problems Encountered during Wound Repair in the Horse/How the Horse Differs

Horses respond to danger with a fight-or-flight instinct, which predisposes them to massive skin wounds. In contrast to other species, problems in the wound repair process are frequent and lead to extensive scarring. This adversely affects function, often through lameness. Because most horses are destined to an athletic career, defective wound repair represents an important economic burden to the equine industry. It was recently reported that roughly 7% of injuries leading to the retirement of race horses are the direct result of a wound.[1]

Wounds in horses most often repair by second intention because of massive tissue loss, extreme contamination, skin tension, and/or unacceptable duration from the onset of injury. Indeed, a retrospective study of 422 horses recently determined that complete primary closure was successful in only 24% of traumatic wounds in which it was attempted.[2] To exacerbate this predicament, repair of full-thickness wounds by second intention is subject to numerous difficulties which compromise aesthetic and functional outcome in the horse, including chronic inflammation, development of exuberant granulation tissue, slow epithelialization, and poor wound contraction.

Intriguingly, whereas even extensive wounds of the trunk and head usually heal uneventfully,[3–5] horses display a debilitating impediment to the repair of wounds located on the lower limb. Specifically, horses suffer from chronic non-healing wounds similar to the venous leg ulcers of man (Figure 1.23) or, conversely, from the development of exuberant granulation tissue (Figure 1.24), which in some ways resembles the human hypertrophic scar or keloid. Factors that hamper repair in the horse limb remain obscure, though several have been suggested and studied.

Gene Control

Dermal wound repair involves complex interactions between various cell types, mediators, and extracellular matrix components acting locally and in parallel with numerous systemic factors.[6] Transition between the three

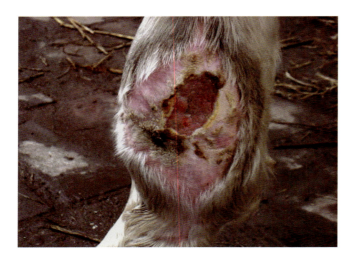

Figure 1.23. Horses may suffer from chronic non-healing wounds similar to the venous leg ulcers of man. This wound on the lateral surface of the fetlock had healed uneventfully 2 years earlier but the scar was damaged, resulting in a new wound. Despite daily cleansing, debridement, bandaging, and antibiotic therapy, repair was sluggish. A biopsy of the indolent wound revealed multifocal inflammation and infection with foci of coccae-like bacteria everywhere in the tissue. Courtesy of Dr. J.M. Wilmink.

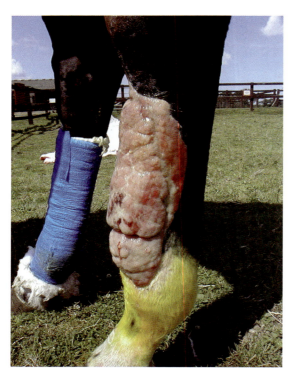

Figure 1.24. Example of a wound over the dorsal surface of the metatarsus, suffering from the development of exuberant granulation tissue, also known as "proud flesh." Notice the absence of an epithelial border, probably obscured by the granulation tissue having spilled over the wound edge. Courtesy of Dr. D. Knottenbelt.

phases of repair entails the activation and/or silencing of many genes,[7] such that a disturbance in gene expression and/or transcription could lead to abnormal scarring, as has been shown in the human and rodent.[8–10] A thorough outline of all contributing molecules in the horse is required if healing is to be positively influenced in this species.

We recently undertook an elaborate series of experiments to satisfy this objective. With our first study we identified a number of genes that had not previously been attributed a role during wound repair in any species.[11] These novel genes, up-regulated during the proliferative phase of body wound repair in horses, may be responsible for some aspects of repair and could be differentially expressed in limb wounds compared to body wounds, in horses compared to ponies, or in wounds that become chronically inflamed or develop exuberant granulation tissue compared to those healing normally. We subsequently cloned full-length cDNAs of selected genes in view of correlating changes in mRNA levels for precise molecules with spatio-temporal protein expression within the repair tissues.[12] Our ultimate objective is to identify the function of key genes in biological processes such as angiogenesis, fibroplasia, epithelialization, and remodeling to positively manipulate repair via molecular targeting.

Inflammatory Response

Wounds to the extremities are often near bony prominences and highly mobile joints and, because of their proximity to the ground, may suffer from significant contamination. Prompt repair is contingent upon the acute inflammatory response to trauma such that any obstruction will retard repair and encourage progression of the wound toward either an indolent or a fibro-proliferative state. The horse displays a deficient yet protracted inflammatory response compared to the pony, especially when wounds are located on the limb,[13,14] analogous to what is observed in a number of diseases characterized by disproportionate scarring (hepatic cirrhosis, glomerulonephritis, pulmonary fibrosis, corneal scarring, and dermal keloids in humans).

Blood Supply/Oxygen Tension

Inferior blood supply could thwart rapid and cosmetic repair of wounds of the limb. Indeed, there is a strong correlation between regional blood supply and the quality of repair. Local microcirculation provides necessary oxygen and other nutrients; thus, any interference will negatively impact wound repair. Intriguingly, it has been determined by laser Doppler velocimetry that cutaneous blood flow in the metacarpal area of the horse exceeds that of thoracic skin.[15] This apparent contradiction supports the notion that dermal repair relies upon more than strictly cutaneous vasculature.

Although the normal wound environment is characterized by low oxygen tension, hypoxia can be detrimental. On the one hand, it enhances the expression of angiogenic mediators[16] which favor collagen synthesis and possibly excessive fibrosis[17] as seen in horse limb wounds. On the other hand, hypoxia may retard repair by increasing the production of matrix metalloproteinase (MMP)-1 which degrades newly-formed collagen and may force the wound into a sluggish state.[18] While indolent wounds also afflict horses with some frequency, few investigators have studied the condition in this species. It was shown that MMP-9 levels in chronic wounds of horses remain elevated late in the healing process, while tissue inhibitors of metalloproteinase (TIMP)-1 levels are lower in chronic than in healing wounds, suggesting that increased proteolysis in chronic wounds retards successful healing.[19]

Granulation tissue is characterized by a great number of blood vessels. We have recently shown that the lumens of microvessels populating limb wounds are occluded significantly more often than those of microvessels within thoracic wounds.[20] It thus appears that despite the presence of numerous vessels within granulation tissue, hypoxia, sustained by occlusion of the microvessels, could predominate. Hypoxia is known to stimulate proliferation of fibroblasts and synthesis of extracellular matrix components by these cells;[21] this helps confirm the relationship between the oxygen tension of a wound and its propensity to become fibro-proliferative.

Fibroblast Growth and Synthesis

The horse activates collagen formation to a greater extent and earlier during wound repair than do other species,[22] predisposing it to the formation of exuberant granulation tissue which preferentially afflicts wounds of the limb. Interestingly, a cranio-caudal pattern of fibroplasia exists in the rat and has been blamed on unequal mitotic activity of fibroblasts due to differences in blood supply, which dictates the availability of nutrients, hormones, growth factors, or mitotic inhibitors.[23] Although an inherent difference in growth characteristics between trunk and limb fibroblasts was suspected of contributing to the development of exuberant granulation tissue in the horse, this hypothesis was not supported by an in vitro study showing that fibroblasts from the limb grow significantly more slowly than those from the trunk.[24] Conversely, in vivo mitotic activity of distal metatarsal wounds of horses remained elevated compared to that present in wounds healing normally on the hindquarters.[5] This may be coupled with deficient cell death, which could result from down-regulation of apoptosis, as occurs in humans suffering from keloids.[25] We recently investigated this hypothesis in the horse and found that the balance of signals was indeed altered against apoptosis in limb versus body wounds.[20]

Fibroblast Phenotype

Wound fibroblasts exhibit a range of phenotypes which reflect the various needs of the wound as repair progresses. Thus, migratory, proliferative, synthetic, and contractile phenotypes succeed one another as the wound matures. Should the synthetic phenotype reign, an imbalance between collagen synthesis and lysis might arise and contribute to the fibro-proliferative nature of some wounds. It has been shown that the local cytokine profile in these wounds is skewed in favor of fibrogenic mediators.[19,26–28] These will encourage migration and proliferation of, as well as collagen synthesis by, wound fibroblasts, in addition to inhibiting extracellular matrix turnover by down-regulating MMPs and up-regulating TIMPs. Indeed, the expression of fibrogenic transforming growth factor beta (TGF-β)1 persists throughout the proliferative phase of repair in wounds of the limb, predisposed to the development of exuberant granulation tissue, while it quickly returns to baseline values in thoracic wounds after the initial inflammatory phase.[26,28]

Epithelial Cover

Epithelialization can be deficient in horse wounds, primarily in those of indolent nature and those in which fibroplasia is excessive. In the former, granulation tissue of deficient quantity and quality hinders the migratory efforts of epithelial cells which require a scaffold upon which to move. In the latter, protruding granulation tissue may physically impede epithelial migration and/or may inhibit epithelial cell mitosis.[29]

The absence of an epithelial cover could in turn up-regulate the synthesis of fibrogenic growth factors[30] and debilitate apoptosis,[31] thus perpetuating the development of granulation tissue. Indeed, it has been shown in humans suffering from hypertrophic scars that epithelial cells are involved in the development of pathological fibrosis by influencing the behavior of underlying dermal fibroblasts; the dermis is thicker in the absence of epithelial cells, while it is thinner in the presence of epithelial cells.[32]

Wound Contraction

Deficient contraction has likewise been blamed for poor repair of limb wounds in horses.[13] Variability in wound contraction between the horse trunk and limb might relate to the innate contraction capacity of the myofibroblast from each site, differing cytokine/growth factor profile, and/or increased local tension in the skin. Furthermore, poor wound contraction is often coupled with the development of exuberant granulation tissue in the horse.

An association may exist between tension in the surrounding skin and excessive synthesis/impeded remodeling of extracellular matrix. Skin on the horse limb is tightly fixed, which after trauma may limit the ability of a wound in this area to contract and may result in increased local skin tension if some contraction does occur. Relief of mechanical stress seems necessary for a wound to progress from granulation tissue to scar.[33] Indeed, cell proliferation and matrix synthesis carry on if the wound tissue is under mechanical tension.

Although not documented in the horse, there may be a relationship between constant mechanical tension (resistance to contraction) in limb wounds and over-expression of fibrogenic cytokines. Transforming growth factor-β is known to enhance fibroblast proliferation and extracellular matrix synthesis;[34] in addition, TGF-β appears to have an anti-apoptotic role in fibroblasts.[35,36] Hence, this growth factor could represent the molecular link between poor contraction and the production of exuberant granulation tissue in horse limb wounds.

Wound Remodeling

The remodeling phase of repair continues indefinitely in an effort to improve the resilience and tensile strength of new tissue. Conversion of granulation tissue to scar tissue occurs via protein synthesis and lysis; proteinases and their inhibitors are the key players during this phase. Equilibrium between these two opposing mechanisms must be preserved for the wound to repair normally. An imbalance in favor of lysis could lead to deficient extracellular matrix, as seen in chronic indolent wounds,[19] while a situation bolstering synthesis might enhance the development of exuberant granulation tissue.

Investigators recently documented greater TIMP-1 mRNA expression in limb wounds than in thoracic wounds of horses, both 1 and 4 weeks following trauma.[27] Because TIMP-1 inhibits collagenolysis, the presence of high levels 4 weeks post-wounding might favor accumulation of extracellular matrix, as is commonly seen in wounds at this location.

Innovative Solutions

Classical wound management includes surgical debridement and lavage coupled with topical medication and wound dressings. While data is not available for the veterinary industry, the estimated market share of topical wound products in the human field was more than 3 billion dollars in 2005 (Figure 1.25).[37] Furthermore, because topical medications are not required to undergo as stringent FDA testing and approval as systemic products, rapid expansion has characterized the market in recent years.

Growth rates for novel technologies in the next decade are expected to skyrocket, galvanized by the introduction of biotechnology-based, full-thickness skin replacements as well as a plethora of growth factor-based products. Although today's scientific breakthroughs may well lead to tomorrow's therapeutic achievements, one must bear in mind that due to the unique nature of wound repair in horses, therapies beneficial to other species may not be suitable. Moreover, while it is imperative that innovations in wound management be provided to the equine practitioner, many commercially available products rely heavily upon anecdotal evidence and still await appropriate evaluation.

Rather than providing a comprehensive review of existing wound medications and dressings (see Chapter 3), the purpose of this chapter is to introduce the novel concepts arising from recent investigations into the physiology of wound repair in the horse.

When we first see a wound, it may be a couple of hours old or perhaps a few weeks old. It is imperative to recall the different phases of repair prior to designing the treatment regimen, and to keep in mind that the approach must be dynamic. Indeed, accelerating and/or improving repair is not as simple as applying a single treatment to the wound and maintaining it for the duration of the healing process. With this in mind, the following sections will address the concepts relevant to each of the three phases.

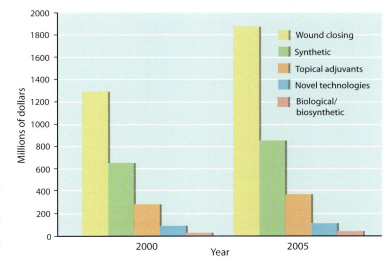

Figure 1.25. The estimated market share of topical wound products in the human field was more than $3 billion in 2005. The average annual growth rate over the past 5 years was especially high, at approximately 14.2%, for the category of biological/biosynthetic dressings. Source: Business Communications Company Inc., Research Division, 25 van Zant Street, Norwalk CT.

Therapy during the Inflammatory Phase

A robust yet transitory inflammatory response to injury cleanses the wound in an effort to stave off infection. Inflammatory cells, along with platelets, may also contribute to initiation of the proliferative phase of repair through the release of cytokines and growth factors. Until recently it was believed that wound repair could not progress normally in the absence of macrophages.[38] Conversely, the latest studies in rodents suggest that depletion of one or more of the inflammatory cell lineages (neutrophil, macrophage, mast cell) might actually enhance repair and have opened the door to innovative inflammation-blocking therapies for reducing fibrosis and scarring.[39] Because this novel approach has yet to be tested in the horse, this section will be modelled on the current veterinary literature.

Given that the inflammatory response to wounding is weak but protracted in horses and correlates with the development of both exuberant granulation tissue and chronic indolent wounds, it has been suggested that normalizing the inflammatory response might enhance certain aspects of repair in this species.[40] The main objective is thus to boost its intensity while restricting its duration, challenging the routine use of NSAIDs, which can exert adverse effects on leukocyte migration, infection rate, and wound repair. For example, repair of linea alba incisions in ponies was delayed by the use of high doses of flunixin meglumine in the early period following wounding.[41] That said, a low dose of NSAIDs, given for a limited period, may be beneficial in cases of severe lameness or profuse swelling that could restrict local circulation.[40]

One way a practitioner can reduce the length of the inflammatory phase is by debriding the wound to demarcate non-viable tissue, particularly in cases where necrosis, exposed cortical bone, or frayed tendons are present.

Box 1.1.

Maggot Therapy

Olivier M. Lepage

Maggot therapy (biosurgery) has recently experienced a renaissance in wound management. Maggots have been used for the treatment of equine and human wounds for centuries; they have been described in the Mayan civilization and Aboriginal tribes of Australia and later reported by surgeons during the wars of Napoleon and the American Civil War.[42]

While maggot therapy was often considered a traditional therapy, today it is generally categorized as a "biosurgical" therapy. Sterile maggots are produced by specialized centers such as Zoobiotic Ltd. (Bridgend, UK) and used for human and veterinary medical purposes. Maggot therapy, a form of artificially induced myiasis in a controlled clinical situation, relies on freshly emerged, sterile larvae of the common green-bottle fly *Lucilia sericata*. Naturally seeded maggots cannot be used therapeutically because many common flies will devour live tissue along with necrotic tissue in a non-selective manner.

The beneficial action of maggots on wound healing is attributed to a debridement effect via the production of potent proteolytic enzymes;[43] a single maggot reportedly consumes up to 75 mg of necrotic tissue per day.[44] Interestingly, maggot secretions fulfil the definition required of an antiseptic.[45] During the process of dissolving fibrin and necrotic tissue, maggots also destroy and digest bacteria,[45] including MRSA.[46] The action of maggots against MRSA is of particular interest with regard to the prevalence of antibiotic resistance because it limits the spread of infection from the wound both systemically and from patient to patient. However, in vivo, maggots seem to be less effective against gram-negative infected wounds.[47]

Sterile maggots can be applied to a wound in a direct (free-range) or indirect (contained) manner. In the direct contact manner, larvae (e.g., LarveE®, ZooBiotic Ltd.) are applied directly onto the wound with a hydrocolloid dressing stuck on the surrounding healthy skin (Figure 1.26). After the maggots are placed on the wound, a nylon mesh is fixed to the hydrocolloid dressing to cage the maggots within the wound and prevent them from escaping. In this approach the maggots should not be applied to wounds communicating with the thoracic or abdominal cavities.

In the indirect contact manner, maggots are supplied within a closed polyester net with absorbent hydrophilic polyurethane foam (e.g. LarveE® BioFOAM™, ZooBiotic Ltd.) (Figure 1.27a). This new development in maggot therapy has obvious practical and an aesthetic advantages compared to free-ranging maggots. The manufacturer declares that tiny pieces of foam within the net provide a physical environment that appears to markedly stimulate the activity and development of the maggots while assisting with exudate management[48] (Figure 1.27b). However, an in vivo study of 64 patients suffering from gangrenous or necrotic tissue showed that a better outcome is achieved with the free-range technique.[49] Moreover, maggots should be applied in the free range manner where cavities or areas of undermining are present.

In horses, maggot debridement therapy is described as an alternative approach to the management of septic navicular bursitis, hoof infections and necrosis in cases of complicated laminitis,[50] infected abscesses with distal phalanx osteomyelitis, and other hoof disease.[42] This therapy has also been used in supraspinous bursitis (Figure 1.28a), a pathology rarely encountered in equids in the developed world, but which remains one of the dominant pathologies among working animals in West Africa.[51] These cases are typically treated with a combination of Ivermectin, antibiotics, NSAIDs, local drainage, and hydrotherapy. When treating this type of wound with maggots, the practitioner can create or use existing openings at either end of the necrotic cavities to ensure free drainage of exudate and afford the maggots an adequate supply of oxygen.[52] Zinc paste is placed along the margins of these openings to protect normal tissue from scald and to limit migration of the maggots beyond the wound edges; the wounds are left open. No occlusive or film dressings should be applied overtop, because they may cause the maggots to suffocate. The nets with maggots are changed every 2 to 3 days until complete wound debridement and pink granulation tissue is observed without evidence of infection (Figure 1.28b).

From these observations in equine medicine and various evidences in human medicine,[53] maggot therapy can be recommended for the following beneficial effects on a wound: debridement, disinfection, potent antibacterial action, and enhanced angiogenesis. Following use, maggots contain viable bacteria which they may continue excreting;[45] therefore, they must be disposed of. (The author places the dressings and maggots in plastic bags dedicated to medical waste, which are then incinerated.)[52]

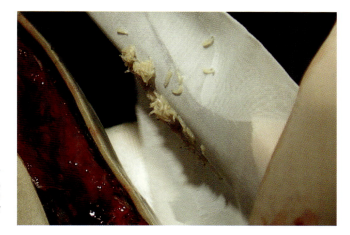

Figure 1.26. Maggots applied in the direct contact manner (free-range maggots). Larvae are applied directly onto a chronic, infected, and ulcerative wound of the canon bone of a foal. Note the hydrocolloid dressing adhered to the surrounding healthy skin. Courtesy of Dr. O.M. Lepage.

A general strategy for accelerating repair may be via the recruitment and/or activation of macrophages following injury. According to this premise, activated macrophage supernatant was applied to distal limb wounds of ponies, under the assumption that the secreted cytokines would boost the inflammatory response.[54] Although the supernatant effectively inhibited proliferation of dermal fibroblasts in vitro, no significant effects on repair could be determined in vivo.

The effect of a protein-free dialysate of calf blood, (Solcoseryl®, Solco Basle Ltd., Birsfelden, Switzerland) was studied in open wounds of horses and ponies.[55] During the first month following wounding, the dialysate provoked a greater inflammatory response, which accentuated fibroplasia and wound contraction. Beyond this

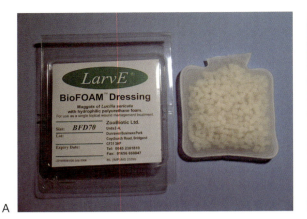
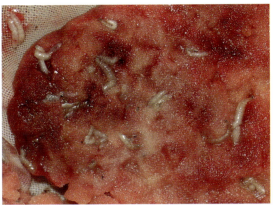

Figure 1.27. (A) Maggots supplied within a closed polyester net containing absorbent hydrophilic polyurethane foam (e.g., LarveE® BioFOAM™, ZooBiotic Ltd.) to be used in an indirect contact (contained) manner. (B) Pieces of foam within the net provide a physical environment to stimulate the activity and development of the larvae while assisting with exudate management. Courtesy of Dr. O.M. Lepage.

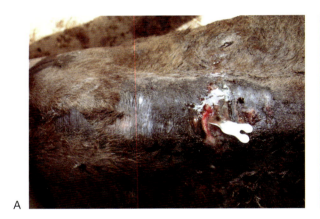
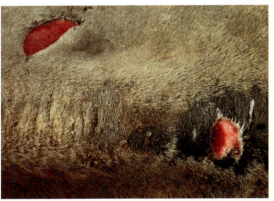

Figure 1.28. Dorsal view of a supraspinous bursitis in a donkey. (A) A 14 cm probe is placed in a naturally-occurring fistula. (B) Dorsal view of the same supraspinous bursitis following 3 days of treatment with maggots placed into the infected cavity in a indirect contact manner. The exudate at the original fistulous tract has cleared, and pink granulation tissue, without evidence of infection, is present at the site of the surgical incision. Courtesy of Dr. O.M. Lepage.

time its effects became deleterious, delaying epithelialization, possibly via protracted inflammation. This inflammatory stimulant could thus be used during the early inflammatory phase of repair, but treatment should cease when epithelialization commences.

Honey and sugar are attractant for tissue macrophages and may exert an antibacterial effect when applied to contaminated wounds. Honey has been shown to up-regulate the expression by monocytes of some inflammatory cytokines [tumor necrosis factor-alpha (TNF-α), interleukin (IL)-1β, IL-6], which may be the mechanism whereby it enhances fibroplasia and epithelialization (Figures 1.29a,b).[56] Standardized honey products are commercially available for wound care [Manuka honey–impregnated tulle dressing, Advancis Medical, Nottingham, UK (Figure 1.30); Meloderm UMF® 16+ irradiated active Manuka honey, Surrey, UK; Vetramil® BFactory BV, Wageningen, Netherlands].

At the wound site the enzymes (inhibine) contained within the honey exert a strong antibacterial effect via acidification and the slow release of hydrogen peroxide, a mild disinfectant, and glucolactone/gluconic acid, a mild antibiotic. Honey also provides antioxidants, which protect wound tissues from the damage imparted by free oxygen radicals released from inflammatory cells. Honey used for the treatment of wounds should ideally be unpasteurized and not heated above 37°C to prevent inactivation of glucose oxidase. It is recommended to

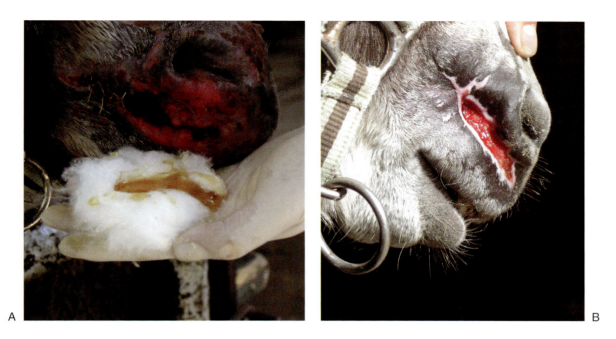

A   B

Figure 1.29. (A) This donkey was presented with a deep bite wound to the nostril/lip area. The wound was initially debrided by sharp scalpel incision, then lavaged. In view of massive contamination and the presence of residual necrotic tissue, the wound was subsequently treated with a honey dressing to aid with continued debridement. (B) Same wound, 22 days later. Courtesy of Dr. D. Frappier.

Figure 1.30. Manuka honey–impregnated tulle dressing from Advancis Medical, Nottingham, UK. Courtesy of Dr. D. Knottenbelt.

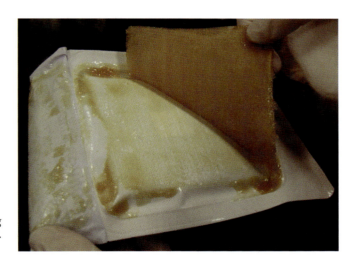

use 30 ml of honey for each 10 cm × 10 cm dressing pad. Dressings should be changed daily or when there is exudate on the outer layer of the bandage.

A synthetic form of sugar, Maltodextrin N.F., is commercially available (Intracell®, McLeod Pharmaceutical, Fort Collins, CO). When applied to the wound surface it mixes with exudate to form a semi-permeable barrier which maintains moisture while protecting the wound from environmental contamination. It is alleged to attract both inflammatory and mesenchymal cells, thus accelerating fibroplasia and epithelialization. While purported by the manufacturer to prevent the development of proud flesh, no scientific studies have evaluated the efficacy of either natural or synthetic sugar in the management of horse wounds.

High levels of serotonin present during the early inflammatory phase are thought to impair macrophage activation. Ketanserin antagonizes this serotonin-induced suppression, enabling a stronger and more effective inflammatory response which should translate into better control of infection and a superior orchestration of the later phases of repair when mediators released by the activated macrophage are required. Vulketan gel® (Jannsen Animal Health, Toronto, Canada), whose active ingredient is ketanserin, was tested against an antiseptic and a debriding agent in a large, multi-center randomized controlled field study of equine lower limb wounds. Vulketan gel® was 2 to 5 times more likely to result in successful closure, by minimizing infection and limiting the development of exuberant granulation tissue.[57]

Topical therapies, as described above, are habitually used in combination with wound dressings. The market for synthetic dressings constitutes the second largest for the entire advanced wound care business in the human field. Traditional gauze-type dressings adhere to the wound surface, causing pain and tissue injury upon removal. An in vitro model using equine wound fibroblasts and epithelial cells to evaluate cell-dressing interactions found that modern gelling dressings overcame the adherence problem.[58]

Despite this significant improvement, the use of contemporary dressings may give rise to other concerns. Indeed, while in other species the rate and quality of repair are enhanced by a moist environment such as that present under certain bandages, synthetic fully occlusive dressings may significantly prolong healing times in horse wounds. In a study performed on equine limb wounds, a hydrogel sheet dressing (BioDres®, DVM Pharmaceuticals Inc, Miami, FL) led to excess accumulation of wound exudate and an increased need to trim granulation tissue, such that the authors recommended discontinuing its use once fibroplasia commenced.[59]

Other hydrogel dressings are marketed for veterinary use, some of which boast properties compatible with the objectives of the inflammatory response to injury. For example, hydrogels containing an acetylated mannan (CarraVet®, Veterinary Products Laboratories, Phoenix, AZ; Carrasorb®, Carrington Laboratories, Irving TX) activate macrophages, encouraging their release of angiogenic and fibrogenic cytokines which synchronize the ensuing phases of repair. Although not yet tested in horses, acemannan-containing hydrogels appear beneficial in the management of dog foot pad wounds.[60,61]

A fair proportion of wounds located on the limbs of horses develop signs of chronic inflammation, whether infected or not. Chronic wounds appear trapped at some critical stage, probably during inflammation. Current management focuses on three main issues with the objective of magnifying the intensity of the inflammatory response while abridging its duration: (1) identification of the obstruction to healing; (2) removal of the obstruction by debridement or other suitable means; and (3) creation of a favorable wound environment. Suggested therapy for chronic wounds includes a combination of proteinase inhibitors and anti-inflammatory agents followed by the application of cytokines/growth factors. As opposed to more conventional therapies, gel that contains tri-peptide copper complex, as well as calcium alginate and oxidized regenerated cellulose/collagen dressings, proffer features which may directly contribute to these objectives.

Tri-peptide copper complex (Iamin 2% gel®, ProCyte Corporation, Redmond, WA) in topical or injectable form stimulates several biological activities inherent to wound repair. Initially isolated from human plasma, this complex has been variably described as a chemotactic agent, a growth factor, and a potent activator of wound repair. Its properties in acute wounds include improved angiogenesis (copper), increased epithelialization and collagen deposition, and accelerated wound contraction. The Iamin 2% gel® was tested in ischemic wounds in rats, where it significantly improved the wound environment by decreasing the concentration of inflammatory cytokines and various MMPs, thereby accelerating repair.[62] It has been injected into dog foot pad wounds zero, 3, and 6 days post-wounding and has been found to increase the type I collagen content of wound biopsies at 6 and 14 days compared to saline.[61]

Calcium alginate dressings (Curasorb®, Ken Vet, Greeley, CO; Nu-Derm®, Johnson and Johnson Products Inc., New Brunswick, NJ) exert their bioactivity via the stimulation of macrophages within a chronic wound. In addition to providing a moist environment conducive to cell growth and migration based on their hydrophilic nature, these dressings generate a pro-inflammatory signal which promotes fibroplasia via a cascade of mediators released from the activated macrophage.[63]

An oxidized regenerated cellulose (ORC)/collagen dressing (Promogran®, Johnson and Johnson Products Inc., New Brunswick, NJ) has been developed for wounds that have not progressed beyond the inflammatory phase. It is designed to inactivate key MMPs in the wound fluid, thereby limiting degradation of proteins such as collagen and various cytokines/growth factors critical to repair. Furthermore, the dressing binds growth factors within the wound bed to then release them in an active form as the dressing matrix is slowly broken down. A study in diabetic rats found faster epithelialization of full-thickness wounds treated with ORC/

collagen than with hydrocolloid dressing alone. This was accompanied by higher levels of various growth factors, including platelet-derived growth factor (PDGF), keratinocyte growth factor (KGF or FGF-7), and insulin-like growth factor-I (IGF-I).[64] The use of this product has not been described in the veterinary literature.

Finally, while pro-apoptotic drugs are not available to the veterinary market, it is worthy to mention their use in the human field for facilitating the resolution of a cellular response which has become chronic (e.g., inflammation). Although this approach has not yet been integrated into equine wound management strategies, the literature justifies a clinical study.[9,20,25,65]

Therapy during the Proliferative Phase

The therapeutic goal during the proliferative phase of repair of wounds in the horse is to enhance cell migration and proliferation, necessary to angiogenesis, fibroplasia, and epithelialization, while restraining the synthetic activity of fibroblasts to prevent excessive generation of extracellular matrix components.

As the acute inflammatory response to wounding begins to resolve, it might be advantageous to use chemoattractant agents specific to mesenchymal cells—for example epithelial cells—and to provide a support to migration should the natural one be lacking. These methods are not mutually exclusive; rather, molecule-based and scaffold-based therapies should be viewed as synergistic.

Therapies based on bioactive molecules principally depend on cytokines and growth factors, many of which have recently been identified, isolated, and purified. Several of these are known to variably stimulate attachment, migration, proliferation, and differentiation of endothelial cells, epithelial cells, and fibroblasts, important to wound repair. For instance, while most of these mediators are pleiotropic, fibroblast growth factor (FGF) and vascular endothelial growth factor (VEGF) are potent facilitators of angiogenesis; KGF, TGF-α, and epithelial growth factor (EGF) promote epithelialization; and PDGF and TGF-β are principally chemotactic and mitogenic for fibroblasts. These powerful mediators can be used in a purified form in an effort to augment wound repair in a range of tissues and organs.

Despite the likelihood that cytokine bioactivity is conserved across species, thorough data to uphold this claim is limited.[66,67] Thus, while in 1998 the FDA approved marketing of recombinant human PDGF (Regranex®, Ethicon Products, Somerville, NJ) for use in chronic non-healing ulcers of diabetic human patients,[68] the aforementioned reason along with a prohibitive price tag and limited in vivo efficacy in wounds in which the healing impairment is not due to the relative lack of PDGF, curtails its use in the veterinary field.

The first study to evaluate the effectiveness of bioactive molecules during wound repair in the horse focused on cell extracts and supernatants from human and porcine epithelial cells, which were topically applied to chronic granulomas of the limb. Although the active ingredient was not identified (rather it was given the generic term "epidermis-derived factor"), the investigation provided promising results in that fibroplasia was reined in, which concomitantly accelerated epithelialization.[69] Subsequent studies examined the effects of specific growth factors on equine wound repair. Recombinant human TGF-β1 was applied in concentrations of 50 ng/wound or 500 ng/wound to 4 cm² full-thickness wounds located on the distal limb. The treatment had no effect on the total area of the wound; the granulation tissue; or epithelialization, histological assessment, or subjective clinical assessment of wounds.[70] The authors suggested that inappropriate dosage/administration schedule or an inadequate delivery system may have precluded significant effects.

Conversely, promising results were achieved when TGF-β3, the anti-fibrogenic isoform of TGF-β, was applied to wounds created at the distal aspect of the limb in horses. Granulation tissue had a healthier appearance and did not become exuberant despite the use of bandages. Preliminary results from this study are encouraging, although the limited number of subjects obviated statistical significance.[71]

The complex mechanism of action of cytokines has not yet been fully elucidated. Because these molecules network both spatially and temporally among themselves but also with cells and the surrounding matrix, addition of an isolated cytokine might disturb the fine balance. Furthermore, the exogenous cytokine may not exert its anticipated impact because interaction with endogenous counterparts could abrogate its in vivo effect. As such, it may be illusory to expect an individual bioactive molecule to enhance repair. Indeed, because the process is dynamic, combination therapy, as is the case with dressings that must vary to suit the phases of repair, may be necessary. A therapeutic option is to use a physiologically natural mixture of cytokines intended to modulate the wound environment.

We recently accelerated wound repair in diabetic rats with topical application of elk velvet antler extracts.[72] Velvet antler contains a blend of cytokines, and a soluble extract enhances dermal fibroblast growth *in vitro*.[73] We suggest that such an extract (e.g., BioSynergy IGF-1 LipoSpray, BioSynergy Health Alternatives Products, New Zealand) may be an economical adjunct to the conventional treatment of compromised wounds in horses. It might help regulate the various phases of repair via the blend of growth factors that it provides.

Box 1.2.

Platelet-Rich Plasma

Reprinted from volume 22 of the NAVC proceeding, with permission from the North American Veterinary Conference, 2008.

In an effort to provide combination therapy, investigators have turned to platelet-rich plasma (PRP), which is, by definition, a volume of the plasma fraction of autologous blood having a platelet concentration above baseline.[74] Other terms used in the literature to describe platelet preparations include platelet concentrate, platelet gel, and platelet releasate. PRP represents a concentrated form of platelets, clotting factors, and multiple cytokines/growth factors released from platelet α-granules at sites of tissue injury upon hemorrhage and clotting. Growth factors liberated upon platelet degranulation include, among others, PDGF and TGF-β.

The principal therapeutic advantage of PRP over isolated growth factors is that it represents a natural mixture of stimulatory and inhibitory mediators designed to have synergistic biologic effects in a wound healing environment.[75] Autologous PRP enjoys a wide range of clinical applications, with most studies endorsing a place in the surgeon's armamentarium. The use of PRP has been reported in the treatment of chronic wounds[76–78] and more recently was shown to accelerate closure of experimental acute skin wounds in man.[79]

Normal horse blood contains approximately 165,000 platelets/μl which remain in the circulation for an average of 10 days before removal by macrophages of the reticuloendothelial system.[80] The active secretion of proteins by platelet α-granules begins within 10 minutes of clotting, with more than 95% of the pre-synthesized cytokines/growth factors secreted in the first hour. After this initial burst, platelets synthesize and secrete additional proteins for the balance of their life (5–10 days).[74]

The literature suggests that PRP should achieve a 3- to 5-fold increase in platelet concentration, over baseline, to ensure a therapeutic effect.[81] There are various methods to produce PRP: tube (manual), buffy coat (semi-automated), and apheresis (automated). When anticoagulated blood is centrifuged, three layers become evident: the bottom layer comprised of red blood cells, the middle layer comprised of platelets and white blood cells (the buffy coat), and the top plasma layer. The use of acid-citrate-dextrose anticoagulant, as well as low G forces during centrifugation, preserve the integrity of the platelet membrane. A recent study concluded that the buffy coat method was faster (requires approximately 15 minutes for setup and processing) and less expensive than the apheresis method in obtaining equivalent numbers of platelets and concentrations of TGF-β from equine blood.[80]

A number of small, compact office systems are commercially available to produce approximately 6 mL of PRP from 45–60 mL of whole blood. Two such buffy coat systems have been used in the horse (SmartPReP2 system, Harvest Technologies, Plymouth MA[82]; Sequire Kit, PPAI Medical, Fort Myers FL[80]). A standard laboratory centrifuge (we spin whole blood at 1,200–1,600 G for 8 minutes) along with a commercially designed platelet sequestration tube (RegenLab, Mollens, Switzerland) can also be used to produce PRP (Figure 1.31a), though this entails transfers which may compromise sterility (not a problem when using the PRP on open wounds).

The yield of PRP using this method is approximately 10% of the volume of whole blood drawn, with platelet numbers 4.7× greater than those of whole blood and TGF-β1 protein concentrations increased 3-fold.[83] A double centrifugation tube (manual) method for concentrating equine platelets has recently been validated.[84] Citrated blood is placed in a polypropylene tube and centrifuged first at 120 G for 5 minutes; the 50% fraction closest to the buffy coat is aspirated with a 9 cm, 18 gauge spinal needle attached to a 20 mL syringe; this fraction is transferred to a new polypropylene tube then centrifuged a second time at 240 G for 5 minutes. Following this method, the lower 25% fraction of the sample showed platelet concentrations 71% higher than those of citrated whole blood while TGF-β1 concentrations were 44% higher.[84] Processing of PRP in this manner takes approximately 20 minutes.

Once the PRP is prepared, it is stable in the anticoagulated state for 8 hours or longer. Because clotting induces immediate release of secretory proteins from the platelets, these should be activated just prior to delivery of PRP to the wound surface. The most common way of accomplishing this is to add a solution of thrombin reconstituted in 10% $CaCl_2$ to the PRP.[74] We activate 1.5 mL of PRP by adding 50 IU of lyophilized human thrombin reconstituted in 0.5 mL of 10% $CaCl_2$.[83] If thrombin is difficult to come by, $CaCl_2$ can be used alone, but clotting will take longer (up to 1 hour).

PRP can be delivered to the wound either with a commercial spray applicator or a dual injection system (one syringe contains the PRP while the other contains the thrombin/$CaCl_2$ mix) or it can be activated with thrombin/$CaCl_2$ directly in the centrifuge tube after which the resulting gel is applied manually to the wound. The latter method is preferred when treating vertical wounds (i.e., limb wounds in horses) because clotting does not occur instantaneously with the spray applicator or dual injection system, such that the PRP runs off the wound before it has a chance to form a more adherent, gel-like substance.[83] While no specific guidelines are currently available, we apply 0.25 mL of PRP/cm^2 of wound surface area at the time of injury and again 1 week later (Figure 1.31b).[83]

Using an in vitro system, inactivated PRP was shown to exert positive anabolic effects on equine suspensory ligament fibroblasts;[85] likewise, equine superficial digital flexor tendon explants cultured in media consisting of 100% PRP showed enhanced expression of anabolic, but not catabolic, genes[82] supporting the use of autologous PRP as a treatment for desmitis and tendonitis. A recent study reports clinical benefits to using autologous PRP intra-articularly in 23 horses suffering from joint disease (degenerative joint disease, *osteochondritis dissecans*, or intra-articular fractures of the distal phalanx) and intralesionally or perilesionally in 62 horses with tendinous or ligamentous problems.[86]

We are currently investigating the effect of topical application of autologous PRP to acute full-thickness skin wounds located on the distal aspect of the limb in horses. Eighteen wounds were treated twice (at 1-week interval) with PRP while the same number of wounds served as controls. Preliminary data suggest that PRP favors fibroplasia, indicating that this therapy may be most useful for acute avulsive wounds in which a large deficit must be filled with new tissue.[83] While more than one application may be necessary in extensive or slowly healing wounds, PRP should be discontinued as soon as a healthy bed of granulation tissue fills the defect. Based on our experience and the literature, it can be conjectured that the use of PRP might also be of benefit in chronic wounds following thorough debridement.

An equine-specific wound healant that contains a heterologous source of activated platelets is commercially available to equine practitioners. Lacerum™ (PRP Technologies, Roanoke, IN) has a platelet concentration averaging $4.9 \times 10^{11}/l$ and is stored frozen ($-12°C$ to $-30°C$). To prepare the Lacerum™ gel it is thawed, immediately after which the platelets are activated with thrombin and ascorbic acid. A preliminary study evaluating the effect of Lacerum™ on full-thickness, 6.25 cm^2, distal limb wounds reports accelerated epithelial differentiation, though only one horse was enrolled in the study, which was conducted by the company.[87]

In conclusion, scientific data supporting the use of autologous PRP in horses to assist repair and regeneration of injured tissues is forthcoming. This promising technology is readily accessible to equine practitioners and necessitates minimal investment or expertise.

Various naturally occurring or synthetic materials have been developed in an effort to encourage the ingrowth of mesenchymal cells during the proliferative phase of repair, particularly in indolent wounds. These are collectively referred to as scaffold-based therapies, of which collagen membranes and sponges, amnion, skin grafts, and extracellular matrices have been evaluated in horses. It has been theorized that besides accelerating wound closure, this approach might limit the development of exuberant granulation tissue in limb wounds.

Collagen may function as a substrate for hemostasis; a template for cellular attachment, migration, and proliferation; and/or a scaffold for more rapid transition to mature collagen. A porous bovine collagen membrane was shown to generate a strong inflammatory response in full-thickness limb wounds of horses, which may augment the cytokine/growth factor content of wound tissues, although it did not significantly alter the

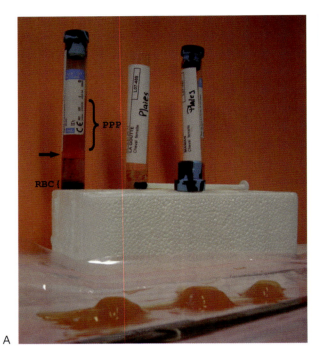 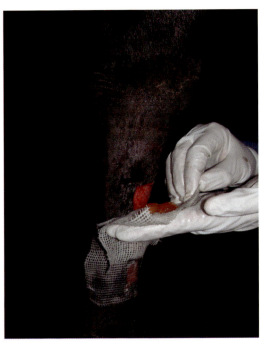

Figure 1.31. (A) Platelet-rich plasma (PRP) is prepared by centrifuging autologous whole blood to separate the red blood cells (RBC), most visible at the bottom of the tube to the left, from the buffy coat (arrow) containing the platelets and white blood cells and the supernatant consisting of platelet-poor plasma (PPP). The orange jelly-like masses in the foreground are activated PRP (PRP gel), which will be applied to the wound. (B) PRP gel being applied to a wound on the metacarpus, using a paraffin-strip non-adherent dressing (Jelonet®; Robinson Healthcare, UK).

total wound, epithelialization, or contraction areas.[88] Conversely, the use of hydrolyzed bovine collagen dressings in dog wounds significantly increased the rate of epithelialization.[89]

Although the value of creating a moist environment in wounds on the limbs of horses through the use of occlusive dressings is debatable,[59] two equine studies have shown the benefits of amnion, a biological non-adherent wound dressing material. Compared to a synthetic semi-occlusive control dressing, amnion significantly reduced the time to complete healing of full-thickness wounds to the distal limb.[90] It likewise accelerated closure of amnion-dressed pinch-grafted wounds in ponies.[91] As such, the use of amnion dressings should be considered in wounds predisposed to the development of exuberant granulation tissue and subsequent delays in epithelialization.

The value of skin grafting is acknowledged in cases of limb wounds in which there is a healthy granulation bed but an impediment to epithelialization. Grafts exert a significant inhibitory effect on endothelial cell and fibroblast growth as well as on the synthetic activity of dermal fibroblasts, while enhancing proliferation and migration of epithelial cells. It is proposed that the inhibitory effect of grafts on fibroblast proliferation and collagen synthesis may be regulated by a soluble epithelial-derived product which potentiates apoptosis of underlying cells during scar establishment.[31,92] It is recommended that the graft be obtained from a site which normally heals well and in which contraction is prominent (e.g., lateral cervical, abdominal or pectoral), although this was not supported by Schumacher, et al.[93] They found that punch grafts obtained from the lateral cervical region and inserted into wounds located on the distal portion of the forelimb of horses 14 days after their creation did not significantly affect the rate constant of each phase of repair (expansion, contraction, epithelialization) over 32 days, when compared to no treatment.[93]

A proteinaceous material composed principally of collagen, proteoglycans, glycoproteins, and growth factors is secreted by the resident cells of each tissue. This extracellular matrix provides the structural framework and dictates the form and function of cells within the organ. Resorbable extracellular matrix scaffolds derived from the submucosa of porcine small intestine (Vet BioSist®, Cook Veterinary Products, Bloomington, IN) or bladder (ACell Vet®, Jessup, MD) are commercially available to veterinarians to be used as biologic dressings to ameliorate wound repair by facilitating tissue in-growth and reducing scarring.

While extracellular matrix products are touted as assisting constructive remodeling of damaged tissue via the recruitment of bone marrow–derived stem cells and the release of a host of cytokines, a limited number of veterinary studies have verified these claims. Vet BioSist® was compared to a non-biological non-adherent synthetic dressing, an allogeneic split-thickness skin graft, and an allogeneic peritoneal dressing in the treatment of small, granulating wounds on the distal limb of horses.[94] In this experiment no differences in bacterial proliferation, inflammatory reaction, vascularization, or overall healing could be discerned between the biocompatible extracellular matrix and the other treatments. Likewise, no positive effect of Vet BioSist® on healing time, inflammation, epithelialization, angiogenesis, and wound contraction could be detected when the product was applied to wounds with exposed bone in dogs.[95] It is possible that enhancement of repair was not evident because of the mild nature of the wounds in these studies, since extracellular matrix scaffolds are not intended for applications in which natural healing results in near normal tissue structure and function. For more information, see The Extracellular Matrix as a Biologic Scaffold for Wound Healing in Veterinary Medicine in Chapter 3.

More recently, augmentation of the wound's natural population of mesenchymal cells has been proposed to enhance the repair of tissues, including skin. While stem cells were first identified as pluripotent cells in embryos (ESC), it is now clear that they are also present in many, if not all, tissues in adult animals where they contribute to the maintenance of tissue renewal and homeostasis.[96] Compared to ESCs, adult stem cells have a more restricted differentiation capacity. The adult bone marrow mesenchymal stem cell (MSC) has been a favored target of investigation because it harbors a heterogeneous population of stem cells which appear to have very broad development capabilities (mesodermal, endodermal, and neuroectodermal). That said, multipotent adult progenitor cells are not confined to the bone marrow. Stem cells outside the bone marrow are generally referred to as "tissue stem cells" and have been isolated from muscle, brain, and skin, specifically from the bulge area of the hair follicle.

There are at least four ways of using MSCs therapeutically: local implantation for localized disease, systemic transplantation, combining stem cell therapy with gene therapy, and using MSCs in tissue engineering protocols. In the treatment of wounds, Nakagawa, et al. suggested that human MSCs together with bFGF in a rat skin defect model accelerated wound healing and showed that the MSCs transdifferentiated into epithelium.[97] Falanga, et al. showed that autologous bone marrow–derived cultured MSCs delivered in a fibrin spray accelerated healing of experimental wounds in diabetic mice and chronic, non-healing cutaneous wounds of man.[98] Interestingly, that study showed a strong direct correlation between the number of cells applied (greater than 1×10^6 cells per cm^2 of wound area) and the subsequent decrease in size of the chronic wound. To date, no studies have been reported on the use of MSCs in the treatment of skin wounds in horses, though reports have been published on the use of equine MSCs in articular cartilage and in tendon defects.

Because the fibroblastic response of wounds in horses tends to be vigorous, which subsequently delays wound contraction and epithelialization, an important therapeutic goal during the proliferative phase of repair in this species is to restrain proliferation and the synthetic activity of the wound fibroblast. Indeed, once the wound bed has filled with granulation tissue, fibroplasia is no longer necessary nor desirable. While proud flesh in the horse differs from the human keloid in that the latter possesses an epithelial cover, it is tempting to speculate that the two conditions are governed by similar underlying mechanisms. For this reason, approaches used to either prevent or treat keloids in people may be of interest to the equine practitioner.

We recently investigated one such therapy, the silicone gel dressing (CicaCare®, Smith-Nephew, Hull, UK), in the treatment of horse limb wounds.[99] Silicone dressings have been used since the early 1980s as a complement to surgery or a substitute to administration of corticosteroids for the management of dysregulated dermal scarring in man.[100,101] This synthetic, non-adherent occlusive dressing appears to surpass other local therapies in minimizing the amount of scar tissue that develops (Figure 1.32). Plastic and reconstructive surgeons use the dressing on mature scars but also to prevent recurrence of keloids following their removal,[101] as well as on wounds in patients predisposed to excessive scarring.[102] It is suggested that the dressing occludes microvessels and gradually decreases oxygen tension within the tissues until a point of anoxia, when fibroblasts undergo apoptosis rather than proliferating and secreting extracellular matrix components.[103]

In our study, the silicone dressing prevented the formation of exuberant granulation tissue when compared to a control dressing. Microvessels were occluded significantly more often in wounds dressed with the silicone gel, principally as a result of endothelial cell hypertrophy.[104] The dressing also diminished the expression of an

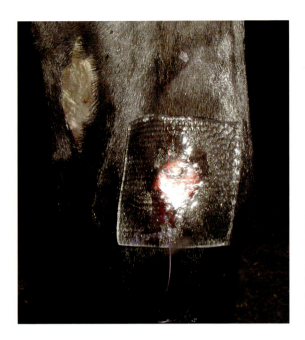

Figure 1.32. The silicone gel dressing (CicaCare®, Smith-Nephew, Hull, UK) can be used to curb excessive scarring in horse limb wounds predisposed to the development of exuberant granulation tissue. This wound on the medial surface of the distal radius dehisced after primary closure following a transphyseal bridging procedure for a valgus deformity in a foal. The wound needed to heal by second intention and the threat of exuberant granulation tissue was limited by using a silicone gel dressing on the open wound. Courtesy of Centre Hospitalier Universitaire Vétérinaire, Université de Montréal.

apoptosis inhibitor, although greater apoptosis was not confirmed quantitatively. We thus propose that the silicone dressing could be integrated in a management strategy designed to improve the repair of limb wounds in horses.

While topical application of imiquimod 5% cream (Aldara® 3M Pharmaceuticals, St. Paul, MN) to keloids in man was shown to alter the expression of genes associated with apoptosis,[105] equivalent therapy has so far only been used to treat sarcoids in the horse.[106]

Therapy during the Remodeling Phase

A high level of wound contraction is a desired feature of repair in the horse. This process reduces the size of a wound while enhancing its tensile strength and cosmetic appearance because less of the original wound area must be covered by newly-formed, inferior quality epithelium.[40] Wound retraction and subsequent contraction exhibit an altered pattern in horse wounds, particularly those located on the limb, where skin is more tightly fixed. Wound contraction results from the action of specialized wound fibroblasts (myofibroblasts), which in theory relies upon local tissue conditions in addition to the innate contraction capacity of the cells. Myofibroblast differentiation is regulated by at least one cytokine (TGF-β1), an extracellular matrix component (fibronectin), as well as the presence of mechanical tension.[107] Whereas poor contraction in limb wounds has been ascribed to local environmental factors such as inflammatory mediators (Figure 1.33),[108] other investigators deduced that a deficient inherent contractile capacity of the specialized fibroblast was at fault.[109]

Regardless of the grounds for defective contraction in limb wounds of horses, one therapeutic objective during the remodeling phase of repair is to temporarily promote the activity of myofibroblasts to accelerate wound closure. Once this aim has been achieved, the myofibroblast should be eliminated. Disappearance is critical because myofibroblasts not only promote contraction but also synthesize high levels of extracellular matrix components and MMPs, thereby leading to excessive scarring and functional impairment of the affected organ.[107]

Factors regulating granulation tissue contraction have not been fully elucidated but appear to include TGF-β1, which promotes a dose-dependent increase in the contractile force of cultured myofibroblasts.[110] Thrombospondin-treated sponges, via activation of latent TGF-β, increased fibroblast numbers and augmented wound contraction when implanted subcutaneously into rats,[111] while a TGF-β antagonist reduced contraction in pig burn wounds.[112] It is thus felt that bioactive molecule-based therapies hold some promise and should be further investigated as potential catalysts of wound contraction.

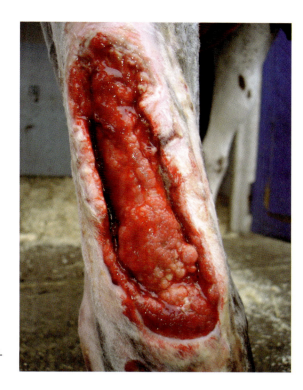

Figure 1.33. Poor wound contraction is often found in limb wounds suffering chronic inflammation. Courtesy of Dr. O.M. Lepage.

In the horse, some dressings are touted as facilitating wound contraction (silicone gel dressing, amnion). Although not proven, this may relate to their ability to modify the pH of the wound environment, thus altering myofibroblast contractility.[113] Dart and colleagues recently evaluated the effect of recombinant equine growth hormone (reGH) on the healing of equine limb wounds to verify whether the protein could exert a beneficial effect on repair in this species as it had in laboratory animals.[114] It was found that intramuscular injections of reGH exerted a negative impact on the process of wound contraction.[115] Wound healing studies on transgenic mice over-expressing GH have since confirmed that wound closure is severely delayed in these animals as a result of impaired wound contraction. The latter is ostensibly related to a reduced number of myofibroblasts at the wound site, in which contractile activity is attenuated, apparently as a result of GH inhibition of TGF-β-induced myofibroblast differentiation.[116]

Because myofibroblasts synthesize elevated levels of extracellular matrix components, thereby favoring excessive scarring, it is imperative to eliminate these players once wound contraction has proceeded appropriately. Indeed, it has been shown that defective apoptosis impedes myofibroblast disappearance during pathological scar formation in man.[117] On this basis, the myofibroblast may represent an important target for improving the evolution of such diseases as hypertrophic scars or keloids in humans and proud flesh in the horse.

For example, it has been shown that fibrosis of the liver, such as in hepatic cirrhosis, can be remodeled by decreasing the expression of type I collagen and TIMP, activating various MMPs, and inducing apoptosis of cells that possess a myofibroblast phenotype.[118] It is postulated that remodeling of extracellular matrix by MMPs exerts an impact by interfering with myofibroblast adhesion to the matrix, as implied by a study showing regression of granulation tissue under a vascularized skin flap.[119] The latter demonstrated that placement of a vascularized flap over the granulation tissue covering a wound encouraged tissue remodeling and concomitantly decreased expression of TGF-β1, β1-procollagen, α-smooth muscle actin, and TIMP-1, while increasing expression of MMP-2, MMP-13, and inducible nitric oxide synthase (iNOS). Remodeling could thus relate to a decrease in expression of the trophic factor TGF-β1 and increased extracellular matrix degradation due to an alteration in the balance between MMPs and their inhibitor, TIMP-1. Furthermore, increased iNOS expression could favor apoptosis through the generation of free radicals. While such an extensive investigation has not been conducted in the horse, clinical impressions certainly support the use of full-thickness grafts in poorly healing wounds on the limbs.

Finally, physical anchorage of the extracellular matrix is a positive modulator of granulation tissue survival.[120] A change in physical stress on wound granulation tissue may favor myofibroblast apoptosis as suggested by in vitro studies of fibroblasts in collagen lattices.[121] In vivo, releasing the wound edges (desplinting) leads to a marked increase in apoptosis[120] as does covering the wound with a skin flap, which reduces tension and thereby causing fibroblasts to regress coincident with a decrease in TGF-β expression.[119] This further justifies the use of grafts in large, granulating limb wounds in horses.

Conclusion

In conclusion, the horse is characterized by significant physiological differences in its response to trauma. Consequently, while much data is available for the human wound patient, equine practitioners must be cautious about extrapolating to the horse. It is thus imperative to support continued research in the field of veterinary wound repair and regeneration to gain a more precise understanding of the mechanisms underlying these processes in the horse in view of developing and implementing rational therapeutic approaches. Until this ultimate objective is reached, one can simply recommend that practitioners "use what we know and know what to use!"

References

1. Perkins NR, Reid SW, Morris RS: Profiling the New Zealand Thoroughbred racing industry. 2. Conditions interfering with training and racing. NZ Vet J 2005;53:69
2. Wilmink JM, van Herten J, van Weeren PR, et al: Retrospective study of primary intention healing and sequestrum formation in horses compared to ponies under clinical circumstances. Equine Vet J 2002;34:270
3. Jacobs KA, Leach DH, Fretz PB, et al: Comparative aspects of the healing of excisional wounds on the leg and body of horses. Vet Surg 1984;13:83
4. Knottenbelt DC: Equine wound management: are there significant differences in healing at different sites on the body? Vet Dermatol 1997;8:273
5. Wilmink JM, Stolk PWTH, Van Weeren PR, et al: Differences in second-intention wound healing between horses and ponies: macroscopic aspects. Equine Vet J 1999;31:53
6. Soo C, Sayah DN, Zhang X, et al: The identification of novel wound-healing genes through differential display. Plast Reconstruct Surg 2002;110:787
7. Cole J, Tsou R, Wallace K, et al: Early gene expression profile of human skin to injury using high-density cDNA microarrays. Wound Repair Regen 2001;9:360
8. Russell SB, Trupin JS, Myers JC, et al: Differential glucocorticoid regulation of collagen mRNAs in human dermal fibroblasts. Keloid-derived and fetal fibroblasts are refractory to down-regulation. J Biol Chem 1989;264:13730
9. Sayah DN, Soo C, Shaw WW, et al: Down-regulation of apoptosis-related genes in keloid tissues. J Surg Res 1999;87:209
10. Tsou R, Cole JK, Nathens AB, et al. Analysis of hypertrophic and normal scar gene expression with cDNA microarrays. J Burn Care Rehabil 2000;21:541
11. Lefebvre-Lavoie J, Lussier JG, Theoret CL: Profiling of differentially expressed genes in wound margin biopsies of horses, using suppression subtractive hybridization. Physiol Genomics 2005;22:157
12. Miragliotta V, Ipina Z, Lefebvre-Lavoie J, et al: Equine CTNNB1 and PECAM1 nucleotide structure and expression analyses in an experimental model of normal and pathological wound repair. BMC Physiol 2008;31:1
13. Wilmink JM, van Weeren PR, Stolk PW, et al: Differences in second-intention wound healing between horses and ponies: histological aspects. Equine Vet J 1999;31:61
14. Wilmink JM, Veenman JN, van den Boom R, et al: Differences in polymorphonucleocyte function and local inflammatory response between horses and ponies. Equine Vet J 2003;35:561
15. Manning TO, Monteiro-Riviere NA, Bristol DG, et al: Cutaneous laser-Doppler velocimetry in nine animal species. Am J Vet Res 1991;52:1960
16. Semenza GL: Regulation of hypoxia-induced angiogenesis: a chaperone escorts VEGF to the dance. J Clin Invest 2001;108:41
17. Le AD, Zhang Q, Wu Y, et al: Elevated vascular endothelial growth factor in keloids: relevance to tissue fibrosis. Cells Tissues Organs 2004;176:87
18. Kan C, Abe M, Yamanaka M, et al: Hypoxia-induced increase of matrix metalloproteinase-1 synthesis is not restored by reoxygenation in a three-dimensional culture of human dermal fibroblasts. J Dermatol Sci 2003;32:75
19. Cochrane CA: Models in vivo of wound healing in the horse and the role of growth factors. Vet Dermatol 1997;8:259

20. Lepault E, Céleste C, Doré M, et al: Comparative study on microvascular occlusion and apoptosis in body and limb wounds in the horse. Wound Repair Regen 2005;13:520

21. Falanga V, Zhou L, Yufit T: Low oxygen tension stimulates collagen synthesis and COL1A1 transcription through the action of TGF-beta1. J Cell Physiol 2002;191:42

22. Chvapil M, Pfister T, Escalada S, et al: Dynamics of the healing of skin wounds in the horse as compared with the rat. Exp Mol Pathol 1979;30:349

23. Määrtson M, Viljanto J, Laippala P, et al: Cranio-caudal differences in granulation tissue formation: an experimental study in the rat. Wound Repair Regen 1999;7:119

24. Miller CB, Wilson DA, Keegan KG, et al: Growth characteristics of fibroblasts isolated from the trunk and distal aspect of the limb of horses and ponies. Vet Surg 2000;29:1

25. Ladin DA, Hou Z, Patel D, et al: P53 and apoptosis alterations in keloids and keloid fibroblasts. Wound Repair Regen 1998;6:28

26. Theoret CL, Barber SM, Moyana TN, et al: Expression of transforming growth factor β1, β3 and basic fibroblast growth factor in full-thickness skin wounds of equine limbs and thorax. Vet Surgery 2001;30:269

27. Schwartz AJ, Wilson DA, Keegan KG, et al: Factors regulating collagen synthesis and degradation during second-intention healing of wounds in the thoracic region and the distal aspect of the forelimb of horses. Am J Vet Res 2002;63:1564

28. van den Boom R, Wilmink JM, O'Kane S, et al: Transforming growth factor-beta levels during second-intention healing are related to the different course of wound contraction in horses and ponies. Wound Repair Regen 2002;10:188

29. Shakespeare V, Shakespeare P: Effects of granulation-tissue–conditioned medium on the growth of human keratinocytes in-vitro. Br J Plast Surg 1991;44:219

30. LePoole IC, Boyce ST: Keratinocytes suppress TGF-b1 expression by fibroblasts in cultured skin substitutes. Br J Dermatol 1999;140:409

31. Greenhalgh DG: The role of apoptosis in wound healing. Internat J Biochem Cell Biol 1998;30:1019

32. Bellemare J, Roberge CJ, Bergeron D, et al: Epidermis promotes dermal fibrosis: role in the pathogenesis of hypertrophic scars. J Pathol 2005;206:1

33. Grinnell F, Zhu M, Carlson MA, et al: Release of mechanical tension triggers apoptosis of human fibroblasts in a model of regressing granulation tissue. Exp Cell Res 1999;248:608

34. Sporn MB, Roberts AB: Introduction: what is TGF-beta? Ciba Found Symp 1991;157:1

35. Chodon T, Sugihara T, Igawa HH, et al: Keloid-derived fibroblasts are refractory to Fas-mediated apoptosis and neutralization of autocrine transforming growth factor-beta1 can abrogate this resistance. Am J Pathol 2000;157:1661

36. Jelaska A, Korn JH: Role of apoptosis and transforming growth factor beta1 in fibroblast selection and activation in systemic sclerosis. Arthritis Rheum 2000;43:2230

37. http://www.bccresearch.com/editors/RC-077N.html

38. Leibovich SJ, Ross R: The role of the macrophage in wound repair: a study with hydrocortisone and antimacrophage serum. Am J Pathol 1975;78:71

39. Martin P, Leibovich SJ: Inflammatory cells during wound repair: the good, the bad and the ugly. Trends Cell Biol 2005;15:599

40. Wilmink JM, van Weeren PR: Treatment of exuberant granulation tissue. Clin Tech Equine Pract 2004;3:141

41. Schneiter HL, McClure JR, Cho DY: The effects of flunixin meglumine on early wound healing of abdominal incisions in ponies. Vet Surg 1981;16:101 (abstr)

42. Jurga F, Morrison SE: Maggot debridement therapy. Alternative therapy for hoof infection and necrosis. Hoofcare and Lameness 2004;78:28

43. Casu RE, Pearson RD, Jamey JM, et al: Excretory/secretory chymotrypsin from Lucilia Cuprina: purification, enzymatic specificity and amino acid sequence deduced from mRNA. Insect Mol Biol 1994;3:201

44. Wollina U, Karte K, Herold C, et al: Biosurgery in wound healing—the renaissance of maggot therapy. J European Acad Dermatol Venereol 2000;14:285

45. Daeschlein G, Mumcuoglu KY, Assadian O, et al: In vitro antibacterial activity of Lucilia sericata maggot secretions. Skin Pharmacol Physiol 2007;20:112

46. Bexfield A, Nigam Y, Thomas S, et al: Detection and partial characterization of two antibacterial factors from the excretions/secretions of the medicinal maggot *Lucilia sericata* and their activity against methicillin-resistant *Staphylococcus aureus* (MRSA). Microbes Infect 2004;6:1297

47. Steenvoorde P, Jukema GN: The antimicrobial activity of maggots: in-vivo results. J Tissue Viabil 2004;14:97

48. Lodge A, Jones M, Thomas S: Maggots "n" chips: a novel approach to the treatment of diabetic ulcers. Br J Community Nurs 2006;11:23

49. Steenvoorde P, Jacobi CE, Oskam J: Maggot debridement therapy: free-range or contained? An in-vivo study. Adv Skin Wound Care 2005;18:430

50. Morrison SE: How to use sterile maggot debridement therapy for foot infections of the horse therapy. Proceedings 51st Congress of AAEP, Seattle, 2005

51. Doumbia A: Fistulous withers: a major cause of morbidity and loss of use amongst working equines in West Africa. World Equine Vet Assoc Proceedings 2006, p. 338
52. Lepage OM. Université de Lyon, Ecole Nationale Vétérinaire de Lyon, Equine Department, Personal communication, 2007
53. Nigam Y, Bexfield A, Thomas S, et al: Maggot therapy: The science and implication for CAM, Part II—maggots combat infection. Evid Based Complement Alternat Med 2006;3:303
54. Wilson DA, Adelstein EH, Keegan KG, et al: In vitro and in vivo effects of activated macrophage supernatant on distal limb wounds of ponies. Am J Vet Res 1996;57:1220
55. Wilmink JM, Stolk PW, van Weeren PR, et al: The effectiveness of the haemodialysate Solcoseryl for second-intention wound healing in horses and ponies. J Vet Med A. Physiol Pathol Clin Med 2000;47:311
56. Tonks AJ, Cooper RA, Jones KP, et al: Honey stimulates inflammatory cytokine production from monocytes. Cytokine 2003;21:242
57. Engelen M, Besche B, Lefay MP, et al: Effects of ketanserin on hypergranulation tissue formation, infection, and healing of equine lower limb wounds. Can Vet J 2004;45:144
58. Cochrane C, Rippon MG, Rogers A, et al: Application of an in vitro model to evaluate bioadhesion of fibroblasts and epithelial cells to two different dressings. Biomaterials 1999;20:1237
59. Howard RD, Stashak TS, Baxter GM: Evaluation of occlusive dressings for management of full-thickness excisional wounds on the distal portion of the limbs of horses. Am J Vet Res 1993;54:2150
60. Swaim SF, Riddell KP, McGuire JA: Effects of topical medications on the healing of open pad wounds in dogs. J Am Animal Hospital Assoc 1992;28:499
61. Swaim SF, Vaughn DM, Kincaid SA, et al: Effects of locally injected medications on healing of pad wounds in dogs. Am J Vet Res 1996;57:394
62. Canapp SO Jr, Farese JP, Schultz GS, et al: The effect of topical tripeptide-copper complex on healing of ischemic open wounds. Vet Surg 2003;32:515
63. Thomas S: Alginate dressings in surgery and wound management—Part 1. J Wound Care 2000;9:56
64. Jeschke MG, Sandmann G, Schubert T, et al: Effect of oxidized regenerated cellulose/collagen matrix on dermal and epidermal healing and growth factors in an acute wound. Wound Repair Regen 2005;13:324
65. Messadi DV, Le A, Berg S, et al: Expression of apoptosis-associated genes by human dermal scar fibroblasts. Wound Repair Regen 1999;7:511
66. Steinbach F, Mauel S, Beier I: Recombinant equine interferons: expression cloning and biological activity. Vet Immunol Immunopathol 2002;84:83
67. Desjardins I, Theoret CL, Joubert P, et al: Comparison of TGF-beta 1 concentrations in bronchoalveolar fluid of horses affected with heaves and of normal controls. J Vet Immunol Immunopathol 2004;101:133
68. Wieman TJ, Smiell JM, Su Y: Efficacy and safety of a topical gel formulation of recombinant human platelet-derived growth factor-BB (becaplermin) in patients with nonhealing diabetic ulcers: a phase III randomised, placebo-controlled, double-blind study. Diabetes Care 1998;21:822
69. Eisinger M, Sadan S, Soehnchen R, et al: Wound healing by epidermal-derived factors: experimental and preliminary clinical studies. Prog Clin Biol Res 1988;266:291
70. Steel CM, Robertson ID, Thomas J, et al: Effect of topical rh-TGF-β1 on second intention wound healing in horses. Aust Vet J 1999;77:734
71. Ohnemus P, von Rechenberg BV, Arvinte T, et al: Application of TGF-β3 on experimentally created circular wounds in horses. Vet Surg 1999;28:216 (abstr)
72. Mikler J, Theoret CL, Haigh J: Effect of topical elk antler velvet administration on cutaneous wound healing in an animal model of streptozotocin-induced diabetes mellitus. J Altern Compl Med 2004;10:835
73. Sunwoo HH, Nakano T, Sim JS: Effect of water-soluble extract from antler of wapiti on the growth of fibroblasts. Can J Animal Sci 1997;77:343
74. Pietrzak WS, Eppley BL: Platelet rich plasma: biology and new technology. J Craniofac Surg 2005;16:1043
75. Badylak SF: Extracellular matrix as a scaffold for tissue engineering in veterinary medicine: applications to soft tissue healing. Clin Tech Equine Pract 2004;3:173
76. Driver VR, Hanft J, Fylling CP, et al: A prospective, randomized, controlled trial of autologous platelet-rich plasma gel for the treatment of diabetic foot ulcers. Ostomy Wound Manag 2006;52:68–70
77. Crovetti G, Martinelli G, Issi M, et al: Platelet gel for healing cutaneous chronic wounds. Transfus Apher Sci 2004;30:145
78. Mazzucco L, Medici D, Serra M, et al: The use of autologous platelet gel to treat difficult-to-heal wounds: a pilot study. Transfusion 2004;44:1013
79. Hom DB, Linzie BM, Huang TC: The healing effects of autologous platelet gel on acute human skin wounds. Arch Facial Plast Surg 2007;9:174
80. Sutter WW, Kaneps AJ, Bertone AL: Comparison of hematologic values and transforming growth factor-β and insulin-like growth factor concentrations in platelet concentrates obtained by use of buffy coat and apheresis methods from equine blood. Am J Vet Res 2004;65:924

81. Gonshor A: Technique for producing platelet-rich plasma and platelet concentrate: background and process. Int J Periodontics Restorative Dent 2002;22:547

82. Schnabel LV, Hussni MO, Miller BJ, et al: Platelet rich plasma (PRP) enhances anabolic gene expression patterns in flexor digitorum superficialis tendons. J Orthop Res 2007;25:230

83. Monteiro S, Lepage OM, Theoret CL: The effects of autologous platelet-rich plasma (PRP) on the repair of wounds on the distal limb in horses. Am J Vet Res, in press 2008

84. Argüelles D, Carmona JU, Pastor J, et al: Evaluation of simple and double centrifugation tube method for concentrating equine platelets. Res Vet Sci 2006;81:237

85. Smith JJ, Ross MW, Smith RKW: Anabolic effects of acellular bone marrow, platelet rich plasma and serum on equine suspensory ligament fibroblasts in vitro. Vet Comp Orthop Traumatol 2006:19:43

86. Prades M, Abellanet I, Carmona JU, et al: Platelet rich plasma: a realistic alternative in tissue repair. Eur College Vet Surg proceedings 2006, p.211

87. Carter CA, Jolly DG, Worden CE Sr, et al: Platelet-rich plasma gel promotes differentiation and regeneration during equine wound healing. Exp Mol Pathol 2003;74:244

88. Yvorchuk-St Jean K, Gaughan E, St Jean G, et al: Evaluation of a porous bovine collagen membrane bandage for management of wounds in horses. Am J Vet Res 1995;56:1663

89. Swaim SF, Gillette RL, Sartin EA, et al: Effects of a hydrolyzed collagen dressing on the healing of open wounds in dogs. Am J Vet Res 2000;61:1574

90. Bigbie RB, Schumacher J, Swaim SF, et al: Effects of amnion and live yeast cell derivative on second-intention healing in horses. Am J Vet Res 1991;52:1376

91. Goodrich LR, Moll DH, Crisman MV, et al: Comparison of equine amnion and a nonadherent wound dressing material for bandaging pinch-grafted wounds in ponies. Am J Vet Res 2000;61:326

92. Desmoulière A, Redard M, Darby I, et al: Apoptosis mediates the decrease in cellularity during the transition between granulation tissue and scar. Am J Pathol 1995;146:56

93. Schumacher J, Brumbaugh GW, Honnas CM, et al: Kinetics of healing of grafted and nongrafted wounds on the distal portion of the forelimbs of horses. Am J Vet Res 1992;53:1568

94. Gomez JH, Schumacher J, Lauten SD, et al: Effects of 3 biologic dressings on healing of cutaneous wounds on the limbs of horses. Can J Vet Res 2004;68:49

95. Winkler JT, Swaim SF, Sartin EA, et al: The effect of a porcine-derived small intestinal submucosa product on wounds with exposed bone in dogs. Vet Surgery 2002;31:541

96. Cha J, Falanga V: Stem cells in cutaneous wound healing. Clin Dermatol 2007;25:73

97. Nakagawa H, Akita S, Fukui M, et al: Human mesenchymal stem cells successfully improve skin-substitute wound healing. Br J Dermatol 2005;153:29

98. Falanga V, Iwamoto S, Chartier M, et al: Autologous bone marrow–derived cultured mesenchymal stem cells delivered in a fibrin spray accelerate healing in murine and human cutaneous wounds. Tissue Eng 2007;13:1299

99. Ducharme-Desjarlais M, Lepault E, Celeste C, et al: Determination of the effect of a silicone dressing (CicaCare®) on second intention healing of full-thickness wounds of the distal limb of horses. Am J Vet Res 2005;66:1133

100. Carney SA, Cason CG, Gower JP, et al: CicaCare® gel sheeting in the management of hypertrophic scarring. Burns 1994;20:163

101. Gold MH: A controlled clinical trial of topical silicone gel sheeting in the treatment of hypertrophic scars and keloids. J Am Acad Dermatol 1994;30:506

102. Gold MH, Foster TD, Adair MA, et al: Prevention of hypertrophic scars and keloids by the prophylactic use of topical silicone gel sheets following a surgical procedure in an office setting. Dermatol Surg 2001;27:641

103. Kischer CW, Shetlar MR, Shetlar CL: Alteration of hypertrophic scars induced by mechanical pressure. Arch Dermatol 1975;111:60

104. Dubuc V, Lepault E, Theoret CL: Endothelial cell hypertrophy is associated with microvascular occlusion in limb wounds of horses. Can J Vet Res 2006;70:206

105. Jacob SE, Berman B, Nassiri M, et al: Topical application of Imiquimod 5% cream to keloids alters expression of genes associated with apoptosis. Br J Dermatol 2003;149:62

106. Nogueira SA, Torres SM, Malone ED, et al: Efficacy of Imiquimod 5% cream in the treatment of equine sarcoids: a pilot study. Vet Dermatol 2006;17(4):259

107. Desmouliere A, Chaponnier C, Gabbiani G: Tissue repair, contraction, and the myofibroblast. Wound Repair Regen 2005;13:7

108. Wilmink JM, Nederbragt H, van Weeren PR, et al: Differences in wound contraction between horses and ponies: the in vitro contraction capacity of fibroblasts. Equine Vet J 2001;33:499

109. Cochrane CA, Pain R, Knottenbelt DC: In-vitro wound contraction in the horse: differences between body and limb wounds. Wounds 2003;15:175

110. Vaughan MB, Howard EW, Tomasek JJ: Transforming growth factor-beta-1 promotes the morphological and functional differentiation of the myofibroblast. Exp Cell Res 2000;257:180

111. Sakai K, Sumi Y, Muramatsu H, et al: Thrombospondin-1 promotes fibroblast-mediated collagen gel contraction caused by activation of latent transforming growth factor beta-1. J Dermatol Sci 2003;31:99

112. Huang JS, Wang YH, Lin TY, et al: Synthetic TGF-beta antagonist accelerates wound healing and reduces scarring. FASEB J 2002;16:1269

113. Pipelzadeh MH, Naylor IL: The in vitro enhancement of rat myofibroblast contractility by alterations to the pH of the physiological solution. Eur J Pharmacol 1998;357:257

114. Garrel DR, Gaudreau P, Zhang LM, et al: Chronic administration of growth hormone-releasing factor increases wound strength and collagen maturation in granulation tissue. J Surg Res 1991;51:297

115. Dart AJ, Cries L, Jeffcott LB, et al: The effect of equine recombinant growth hormone on second intention wound healing in horses. Vet Surg 2002;31:314

116. Thorey IS, Hinz B, Hoeflich A, et al: Transgenic mice reveal novel activities of growth hormone in wound repair, angiogenesis, and myofibrolast differentiation. J Biol Chem 2004;279:26674

117. Moulin V, Larochelle S, Langlois C, et al: Normal skin wound and hypertrophic scar myofibroblasts have differential responses to apoptotic inductors. J Cell Physiol 2004;198:350

118. Issa R, Zhou X, Constandinou CM, et al: Spontaneous recovery from micronodular cirrhosis: evidence for incomplete resolution associated with matrix cross-linking. Gastroenterol 2004;126:1795

119. Darby IA, Bisucci T, Pittet B, et al: Skin flap-induced regression of granulation tissue correlates with reduced growth factor and increased metalloproteinase expression. J Pathol 2002;197:117

120. Carlson MA, Longaker MT, Thompson JS: Wound splinting regulates granulation tissue survival. J Surg Res 2003;110:304

121. Grinnell F: Fibroblast biology in three-dimensional collagen matrices. Trends Cell Biol 2003;13:264

2 Factors That Influence Wound Infection and Healing

2.1 Selected Factors That Negatively Impact Healing

Ted S. Stashak, DVM, MS, Diplomate ACVS

Introduction

A myriad of factors are known to influence wound healing. This chapter will focus on selected factors that have a negative impact on healing and, where applicable, a remedy will be suggested. The subject will be approached in the order in which a case involving a wound would be assessed. Infection, which represents a major cause of delayed wound healing, will be discussed in detail in the first portion of this chapter, and the management practices to reduce the risk of infection will be covered in the second portion.

Patient Factors

Age and Physical Status

The patient's age and physical status may influence the rate of wound healing. For example, wounds in young human patients heal more rapidly than do those of older patients.[1] Older humans, besides showing a sluggish inflammatory response to injury, also exhibit tardy formation of granulation tissue and delayed wound contraction. They consequently also appear more susceptible to infection.[2] Conversely; rapid (scarless) healing is seen in fetuses. Although there currently is no similar data for the horse, in the author's experience it appears that young horses heal more readily and with fewer complications than do older horses.

Human patients suffering from systemic infection or diseases of the liver, kidney, or cardiovascular system, as well as animals with endocrine imbalances, exhibit delays in wound healing.[1,3] However, as Theoret points out, since horses, compared to companion animals, are less commonly affected by these diseases, they are generally not a concern.[4] An exception may be horses suffering from Cushing's disease (Pars intermedia dysfunction) in which high endogenous cortisol can suppress inflammation sufficiently to delay healing.[5] Also, since high concentrations of glucocorticoids are known to be immunosuppressive, it is logical that horses suffering from this malady may be more susceptible to wound infection.

Anemia/Blood Supply/Oxygen Tension

Because most of the oxygen in blood is carried by hemoglobin, it is intuitive that anemia should be an important factor in reduced oxygen delivery and impaired wound healing; this concept however, is unfounded. Data suggest that normovolemic anemia with a packed cell volume (PCV) >20, unrelated to malnutrition, cancer, or chronic infection, does not appear to affect wound healing.[6] However, hypovolemia associated with hemorrhage and anemia or shock can greatly impair healing if not corrected.[7,8] Decreased perfusion of the wound appears to be the cause of altered healing.[9]

Local tissue hypoxia that results from insufficient blood volume in hypovolemic patients inhibits many of the responses that initiate healing.[10] An oxygen gradient exists between the nearest functioning capillary and the wound edge. The oxygen tension near a wound capillary is between 60 and 90 mm Hg; however, near the advancing edge of granulation tissue the oxygen tension approaches 0 mm Hg. This decrease is caused by the diffusion gradient and the consumption of oxygen by cells at the wound margin. Since the activities of the new fibroblasts (migration, proliferation, and protein synthesis) rely on the rate at which new capillaries are formed, the wound tensile strength is limited by perfusion and tissue oxygen tension.

The maturity and fragility of the new blood vessels forming in an acute wound appear to be affected by oxygen tension. New vessels forming in a hypoxic environment (13% inspired oxygen) are immature and bleed easily. Conversely, new vessels forming in a hyperoxic environment (50% inspired oxygen) are mature and form at a more rapid rate than do vessels in either a normoxic (21% inspired oxygen) or hypoxic environment.[10]

Reduced oxygen tension, besides inhibiting fibroblastic replication and migration, development of collagen, and tensile strength, also renders the wound more susceptible to infection by altering cellular phagocytic mechanisms.[2,7,8] When leukocytes ingest organisms and wound debris, more oxygen is consumed. Lack of sufficient oxygen slows the activity of leukocytes and decreases superoxide release, making the wound more susceptible to infection.[7,8,10] Correction of hypovolemia, and possibly the use of hyperbaric oxygen (HBO) therapy, should reduce the incidence of wound infection and allow healing to progress normally.

Malnutrition and Protein Deficiency

Wound healing is impaired in humans with mild to moderate short- or long-term protein energy malnutrition.[11] It appears that the direction the patient is moving toward metabolically (positive or negative) at the time of injury or surgery is most important, since the adverse effect of protein energy malnutrition occurs well in advance of the external evidence of weight loss. Impaired nutrition can alter growth factor synthesis and fibroblastic proliferation, and limit hydroxyproline and collagen deposition, as well as impair immune functions and oxygen transport in healing patients. Insufficient lipid levels, important to inflammation and membrane stabilization, have also been shown to adversely affect wound healing.[2]

The impairment in wound healing is easily reversed by providing adequate nutrition. Although this has not been proven in horses, it seems logical that there would be an effect of inadequate nutrition on wound healing in this species as well. Therefore, it is recommended that animals be offered balanced nutrition in adequate amounts prior to elective surgery and/or after wounding and emergency surgery.

Hypoproteinemia alone adversely affects wound healing primarily by altering fibroplasia, angiogenesis, remodeling, and gain in tensile strength, consequently prolonging the repair phase of healing.[1] The impairment in wound healing from hypoproteinemia is seen well in advance of alterations in the plasma protein levels. As an example, albumin fractions are depleted almost immediately following withdrawal of protein from the diet. Since albumin is the major oncotic pressure stabilizer in the intravascular compartment, it is not surprising that a decreased serum concentration is associated with poor healing outcomes.[2] Even though the alteration in healing is not strongly correlated to plasma protein levels, when these levels fall to 6 g/dl, healing is retarded. Below 5.5 g/dl, a 70% incidence of wound disruption is expected, and below 2 g/dl, wound healing is disrupted, edema occurs, and death ensues.[12]

Because fats can be synthesized from carbohydrates, and carbohydrates can be synthesized from protein—but protein can only be produced from protein or its digested byproducts (amino acids and peptides)—a protein-rich diet is required to counteract the adverse effects on wound healing. Feeding D-L methionine to protein-deficient animals reverses the retardation in wound healing.[1] D-L methionine is converted to cysteine, which serves as an important cofactor in collagen synthesis and it may also be involved in disulfide cross-linking as collagen matures.

D-L methionine powder is commercially available from Butler Animal Health Supply, (phone: [888] 838-2247); it also can be purchased from many animal feed stores in the USA. Specialty dosage formulations can be obtained from Optimal Compounding Services (phone: [888] 832-4993). Plumb recommends the following dosage regime: 22 mg/kg/daily for 1 week; 11 mg/kg/daily for 2 weeks; and 5.5 mg/kg/daily for 1 week.[13]

Experimentally, animals placed on high-protein diets have a more rapid gain in wound tensile strength with less edema formation when compared to animals receiving a protein-deficient diet.[12]

Dehydration

Dehydration of the patient as well as the wound can negatively affect wound healing. The poor perfusion of peripheral tissues in the dehydrated patient is thought to be the reason that healing is delayed in these subjects.[1] This problem can easily be rectified by hydrating the patient. Wound dehydration will be discussed later under "nature of the wound."

Wound Factors

Trauma

Excessive trauma, associated with the wound or at a site or sites remote from the wound (e.g., multiple lacerations or multiple fractures) can negatively affect repair and make the wound more susceptible to infection (Figures 2.1a,b).[1] When the effects of simultaneous trauma from either fracture or muscle contusion elsewhere on the body were examined, a delay in wound tensile strength was observed out to 15 days post-trauma. A delay in gain of wound tensile strength was also observed at the other sites when a second wound was made within 14 days of the first, and the degree and loss in gain of wound tensile strength was proportional to the severity of trauma.[1] Whether the excessive trauma is associated with one or multiple wounds, the decrease in healing and reduction in gain in tensile strength appear to result from prolonged inflammation and reduced capillary perfusion.

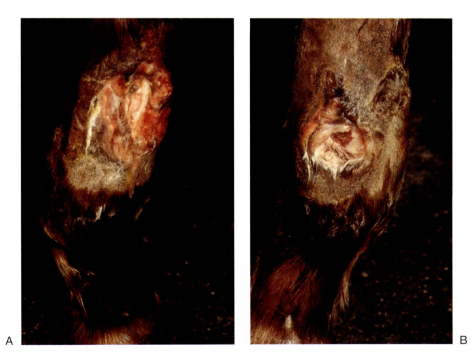

Figure 2.1. Example of excessive trauma to the distal metacarpal region from an entrapment injury that occurred 4 days earlier. The nature of this injury makes the wounds highly susceptible to infection. (A) Lateral view; note the exposed metacarpus, with a missing piece of cortical bone and the extensive "crushed" soft tissue. (B) Medial view; note the missing cortex of the bone (center of the wound) and a lesser amount of soft tissue injury compared to the lateral side.

As surgeons, we can reduce local tissue trauma by using scalpel dissection rather than scissors—which crush tissue—or blunt dissection—which tears tissue. Furthermore, tissue trauma in the surgically created wound can be reduced by reducing surgery time ("time equals trauma"),[1] using non-cytotoxic isotonic/iso-osmolar lavage solutions, reducing fluid accumulation in tissues, and apposing tissues with non-reactive suture material. For the traumatic wound destined to heal by second intention, proper cleaning/irrigation, thorough debridement, selecting an appropriate wound dressing, bandaging to achieve immobilization, and using appropriate antibiotics are considered most important.

Age of Wound

A chronic wound (slow or non-healing) is often associated with an underlying problem that has exerted a negative impact on the normal progress in repair.[14] Chronic inflammation from foreign bodies, necrotic tissue, repetitive mechanical trauma, and the application of caustic agents is a common cause (Figure 2.2). The goal in treating a chronic wound is to eliminate the causal agent/agents and convert the wound environment to one that closely resembles that of the acute wound; this is best done by wound debridement. In a case in which repeated mechanical trauma is the underlying cause, the use of appropriate bandaging/splinting techniques to immobilize the region is most important to ensure a successful outcome. For more information regarding bandaging and splinting techniques, see Chapter 16.

Previous Treatments

What the horse was previously treated with can negatively impact healing. Unfortunately, substances such as lye, gentian violet, pine tar, and other caustic agents are still used for wound treatment by horse owners. Generally, wounds treated with these substances should not be managed by primary suture closure, even after

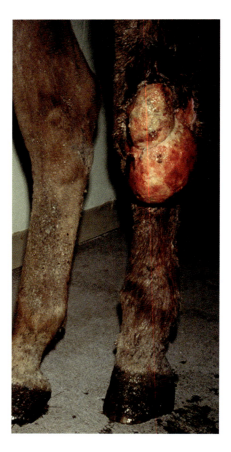

Figure 2.2. Example of a large fibrogranuloma on the dorsal surface of the hock that likely resulted from continued mechanical trauma from unrestricted movement of the joint during the repair phase.

thorough irrigation and debridement because the tissue damage is more extensive than can be visualized, thus they are more susceptible to infection. It is generally better to delay closure until a healthy appearing bed of granulation tissue forms.

Location

Wounds of the distal extremities (carpus/tarsus and below) of horses heal more slowly and are more problematic than wounds of the upper body and head regions. Specifically, delays in epithelialization and contraction, as well as the propensity to develop exuberant granulation tissue (EGT), commonly afflict full-thickness wounds of the distal limbs.[15–17] Although the causes of problematic healing in the horse's distal limbs have yet to be completely clarified, several have been proposed. Better blood supply, a greater amount of adnexal structures, and the thinner epidermis covering the head and neck contribute to the more rapid and cosmetic repair occurring in these regions.[18] Wounds of the distal extremities have an absence of underlying musculature, may be near highly mobile joints and bony prominences, and are often more contaminated than are body wounds.[19,20]

Differences between growth characteristics of trunk and limb fibroblasts and a tardy and prolonged inflammatory response are believed to contribute to the development of EGT, especially in limb wounds, in the horse. A study showed that fibroblasts isolated from the horse distal limb grow significantly more slowly than those of the trunk.[15] The horse displays a deficient and protracted inflammatory response compared to the pony, especially in wounds involving the distal extremities.[21] Furthermore, leukocytes from horses appear to be poorly equipped to kill bacteria compared to those of ponies.[22] Horses also appear to suffer an imbalance between collagen synthesis and lysis during the repair of limb wounds, resulting in excessive scarring in this location. Moreover, their local cytokine profile is skewed in favor of fibrogenic mediators.[17,23–25] Deficient contraction of limb wounds compared to body wounds may be due to a poor arrangement of myofibroblasts, precluding an ordered contractile activity.[21,26] Cytokine profiles may also negatively affect contractility.[26] For more information, see Differences in Wound Healing between Horses and Ponies in Chapter 1.

Wounds subjected to excessive movement, such as those located over highly moveable joints or those oriented perpendicular to lines of skin tension (e.g., perpendicular to the limb's long axis), are often slow to heal, and they usually form a disproportionate amount of scar tissue (Figure 2.2).[27] Movement can also occur between healing skin and underlying tendon or muscle or between the heel bulbs, causing the wound edges to gape during weight bearing (Figures 2.3a–c).[19] Stabilizing the wound site using special suturing techniques and bandages, splints, and casts can reduce the detrimental effects of movement. For more information regarding the specific techniques to reduce movement of a wound, see chapters 4 and 16.

Wounds located over synovial structures (e.g., tendon sheaths, bursa, and joints) must be examined closely to rule out their involvement. Early closure of wounds without employing an appropriate treatment plan may result in a septic synovial cavity that can limit function and may be life threatening. For more information regarding the appropriate examination procedures and the management of open synovial cavities, see the second section of this chapter as well as chapter 9.

Wounds overlying bony prominences often heal more slowly than those in other regions because of the increased tissue tension and movement, as well as pressure applied to the region while the horse is in recumbency. Reducing pressure at the site by either using appropriate padding techniques or preventing the horse from lying down will allow many of these wounds to heal by second intention. Successful primary intention healing, on the other hand, often requires the use of reconstructive approaches and tension-reducing suturing techniques to close the wound. Preventing the horse from lying down and applying protective padding is also important to a successful outcome in these cases.

Nature of the Wound

Type

Degloving injuries that damage (strip off) the periosteum and the paratendon are more susceptible to infection and subsequent osteomyelitis or septic tendonitis because of loss of blood supply (Figures 2.4a,b). In these cases, soft tissue coverage of the site should be achieved as soon as possible because of the increased risk of bony sequestration, tendon degeneration, and uncontrollable bone and soft tissue infection if the blood supply

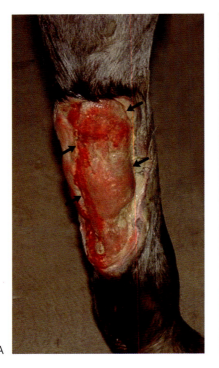
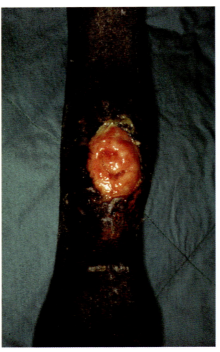
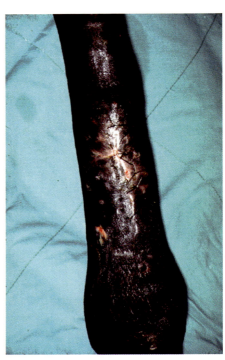

A   B,C

Figure 2.3. Examples of wounds in which movement between the healing skin and underlying tendon will either delay or prevent healing. (A) This horse sustained a smooth wire laceration to the right hind limb 1 month previously. Note the cleft between the granulation tissue (GT) and the surrounding skin (arrows). Bandage splinting would facilitate healing of this wound. (B) This horse sustained a transverse laceration of the plantar surface of the mid-metatarsal region 1 year earlier. Note the centrally located knob of GT surrounded by a ring of GT. The centrally located GT comes from the superficial digital flexor tendon, while the concentric ring of GT emanates from the subcutaneous tissue. Upon weight-bearing, the central knob of GT descends below the concentric ring of GT while the opposite effect is seen upon fetlock flexion. (C) Healed wound B following excision of the GT, appositional skin suturing, and immobilization in a lower limb cast for 2 weeks.

is not quickly re-established.[28] In some cases all that is needed is to suture the vascularized soft tissues into a position so they can supply the oxygen and metabolites required by the bone devoid of periosteum or the tendon devoid of paratendon (Figures 2.5a,b).

Wounds in which a flap of tissue is at odds with the distribution of blood vessels in the extremities often experience delays in healing and are more susceptible to infection (Figure 2.6a).[28] In most cases it is best to delay suturing these wounds until a healthy bed of granulation tissue forms; this will ensure a good blood supply to support the healing of the skin flap following suturing. Stabilizing the flap into a somewhat normal position using a few large sutures, while awaiting definitive treatment, will prevent skin flap retraction (Figure 2.6b).

Puncture wounds appear to be more susceptible to infection because the puncture tract often closes, entrapping bacteria deep in the tissue, creating an optimum environment for their survival. Opening the tract to allow it to drain, flushing the tract, and packing it open will often reduce the chances of infection becoming established.

Crush or entrapment injuries often are slow to heal and are more susceptible to infection because of the alteration to the wound's vascular supply (Figures 2.1, 2.7a,b). Delaying closure of these wounds until a healthy bed of granulation tissue develops usually obviates the problems associated with these types of injuries. For more detail, refer to the cause of the injury under the heading of infection.

Degree of Contamination

Wounds may be classified according to contamination and increasing risk of infection. A clean wound is one created surgically under aseptic conditions in situations where a contaminated site is not entered. Wounds are considered clean, clean contaminated, contaminated, or dirty contaminated/infected (see Table 2.1).

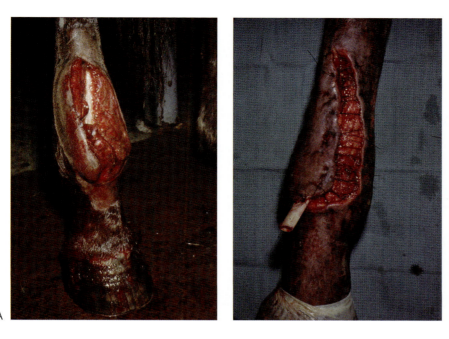
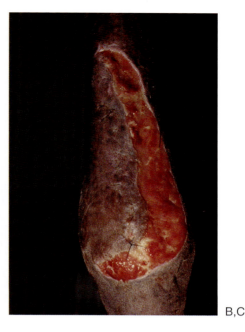

A
B,C

Figure 2.4. (A) Example of a degloving injury (~4 hours old) that stripped the periosteum off the metatarsus. Soft tissue coverage of the site should be achieved as soon as possible because of the increased risk of bony sequestration and uncontrollable bone and soft tissue infection if the blood supply is not quickly re-established. (B) Following wound irrigation and layered debridement, the exposed bone was covered with soft tissues which were held in place with vertical mattress interrupted sutures. Note that a Penrose drain was placed underneath the skin flap to prevent accumulation of blood and serum; the drain was removed at bandage change 2 days after surgery. Complete reconstruction of the site was not considered in this case due to economic constraints imposed by the owner. (C) Healing wound 2 weeks postoperatively, just prior to suture removal. Bandaging continued until second intention healing of the remaining open wound was achieved.

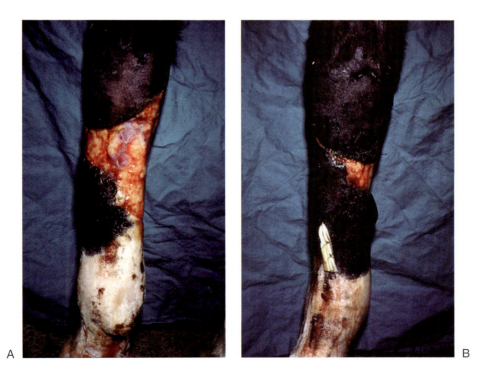

A
B

Figure 2.5. Laceration of the palmarolateral aspect of the right proximal metacarpal region. (A) At presentation ~6 hours following injury. After cleansing the wound it was noted that the paratendon had been stripped off the flexor tendons. (B) The skin flap is positioned and stabilized with sutures to cover the tendons devoid of paratendon. Note the drain placed under the skin flap and exiting distally. A bandage splint was used to immobilize the limb.

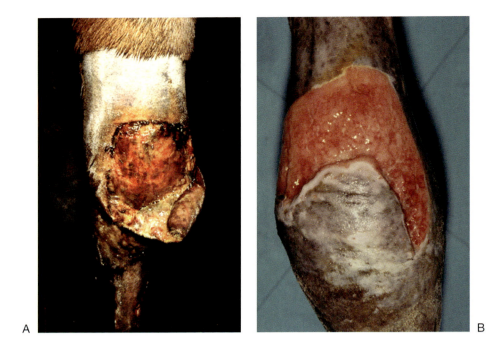

A   B

Figure 2.6. Example of a flap wound over the dorsal carpal region. The flap is positioned such that it is at odds with the limb's major distribution of blood vessels. (A) At presentation ~6 hours after injury. Note the absence of subcutaneous tissue at the proximal limit of the flap. Upon palpation, the tip of the flap felt cool. Following cleansing of the wound, the skin flap was elevated into its normal position, after which a bandage splint was applied. (B) Five days following injury. The skin flap has retracted and a healthy bed of granulation tissue has formed. This flap should have been stabilized, in as normal a position as possible, using a few large tension sutures. This would have prevented retraction of the skin flap, which will complicate delayed closure of the wound.

Table 2.1. Classification of operative wounds based on degree of microbial contamination.

Wound classification	Description
Clean	Elective, non-emergency, non-traumatic, non-inflamed operative wounds in which the respiratory, gastrointestinal, biliary, genitourinary, and oropharyngeal tracts are not entered.
Clean contaminated	Urgent or emergency case that is otherwise clean. Operative wounds in which the respiratory, gastrointestinal, biliary or genitourinary tracts are entered under controlled conditions, with minimal spillage.
Contaminated	Operations on traumatic wounds <4 hours duration without purulent discharge or chronic open wounds to be grafted. Procedures in which there is spillage of gastrointestinal contents or bile or infected urine. Procedures in which there is a major break in aseptic technique.
Dirty contaminated/infected	Operations on traumatic wounds with purulent discharge, devitalized tissue, or foreign bodies or wounds that are >4 hours duration. Procedures in which there is a preoperative perforation of a viscous, biliary, or genitourinary tract, or fecal contamination.

Adapted from Gottrup F, Melling A, Hollander DA: An overview of surgical site infections: etiology, incidence and risk factors. J European Wound Management Assoc 2005;5:11

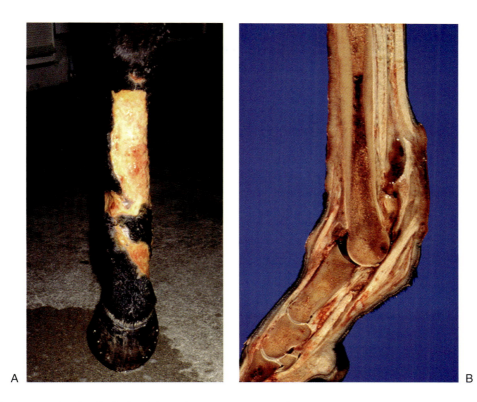

Figure 2.7. This horse sustained a degloving injury due to entrapment of the right hind limb 6 weeks earlier. The injury exposed the metatarso-phalangeal (fetlock) joint capsule and stripped the periosteum from the dorsal and lateral surfaces of the metatarsus as well as the paratendon associated with the flexor tendons on the medial side. Despite proper wound care, including wound irrigation and debridement, bandage changes at four-day intervals, and continued administration of broad spectrum antibiotics, the horse became non-weight bearing. (A) Horse at presentation. Radiographs revealed septic arthritis of the fetlock joint with subluxation and extensive septic osteitis of the metatarsal bone. (B) Post-mortem saggital section of the distal limb, illustrating the effects of chronic infection 6 weeks following injury. Note the plantar subluxation of the fetlock joint and the loss of integrity of the flexor tendons. It is presumed that the inability of the referring veterinarian to control the infection was due to altered blood supply associated with the injury.

As would be expected, the greater the contamination the greater the risk for infection. Dirty wounds have a 25-fold greater infection rate than do clean wounds.[29] Wounds contaminated with fecal material and dirt run a high risk of infection despite therapeutic intervention; indeed, feces may contain up to 10^{11} microorganisms per gram.[30] Specific infection potentiating fractions (IPFs) found in the organic and inorganic components of soil increase the wound's susceptibly to infection. These highly charged fractions reduce the effects of white blood cells, decrease humoral factors, and neutralize antibodies. Consequently, as few as 100 microorganisms can cause infection in wounds contaminated with soil.[31]

The metabolic impact of contaminating bacteria (bioburden) on tissues can significantly impair healing.[29] Contaminating bacteria compete with healing tissues for oxygen and nutrients, while their byproducts are deleterious to the normal balance in a healing wound. Contamination of the wound with large numbers of bacteria predisposes the patient to delayed healing and sets up an environment for infection to develop. Following the management practices outlined later in this chapter will markedly reduce the risk of infection becoming established in a wound.

Wound Fluids

Wounds with pockets that allow exudate or seroma/hematoma to accumulate are often slower to heal and are susceptible to infection. While persistent contact with inflammatory products present in the exudate during the repair phase is believed to cause the delay in repair, accumulation of seroma/hematoma further provides an excellent medium for bacterial growth, thus making the wound more susceptible to infection. Expanding fluid pressure from the exudate/seroma/hematoma may also be great enough to alter the local blood supply.[19,28] Drainage of the fluid-filled pocket followed by bandaging, where applicable, is usually all that is needed. For more information regarding the use of drains, see Chapter 4; for information regarding bandaging techniques, see Chapter 16.

Experiments have identified differences between acute and chronic wound fluids in humans.[32,33] Metalloproteinases, essential in the various phases of healing but detrimental in the case of persistent up-regulation, were found to be 5 to 10 times higher in chronic wound fluid. Serine proteinases that degrade fibronectin and impede collagen synthesis and epithelialization were also found to be increased in chronic wound fluids. Interestingly, when a chronic wound reverts to active healing, the levels of metalloproteinase activity decrease significantly, which parallels the processes observed in normally healing acute wounds.[34] Whether the nature of the wound fluid is a contributing factor or a consequence of delayed healing in horses is unknown but should be further studied. Debridement of the chronic wound is usually all that is needed to jumpstart healing. For more information regarding the approaches to wound debridement, see Management Practices that Influence Wound Infection and Healing later in this chapter.

Wound Dehydration

Wound dehydration results in desiccation of the marginal epithelial cells, which retards epithelialization and thus delays healing. Creating a moist wound healing environment can correct this problem. For more information regarding the selection of wound dressings, see Chapter 3.

Infection

Definition and Effects

Infection is defined as the presence of replicating microorganisms in a wound, leading to subsequent host injury.[35] It should be distinguished from wound contamination in which microorganisms are not replicating, as well as wound colonization in which replicating microorganisms do not result in host injury but rather impose a metabolic load on the healing wound.[29] Interestingly, some studies in dogs suggest that the organisms which infect may be a subset of those organisms that colonize the wound site.[36,37] Although not discussed in either Allaker's or Pedersen's papers, it is conjectured by this author that colonizing bacteria may impart a significant bioburden on the wound, rendering it more susceptible to infection.

Infection is considered to be a major cause of delayed wound healing, reduced gain of tissue tensile strength, as well as dehiscence following wound closure.[29,38] Potential pathogenic bacteria bind to extracellular matrix proteins (e.g., fibronectin), which may limit the latter's availability for promoting migration of mesenchymal cells and consequently bear a direct negative effect on wound healing.[39] Additionally, bacteria that produce exotoxins (e.g., *Clostridium spp, S. pyogenes, S. aureus*) cause more tissue damage, creating a microenvironment conducive to their survival. Those with thick capsules (e.g., *S. pyogenes, S. aureus, and Klebsiella pneumoniae*) are more resistant to phagocytosis by leukocytes. During the process of bacterial degradation, released endotoxins can activate coagulation pathways which may cause thrombosis of the microvasculature or systemic organ or immune dysfunction, and activate macrophages to release more inflammatory mediators.[40]

Risk Factors

Whether infection develops depends on many factors including: (1) dose of microorganisms (we have the most influence over this), (2) wound microenvironment/degree of contamination, (3) virulence and pathogenicity of the microorganisms, (4) functional capacity of the host, and (5) mechanism of injury.[28,39,41,42]

Generally, when bacterial numbers exceed 10^6 organisms per gram of tissue or per milliliter of exudate, in an open wound, the wound becomes infected.[43] A significant increase in failed delayed wound closure, due to infection, is seen in wounds containing >10^5 organisms per gram of tissue.[44] An exception is with *beta-hemolytic Strep sp.*, where merely 10^3 organisms per gram of tissue can produce infection.[29]

Contaminated wounds with lesser concentrations of bacteria may become infected when: (1) foreign bodies are present (e.g., wood, dirt, sutures, glove powder, etc.), (2) necrotic tissue is present, (3) a hematoma forms,

(4) local tissue defenses are impaired (e.g., burn patients or immune-suppressed patients), or (5) the vascular supply is diminished.[28,40,45]

As mentioned previously under Contamination, dirty wounds have a 25-fold greater infection rate than do clean ones.[29] Wounds contaminated with dirt have a higher risk of infection because the IPFs in soil decrease the protective effects of white blood cells and humoral factors and neutralize antibodies. Feces may contain up to 10^{11} microorganisms/gram.[30] Foreign bodies such as environmental organic material—which is common in the grossly contaminated wound—bone sequestrum, suture material, glove powder, or a bone plate and screws promote infection by providing protective surface areas for bacteria to grow. In general, the smaller the initial inoculum of microorganisms, the longer it takes to reach the point of clinical infection and the greater the chances that host defenses will curtail its onset.[28]

Hemoglobin, liberated upon hemorrhage into a wound, suppresses local tissue defenses. The ferric ion from hemoglobin also inhibits the natural bacteriostatic properties of serum and the intraphagocytic killing capabilities of bacteria by the granulocyte.[29] The ferric ion also can increase the virulence and replication of infecting bacteria. Hematoma formation is believed to be a leading factor in decreasing local wound resistance to infection.[46] Although the use of drains is somewhat controversial because they represent a foreign body within the wound, if drainage of a hematoma from "dead space" is needed the consequences of not using a drain are considerably more serious than those associated with the drain.[46]

The cause of injury also influences the wound's susceptibility to infection. In general, the greater the magnitude of impact, the more severe the soft tissue damage and the greater the alteration in blood supply. Wounds created by impact injury are believed to be 100 times more susceptible to infection than those caused by shearing forces.[47] See the Historical Considerations section later in this chapter for a more complete discussion.

Mechanisms Involved in Delaying Wound Healing

Bacterial infection delays healing by: (1) mechanically separating the wound edges via accumulation of exudate; (2) reducing the vascular supply, a result of mechanical pressure and a tendency for microthrombi to form in small vessels adjacent to the wound; (3) increasing cellular responses with prolongation of the inflammatory phase of wound healing; (4) producing proteolytic enzymes that digest collagen; (5) microorganisms binding to extracellular matrix proteins which may limit their availability for promoting mesenchymal cell migration; and (6) releasing endotoxins which inhibit growth factor and collagen production.[38–40] Thus, bacterial injury to wound tissues results in cellular and vascular responses typical of inflammation.[28]

Suture Material and Pattern

Suturing technique, as well as the material selected, may have a negative impact on healing. When simple interrupted sutures were compared to simple continuous sutures, wounds sutured in a simple interrupted fashion had less edema, increased microcirculation, and a 30%–50% greater tensile strength after 10 days.[48] These results support the use of an interrupted suture pattern rather than a continuous suture pattern when impaired healing is anticipated and excessive tension is present.

When the effects of suture tension (normal tension versus reduced tension) on skin healing were examined, it was found that wounds in which edges were loosely approximated were stronger at 7, 10, and 21 days postoperatively than those secured tightly with sutures.[49] It is recommended that wound edges just be apposed, whereas over-reduction of tissues should be avoided. When excessive tension is generated by closure, the use of tension suturing techniques is indicated. For more information regarding tension suturing techniques, see Chapter 4.

Because each passage of a suture through tissue creates a small wound, patterns with a single passage such as the simple interrupted pattern create less inflammation than those requiring a greater number of penetrations (e.g., vertical mattress and far-near-near-far suture patterns).

Generally, the synthetic absorbable and nonabsorbable suture materials cause less reaction than do natural products (e.g., surgical gut, cotton, and silk). A monofilament design induces less reactivity than do twisted and braided sutures. For more information regarding the selection of suture material and suture patterns, see Chapter 4.

Wound Dressings and Bandages

Dressings play an important role in healing and therefore it is not surprising that selection of an inappropriate dressing for a given phase of healing can negatively impact the rate of repair. For example, the continued use of a debridement dressing during the repair phase can markedly delay healing. See Chapter 3 for more information regarding the effects of wound dressings on the various stages of healing.

Bandages applied too tightly or loosely can also exert a negative impact on healing. While tight bandages can result in a reduction of wound perfusion, loose bandages may allow too much movement at the wound site, resulting in disruption. Reduction in wound perfusion is known to delay healing and make the wound more susceptible to infection.[1,27] Too much movement at the wound site results in increased inflammation and causes a delay in wound healing. For more information regarding the appropriate application of bandages, see Chapter 16.

Neoplastic Transformation

Neoplastic transformation at a wound site, although uncommon, should be considered in any non-healing chronic granulating wound. Both sarcoid and squamous cell carcinoma transformation have been reported following wounding in horses.[19,50,51] It appears the transformation can occur at any wound site on the body. While sarcoid transformation is more likely to occur in a horse with a sarcoid at another site on its body, no such relationship has been established for squamous cell transformation. A typical history for neoplastic transformation includes failure of a granulating wound to heal following repeated attempts to debride the granulation tissue (Figure 2.8) or dehiscence of a sutured wound in the absence of an identifiable cause. See Chapter 14 for more information regarding sarcoid transformation.

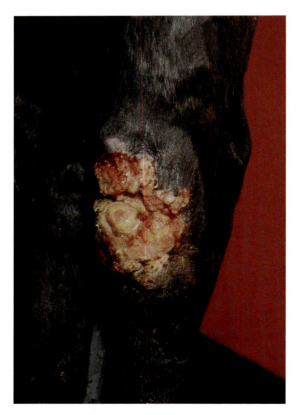

Figure 2.8. Example of a wound that would not heal following repeated attempts to excise the granulation tissue. Histological examination of the tissue revealed a squamous cell carcinoma.

Conclusion

The rate of wound repair is determined by many factors, some of which already exist at the time of presentation. Thus, our role as clinicians is to recognize the factors that negatively impact repair and correct and prevent as many of these as possible. In doing so we can best fulfill the therapeutic goal of wound management, which is to return the horse to normal function as soon as possible while achieving a cosmetic outcome.

References

1. Peacock EE: Collagenolysis and the biochemistry of wound healing. In E Peacock ed. *Wound repair (3rd edition)*. Philadelphia: WB Saunders, 1984, p.102
2. Stotts NA, Wipke-Tevis DD: Cofactors in impaired wound healing. In D Krasner, G Rodeheaver and G Sibbald ed. *Chronic wound care: a clinical source book for the healthcare professional (3rd edition)*. Wayne PA: HMP Communications, 2001, p.265
3. Stashak TS: Selected factors that affect wound healing. In T Stashak ed. *Equine wound management (1st edition)*. Philadelphia: Lea and Febiger, 1991, p.19
4. Theoret C: Wound repair. In JA Auer, JA Stick eds. *Equine surgery (3rd edition)*, Philadelphia: Saunders/Elsevier, 2006, p.44
5. Knottenbelt DC: Factors that prevent healing of traumatic wounds in horse. Proc North Am Vet Conf 2007;21:123
6. Heughan C, Grislis G, Hunt T: The effect of anemia on wound healing. Ann of Surg 1974;179:163
7. Jonsson K, Jensen JA, Goodson WH, et al: Assessment of perfusion in postoperative patients using tissue oxygen measurements. Br J Surg 1987;74:263
8. Hunt TK, Hopf W, Hussain Z: Physiology of wound healing. Adv Skin Wound Care 2000;13:6
9. Taylor DEM, Cooper GJ, Evans VA, et al: Effect of hemorrhage on wound healing and its possible modification by 1-ethoxysilatrane. J Royal Coll Surg Edinburgh 1986;31:13
10. Hopf HW, Rollins MD: Wounds: an overview of the role of oxygen. Antioxid Redox Signal 2007;9:1183
11. Haydock DA, Graham LH: Impaired wound healing in surgical patients with varying degrees of malnutrition. J Parenterol Enteral Nutr 1986;10:550
12. Noffsinger GR, McMurray BL, Jones TJ: Proteins in wound healing. J Vet Med Assoc 1957;30:481
13. Plumb DC: *Plumb's veterinary drug handbook*. Ames Iowa: Blackwell, 2005, p.504
14. Kane DP. Chronic wound healing and chronic wound management. In D Krasner, G Rodeheaver, and G Sibbald. *Chronic wound care: a clinical source book for healthcare professionals. 3rd ed*. Wayne, PA: HMP Communications, 2001, p.7
15. Bacon Miller C, Wilson DA, Keegan KG, et al: Growth characteristics of fibroblasts isolated from the trunk and distal aspect of the limb of horses and ponies. Vet Surg 2000;29:1
16. Wilmink JM, Stolk PWTH, Van Weeren PR, et al: Differences in second-intention wound healing between horses and ponies: macroscopic aspects. Equine Vet J 1999;31:53
17. Theoret CL, Barber SM, Moyana TN, et al: Expression of transforming growth factor β1, β3, and basic fibroblast growth factor in full-thickness skin wounds of equine limbs and thorax. Vet Surg 2001;30:269
18. Moy LS: Management of acute wounds. Dermatol Clin 1993;11:759
19. Knottenbelt DC: Equine wound management: are there significant differences in healing at different sites on the body? Vet Dermatol 1997;8:273
20. Cochrane CA, Pain R, Knottenbelt DC: In vitro wound contraction in the horse: differences between body and limb wounds. Wounds 2003;15:175
21. Wilmink JM, van Weeren PR, Stolk PW, et al: Differences in second-intention wound healing between horses and ponies: histological aspects. Equine Vet J 1999;31:61
22. Wilmink JM, Veenman JN, van den Boom R, et al: Differences in polymorpho-nucleocyte function and local inflammatory response between horses and ponies. Equine Vet J 2003;35:561
23. Schwartz AJ, Wilson DA, Keegan KG, et al: Factors regulating collagen synthesis and degradation during second-intention healing of wounds in the thoracic region and the distal aspect of the forelimb of horses. Am J Vet Res 2002;63:1564
24. van den Boom R, Wilmink JM, O'Kane S, et al: Transforming growth factor-beta levels during second-intention healing are related to the different course of wound contraction in horses and ponies. Wound Repair Regen 2002;10:188
25. Cochrane CA: Models in vivo of wound healing in the horse and the role of growth factors. Vet Dermatol 1997;8:259
26. Wilmink JM, Nederbragt H, van Weeren PR, et al: Differences in wound contraction between horses and ponies: the in vitro contraction capacity of fibroblasts. Equine Vet J 2001;33:499
27. Stashak TS: Principles of reconstructive surgery. In T Stashak ed. *Equine wound management (1st edition)*. Philadelphia: Lea and Febiger, 1991, p.70

28. Stashak TS: Current concepts in wound management in horses: parts I-III. Proc North Am Vet Conf 2003,17:231
29. Robson MC: Wound infection: A failure of wound healing caused by an imbalance of bacteria. Surg Clin North Am 1997;77:637
30. Stashak TS: Wound Infection: contributing factors and selected techniques for prevention. Proc Am Assoc North Equine Pract 2006;52:270
31. Rodeheaver G, Pettry D, Turnbull V, et al: Identification of the wound infection-promoting factors in soil. Am J Surg 1974;128:8
32. Wysocki AB, Staiano-Coico L, Grinnell F: Wound fluid from chronic leg ulcers contains elevated levels of metalloproteinases MMP-2 and MMP-9. J Invest Dermatol 1991;101:64
33. Rao CN, Ladin DA, Liu YY, Chilikuri K, et al: Alpha 1-antitrypsin is degraded and non-functional in chronic wounds but intact and functional in acute wounds: the inhibitor protects fibronectin from degradation by chronic wound fluid enzymes. J Invest Dermatol 1995;105:572
34. Trengrove NJ, Stacey MC, MacAuley S, et al: Analysis of the acute and chronic wound environments: the role of proteases and their inhibitors. Wound Rep Regen 1999;7:442
35. Dow G: Infection in chronic wounds. In D Krasner, G Rodeheaver, and G Sibbald, eds. *Chronic wound care: a clinical source book for the healthcare professional (3rd edition)*. Wayne PA: HMP Communications, 2001, p.343
36. Allaker RP, Garrett N, Kent L, et al: Characterization of *Staphylococcus intermedius* isolates from canine pyoderma and from healthy carriers by SDS-PAGE of exoproteins immuno-blotting and restriction endonuclease digest analysis. J Med Microb 1993;39:429
37. Pedersen K, Wegener HC: Antimicrobial susceptibility and rRNA gene restriction patterns among *Staphylococcus intermedius* from healthy dogs and from dogs suffering from pyoderma or otitis externa. Acta Vet Scand 1995;36:335
38. Bucknell T: The effect of local infection upon wound healing: an experimental study. Br J Surg 1980;67:851
39. Maheshwari RK, Kedar VP, Bharttiya D, et al: Interferon enhances fibronectin expression in various cell types. J Biol 1990;4:117
40. Brumbaugh GW: Use of antimicrobials in wound management. Vet Clin North Am; Equine Pract 2005;21:63
41. Dunning D: Surgical wound infection and the use of antimicrobials. In D Slatter, ed. *Textbook of small animal surgery (3rd edition)*. Philadelphia: WB Saunders, 2003, p.113
42. Baxter GM: Management of wounds. In P Colahan, I Mayhew, A Merritt, and J Moore, ed. *Equine medicine and surgery, (vol 2., 5th edition)*. Philadelphia: Mosby, 1999, p.1808
43. Noyes H, Chi N, Linah L, et al: Delayed topical antimicrobials as adjuncts to systemic antibiotic therapy of war wounds: bacteriologic studies. Mil Med 1967;132:461
44. Robson M, Heggers J: Bacterial quantification of open wounds. Mil Med 1969;134:19
45. Swaim SF: Management of contaminated and infected wounds. In S Swaim, ed. *Surgery of traumatized skin: management and reconstruction in the dog and cat (1st edition)*. Philadelphia: WB Saunders Co, 1980, p.119
46. Cruse PJ, Foord R: The epidemiology of wound infections: a 10-year prospective study of 62,939 wounds. Symposium on surgical infections. Surg Clin of North Am 1980;60:27
47. Edlich RF, Rodeheaver GT, Morgan RF, et al: Principles of emergency wound management. Ann Emerg Med 1988;17:1284
48. Speer DP: The influence of suture techniques on early wound healing. J Surg Res 1979;27:385
49. Brunius U, Ahren C: Healing of skin incisions suturing reduced tension of the wound area. Acta Chir Scand 1969;135:383
50. Schumacher J, Watkins JP, Hardy SB et al: Burn-induced neoplasia in two horses. Equine Vet J 1986;18:410
51. Baird AN, Frelier PF: Squamous cell carcinoma originating from an epithelial scar in a horse. J Am Vet Med Assoc 1990;12:1999

2.2 Management Practices That Influence Wound Infection and Healing

Ted S. Stashak, DVM, MS, Diplomate ACVS

Introduction

Preserving life, preventing infection, and creating an optimum environment for wound healing to continue should be major objectives when a veterinarian is presented with a patient suffering a traumatic wound.[1] On initial examination, a minor wound should not divert attention from a more serious problem such as hemorrhagic shock, exhaustion, or cerebral contusion associated with head injuries.[2] Thus, a rapid assessment of the wound should be followed by a thorough physical examination. Hemorrhage should be controlled and therapy directed toward returning the patient to function and obtaining a cosmetic outcome as quickly as possible.[3]

This section will review wound management practices that influence wound infection and healing. The subject will be approached in the order in which a case involving a wound would be evaluated and managed. Because infection is a major cause of delayed healing and wound dehiscence following suturing, the management practices that reduce the incidence of infection will be discussed in detail.

Historical Considerations

Duration since Injury

Historically, it was accepted that wounds treated within 6 to 8 hours after injury could be safely sutured with little risk of infection. This temporal relationship, referred to as the "golden period," was suggested as a result of research performed in laboratory animals, indicating that bacterial contaminants took longer than 6 to 8 hours to reach sufficient numbers to cause infection in a sutured wound. Subsequent experiments using quantitative bacterial analysis documented a very high incidence of infection in sutured wounds containing 10^5 organisms per gram of tissue.[4] Others found that it took only 3 hours for some bacteria to proliferate to infective levels of 10^6 organisms per gram of tissue.[5]

As we know today, many factors, including the virulence of the organism, location and type of wound, degree and type of contamination, patient's immune status, mechanism of injury, and how the wound is managed, play a role in the susceptibility of any given wound to infection. Therefore, although rough guidelines regarding the time from injury to treatment can be followed, the most important criteria in deciding on the treatment of any given wound should come from the physical examination of the wound and the patient.

Cause of Injury

The cause of injury can greatly influence the wound's susceptibility to infection. Lacerations caused by sharp objects (e.g., metal or broken glass) are generally resistant to infection (Figure 2.9). Conversely, shear wounds from barbed wire, sticks, nails, and bites are more prone to infection because of the greater soft tissue damage. Wounds caused by entrapment (e.g., limb caught in cattle guard) or impact from collision with solid objects or from a kick are very susceptible to infection because of the greater magnitude of soft tissue injury. The greater the energy upon impact, the greater the soft tissue damage and alteration in blood supply. Entrapment injuries in which the distal limb becomes caught for some time can be particularly difficult to treat because of the massive soft tissue damage, subsequent vessel thrombosis, and infection that often becomes established (Figures 2.7a,b). Wounds created by impact are believed to be 100 times more susceptible to infection than those caused by shearing forces (Figure 2.10).[6]

Previous Treatments

Prior treatment of wounds with caustic chemicals (e.g., lye) and other cytotoxic agents (e.g., detergent antiseptic soap, full strength antiseptics, hydrogen peroxide) has a negative effect on repair and makes the wound more susceptible to infection.[3,7] Generally, wounds treated in this fashion should not be managed by primary suture closure even after thorough irrigation and debridement because the tissue damage is more extensive than can be visualized; thus they are more susceptible to infection. It is generally better to delay closure until a healthy appearing bed of granulation tissue has formed.

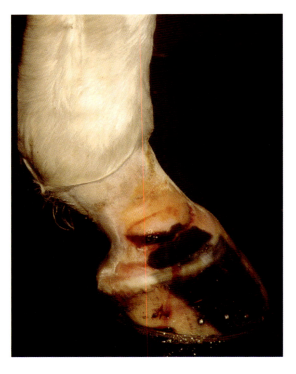

Figure 2.9. Example of a sharp laceration involving the lateral pastern region. This type of wound would be expected to have a reduced chance of developing infection following appropriate treatment. However, because of the wound location, it would be important to rule out the involvement of the proximal interphalangeal joint; techniques for doing this will be illustrated later.

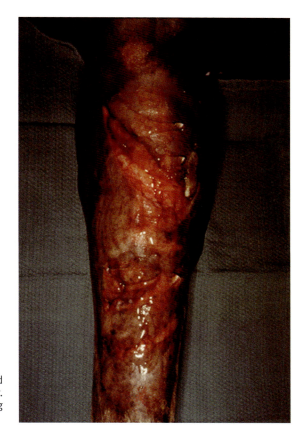

Figure 2.10. Example of wounds to the plantar hock region of the left hind limb caused by the horse repeatedly kicking the wall of a horse trailer. This type of impact injury alters the blood supply to the region, making the wounds very susceptible to infection.

Horses sustaining deep penetrating wounds (e.g., puncture wounds or snake bites) are more vulnerable to developing tetanus. If a tetanus toxoid booster has not been administered within the past year, then it should be given at this time and penicillin therapy should be initiated.[1] Tetanus antitoxin should only be given to horses and foals lacking a history of tetanus vaccination or exhibiting clinical signs of tetanus. In these cases, tetanus toxoid should be administered concurrently but in a site separate from where the antitoxin is given. A caveat to the administration of antitoxin, particularly in adult horses, is the possibility of developing serum hepatitis (Theiler's disease) 4 to 10 weeks following administration.[1]

Management Practices

The following section will review management approaches that influence healing and will help reduce the incidence of infection.

General Anesthesia and Duration of Surgery

The depth and duration of anesthesia, and the duration of surgery, have independently been shown to be significant risk factors for the development of postoperative infection.[7-10] Excessive depth of anesthesia reduces tissue perfusion and oxygenation, causing acidosis and an impaired resistance to infection. Prolonged anesthesia impairs the alveolar macrophage function and depresses systemic leukocyte migration and function.[11,12] Wound infection rates have been shown to increase by 0.5% per minute after the initial 60 minutes of anesthesia.[10] This translates to a 30% greater risk of postoperative infection for each additional hour of anesthesia. Practical recommendations include reducing the depth and duration of anesthesia and ensuring proper hydration of the anesthetized patient. Propofol should be avoided because it has been shown to increase infection rates 3.8 times in clean wounds.[13]

Reducing the surgery time is also logical; wound infection rates doubled after 90 minutes of surgery and nearly tripled when surgery exceeded 120 minutes.[8,14] Finally, one should limit the use of electrocautery because excessive use has been shown to double infection rates.[15] However, if bleeding vessels are grasped with fine non-serrated tissue forceps and electrocautery is used, the infection rate is not increased over that of other methods of hemostasis.[15]

Wound Anesthesia

Many wounds can be cleaned, explored, and repaired in the standing horse using a combination of sedation and/or tranquilization and local anesthesia. Local anesthesia can be accomplished by regional, perineural, or intralesional infiltration of a local anesthetic agent. Intralesional injection should only be performed after cleaning the wound to minimize the chances of disseminating bacteria deeper in the wound. Two percent mepivacaine or lidocaine is the most commonly used for local anesthesia.

Studies evaluating the effects of 2% anesthetic solutions on healing have inconsistently reported that they may inhibit collagen synthesis, platelet aggregation, and leukocyte function and may cause vasoconstriction and thrombosis in microvessels.[16–20] Adding epinephrine to the local anesthetic causes vasoconstriction, which exacerbates these effects. However, no negative effects on healing were found following intralesional injection of 0.5% lidocaine compared to intralesional injection of saline. In fact, 0.5% lidocaine treatment resulted in stronger wounds out to 12 days compared to those treated with 2% lidocaine.[21]

Although it has been recommended that 2% local anesthetic solutions be injected into a site well removed from the wound in an effort to avoid their potential negative effects on healing, intralesional administration appears safe and effective.[1,2] To avoid any potential negative side effects on healing and because 0.5% is apparently equally as effective as a 2% solution of lidocaine in providing local anesthesia,[22] some practitioners routinely dilute 2% anesthetic solution with sterile water to make a 0.5% solution.

Wound Preparation

Proper wound preparation includes removal of hair adjacent to the wound and wound cleansing (lavage/irrigation).[3]

Hair Removal

Although clipping the hair prior to the induction of general anesthesia is most applicable for elective surgery, two comprehensive small animal studies have shown that it is preferable to avoid this practice because it significantly increases infection rates.[8,10] "Nipping" of the skin at its creases by the clipper blades, producing gross cuts in which bacteria can colonize, was incriminated.[23] The author has speculated that clipping may compromise the natural seal (infundibulum) at the hair shaft/epidermal junction, allowing bacteria that normally reside within the hair follicles and sebaceous glands to come to the surface and contribute to colonizing bacterial numbers.[3]

Prior to hair removal, the wound must be protected with sterile moist gauze sponges and the hair dampened with water or coated lightly with KY water-soluble jelly to prevent it from falling into the wound. A wide area of hair around the wound must be clipped, while the wound edges should be shaved using a recessed head razor, which will minimize damage to the infundibulum at the hair shaft epidermal junction and thus reduce skin contamination from bacteria located in the hair follicle and sebaceous glands.[24] Following hair removal, sponges used to pack the wound should be discarded and replaced with new ones. The clipped area of skin should be scrubbed at least 3 times with antiseptic soap and rinsed between scrubs with sterile 0.9% saline solution. (Antiseptic skin preparation will be discussed in greater detail later).

Wound Cleansing/Irrigation

Wound cleansing is one of the most important components of effective management. In the strictest sense, wound cleansing is the use of fluids to gently remove loosely adhered contaminants (including bacteria) and devitalized tissue from the wound surface. If contaminants cannot be removed with gentle wound cleansing, then more specific cleansing and debridement techniques should be used.[7]

Irrigation is recommended for all wounds. In clean, acute (<3 hours duration) wounds, water or saline may be all that is needed for adequate cleansing. For field use, an acceptable saline solution can be made by adding 2 teaspoons (10 ml) of salt to 1 liter or 8 teaspoons (40 mL) to 4 liters (~1 gallon) of boiling water.[7] Although tap water is effective for irrigation, it should be discontinued after a healthy bed of granulation tissue has formed.[25] Irrigation solutions are often combined with antiseptics and antibiotics; the justification for this will be discussed later. Additionally, a commercial wound cleanser may be used if enhanced wound cleansing is needed; this is also discussed later.

Because bacteria and contaminants initially adhere to the wound surface via an electrostatic charge, adequate fluid pressure is required to dislodge them from the wound. The irrigation solution is most effective when delivered at an oblique angle by a fluid jet at a pressure of at least 7 pounds per square inch (PSI) of pressure. Pressure equal to or above 7 PSI cannot be achieved by gravity flow or lavage with a bulb syringe.[26,27] Pulsating pressures of 10–15 PSI have been shown to be 80% effective in removing adherent bacteria from wounds.[27] Increasing the lavage pressure to 20–25 PSI does not significantly improve the result obtained with 15 PSI.[7] Although 70 PSI was found to be more effective than 25 or 50 PSI in removing wound tissue fragments and debris,[28] this amount of pressure is not recommended because it causes fluid dispersion into wound tissue.[29] Thirty PSI delivered from a single orifice has also been shown to penetrate and damage tissue.[30] A study comparing the effects of saline irrigation at 15 PSI versus 20 PSI, on penetration of partial thickness wounds, found that 20 PSI penetrated the entire wound depth. In contrast, irrigation with 15 PSI resulted in superficial (10–15%) penetration of the wound tissue.[31] Results of these studies suggest that wounds are best irrigated with pressures from 7–15 PSI and not exceeding 15 PSI.[7]

As for the methods of delivery, pulsatile pressures (7–15 PSI) can be achieved by delivering the fluids with: (1) a 35 or 60 cc syringe with a 19 gauge needle; (2) a spray bottle (Figure 2.11a); (3) a "Water Pik"; (4) a Stryker inter-pulse irrigation system™ (Stryker Instruments, Kalamazoo, MI); or (5) an Equine Hydro–T™ (Innovative Products International, Three Forks, MT) (Figures 2.11b,c), though the superiority of a pulsatile fluid stream compared to a continuous stream has not been established.[26]

A "Water Pik" at a low-intermediate setting (10–15 PSI) delivers 40–50 ml/min.[3] It appears to be most effective for irrigating heavily contaminated avulsion wounds involving the teeth. The spray bottle or the Stryker inter-pulse irrigation system™ are preferred for irrigation of most wounds. The Hydro-T™ can deliver tap water

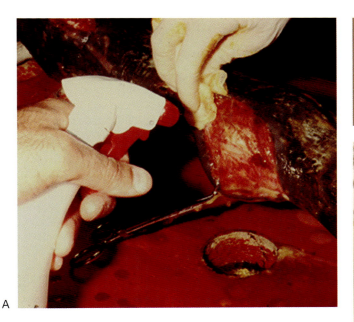
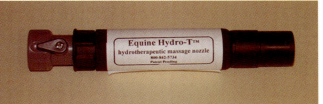

Figure 2.11. Examples of two irrigation devices that can deliver fluid to a wound at a pressure of 7–15 PSI. (A) Spray bottle. (B) Equine Hydro–T™. (C) The three rows of three holes in the head of the Equine Hydro–T™ allow delivery of a soft spray of water.

to the wound, in a pulsatile stream, at ~15 PSI. Irrigation with tap water should be discontinued once a bed of granulation tissue has developed.[25] Care must be taken when using pressure irrigation to ensure that contaminants are not driven deeper into the tissues and that fascial planes are not inadvertently separated.[24]

The clinical benefits of wound irrigation have been established in several studies. An experimental study comparing irrigation with a bulb syringe to fluid delivery at 8 PSI using a 35 ml syringe and a 19 gauge needle found a significant reduction in bacterial load and a reduced incidence of infection with the latter method.[32] A study of 335 humans suffering a traumatic wound <24 hours old showed that wound irrigation with at least 13 PSI, using a 12 ml syringe and a 22 gauge needle, significantly decreased wound inflammation and infection rate compared to irrigation with a standard bulb syringe.[33]

The ability of low-pressure irrigation (15 PSI) to remove bacteria decreases as the wound ages.[7] In acute wounds the majority of bacteria reside on the surface. Bacteria invade wound tissues as time passes; therefore they are not removed with irrigation alone and debridement is required. Although the exact time required for bacteria to invade wound tissues has not been established, it is proposed to range from 3 to 6 hours.[24,34]

The volume of irrigation fluid needed to effectively cleanse a wound depends upon its size and degree of contamination. At minimum, the gross contaminants should be removed and irrigation should be discontinued before the tissue becomes waterlogged.[3]

Antiseptics. Povidone-iodine (PI) and chlorhexidine diacetate (CHD) are the two antiseptics most commonly added to irrigation solutions.[24] Although there is some controversy, the literature supporting their use in the clinical situation is compelling. PI (1%) solution used for wound lavage of abdominal incisions following closure of the peritoneum was shown to surpass saline in reducing post-surgical wound infection.[35] PI (0.5%) powder sprayed on contaminated incisional wound beds following gastrointestinal surgery significantly reduced infection rates to 9.9% compared to 24.4% for nonsprayed controls. Bacterial contamination (established by cultures) at the time of surgery was associated with 52% infection rates in control groups while this was reduced to 11% in the PI-treated group.[36] Irrigation with (1%) PI solution does not appear to affect gain of tensile strength in healing wounds.[37]

Antiseptics are best used when diluted with sterile isotonic crystalloids such as saline or lactated Ringer's solution. PI solution diluted to 0.1% to 0.2% (10–20 ml/l) and CHD diluted to 0.05% (1:40 = 25 ml of the 2% concentrate diluted with 975 ml of sterile isotonic crystalloid) concentrations are considered best for wound lavage. These dilutions were also shown to be effective in reducing bacterial numbers in wounds of dogs[38,39] and have been shown to kill many bacteria within 15 seconds.[40] Conversely, CHD concentrations >0.05% have been shown to delay wound healing.[41]

Faster wound contraction was reported in dog wounds treated with dilute CHD or PI compared to a saline control.[38] An in vitro study comparing sterile saline to diluted solutions of PI and CHD delivered at 14 PSI to a bone surface contaminated with a fixed number of bacteria showed that the antiseptic solutions reduced the bacterial numbers 19-fold compared to saline controls.[42] Antiseptics appear most effective in reducing bacterial numbers in acute contaminated wounds and not in chronic wounds or those with established infection.[7] For more information regarding the topical effects of antiseptics, see Topical Wound Treatments and Wound Care Products in Chapter 3.

Antibiotics. The addition of antibiotics to an irrigation solution has been shown to effectively reduce the numbers of bacteria in a wound.[43] Experimentally, 1% neomycin solution was found to be effective in preventing infection in wounds contaminated with feces.[44] In a double-blind study performed on 260 sutured lacerations, penicillin sprayed on the wound before closure prevented three out of four infections.[45] For more information regarding the topical effects of antibiotics, see Topical Wound Treatments and Wound Care Products in Chapter 3.

Commercial Wound Cleansers. Commercial wound cleansers may be used when enhanced cleansing is required. However, most ionic and many nonionic surfactants present in wound cleansers have been shown to be toxic to cells, to delay healing, and to inhibit the wound's defenses against infection.[6,7] Nonetheless, the following products appear to exert minimal toxicity: Constant Clens™ (Covidien Animal Health/Kendall, Dublin, OH), ShurClens™ (Convatec ER Squibb and Sons, LLC, Princeton, NJ), and Equine Vet™ (Carrington Labs, Irving, TX).[46,47] Equine Vet™ is a relatively new wound cleansing product containing acemannan, a healing stimulant derived from the aloe vera plant.[48] The products come with an adjustable spray nozzle that can deliver a fluid stream of approximately 12 PSI at a distance of 15 cm. Vetricyn™ (www.oculusis.com) is a new cleansing solution that is the veterinary formulation of Microcyn™. It is a stable, nonirritating super-oxidized solution with a broad antimicrobial spectrum, packaged in a spray bottle. Vetricyn does not contain a surfactant and is thus not toxic.

Antiseptics should not be added to wound cleansers because this will increase the cytotoxic index.[49] In a heavily contaminated wound, the wound bed can be gently cleansed with a wound cleanser and scrubbed with sterile gauze sponges, followed by thorough lavage with a sterile salt solution. The coarseness of the scrubbing device should be as minimal as possible while still providing a cleansing action. Wounds scrubbed with coarse sponges were shown to be significantly more susceptible to infection.[49] An advantage to using a commercial wound cleanser is that the surfactant significantly reduces the coefficient of friction between the scrubbing device and wound tissue.[49]

Antimicrobial cleansers that are formulated to remove fecal contamination from intact skin (e.g., Dermal wound cleanser™ [Smith & Nephew, Hull, UK], MicroKlenz™ [Carrington Labs, Irving, TX]) are more cytotoxic than wound cleansers and therefore should not be used in a wound.[49] Antiseptic soap, detergents, and alcohol should not be allowed to contact raw tissue.[50] See Chapter 3 for a more complete discussion of wound cleansers.

Antiseptic Skin Preparation

Patient

The two most commonly used antiseptic surgical scrubs for preparation of the patient's skin are PI and chlorhexidine gluconate (CHG). Rinsing with saline or 70% isopropyl alcohol, following scrubbing, does not appear to alter the antimicrobial effect of PI surgical scrub. However, rinsing with 70% alcohol reduces the residual effect and antiseptic quality of CHG.[51] Therefore, a saline rinse is recommended.

A disadvantage to PI surgical scrub is the occasional skin reaction exhibited by horses. This phenomenon has been most commonly observed, by the author, in elective surgery patients when the limb is clipped and aseptically prepared with PI scrub, rinsed with 70% isopropyl alcohol, after which the skin is sprayed with PI solution and bandaged many hours before surgery. Skin reactions include subcutaneous edema and skin wheal formation.[3]

A disadvantage to the use of detergent forms of chlorhexidine is that short exposure to the eye, even in small concentrations, may lead to corneal opacification and ocular toxicity.[52–54] Another disadvantage of CHG and saline rinse is this combination's apparent inability to adequately clean the skin, particularly dirty, oily skin. The oily appearance is presumed to be from sebaceous secretion. In this case the author recommends performing the initial skin preparation with PI and 70% isopropyl alcohol followed by the use of CHG and saline.

Despite the associated mechanical effects of scrubbing the wound, which can be helpful in removing wound debris, these antiseptic soaps are very cytotoxic and therefore should not be used for cleansing the wound itself.[7] Moreover, PI surgical scrub was shown to be ineffective in reducing bacterial levels in wounds.[49]

Even with the high bactericidal rate of these antiseptics, 20% of the bacterial population in the skin resides protected within hair follicles, sebaceous glands, and crevices of the lipid coat of the superficial epithelium.[55]

Surgeon

Cultures of hand swabs taken immediately following standard surgical hand preparation and following 4 hours spent in surgical gloves revealed that: (1) alcohol (70% ethyl) and CHG (4%) were effective surgical scrubs with good residual effect, (2) PI had short-term antibacterial effects, (3) triclosan was not effective, and (4) 70% ethanol (V/V) had low antibacterial effectiveness.[56,57]

A waterless skin preparation (Avagard™, 3M Animal Care Products, St. Paul, MN) appears to have many desirable qualities. Avagard contains 1% CHG and 61% ethyl alcohol in an emollient. A study comparing Avagard to 4% CHG or 7% for hand and arm preparation, over 5 days, and under surgical gloves for 6 hours, found Avagard™ superior in antiseptic quality and less irritating than the PI and CHG antiseptic scrubs.[57]

Wound Exploration

A wound is explored to document its extent and to identify if a bone or a synovial structure is exposed and if foreign bodies are present. After the wound is cleansed and free of debris, it can be explored digitally using a sterile glove from which the talcum powder has been rinsed off the outer surface. Talcum powder left in a wound represents a foreign body, which increases the wound's susceptibility to infection.[3]

If the wound has a small opening, precluding the insertion of a finger, a sterile probe can be used to identify the depth of the wound, whether a foreign body is present, or if bone has been contacted. Once the depth of the wound has been reached with the probe, a radiograph can be taken to identify its location in relation to bone or a synovial cavity (Figures 2.12a,b). If the probe seems to be close to a synovial structure/structures, then a contrast radiographic exam should be done. To do this, a Foley catheter may be inserted into the wound tract, the balloon tip inflated, and contrast dye injected (Figures 2.13a,b, 2.14a,b). It is important that, for puncture wounds adjacent to or overlying a synovial cavity, the limb be flexed and extended, passively, during the injection of contrast material. This allows thorough penetration of contrast material within the fascial planes.

If the appearance of fluid at the wound site suggests a synovial origin, this should be confirmed by stringing it between the thumb and forefinger. A definitive diagnosis requires that a sample of the fluid be submitted for cytological examination. If synovial penetration is suspected and suspicious-looking fluid is not present at the wound site, a needle should be placed into the synovial cavity at a site away from the wound (Figure 2.15). If synovial fluid can be retrieved, it is submitted for cytology and culture/sensitivity. Following this, sterile saline solution is injected into the synovial structure; if the synovial capsule has been breached by trauma, fluid will flow from the wound. For more information on the management of wounds involving synovial structures, see Chapter 9.

Radiography can be useful in documenting fractures, joint subluxation/luxation, and radiodense foreign bodies. Contrast radiography is also useful in identifying a foreign body/bodies (e.g., wood fragments) within a wound or synovial cavity that is not seen on routine radiographic exam (Figures 2.16a,b,c,d,e, 2.17a,b). Ultra-

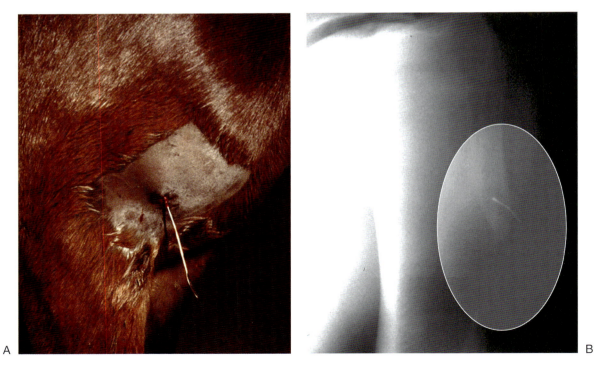

A   B

Figure 2.12. This horse had a history of recurrent drainage from a tract following a puncture wound occurring ~2 months earlier. The wound apparently healed only to break open and drain after antibiotic treatment was discontinued. (A) A sterile probe was used to identify the direction and depth of the draining tract. The probe appeared to contact bone at the depth of the tract. (B) Radiography revealed focal bone lysis of the deltoid tuberosity of the humerus, indicating osteomyelitis (oval).

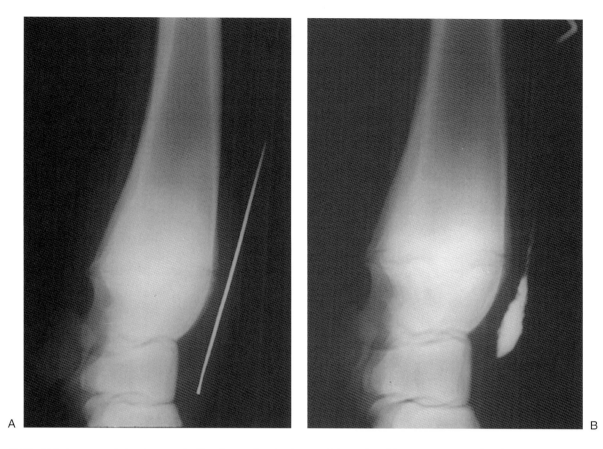

Figure 2.13. This horse sustained a penetrating laceration to the cranial antebrachium, ~15 cm proximal to the antebrachiocarpal joint. Digital palpation was of little value because the hole in the skin was so small. (A) Lateral radiograph with a 20 cm long sterile probe inserted into the wound tract. The radiograph could not rule out the involvement of a carpal joint or an extensor tendon sheath. (B) Contrast study excluded the involvement of a carpal joint or an extensor tendon sheath.

sound is most useful in identifying injury to soft tissue support structures, gas accumulation, and muscle separation, and radiographically unapparent foreign bodies (Figures 2.18a,b).[3]

Arthroscopy or tenoscopy can be valuable in revealing radiographically occult lesions, particularly those involving cartilage, and in identifying foreign bodies within the joint or tendon sheath (e.g., hair, dirt, or other foreign bodies) (Figure 2.19).

Wound Debridement

Wound debridement is a very important component of wound care. Properly implemented, it effectively removes necrotic and ischemic tissues as well as those contaminated with foreign bodies and bacteria. In doing so, debridement creates a new environment which favors blood supply and healing while reducing the risk of infection.[3] Debridement can be accomplished with a scalpel, CO_2 laser, or hydrosurgical unit; with enzymes or chemicals; or with debridement dressings. The discussion that follows will cover the various techniques for wound debridement.

Sharp

The standard approach is sharp debridement, converting a contaminated wound to a clean one. Techniques of sharp debridement include: (1) excisional (layered), (2) en block, (3) simple or piecemeal, and (4) staged. Sharp layered debridement begins with removal of the most superficial tissues and continues deeper into the

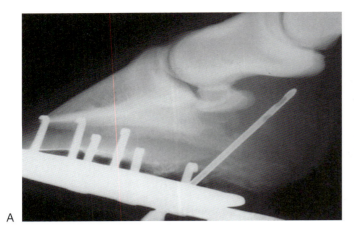

A

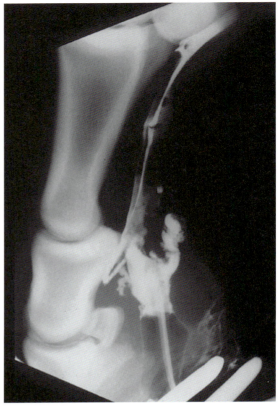

B

Figure 2.14. This horse sustained a penetrating wound to the central one-third of the frog approximately 1 week earlier. The horse was non-weight–bearing at presentation. Examination of the foot revealed a sharp piece of wood embedded in the central sulcus of the frog. Following removal of the wood, a teat cannula was used to identify the depth and direction of the wound tract. (A) Radiograph of a teat cannula in the wound tract. Note the tip close to the proximopalmar border of the middle phalanx, indicating that the digital flexor tendon sheath was likely penetrated. (B) Contrast radiograph identifying involvement of the synovial sheath.

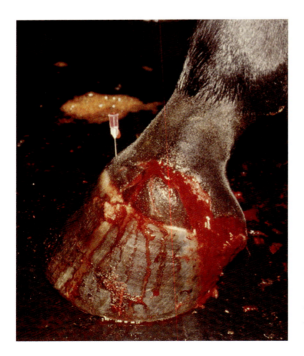

Figure 2.15. A sterile needle has been placed in the distal interphangeal (coffin) joint at a site remote to the wound. Reprinted from Proceedings of the American Association of Equine Practitioners, 52, Stashak TS, Wound infection: Contributing factors and selected techniques for prevention, pp. 270–280, Copyright (2006), with permission from American Association of Equine Practitioners.

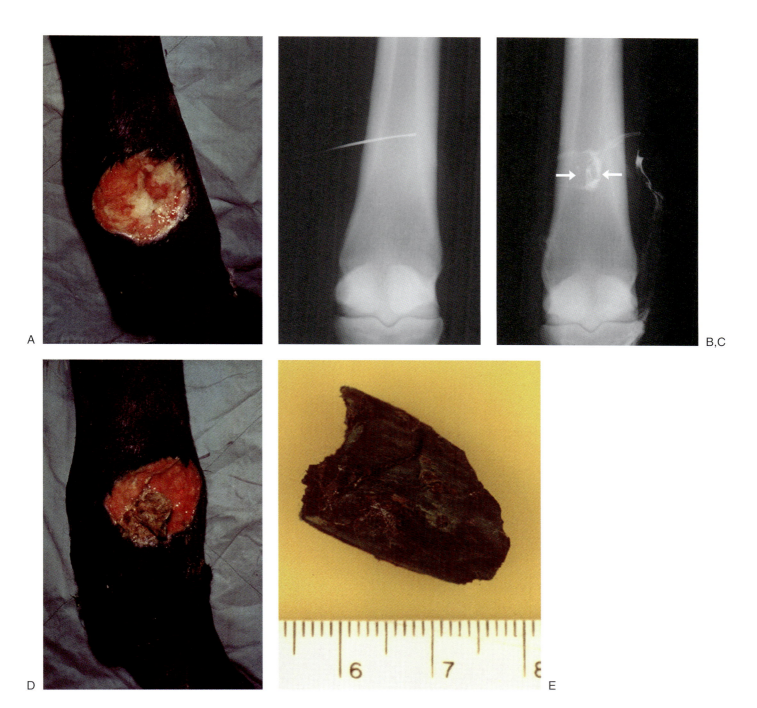

Figure 2.16. This horse sustained a penetrating wound to the lateral surface of the right metatarsal region 1 year earlier. A piece of wood was removed from the initial wound site. Following this, two additional surgeries were performed to determine the cause of continued drainage from the wound site. (A) Wound at presentation. A similar granulating wound was present on the medial side of the limb. (B) A sterile probe was used to explore the wound. (C) Contrast radiography revealed a filling defect (arrows) distal to the wound tract. (D) A piece of wood was removed from a pocket just distal to the tract. (E) The piece of wood.

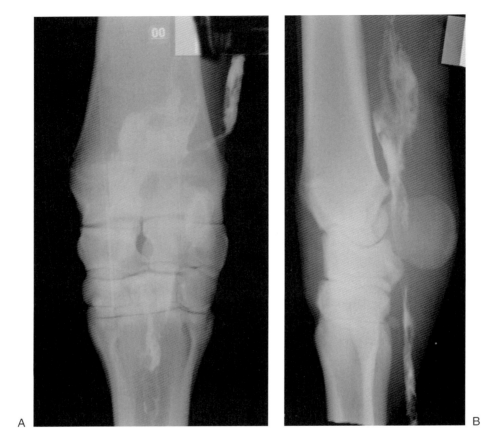

Figure 2.17. This horse sustained a penetrating wound to the lateral aspect of the distal antebrachium 3 weeks earlier. Initial exploration revealed several pieces of wood in the wound, which were subsequently removed. Following debridement and lavage, the wound was sutured and the horse was placed on antibiotic therapy. The horse became non-weight–bearing within 7 days and the wound broke open and drained 10 days postoperatively. The antibiotic regime was changed but no improvement was seen. (A) Craniocaudal contrast radiographic study revealing multiple filling defects (a result of pieces of wood) in the carpal canal. (B) Lateral radiographic view identifying multiple filling defects in the carpal canal.

wound until its depths are reached and all contaminants have been removed (Figures 2.20a,b). En block debridement is used primarily for companion animals, in regions where there is a lot of loose skin. For this reason it will not be addressed in this presentation. Piecemeal debridement is helpful for large wounds, usually involving the body. Beginning at one wound margin and advancing toward the other, all devitalized tissue and foreign material are sharply removed a little at a time (Figure 2.21).

Staged debridement is used over a number of days. The advantage of this approach is that it limits inadvertent removal of viable tissue. Tissue color and attachment are the criteria governing staged surgical debridement. White, tan, black, or green tissue that is poorly attached should be debrided. Pink to dark purple tissue that is well attached should be left in place and debrided later if need be (Figure 2.22).[1] Exposed cortical bone devoid of periosteum should be debrided in an effort to promote the formation of granulation on its surface and reduce the incidence of sequestrum formation (Figure 2.22).

Debridement of bone is best accomplished with a hip arthroplasty rasp (Figures 2.23a,b), but a bone rasp, bone chisel, or osteotome can be used. If exposed bone is debrided to a point at which it oozes a yellow-colored fluid, granulation tissue will soon proliferate from its surface.[3,58] A hydrogel dressing containing acemannan (Carrasorb®, Carrington Laboratories, Irving, TX) can be used to accelerate fibroblast migration and formation of granulation tissue over exposed bone.[59]

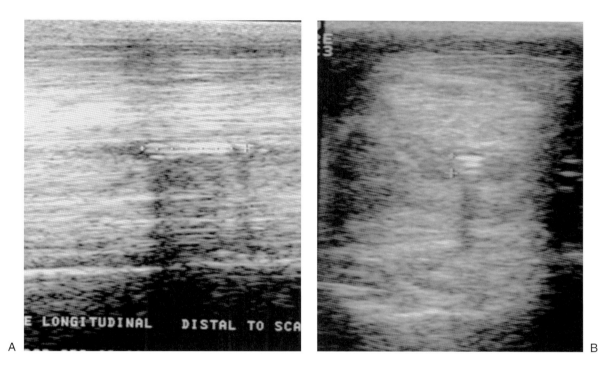

A

B

Figure 2.18. The same horse as in Figure 2.17, illustrating the value of ultrasonography in identifying a piece of wood that was not seen using contrast radiography. (A) Longitudinal ultrasound image, in the mid-metacarpal region, identifying a hyperechoic density (cursor) located at the distal extent of the carpal canal between the carpal check ligament and the deep digital flexor tendon. (B) Transverse ultrasound image of the same; note the hyperechoic density (cursor). Reprinted from Proceedings of the American Association of Equine Practitioners, 52, Stashak TS, Wound infection: Contributing factors and selected techniques for prevention, pp. 270–280, Copyright (2006), with permission from American Association of Equine Practitioners.

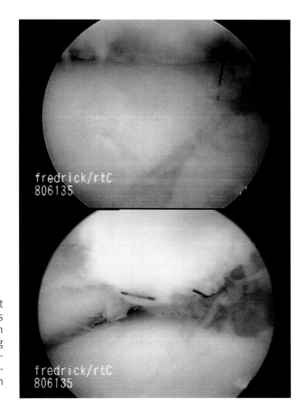

Figure 2.19. Arthroscopic view of the distal interphalangeal (coffin) joint that had sustained a penetrating wound 24 hours earlier. Note the pieces of hair and debris in the joint. These foreign bodies would not have been identified, and it is unlikely they would have been removed by flushing alone without arthroscopic visualization. Reprinted from Clinical Techniques in Equine Practice, 3, Baxter GM, Management of Wounds Involving Synormal Structures In Horses, pp. 204–214, Copyright (2004), with permission from Elsevier, Inc.

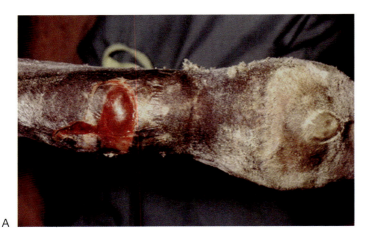
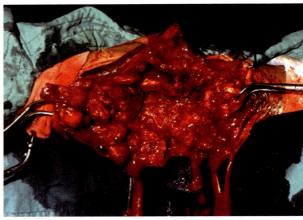

A   B

Figure 2.20. This horse sustained a laceration of the superficial and deep digital flexor tendons 4 days earlier. Treatment included superficial cleansing of the wound, bandage splinting, and the administration of penicillin G and phenylbutazone. (A) The horse under general anesthesia after removal of the splint bandage. (B) Following layered debridement and irrigation. During debridement, dirt and plant awns were found embedded in the wound, the superficial and the deep digital flexor tendons were completely transected, and the suspensory ligament had a superficial laceration.

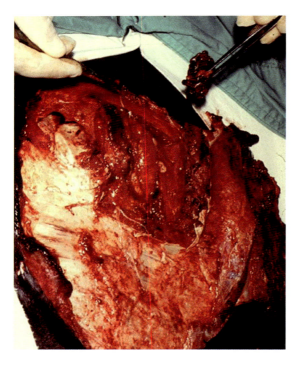

Figure 2.21. Example of piecemeal debridement being used for a large wound in the lateral thoracic region in a horse. Reprinted from Proceedings of the American Association of Equine Practitioners, 52, Stashak TS, Wound infection: Contributing factors and selected techniques for prevention, pp. 270–280, Copyright (2006), with permission from American Association of Equine Practitioners.

CO_2 Laser

A CO_2 laser can replace a steel scalpel, with the advantages that it removes a substantial portion of the bioburden in the wound, facilitates contraction of collagen fibers, photoablates exuberant granulation tissue, reduces postoperative pain, and causes minimal hemorrhage.[60] See Chapter 15 for more information.

Hydrosurgical Debridement

Hydrosurgical debridement can be accomplished with a Versajet™ Hydrosurgery System (Smith & Nephew, Hull, UK). The unit consists of a power console and a reusable handpiece. The console is activated by

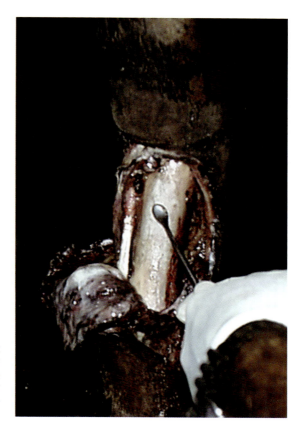

Figure 2.22. Example of a degloving wound in which staged debridement would be recommended. White, tan, black, or green tissue that is poorly attached is debrided. Pink to dark purple tissue that is well attached is left in place and debrided later if need be. The bone that appears chalky white and is devoid of periosteum is also being debrided with a hip arthroplasty rasp.

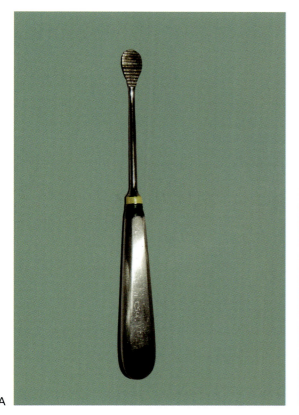

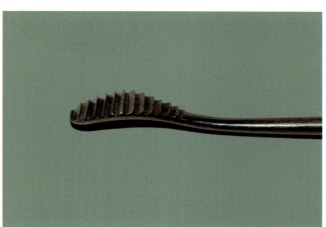

A   B

Figure 2.23. A hip arthroplasty rasp is very effective for debriding the surface of bone stripped of its periosteum. (A) Underside (bottom) view. Note the serrated spatula-shaped head. (B) Side view. Close-up of the head; the curved shape facilitates bone contact. Reprinted from Proceeding of the American Association of Equine Practitioners, 52, Stashak TS, Wound infection: Contributing factors and selected techniques for prevention, pp. 270–280, Copyright (2006), with permission from American Association of Equine Practitioners.

a foot pedal and comes with a sterile bag to hold the irrigant fluid as well as a receptacle to collect the waste effluent (Figure 2.24). The handpiece is available with variable operative window diameters (8 mm and 14 mm) and with a choice of a 15° or 45° angle tip (Figure 2.25).[61]

The system generates a high-velocity stream of sterile saline, which jets out the operative window of the handpiece. This creates a localized Venturi (suction) effect, enabling the surgeon to hold, cut, and remove wound debris and necrotic tissue while irrigating the wound. The handpiece can be oriented in variable positions to achieve the desired effect. When the tip is oriented obliquely to the tissue, wound irrigation and contaminant removal is the primary effect. When the tip is oriented parallel to the tissue, the result is controlled excision with concomitant aspiration. A variable power setting on the console adjusts the speed and depth of debridement. The advantage to this system is that it combines wound irrigation with lavage and selectively removes only nonviable tissue (Figures 2.26a,b).[61]

Proteolytic Enzymes

Proteolytic enzymes can be used to debride the wound's proteineous coagulum and bacterial biofilm which harbor contaminants and bacteria, thus limiting the access of topical antibiotics/antiseptics and systemic antibiotics. Proteolytic enzymes are appropriate when surgical debridement could result in damage to or removal of tissue needed for reconstruction of a wound, as well as for wounds that closely approximate nerves and/or vessels. An in vitro study comparing the effectiveness of different dressings for removing fibrin from blood clots of horses found that dressings containing collagenase and papain/urea were significantly less effective as debriding agents than were saline-soaked gauze or hydrofiber dressings.[62] Nonetheless, some papain/urea–

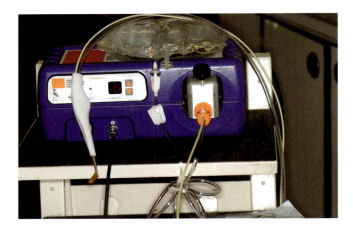

Figure 2.24. Versajet™ Hydrosurgery System power console and reusable handpiece. A sterile bag to hold the irrigant fluid is on top of the console and the receptacle to collect the waste effluent is just out of view at the bottom. Courtesy of Dr. D. Knottenbelt.

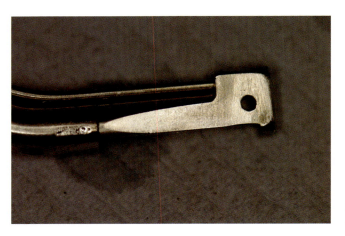

Figure 2.25. Close-up view of the tip of the Versajet™ Hydrosurgery System. Courtesy of Dr. D. Knottenbelt.

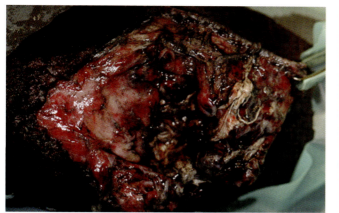
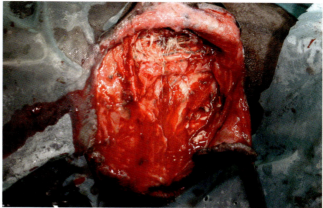

A

B

Figure 2.26. (A) Example of a heavily contaminated wound. (B) The same wound as in (a) following hydrosurgical lavage. Courtesy of Dr. D. Knottenbelt.

based and collagenase preparations have been shown to stimulate angiogenesis and granulation tissue and to accelerate epithelialization, thus they are believed to be effective in stimulating healing of a chronic wound.[63,64]

Enzymatic debridement should be used with caution because bacteremia has been reported in human patients following enzymatic debridement of infected wounds.[65] While the authors did not postulate as to the cause of bacteremia, it is conjectured by this author that the enzymes dissolved the biofilm, freeing the entrapped bacteria to invade the exposed capillaries. For more information regarding enzymatic debridement of wounds, see Chapter 3.

Dressing

Debridement dressings include: (1) adherent open mesh gauze, (2) antimicrobial gauze dressing (Kerlix AMD™ Covidien Animal Health/Kendall, Dublin, OH), (3) hypertonic saline gauze dressing (Curasalt™ Covidien Animal Health/Kendall, Dublin, OH), (4) alginate dressings, and (5) occlusive dressings. Open mesh gauze can be applied either dry or can be wetted (to achieve wet-to-dry debridement). Kerlix AMD™ is an excellent choice for heavily contaminated wounds because it is impregnated with a broad-spectrum antiseptic that has been shown to kill bacteria on the surface of the wound and prevent strike through. Curasalt™ is best used for necrotic, heavily infected exuding wounds. Occlusive dressings promote moist wound healing and "autolytic cellular debridement" and are best used for clean wounds.[66]

An in vitro study comparing the effectiveness of various dressings for debriding fibrin from blood clots of horses found that dressings hydrated with saline were better debriding devices than those hydrated with water because of their greater osmolarity.[62] Gauze and hydrofiber dressings hydrated with saline were significantly (47%) more effective in breaking down protein (primarily fibrin) than were dressings impregnated with collagenase or papain/urea or hydrogel dressing.[62] Dressings reached a plateau in their rate of protein breakdown within 24 hours. Although this study did not consider the in vivo cellular effect on debridement, it did suggest that gauze, hydrofiber, and alginate dressings, wetted with saline, would be most effective in debriding wounds with a proteinaceous coagulum or those that have formed scabs. See Chapter 3 for more information about debridement dressings.

Chemical Debridement

For information regarding chemical debridement of wounds, see Topical Wound Treatments and Wound Care Products in Chapter 3.

Biosurgical Debridement

For information regarding biosurgical debridement (maggot therapy) of wounds, see Wound repair: Problems in the Horse and Innovative Solutions in Chapter 1.

Antibiotics

The ultimate aim of antibiotic therapy is to inflict insult upon infecting bacteria sufficient to kill the organism or render it susceptible to inactivation by natural host defenses. Where an "educated guess" approach is often used to design an antimicrobial regime in a non-infected wound, culture and sensitivity should direct the antimicrobial selection when dealing with an infected wound.

Systemic Administration

In a surgically created wound, antibiotics are generally not needed if the patient is in good health and has an adequate immune status, and if the surgery lasts <1 hour and is performed in a clean environment. Antibiotics are generally recommended in any situation where there is vascular compromise, an enterotomy is performed, or the surgery is expected to exceed 60 minutes.[3,10] Administration of perioperative antibiotics is usually initiated <2 hours before surgery and continued for 24 hours.

A study evaluating infection rates (IR) in 1,573 clean wounds found a 4.4% IR in patients not given perioperative antibiotics, a 2.2% IR in patients receiving perioperative antibiotics <2 hours before surgery out to 24 hours (control antibiotic protocol), a 6.3% IR in patients receiving antibiotic >2 before surgery and for longer than 24 hours after surgery, and an 8.2% IR in patients given antibiotics after surgery only.[9] Although the reasons for the increased IR in patients given antibiotics outside the protocol (6.3%) or only after surgery (8.2%) were not discussed, it is conjectured by this author that administering antibiotics for longer than 24 hours postoperatively may have been selected for bacteria resistant to the antibiotic in use. Supporting this hypothesis is the work done by Dunowska (2006), who found that administering antibiotics for 3 days allowed for selection of resistant bacteria, not only in treated horses but also in other hospitalized patients.[67] Administering the antibiotic after surgery may have allowed bacteria trapped in the fibrin clot within the wound to proliferate while those bacteria not contained in the clot would be killed.

A study performed on 136,231 human patients undergoing orthopedic surgical procedures supports the use of short-term perioperative antibiotics. The study found that the incidence of surgical site infection was not decreased by extending the chemoprophylaxis for >24 hours after surgery. Infection rates were further reduced from 2.5% to 1.4% by using a combination antibiotic therapy.[68]

The decision whether to administer antibiotics is straightforward for the traumatic wound; the selection depends on type and location of the wound. If systemic administration is selected, the intravenous (IV) route is preferred initially because the effect is predictable. Intramuscular (IM) absorption is prolonged and variable and depends on site selection and the expected amount of exercise. For example, less absorption would be expected if the IM injection were made in the caudal thigh muscle in a horse that was reluctant to move. Oral administration is often used once adequate blood levels have been achieved.

For superficial wounds, penicillin alone or in combination with trimethoprim sulfa is usually effective. Deeper wounds, including those involving synovial cavities, are usually best treated with penicillin or cefazolin with an aminoglycoside such as gentamicin or amikacin; the combination appears synergistic. Ceftiofur or enrofloxacin are generally reserved for infections caused by bacteria that are resistant to penicillin and aminoglycosides. Enrofloxacin is not recommended for foals because it can result in a rapid onset of noninflammatory arthropathy in immature animals.[69] For deep fascial cellulitis/septic myositis due to Clostridia or pyonecrotic processes, high doses of penicillin (penicillin G or ampicillin) with metronidazole are recommended.

A minimum course of 3 to 5 days of antibiotic therapy is generally recommended in contaminated wounds without signs of infection. 7 to 10 days is usually the minimum duration for wounds with an established soft tissue infection. In cases of established synovial cavity infection, 10–21 days is recommended, while established bone infection will require antibiotic therapy lasting 3 to 6 months. Although antibiotics are important in the prevention and treatment of infections, wounds contaminated with 10^9 micro-organism/g of tissue will develop infection despite an appropriate antibiotic regimen.[6]

For a more complete discussion of the use of systemic antibiotics, including selection, dosage, route of administration, and duration of treatment, see Chapters 9 and 12.

Topical Application

The application of topical antibiotics remains somewhat controversial. Application <3 hours after wounding is generally accepted as the best, though it is unlikely to occur in many cases. However, if the wound is thoroughly debrided, a new wound is created; therefore, the topical application of an antimicrobial is appropriate following debridement.[3] In a double-blind study on 260 sutured lacerations in humans, penicillin sprayed on the wound before closure prevented three out of four infections.[45]

The vehicle carrying the antibiotic is also an important consideration. A study evaluating the effect of gentamicin cream versus gentamicin solution on wound healing found the latter to enhance contraction and epithelialization.[70] The antibiotic itself has been shown to exert an effect on wound healing. For example, Neosporin has been shown to increase epithelialization by 25%; in this case it is the combination of antibiotics contained in Neosporin rather than the vehicle that accelerates wound healing.[71] Silvadine has been shown to increase healing by 25% in laboratory animals; however, this same effect was not found in horses.[72] Furacin ointment applied to a wound under a bandage has been shown to significantly decrease the rate of wound contraction in horses.[25] The antibiotic furacin appears to be the cause of delayed healing in laboratory animals.[71]

Finally, solutions are best used in wounds that are to be sutured; they are usually delivered prior to wound closure. Ointments or creams are best used for bandaged open wounds.[3]

Anti-inflammatory Drugs

Nonsteroidal Anti-Inflammatory Drugs (NSAIDs)

Inhibition of either cyclooxygenase (COX)-1 (constitutive) or COX-2 (induced by lipopolysaccharide, nitric oxide, and various cytokines) is the basis for the mechanism of action of NSAIDs. Cell membrane phospholipid-derived arachidonic acid generates various eicosanoids, which mediate inflammation and induce fibroblast proliferation and collagen production. While COX-1 is responsible for the production of prostaglandins involved in normal physiologic function, COX-2 is found in all stages of the inflammatory response and its up-regulation is believed to be accountable for persistent inflammation and many of the cytotoxic effects of inflammation.[73]

That said, inflammation is beneficial in that it protects the wound against infection and is a necessary precursor to the subsequent events leading to the proliferative phase of repair. Accordingly, it is not surprising that controversy surrounds the use of NSAIDs in the early phase of healing, when the normal inflammatory response should not be inhibited. For example, high doses of NSAIDs administered immediately following incision of the linea alba in ponies delayed repair,[74] while suppression of inflammation by COX-2 inhibition reduced the extent of granulation/scar tissue without compromising tensile properties of mouse wounds.[75] Although it is thought that NSAIDs have little effect on the ultimate course or quality of repair, when administered at pharmacological doses, it may be that selective anti-inflammatory agents, such as COX-2 inhibitors, can be fine-tuned to suppress the imbalances of inflammation and consequently lead to a more ideal healing response.

In contrast, chronic inflammation is characterized by excessive and persistent neutrophil and macrophage activity and may forestall the normal repair sequence, leading to a number of diseases typified by disproportionate scarring. In these cases, NSAIDs, in particular COX-2 selective inhibitors, may be effective in the prevention of excessive scarring.[76]

Corticosteroids

Topical and systemic administration of corticosteroids appear to retard wound repair, depending on the specific glucocorticoid used and the timing, concentration, and duration of therapy.[77] Cortisone stabilizes lysosomal membranes and consequently inhibits the normal inflammatory response to trauma. This leads to a delay in repair, although ultimate wound strength does not seem affected. Other mechanisms whereby glucocorticoids may alter various phases of repair include angiostasis,[78] decreased rate of fibroblast proliferation with consequent inhibition of protein synthesis, possible down-regulation of fibrogenic TGF-β[79], and inhibition of keratinocyte growth factor (KGF) production within fibroblasts, which may impair epithelialization.[80]

Traumatic wounds involving the distal extremity of horses appear predisposed to an excessive fibroblastic response, leading to the development of exuberant granulation tissue. Because corticosteroids limit proliferation of both fibroblasts and endothelial cells, topical application may be beneficial in this particular situation. Results from a controlled trial and a clinical report indicate a positive effect following the topical application of glucocorticoids in the management of exuberant granulation tissue in the distal limbs of horses.[81,82] Generally, one application at the first sign of excessive fibroplasia is often all that is needed, since continued application may exert negative effects on wound contraction and epithelialization.

Conclusion

The therapeutic goal of wound management should be to prevent infection, heal the wound, and rapidly return the horse to normal function, while achieving a cosmetic outcome. Selection of the treatment is based on a number of interrelated factors: duration since injury, location, depth and configuration of the wound, degree of contamination and severity, and nature of the trauma. Other factors influencing management design include economics, patient temperament, physical status, and intended use of the horse. Strict guidelines dictating whether a wound may be sutured primarily do not exist; such a decision can only be rendered following a thorough evaluation of the patient and the wound. For information regarding approaches to wound closure, see Chapter 4.

References

1. Wilson DA: Principles of early wound management. Vet Clin Equine Pract 2005;21:45
2. Stashak TS: Selected factors that affect wound healing. In T Stashak ed. *Equine wound management (1st edition)*. Philadelphia: Lea and Febiger, 1991, p.19
3. Stashak TS: Current concepts in wound management in horses: parts 1-III. Proc North Am Vet Conf 2003;17:231
4. Noyes H, Chi N, Linah L, et al: Delayed topical antimicrobials as adjuncts to systemic antibiotic therapy of war wounds: bacteriologic studies. Mil Med 1967;132:461
5. Robson M, Heggers J: Bacterial quantification of open wounds. Mil Med 1969;134:19
6. Edlich RF, Rodeheaver GT, Morgan RF, et al: Principles of emergency wound management. Ann Emerg Med 1988;17:1284
7. Rodeheaver GT: Wound cleansing, wound irrigation, wound disinfection. In: D Krasner, G Rodeheaver, and G Sibbald, ed. *Chronic wound care (3rd edition)*. Wayne PA: HMP Communications, 2001, p.389
8. Brown DC, Conzemius MG, Shofer FS, et al: Epidemiologic evaluation of postoperative wound infections in dogs and cats. J Am Vet Med Assoc 1997;210:1302
9. Nicholson M, Beal M, Shofer F, et al: Epidemiologic evaluation of postoperative wound infection in clean contaminated wounds: a retrospective study of 239 dogs and cats. Vet Surg 2002;31:577
10. Beal MW, Brown CB, Shofer FS: The effects of perioperative hypothermia and the duration of anesthesia on postoperative wound infection rate in clean wounds: a retrospective study. Vet Surg 2000;29:123
11. Kotani N, Hashimoto H, Sessler DI, et al: Intraoperative modulation of alveolar macrophage function during isoflurane and propofol anesthesia. Anesthesiol 1998;89:1125
12. Ciepichal J, Kubler A: Effect of general and regional anesthesia on some neutrophil functions. Arch Immunol Ther Exp 1998;46:183
13. Heldman E, Brown DC, Shofer F: The effect of propofol usage with postoperative wound infection rate in clean wounds: a retrospective study. Vet Surg 1999;28:256
14. Smeak DD, Olmstead ML: Infections in clean wounds: the roles of the surgeon, environment, and host. Cont Ed 1984;6:629
15. Cruse PJ, Foord R: The epidemiology of wound infections: a 10-year prospective study of 62,939 wounds. Symposium on surgical infections. Surg Clin of North Am 1980;60:27
16. Borg T, Modig J: Potential anti-thrombotic effects of local anesthetics due to their inhibition of platelet aggregation. Acta Anaesthesiol Scand 1985;29:739
17. Grant GJ, Ramanathan S, Patel N, et al: The effects of local anesthetics on maternal and neonatal platelet function. Acta Anaesthesiol Scand 1989:33:409
18. Berntsen RF, Simonsen T, Sager G, et al: Therapeutic lidocaine concentrations have no effect on blood platelet function and plasma catecholamine levels. Eur J Clin Pharmacol 1992;43:109
19. Az-ma T, Hardian, Yuge O: Inhibitory effect of lidocaine on cultured porcine aortic endothelial cell-dependent antiaggregation of platelets. Anesthesiol 1995;83:374–381
20. Drucker M, Cardenas E, Ariziti P, et al: Experimental studies on the effect of lidocaine on wound healing. World J Surg 1988;22:394
21. Vasseur PB, Paul HA, Dybdal N, et al: Effects of local anesthetics on healing of abdominal wounds in rabbits. Am J Vet Res 1984;45:2385
22. Ritchie JM, Cohen PJ: Local anesthetics. In L Goodman and A Gillman, ed. *The pharmacological basis of therapeutics (5th edition)*. New York, MacMillan, 1975, p.393

23. Hamilton HW, Hamilton KR, Lone FH: Preoperative hair removal. Can J Surg 1977;20:269
24. Stashak TS: Wound Infection: contributing factors and selected techniques for prevention. Proc Am Assoc Equine Pract 2006;52:270
25. Woollen N, Debowes, RM, Leipold HW, et al: A comparison of four types of therapy for the treatment of full thickness skin wounds of the horse. Proc Am Assoc Equine Pact 1987;33:569
26. Madden J, Edlich RF, Schauerhamer R, et al: Application of principles of fluid dynamics to surgical wound irrigation. Curr Topic Surg Res 1971;3:85
27. Rodeheaver GT, Pettry D, Thacker JG, et al: Wound cleansing by high pressure irrigation. Surg Gynecol Obstet 1975;141:357
28. Grower MF, Bhaskar SN, Horan MJ, et al: Effect of water lavage on removal of tissue fragments from crush wounds. Oral Surg Oral Med Oral Pathol 1972;33:1031
29. Wheeler CB, Rodeheaver GT, Thacker JG, et al: Side effects of high pressure irrigation. Surg Gynecol Obstet 1976;43:775
30. Carlson HC, Briggs RL, Green VA, et al: Effect of pressure and tip modification on the dispersion of fluid throughout cells, and tissues during the irrigation of experimental wounds. Oral Surg Oral Med Oral Pathol 1971;32:347
31. Foresman PA, Etheridge CA, Thacker JG, et al: Influence of a pulsatile irrigation system on bacterial removal from and tissue injury to contaminated wounds (unpublished research report) Charlottesville, VA: University of Virginia Health Sciences Center 1989
32. Stevenson TR, Thacker JG, Rodeheaver GT, et al: Cleansing the traumatic wound by high pressure syringe irrigation. J Am Coll Emerg Phys 1976;5:17
33. Longmire AW, Broom LA, Bursh J: Wound infection following high pressure syringe and needle irrigation. Am J Emerg Med 1987;5:179
34. Baxter G: Management of wounds involving synovial structure in horses. Clin Tech Equine Pract 2004;3:204
35. Viljanto J: Disinfection of surgical wounds without inhibition of normal wound healing. Arch Surg 1980;115:253
36. Grey JG, Lee JR. The effect of topical povidone iodine on wound infection following abdominal surgery. Br J Surg 1981;68:310
37. Mulliken JB, Nancey A, Healey BS, et al: Povidone-iodine and tensile strength of wounds in rats. J Trauma 1980;20:323
38. Sanchez IR, Swaim SF, Nusbaum KE, et al: Effects of chlorhexidine diacetate and povidone iodine on wound healing in dogs. Vet Surg 1988;17:291
39. Amber EI, Henderson RA, Swaim SF, et al: A comparison of antimicrobial efficacy and tissue reaction of four antiseptics on canine wounds. Vet Surg 1983;12:63
40. Berkelman RL, Holland BW, Anderson RL: Increased bactericidal activity of dilute preparations of povidone-iodine solution. J Clin Microbiol 1982;15:635
41. Lee AH, Swaim SF, McGuire JA, et al: Effects of chlorhexidine diacetate, povidone iodine and polydroxydine on wound healing in dogs. J Am Anim Hosp Assoc 1988;24:77
42. Bhandari M, Anthony D, Schemitsch EH: The efficacy of low-pressure lavage with different irrigating solutions to remove adherent bacteria from bone. J Bone Joint Surg 2001;83:412
43. Cutright DE, Bhaskar SN, Gross A, et al: Effect of vancomycin, streptomycin and tetracycline pulsating jet lavage on contaminated wounds. Military Med 1971;136:810
44. Singleton AO, Julian J: An experimental evaluation of methods used to prevent infection in wounds which have been contaminated with feces. Ann Surg 1960;151:912
45. Lindsey D, Nava C, Marti M: Effectiveness of penicillin irrigation in control of infection in sutured lacerations. J Trauma 1982;22:186
46. Wright RW, Orr R: Fibroblast cytotoxicity and blood cell integrity following exposure to dermal wound cleansers. Ost Wound Manag 1993;39:33
47. Forseman PA, Payne DS, Becker D, et al: A relative toxicity index for wound cleansers. Wounds 1993;5:226
48. Tizard I, Busbee D, Maxwell B, Kemp MC: Effects of Acemannan, a complex carbohydrate, on wound healing in young and aged rats. Wounds 1994;6:201
49. Rodeheaver GT, Smith SL, Thacker JG, et al: Mechanical cleansing of contaminated wounds with a surfactant. Am J Surg 1975;129:341–245
50. Lemarie RJ, Hosgood G: Antiseptics and disinfectants in small animal practice. Compend Contin Educ 1995;17:1339
51. Onsuna DJ, DeYoung DJ, Walker RW: Comparison of three preoperative skin preparation techniques part 2: clinical trial in 100 canine patients. Vet Surg 1990;19:20
52. Hamill MB, Osato MS, Wilhelmus KR: Experimental evaluation of chlorhexidine gluconate for ocular antisepsis. Antimicrobial Agents Chemother 1984;26:793
53. Phinney RB, Mondino BJ, Hofbauer JD, et al: Corneal edema related to accidental Hibiclens exposure. Am J Ophthalmol 1988;106:210

54. Nasser RE: The ocular danger of Hibiclens (chlorhexidine). Plast Reconstr Surg 1992;89:164
55. Selwyn S, Ellis H: Skin bacteria and skin disinfection reconsidered. Br Med J 1972;1:136
56. Larson EL, Aiello AE, Heilman JM, et al: Comparison of different regimens for surgical hand preparation. Assn Op Reg Nurs J 2001;73:412
57. Larson EL, Butz Am, Gullette DL, et al: Alcohol for surgical scrubbing? Infect Control Hosp Epidemiol 1990;11:139
58. Lee MJ, Fretz PB, Bailey JV, Jacobs KA: Factors influencing wound healing: lessons from military wound management. Comp Cont Ed 1989;7:850
59. Swaim SF: Personal communication. 2007
60. Sullins KE: Lasers and wound healing: practical uses. Clin Tech Equine Pract 2004;3:182
61. Knottenbelt DC: The value of hydrosurgical debridement in management of contaminated wounds. Proc North Am Vet Conf, 2007;21:133
62. Pain R, Sneddon JC, Cochrane CA: In vitro study of the effectiveness of different dressings for debriding fibrin in blood clots from horses. Vet Record 2006;159:712
63. Raffetto JD, Mendez MV, Marien BJ: Changes in cellular motility and cytoskeletal actin in fibroblasts from patients with chronic venous insufficiency and neonatal fibroblasts in the presence of chronic wound fluids. J Vasc Surg 2001;33:233
64. Herman I: Stimulation of human keratinocyte migration and proliferation in vitro: insights into the cellular responses to injury and wound healing. Wounds 1996;8:33
65. Hummel RP, Kautz PD, MacMillan BG, et al: The continuing problem of sepsis following enzymatic debridement of burns. J Trauma 1974;14:572
66. Stashak TS: Update on wound dressings: indications and best use. Clin Tech Equine Pract 2004;3:148
67. Dunowska M, Morley PS, Traub-Dargatz JL, Hyatt DR, Dargatz DA: Impact of hospitalization and antimicrobial drug use on antimicrobial susceptibility patterns of commensal Escherichia coli isolated from the feces of horses. J Am Vet Med Assoc 2006;228:1909
68. Mini E, Grassi F, Cherubino P, et al: Preliminary results of a survey of the use of antimicrobial agents as prophylaxis in orthopedic surgery. J Chemother 2001;1:73
69. Specht TE, Frederick G: Quinolone-induced arthropathy in immature equidae. J Am Vet Assoc 1991;198:516
70. Lee AH, Swaim SF, Yang ST, et al: Effects of gentamicin solution and cream on the healing of open wounds. Am J Vet Res 1984;45:1487
71. Geronemus RG, Mertz PM, Eaglstein WH: Wound healing: the effects for topical antimicrobial agents. Arch Dermatol 1979;115:1311
72. Berry DB, Sullins KE: Effects of topical application of antimicrobials and bandaging on healing and granulation tissue formation in wounds of the distal aspect of the limbs in horses. Am J Vet Res 2003;64:88
73. Abd-El-Aleem SA, Ferguson MWJ, Appleton I, et al: Expression of cyclooxygenase isoforms in normal human skin and chronic venous ulcers. J Pathol 2001;195:616
74. Schneiter HL, McClure JR, Cho DY, et al: The effects of flunixin meglumine on early wound healing of abdominal incisions in ponies. Vet Surg 1987;16:101 (abstr)
75. Wilgus TA, Vodovotz Y, Vittadini E, et al: Reduction of scar formation in full-thickness wounds with topical celecoxib treatment. Wound Repair Regen 2003;11:25
76. Theoret C: Wound repair. In Jorg Auer and John Stick eds. Equine surgery (3rd edition). Philadelphia: Saunders/Elsevier, 2006, p.44
77. Marks JG Jr, Cano C, Leitzel K, et al: Inhibition of wound healing by topical steroids. Dermatol Surg Oncol 1983;9:819
78. Hashimoto I, Nakanishi H, Shono Y, et al: Angiostatic effects of corticosteroid on wound healing of the rabbit ear. J Med Invest 2002;49:61
79. Beck LS, Deguzman L, Lee WP, et al: TGF-beta 1 accelerates wound healing: reversal of steroid-impaired healing in rats and rabbits. Growth Factors 1991;5:295
80. Chedid M, Hoyle JR, Csaky KG, et al: Glucocorticoids inhibit keratinocyte growth factor production in primary dermal fibroblasts, Endocrinol 1996;137:2232
81. Barber SM: Second intention wound healing in the horse: the effect of bandages and topical corticosteroids. Proc Am Assoc Equine Pract 1989;35:107
82. Blackford JT, Blackford LW, Adair HS: The use of antimicrobial glucocorticosteroid ointment on granulating lower leg wounds in horses. Proc Am Assoc Equine Pract 1991;37:71

3 | Topical Wound Treatments

3.1 Update on Wound Dressings: Indications and Best Use

Ted S. Stashak, DVM, MS, Diplomate ACVS, **and Ellis Farstvedt,** DVM, MS, Diplomate ACVS

Introduction

A wide variety of wound dressings ranging from passive adherent/non-adherent to interactive and bioactive products that contribute to the healing process currently are commercially available.[1] Many newer dressings are designed to create a moist environment which allows wound fluids and growth factors to remain in contact with the wound, thus promoting autolytic debridement and accelerating wound healing. Some dressings contain antimicrobials/antiseptics which are released locally to suppress bacterial growth. Nonetheless, even with substantial advancements in wound dressings it appears that no single material can produce the optimum microenvironment for all wounds or for all stages of the healing process.[2] Consequently, the selection of a wound dressing should be dictated by a precise understanding of the stages of wound healing as well as the condition, location, and depth of the wound.

The purpose of this chapter is to review dressings currently available and their physical characteristics and to describe their best uses as they relate to the condition (clean, contaminated, or infected), location, and depth of the wound and the stage of wound healing. Refer to Table 3.1 for the manufacturer of the various dressings and a summary of their proposed best uses.

Table 3.1. Selected dressings, manufacturers, proposed best uses, and indications.

Dressing	Manufacturer	Proposed best uses and indications
Alginates		
Calcium	Curasorb®, Covidien Animal Health/Kendall, Dublin, OH C-Stat®, R.S. Jackson Inc., Alexandria, VA Nu-Derm®, Johnson and Johnson Products Inc., New Brunswick, NJ Kaltostat®, Convatec ER Squibb and Sons, LLC, Princeton, NJ AlgiSite®, Smith & Nephew, Hull, UK	For moderate to heavily exudative wounds during transition from inflammatory to repair phases of healing. For wounds with substantial tissue loss (e.g., degloving wounds). Traps bacteria in the dressing.
Zinc	Curasorb ZN®, Covidien Animal Health/Kendall, Dublin, OH	Hemostasis: packing sinuses, fistulae, and bleeding tooth sockets
Acemannan	EquineGinate™, Carrington Labs, Irving, TX	May activate macrophages in chronic wounds. Promotes granulation tissue growth over exposed bone.[20]
Activated charcoal	Activate®, 3M Animal Care Products, St. Paul, MN Actisorb®, Johnson and Johnson Products Inc, New Brunswick, NJ CarboFlex™ and Lyofoam®, Convatec, a division of ER Squibb and Sons, Princeton NJ	For heavily infected wounds during inflammatory to repair phase. Absorbs bacteria and reduces odor.
Antimicrobial gauze	Kerlix® Antimicrobial Dressing, Covidien Animal Health/Kendall, Dublin, OH	Inflammatory phase of healing. For wounds with an increased concentration of bacteria. For wounds with an open synovial cavity.
Chitin	N/A	Not used routinely.
Collagens		
Gel	Collasate®, PRN Pharmacal, Pensacola, FL	Not recommended at this time.
Membrane	Collamend™ Veterinary Products Laboratory, Phoenix, AZ Skin Temp® biosynthetic skin dressing, BioCore Inc., Topeka, KS	Not recommended at this time.
Regenerated cellulose	Promogran®, Johnson and Johnson Medical Products, Markham, Canada	Decreases activity of key metalloproteinases.[75] Binds growth factors, making them available for continued healing in chronic wounds.[38]
Powder	HyCure®, Hymed Group Corporation, Bethlehem, PA	No controlled trials. The company boasts accelerated healing.
Antibiotic-impregnated collagen sponge	Collatamp G®, Schering Plough, Kenilworth, NJ	Slow release of gentamicin. Prevents and treats infection.
Equine amnion	N/A	For clean wounds of the distal extremities. Following excision of exuberant granulation tissue. Suppresses formation of exuberant granulation tissue. Accelerates epithelialization.
Equine peritoneum	N/A	Wounds of distal extremities?

Table 3.1. *Continued*

Dressing	Manufacturer	Proposed best uses and indications
Extracellular matrix		
Porcine origin: urinary bladder	ACell Vet®, Inc., Jessup, MD	For large, avulsive wounds of the distal extremities. Results in constructive remodeling.
Porcine origin: small intestine	Vet BioSISt®, Cook Veterinary Products, Bloomington, IN	
Synthetic: contains HA and GAG	EquitrX™, SentrX Animal Care, Inc., Salt Lake City, UT	The company boasts accelerated scar-free healing of skin wounds in horses.
Gauze dressing	Steri-pad™ and Mirasorb™, Johnson and Johnson Products Inc., New Brunswick, NJ Curity™, Covidien Animal Health/Kendall, Dublin, OH	Debrides heavily contaminated, exudative, and necrotic wounds. Applied dry when wound fluids are low-viscosity. Moistened (sterile salt solution ± diluted antiseptic) if wound fluids are high-viscosity and/or the wound surface is dry with scabs.
Hydrocolloid	Duoderm®, ER Squibb and Sons, Princeton, NJ Dermaheal®, Solvay Animal Health, Mendota Heights, MN Comfeel®, Coloplast, Marietta, GA Nu-Derm®, Johnson and Johnson Products Inc., New Brunswick, NJ	For clean wounds. Early inflammatory phase until granulation tissue fills wound in early repair phase. Promotes granulation tissue formation over bone and frayed tendons.[28] Infection may develop under the dressing; if it does, discontinue its use.
Hydrogels		
Sheet non-adhesive	Tegagel dressing™, 3M Center, St. Paul, MN Nu-gel®, Johnson and Johnson Products Inc., New Brunswick, NJ Curagel® and Curafil®, Covidien Animal Health/Kendall, Dublin, OH TrasiGel® and SoloSite®, Smith & Nephew, Hull, UK	For clean, acute, or recently debrided wounds during inflammatory phase. Hydrate dry wounds. Discontinue when granulation tissue fills the wound.
Sheet adhesive	ThinSite®, Tansorbent® , ClearSite®, ConMed®, and AquaSorb®, Wound Care Shop, Indianapolis, IN	For clean, acute, or recently debrided wounds during inflammatory phase. Discontinue when granulation tissue fills the wound. Advantage: sticks to the skin adjacent to the wound.
Containing acemannan	CarraFilm™, CarraGauze™, CarraVet™ Gel, CarraVET® spray-on gel, and EquineVet™ smart gel, Carrington Laboratories, Inc., Irving, TX	Stimulates granulation tissue formation over exposed bone.[21]
Containing HA and chondroitin sulfate	Tegaderm™, 3M Center, St. Paul, MN	Increases epithelialization and granulation tissue formation.
Containing propylene glycol	Solugel®, Johnson and Johnson Medical, North Ryde, Australia	Not clearly defined as yet.
Gauze-impregnated	FasCure®, Ken Vet, Greeley, CO Curafil®, Covidien Animal Health/Kendall, Dublin, OH Aquagauze™, DRoyal, Powell, TN MPM Gel Pad™, MPM Medical, Inc., Irving, TX	Particularly useful in tunneled and undermined wounds because the dressing is able to fill in the dead space and enhance drainage.

Table 3.1. *Continued*

Dressing	Manufacturer	Proposed best uses and indications
Amorphous	Curasol™, Healthpoint, Fort Worth, TX Iamin®, ProCyte, Redmond, WA Hydroactive Gel®, ConcaTec, Princeton, NJ	Can be used to fill a deep wound with irregular contours. Held in place with a secondary dressing that is generally changed daily.
Containing ketanserin	Vulketan gel®, Janssen Animal Health, Toronto, Canada	Prevents exuberant granulation tissue formation and infection in distal limb wounds.[38,39] Best used during the inflammatory and repair phases of healing.
Hypertonic saline	Cursalt™, Covidien Animal Health/Kendall, Dublin, OH	For infected, necrotic, heavily exuding wounds during the inflammatory phase of healing. Only use for the first few days because of nonselective debridement.
Iodine-containing		
Cadexomer iodine (0.9%)—sustained release	Iodosord®, Smith & Nephew, Hull, UK Iodoflex®, Smith & Nephew, Hull, UK	For contaminated wounds early in inflammatory phase. Starch matrix provides good absorption of exudate and allows slow release of iodine. Dressing changes color from brown to white as the iodine is used up.
Povidone iodine (1%) powder	PRN® Wound Dressing, PRN Pharmacal, Pensacola, FL	For contaminated wounds early in inflammatory phase.
Hydrogel	Biozide®, Performance Products Inc., http/www.mwivet.com Oxyzyme™ Wound Dressing, Insense Ltd., UK	For contaminated wounds early in the inflammatory phase Delivers iodine (0.04%) and oxygen to the wound. Not recommended at this time because it is applied without a secondary dressing.
Liquid adhesive		
Butyl cyanoacrylate	Nexaband®, Abbott Laboratories, Abbott Park, IL	Provides protective barrier for small (<10 cm in diameter), clean limb wounds for the entire healing period.[83]
Hydroxyethylated amylopectin	Facilatator®, IDEXX Laboratories, Greensboro, NC	Provides protective barrier for small (<10 cm in diameter), clean limb wounds for the entire healing period. Can be rinsed off.
Maltodextrin	Intracell®, Macleod Pharmaceuticals, Inc., Fort Collins, CO	Debridement powder: for exudating wounds. Gel: for drier wounds. Cleanses and promotes healing in contaminated/infected wounds. Yields glucose to promote healing. Chemotactic to white blood cells.
Particulate dextranomer		
Bead	Debrisan®, Johnson and Johnson Products Inc., New Brunswick, NJ	For debriding sloughing, exuding wounds. Discontinue when a healthy bed of granulation tissue develops.
Flake	Avalon®, Summit Hill Laboratories, Avalon, NJ	Contraindicated for dry wound beds.
Powder	Intrasite®, Smith & Nephew, Hull, UK	The wound bed should be rinsed at bandage change to prevent granuloma formation.

Table 3.1. *Continued*

Dressing	Manufacturer	Proposed best uses and indications
Non-adherent cotton	Gamgee™, 3M Animal Care Products, St. Paul, MN	Non-adherent dressing for highly exudative limb wounds during inflammatory phase of healing.
Omentum	N/A: autogenous source	Limited
Platelet-rich plasma		
Autologous preparation	Harvest Technologies Corp, Grissom Road, Plymouth, MA Magellan™ autologous platelet separator, Medtronic Biologic Therapeutics and Diagnostics, Minneapolis MN Regen PRP-Kit, RegenLab, Mollens, Switzerland	Contains many growth factors. Stimulates healing. Advantages: less hemorrhage at the surgical site and enhanced fibroblastic in-growth in the early phases of wound healing.
Homologous source	Lacerum-A™, PRP Technologies, Roanoke, IN	Contains many growth factors. Stimulates healing of difficult wounds.[85]
	Lacerum™, PRP Technologies, Roanoke, IN	Used for pregnant mares.
Polyurethane semi-occlusive		
Film	Op-Site®, Smith & Nephew, Hull, UK Tegaderm®, 3M Center, St. Paul, MN Bioclusive®, Johnson and Johnson Products Inc., New Brunswick, NJ	Repair phase; however, can be used for all phases if the wound is free of infection/clean.
Foam	Hydrosorb®, Ken Vet, Greeley, CO Hydrosorb® Wound Care Products, Avitar Inc., Canton, MA Sof-Foam®, Johnson and Johnson Products Inc., New Brunswick, NJ	Not routinely used
Sponge	Tielle® hydropolymer adhesive, Johnson and Johnson Products Inc., New Brunswick, NJ	Early in inflammatory phase in exudative wounds. Used to deliver liquid medicants and wetting agents. Dressing is changed daily. Also used during the repair phase.
Poultice pad	Animalintex® Poultice and Hoof Pad, 3M Animal Care Products, St. Paul, MN	Apply wetted-hot for infected hoof wounds. Apply wetted-cold as a poultice.
Protein-free dialysate of calf blood	Solcoseryl®, Solco Basle Ltd., Birsfelden, Switzerland	For deep wounds during early inflammatory phase. Discontinue at the first signs of epithelialization.
Semi-occlusive		
Petrolatum-impregnated	NuGauze®, Johnson and Johnson Products Inc., New Brunswick, NJ Vaseline petrolatum gauze® and Xerofoam®, Covidien Animal Health/Kendall, Dublin, OH Jelonet®, Smith & Nephew, Hull, UK	Repair phase, once a healthy bed of granulation tissue develops. Can be used for the entire healing period in clean, non-infected wounds. Not good for autolytic debridement.
Petrolatum	Adaptic®, Johnson and Johnson Products Inc., New Brunswick, NJ	
Oil emulsion	Curity®, Covidien Animal Health/Kendall, Dublin, OH	
Rayon/polyethylene fabric	Release®, Johnson and Johnson Products Inc., New Brunswick, NJ	

Table 3.1. *Continued*

Dressing	Manufacturer	Proposed best uses and indications
Petrolatum-impregnated gauze with 3% bismuth tribromophenate	Adaptic and Xerofoam®, Johnson and Johnson Products Inc., New Brunswick, NJ	
Perforated polyester film filled with compressed cotton	Telfa®, Covidien Animal Health/Kendall, Dublin, OH	
Adherent film	Mitraflex®, Polymedica Industries Inc., Wheat Ridge, CO	
Silicone	CicaCare®, Smith & Nephew, Hull, UK	Prevents exuberant granulation tissue in distal limb wounds. Accelerates epithelialization. Improves quality of repair tissue.[45] Best used during the repair and remodeling phases of healing.
Silver		
Silver chloride coated nylon dressing	Silverlon®, Argentum, Lakemont, GA	Inflammatory phase with a high bacterial load out to repair phase of healing. Cytotoxic effects relate to the concentration of silver released. Products have shown variable antibacterial activity.
Three-ply gauze with polyethylene net impregnated with nanocrystalline silver	Acticoat® Antimicrobial Barrier, Westaim Biomedical Corp; Ft. Saskatchewan, Canada	
Activated carbon impregnated with silver, enclosed in spun-bound nylon	Actisorb® Silver 220, Johnson and Johnson Products Inc., New Brunswick, NJ	
Hydrocolloid (carboxymethylcellulose) 1.2% ionic silver	Aquacel Silver®, Convatec, a division of ER Squibb and Sons, Princeton, NJ	
Polyurethane membrane containing a surfactant, glycerol, starch copolymer	PolyMem®, Ashton Medical Products, Inc., Dayton, OH	
Hydrocolloid impregnated with Vaseline and silver sulfadiazine	Urgotul SSD®, Urgo, Chenove, France	
Foam dressing with ionic silver	Contreet®, Coloplast Corp., Minneapolis, MN	
Split-thickness allogeneic skin	N/A	For clean wounds in all phases of wound healing.

Modified from Clinical Techniques in Equine Practice; January 2005 issue.

Wound Dressings

Classification

Wound dressings have been broadly classified as: (1) adherent, (2) hydrophilic, (3) non-adherent, (4) absorbent/non-absorbent, or (5) biologic.[1,3,4]

Adherent dressings are frequently made from closely woven or widely open gauze, other cotton materials, or wool. They are considered passive under most circumstances, although a few are considered interactive. Gauze dressings are generally highly absorbent and are still used for heavily contaminated exudative wounds. Hydrophilic dressings, as the name implies, are made from highly absorbent materials that absorb a large amount of fluid from the wound's surface.[4]

Non-adherent dressings have variable absorbency and are subdivided into occlusive, semi-occlusive, and biologic types. By definition, occlusive dressings are nonporous materials that allow low moisture/vapor transmission.[5] Semi-occlusive dressings are moisture and vapor permeable.[6] Synthetic, occlusive, and semi-occulsive materials create a moist wound healing environment and are considered interactive dressings under most circumstances.

Biologic dressings can either be unprocessed (e.g., split thickness skin or amnion) or processed to form an acellular matrix or a cyto-compatible biomaterial or a platelet-rich plasma gel. The biologic dressings are considered bioactive, contributing not only a matrix for repair but also growth factors and cytokines to enhance the healing process.

Absorbent/Adherent and Non-Adherent Dressings

Absorbent dressings can be either the fibrous type (e.g., cotton and cellulose wadding) or fabric type (e.g., gauze) or a combination of fibrous and fabric (e.g., Gamgee™). Many, but not all, of the absorbent dressings adhere to the wound surface, which affects wound debridement.[1] This section will focus on the types of dressings used most frequently in equine practice.

Gauze

Fine and wide meshed weaved cotton gauze (e.g., Steri-pad™, Mirasorb™, Curity™) has been used for many years for debridement of heavily contaminated exudative and necrotic wounds. The material allows egress of fluid and bacteria through the mesh. As the dressing dries, fibrin from the wound bed causes temporary bonding of the dressing to the wound. When the dressing is peeled off the wound fibrin, debris and necrotic tissue are removed. The gauze can be applied dry when wound fluid is copious and of low viscosity.[4]

Application as a wet-to-dry dressing is most commonly used when wound fluid is highly viscous or when the wound surface is dehydrated and scabs have formed (Figure 3.1a). The gauze is wetted with a sterile salt solution, excess fluid is squeezed out, and the dampened dressing is applied to the wound surface. Povidone iodine (PI) 0.01% (10 ml/1,000 ml) or chlorhexidine 0.05% (1:40 dilution) diluted with physiologic saline or physiologic saline solution alone are most commonly used to hydrate the material. Because dilute PI is inactivated by organic debris or blood, it is of little use as an antiseptic when used as a wetting agent.

When a dressing is applied wet it should be considered an interactive dressing because it hydrates the wound surface.[6] When the dressing dries, fibrin adheres it to the wound surface, effecting debridement. The dressing is usually changed after 24 hours and the wound is lavaged with a sterile diluted antiseptic solution which is delivered to the wound surface at a pressure of 10–15 PSI. If further debridement is needed another wet-to-dry dressing is applied. Once the wound appears clean another dressing type is indicated (Figures 3.1b,c).

One to three applications of the wet-to-dry dressing is all that is needed to effectively debride most wounds.[7] The wet-to-dry dressing is still commonly employed in equine practice; it is inexpensive and effective when used properly.[8] Continued use of this approach after the wound has been effectively debrided is contraindicated because of nonselective debridement, which results in stripping off newly formed epidermis.[7]

An in vitro study documenting the effectiveness of different dressings for debriding fibrin in blood clots from horses found that gauze dressing hydrated with normal saline was superior to gauze hydrated with distilled water.[9] In fact, gauze hydrated in saline was the most effective method of debridement when compared to hydrofiber, hydrocolloid, and alginate dressings. The saline gauze and hydrofiber/hydrocolloid dressings had a greater debriding effect early, when the clots were hardest and driest. All dressings tended to reach a

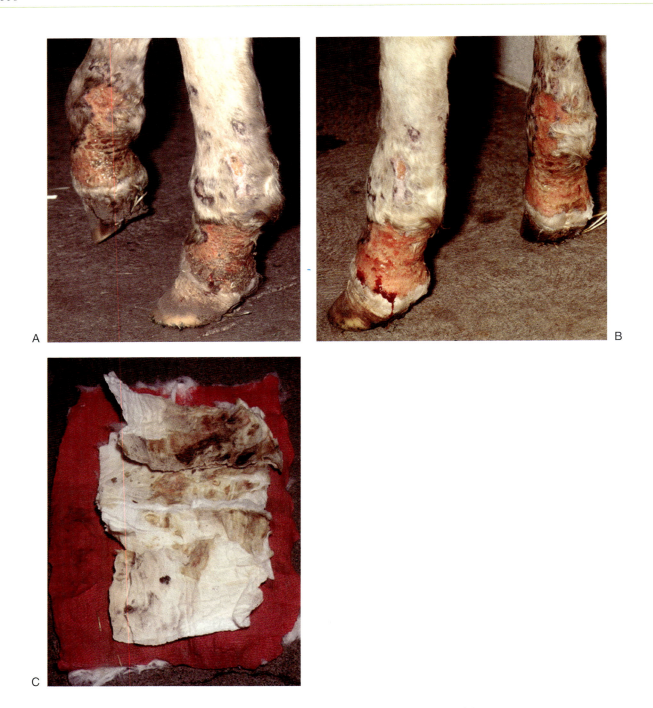

Figure 3.1. (A) A 5-day-old dry wound with scabs. A wet-to-dry gauze dressing was applied. (B) Dressing removed after ~24 hours. Note the healthy-appearing, moist, non-scabbed wound surface. (C) The appearance of the dressing with scabs attached. Reprinted from Clinical Techniques in Equine Practice, 3, Stashak TS, Update on wound dressings, pp. 148–163, Copyright (2004), with permission from Elsevier.

plateau in their rate of protein breakdown within 24 hours. Breakdown of protein, recorded in µg/ml, was the measure used for the debridement effectiveness of the various dressing; the greater the protein breakdown the more effective the dressing. Although this study addressed only one aspect of debridement, leaving out important in vivo autolytic cellular effects, it did confirm that gauze wetted with saline would be a good choice for a dehydrated wound with scabs (Figure 3.1). The reason for saline being more effective than distilled water probably relates to saline's ability to draw water up from the experimental receptor chamber along an osmotic gradient and through the clot, allowing debridement to take place on both sides of the clot.[9] A similar effect has been reported for saline-soaked gauze sponge dressings applied to open ulcers in humans.[10]

Hypertonic Saline Dressing (HSD)

HSD, impregnated with 20% NaCl, is commercially available (Curasalt™). The dressing has a strong osmotic action that affects desiccation of necrotic tissue and bacteria; it therefore is intended for aggressive wound debridement. The debridement is not tissue-specific, however, and must be monitored carefully to avoid collateral tissue damage. The use of this dressing is often limited to the first few days of wound care.[11] A benefit of this osmotic effect is the reduction of interstitial edema, which decreases the pressure on the wound bed capillaries and subsequently improves wound perfusion.[11] The proposed best use for this dressing is for infected, necrotic, heavily exuding wounds (Figure 3.2). Because this type of dressing interacts with the wound surface, it is considered an interactive dressing.[7]

Non-Adherent Cotton (NAC)

NAC, commercially available as (Gamgee™), is a versatile product that can be used as a wound dressing while providing protection, support, and insulation. Gamgee™ is made of a thick layer of absorbent cotton enclosed in a non-woven cover, which makes it non-adherent. The product is soft and easily conforms to the limb and wound surface. Because it is highly absorbent its proposed best use is for highly exudative limb wounds during the inflammatory phase of wound healing.

Hydrophilic Dressings

This group of dressings includes naturally occurring products from a range of polysaccharide materials such as dextranomers, alginates, freeze-dried gels, and chitin. In general, these dressing are highly absorbent (hydrophilic) and best used during the inflammatory phase of wound healing.

Particulate Dextranomers (PDs)

PDs come as beads (e.g., Debrisan®), flakes (e.g., Avalon®), and powders (e.g., Intrasite®). The beads are 100–300 μm in diameter and contain polyethylene glycol and water.[2] Although the beads will absorb the aqueous component (including prostaglandins) of wound exudate and dissolved materials (e.g., low molecular protein and inorganic salts), their pore size precludes the direct absorption of bacteria and viruses.[2] Microorganisms, however, are removed from the wound bed primarily by capillary action between the beads. The beads may be chemotactic, attracting polymorphonuclear and mononuclear cells.

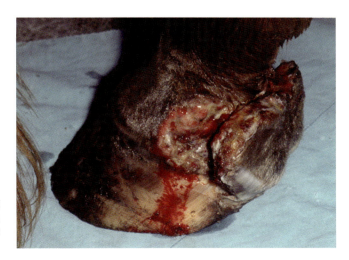

Figure 3.2. A 3-day-old infected heel bulb laceration that would benefit from a one-time application of a hypertonic saline (HS) or maltodextrin dressing. If HS dressing is used it should be applied only once and removed within 24 hours.

The proposed best use for PDs is for debridement of sloughing exuding wounds. They should be discontinued when a healthy bed of granulation tissue develops. They are contraindicated in dry wounds. Because PDs are not biodegradable they should be rinsed from the wound with saline or other sterile salt solutions before the wound dries. This will eliminate particulate residues and prevent the subsequent development of a granuloma.[2]

Maltodextrin (MD)

MD, a D-glucose polysaccharide (Intracell®), is commercially available as a powder or gel containing 1% ascorbic acid. The hydrophilic soluble powder has an affinity for fluids, "pulling" them up through the wound tissues and thus bathing the wound from inside. These fluids can dilute tenacious exudates, which enhances absorption.[12] Once the powder is hydrated it forms a vapor-permeable, hydrophilic film dressing that encourages moist wound healing. MD may also yield glucose from hydrolysis of polysaccharides, providing energy for cell metabolism to promote healing.[13] Additionally, the powder and gel are reported to promote chemotaxis of macrophages, polymorphonuclear cells, and lymphocytes into wounds, thus aiding in the debridement process. Other associated advantages include reduced wound swelling, bacteriostatic and bactericidal effects that reduce infection rates, early granulation tissue formation, and rapid epithelial growth.[12]

The powder should be applied over the wound to a depth of approximately 7 mm. A primary nonadherent semi-occulsive dressing should be applied over the powder, followed by an absorbent wrap and tertiary bandage. Bandages are changed daily and the wound lavaged, after which more powder is applied.

The proposed best use of MD is to debride and promote healing of contaminated and infected wounds (Figure 3.2). The powder is used on exudating wounds and the gel is used on drier wounds. There is also some rationale to the use of MD during the acute inflammatory phase because of its ability to recruit and activate macrophages, which stimulates early formation of granulation tissue as well as rapid epithelial growth. Because of MD's many properties, it is considered a bioactive dressing.

Calcium Alginate (CA)

CA dressings (Curasorb®, C-Stat®, Nu-Derm®, EquineGinate™, Kaltostat®, AlgiSite®) are classified as a fibrous dextranomer. They are available from a variety of sources (see Table 3.1). They are made from salts of alginic acid obtained from *Phaeophyceae* algae found in seaweed. Because the dressing is hydrophilic, it can absorb up to 20–30 times its weight in wound fluid. This process converts the initial dry felt-like material into a hydrophilic gel on the wound surface, which is easily removed. The hydrophilic alginate gel forms via a calcium and sodium ion exchange, providing a moist environment conducive to wound healing.[12] The presence of calcium modifies cell response. All concentrations of calcium produce an initial fall in cell replication; however, intermediate concentrations subsequently stimulate cell division. Reportedly, CA dressings increase epithelialization and fibroplasia.[2] This, however, was not clinically detectable in one study performed in horses.[14] CA dressings also improve clotting. The calcium ion released from the dressing is known to promote the activation of prothrombin in the clotting cascade.[1]

Zinc has been added to an alginate dressing (Curasorb ZN®) to improve the dressing's hemostatic properties.[15] The primary hemostatic use of the dressing is in packing sinuses, fistulae, and bleeding tooth sockets.[1] Additionally, some alginate dressings have the potential to activate macrophages (e.g., EquineGinate™, containing acemannan) within a chronic wound bed, which should subsequently generate a pro-inflammatory signal and promote the formation of granulation tissue.[16]

Moreover, alginates have the ability to jump-start the healing cascade by favoring the balanced release of histamine and serotonin from wound mast cells. Indeed, the first response of the injured blood vessel is serotonin-mediated vasoconstriction, which lasts 5 to 10 minutes, after which histamine-mediated vasodilation ensues and promotes diapedesis of cells, fluid, and protein across the vessel wall into the extravascular space. Coagulated blood and aggregated platelets together form a clot within the wound defect that maintains hemostasis and serves as a scaffold for cell migration.[1]

Because of these attributes, CA dressings are considered bioactive. The alginates have also been cross-formulated with collagen (type 1) and chitosan to increase the possible bioactivity of the material.[1] Chitosan is highly bactericidal and hemostatic and may suppress the formation of exuberant granulation tissue.[17]

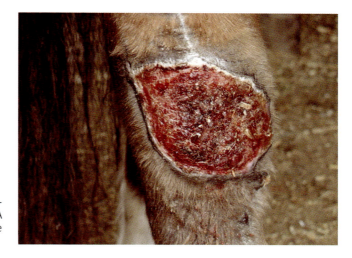

Figure 3.3. Example of a chronic dry wound that needs stimulation to proceed with the formation of granulation tissue. A calcium alginate (CA) dressing, hydrated with saline, would be a good choice for this wound.

The proposed best use for CA dressings is in the moderate to heavily exuding wound during transition from the inflammatory to the repair phases of wound healing. It is also suggested that they are best used for wounds with substantial tissue loss such as degloving injuries,[18] which may relate to the ability of moderate concentrations of calcium to stimulate cell division.

Although the dressing has no inherent antibacterial properties, bacteria may passively become trapped in the gel and be removed during dressing changes.[19] The dressing should be pre-moistened with saline in preparation for application to a chronic dry wound that needs stimulation to proceed with fibroplasia (Figure 3.3). A semi-occlusive non-adherent pad should be placed over the CA dressing, followed by secondary and tertiary bandage layers. An in vitro study documenting the effectiveness of different dressings for debriding fibrin found that alginate dressings immersed in saline was more effective at clot debridement than were hydrofiber or hydrocolloid dressings, but they were not more effective than saline-soaked gauze.[9]

Freeze-Dried Gel (FDG)

A hydrophilic FDG containing acemannan is commercially available (CarraSorb™). Acemannan is the name given to the carbohydrate fraction obtained from the water-soluble gel of the aloe vera (AV) leaf. When acemannan was isolated and purified from the AV gel, it was shown to significantly accelerate healing in experimentally created wounds in rats.[20] Acemannan's potent macrophage activating property and its ability to bind growth factors, prolonging their stimulating effect on granulation tissue formation, were the proposed reasons for this acceleration. CarraSorb™ has also been shown to aggressively promote granulation tissue formation in open wounds and in wounds with exposed bone in dogs.[21] According to the manufacturer, CarraSorb™ also promotes moist wound healing and autolytic debridement.

The dressing should be cut to conform to the wound and hydrated with sterile saline/water before it is applied to a dry wound. Because of its ability to stimulate fibroplasia it is recommended to apply CarraSorb™ only every second or third day.[22]

The best use for CarraSorb™ appears to be during the early inflammatory phase, particularly for moderately exuding wounds and those with exposed bone (Figure 3.4). CarraSorb™ is also effective in reducing wound edema[22] due to its hydrophilic action. To prevent the formation of exuberant granulation tissue, it is recommended that CarraSorb™ be discontinued when granulation tissue fills the wound.

Chitin (C)

C, a polymeric N-acetyl-D glucosamine, is a component of the skeletal material of crustaceans and insects. It is made into various forms including sponge, cotton, flake, and non-woven fabric. A controlled study performed on canine full-thickness skin wounds found that at 21 days the treated wounds tended toward greater epithelialization than did control wounds; however, the scores for epithelialization and granulation tissue

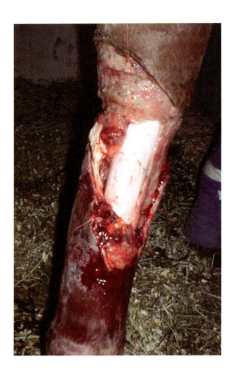

Figure 3.4. Example of a degloving wound of the right metacarpus with exposed bone devoid of periosteum. This wound would benefit from the application of a hydrogel dressing containing acemannan. Courtesy of Dr. C. Rogers.

formation were not statistically significantly different.[23] It is difficult to identify a best use for this product at the time of this writing and to our knowledge C is not being used routinely for wound management in North America.

Chitosan, a byproduct of C, is highly bactericidal and hemostatic and may suppress the formation of exuberant granulation tissue.[17] Its proposed best use is for a heavily contaminated bleeding wound out to the repair phase and for the prevention of hemorrhage following the debridement of granulation tissue.[17]

Occlusive Synthetic Dressings (OSDs)

OSDs are made of nonporous materials that have a low moisture/vapor transmission; thus, they promote "moist wound healing". A moist wound free of infection provides an environment rich in white blood cells, enzymes, cytokines, and growth factors beneficial to wound healing.[24] The enzymes released, primarily from the white blood cells, cause autolytic debridement of the wound which appears to be selective for necrotic tissue.[25] Under these dressings autolytic debridement usually occurs 72–96 hours after wounding (assuming the dressing is applied at the time of wounding), thus cleaning the wound in preparation for the repair phase.[11] Fibroplasia and epithelialization are stimulated by growth factors present in the moist wound.[26] Cytokines, which are signaling peptides, also act locally to stimulate the migration and activation of macrophages and neutrophils within the wound.[27]

Proposed benefits to moist wound healing include:
- Prevention of the formation of a scab, which will otherwise trap white blood cells, preventing them from participating in their important wound healing functions
- Reduction of the environmental pH, which improves oxygenation of the wound by shifting the oxygen/hemoglobin dissociation curve in favor of oxygen release from hemoglobin
- Prevention of bacterial strike-through from the outside environment to the wound surface
- Augmentation of epithelialization, primarily by allowing epithelial cells to freely migrate over the moist wound surface; the moist environment also favors growth factor effects
- Enhancement of bacterial colonization but not infection

Although a moist wound environment favors bacterial colonization and increases bacterial numbers, infection rates are not increased. This is probably due to improved white blood cell function.[28] Reports in the equine literature do not, however, substantiate this latter claim. Several studies indicate that the chance of developing infection is greater in wounds covered with occlusive dressing in horses.[29–31] Additional benefits to moist wound healing appear to be an acceleration (shortening) of the inflammatory and proliferative phases, with more rapid progression into the remodeling phase.[32] OCDs are considered interactive and are commercially available as hydrogels, hydrocolloids, and as silicone dressings.

Hydrogels (HGs) (Polyethylene Oxide Occlusive Dressings)

HGs are a three-dimensional network of hydrophilic polymers with a water content between 90% and 95%.[12] They are made from such materials as gelatin or polysaccharide which is cross-linked with a polymer, while hydrophilic side chains allow HGs to bind up to 3 times their weight in water.[2] Because of their excellent bio-compatibility, the FDA has designated HGs as Class 1 devices, with minimal regulation.[33]

HG products are available as sheets, amorphous gels, and impregnated gauze. The sheets come plain (non-adhesive) or with an adhesive border, eliminating the need for tape to hold them in place. These HGs are believed to possess most of the properties of an ideal wound dressing (e.g., Plain: Curagel®, Curafil®, Tegagel dressing™, Nu-gel®, CarraFilm™, CarrGauze™ containing acemannan, TrasiGel®, SoloSite®; Adhesive: Thin-Site®, Tansorbent®, ClearSite®, ConMed®, AquaSorb®). They are generally used as a primary dressing for shallow, flat wounds.

Most HG sheets come packaged with a protective layer of plastic that is removed before application to the wound. Prior to application, the skin around the wound should be cleaned and dried and the wound surface gently rinsed with a dilute antiseptic solution. The dressing should be cut to the appropriate size for the wound and the thin sheet on one side peeled off. The dressing is then covered with secondary and tertiary bandage layers and should be left in place for 2 days.[7] If the skin surrounding the wound begins to appear macerated because of excess moisture, the dressing should be replaced with a non-adherent semi-occulsive dressing.

When HGs are applied to a dry wound they effectively hydrate it, creating an environment for moist healing. By increasing the moisture content of necrotic tissue and increasing collagenase production, HGs facilitate autolytic debridement.[34] The dressings are considered occlusive even though they are able to absorb some wound fluid into the polymer matrix and possess water vapor permeability comparable to a semi-permeable membrane.[1] Applications to wounds in humans result in almost immediate reduction in pain and a cooling effect that lasts for some 6 hours. Presumably both effects are due to the "airtight" seal created by the dressing over exposed nerve endings.[1] These dressings are easily removed from the wound bed because the moist inter-face between the dressing and the wound limits adherence.

Amorphous HG (e.g., Curasol™, Iamin®, Hydroactive Gel®) can be used to fill a deep wound with irregular contours and is held in place with a secondary dressing that is generally changed daily. These amorphous gels are available in tubes, spray, and foil packets. They are removed from the wound by irrigation.

HG-impregnated gauze (e.g., Aquagauze™, MPM Gel Pad™, Curifil®, FasCure®, Curafil®) is particularly useful in tunneled and undermined wounds because the dressing is able to fill in the dead space.

HGs can also be used to deliver topical wound medications (e.g., metronidazole and silver sulfadiazine). The release mechanism resulting in the diffusion of the medication can be controlled by the extent of cross linkage in the gel.

Both temperature- and pH-sensitive gels have been the subject of recent investigations aiming to develop new products.[1] HGs containing acemannan (e.g., CarraVet™ Gel, CarraVet® spray-on gel, and EquineVet™ smart gel, all with acemannan) reportedly stimulate healing over exposed bone (Figure 3.4).[12] Acemannan is a β-linked acetylated mannan that has the ability to stimulate macrophages to release fibrogenic and angiogenic cytokines, resulting in a positive effect on wound healing. Additionally, it appears that acemannan can bind directly to angiogenic and fibrogenic growth factors which may prolong their stimulatory effect on granulation tissue formation.

Other hydrogels contain hyaluronan and chondroitin sulfate with a chemically cross-linked glycosamino-glycan (GAG) hydro-film (Tegaderm™) which reportedly increases epithelialization and granulation tissue for-mation compared to Tegaderm™ alone.[35] Another HG contains 25% propylene glycol (Solugel®). One study performed in horses evaluating the effects of Solugel® on second intention healing of small (2.5×2.5 cm) full-thickness, distal limb, skin wounds found no beneficial effects when compared to the control saline-soaked gauze dressing.[36]

A study comparing three hydrogels (Exgel®, Intrasite®, and a poloxmer gel containing 3% hydrogen peroxide) to a control occlusive dressing (Tegaderm™) found that Exgel® significantly increased the epithelialization rate (20%) in partial-thickness wounds in domestic pigs, compared to other treatments.[37] In a study performed on full-thickness (2 cm × 2 cm) limb wounds in horses, use of the hydrogel sheet dressing (BioDres®—no longer available) led to an increased requirement to trim exuberant granulation tissue (Figure 3.5) and excess exudate and prolonged wound healing by greater than 2 times that of the controls (Figure 3.6).[31]

The recurrent formation of exuberant granulation tissue was believed to result from prolonged application of the BioDres® dressing, through to the repair phase. This observation brought about the recommendation that the dressing be applied within 6 hours of wounding and maintained to at least 48 hours before changing it.[7] Moreover, use of the dressing should be discontinued at the earliest signs of granulation tissue formation. Generally speaking, these dressings are best used on clean acute wounds during the inflammatory phase of healing (Figure 3.4).

Vulketan gel® is commercially available from Janssen Animal Health. Ketanserin, the active ingredient in Vulketan gel®, is a potent serotonin receptor antagonist. Ketanserin blocks the serotonin-induced macrophage suppression and vasoconstriction present in the early wound environment, thus allowing a strong and effective inflammatory response to occur. This action may translate into a superior control of infection and a better orchestration of the later phases of repair when growth factors released by activated macrophages play an important role.[38]

Vulketan gel® (containing 2.5 mg ketanserin tartrate per mL) was evaluated against an antiseptic (Rivanol™; ASID Veterinär Vertriebs GmbH, D-85716 Unterschleissheim, Germany) and a desloughing cream containing

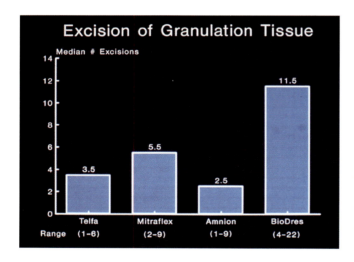

Figure 3.5. Histogram illustrating the number of excisions of exuberant granulation tissue required for wounds dressed with Telfa®, Mitraflex®, Amnion, and BioDres®. The BioDres®-dressed wounds required the most excisions and the amnion-dressed wounds required the least number of excisions. Reprinted from Clinical Techniques in Equine Practice, 3, Stashak TS, Update on wound dressings, pp. 148–163, Copyright (2004), with permission from Elsevier.

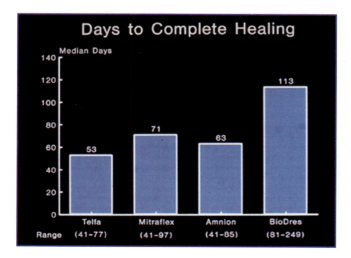

Figure 3.6. Histogram depicting the number of days to complete healing for two semi-occlusive dressings (Telfa® and Mitraflex®), Amnion, and an occlusive dressing (BioDres®). The BioDres®-dressed wounds took the longest to heal while the Telfa-dressed wounds took the shortest time to heal. Reprinted from Clinical Techniques in Equine Practice, 3, Stashak TS, Update on wound dressings, pp. 148–163, Copyright (2004), with permission from Elsevier.

malic, benzoic, and salicylic acids (Dermaflon Crème Elevage™; Pfizer Animal Health, Orsay, France; Dermisol cream™; Pfizer Animal Health, Sandwich, UK) in a multicentric randomized controlled clinical study as a dressing for the prevention of exuberant granulation tissue and infection in equine distal limb wounds.[39]

Treatment was begun in wounds aged 6 to 9 days and continued until the wound healed (success), formed exuberant granulation tissue (failure), or became infected (failure). Treatment was terminated after 6 months in all remaining animals. It was concluded that Vulketan gel® was 2 to 5 times more likely to result in successful closure, by reducing infection and developing exuberant granulation tissue. The proposed best use is during the inflammatory and repair phases of healing. Early in healing it prevents infection; later it prevents the development of exuberant granulation tissue.

Hydrocolloid (HC) Dressings

HC dressings consist of an inner, often adhesive layer, a thick absorbing hydrocolloid "mass," and an outer, thin, water-resistant, bacterial-impervious polyurethane film. The adhesive skin contact layer is composed of an HC dispersed with the aid of a "tackifier" (mineral oil and terpene resin).[2] The HC mass is made of either gelatin, pectin, and carboxymethylcellulose particles suspended in polyisobutylene (Duoderm®, Dermaheal®) or carboxymethylcellulose particles embedded in an elastotic (altered elastic tissue) mesh (Comfeel®).[40] HC dressings tend to adhere to both wet and dry tissues. Some HCs have been shown to bridge the interactive and bioactive classifications by exhibiting fibrinolytic, chemotactic, and angiogenic effects.[2]

Because HCs are able to absorb fairly large amounts of wound fluid they are often referred to as hydroactive dressings.[41] Ultimately, the HC dissolves at the moist interface with the wound producing a yellow-colored fluid. Duoderm® is oxygen-impermeable, which is supposed to promote the rate of epithelialization and collagen synthesis while decreasing the pH of wound exudate, thus reducing bacterial counts. Acceleration of epithelialization has not been documented in all studies, however.

A study in humans comparing epithelialization rates of split-thickness donor sites dressed with Duoderm®, Biomembrane®, and Xerofoam® (a semi-occlusive fine mesh gauze impregnated with bismuth) found that Xerofoam®-dressed wounds healed significantly faster (10.5 days) than did Duoderm®- (15.3 days) and Biomembrane®-dressed wounds (19 days).[6] Although wound fluids beneath the dressing are acidic (pH 6.1) in humans, it is still recommended that these dressings be applied to clean wounds because the moist environment created can be optimal for bacterial growth.[29,30] Some HC dressings (Comfeel plus® and Duoderm®) have, in isolated cases, been associated with an allergic reaction resulting in contact dermatitis in humans.[42]

In a study evaluating the repair of full-thickness skin wounds in dogs out to 28 days, under either a semi-occlusive or one of two occlusive dressings (hydrogel and an HC), it was found that HC-dressed wounds showed the poorest healing based on all of the parameters being evaluated.[30] A study in horses found that Dermaheal® or Duoderm® dressings promoted the formation of granulation tissue from the surface of denuded bone and on the surface of frayed tendons and ligaments.[29] This study also showed that wound infection can develop underneath these dressings. When this happens, application should be discontinued until the wound is healthy.

The best use for these HC dressings in horses appears to be during the early inflammatory phase until granulation tissue fills the wound. The dressing should be applied to a clean wound that is free of infection and discontinued before the development of exuberant granulation tissue. Continuing to dress the wound after granulation tissue forms can result in exuberant granulation tissue and consequently prolonged wound healing.[31] If infection develops, the dressing should be discontinued until the infection is controlled, and then the dressing is reapplied.

Silicone Dressings

A silicone gel sheet dressing (CicaCare®) has been used successfully in reversing hypertrophic scarring in human burn patients, apparently by exerting pressure on the microvasculature of the scar and altering the levels of various growth factors, notably fibrogenic TGF-β.[43,44] The anoxic fibroblasts undergo apoptosis rather than proliferating and secreting extracellular matrix and producing collagen, thus minimizing granulation tissue and ultimately, excess scar.[38]

A study performed in horses determined that the silicone dressing greatly surpassed a non-adherent semi-permeable dressing (Melolite®) in preventing the formation of exuberant granulation tissue in experimentally-created distal limb wounds. Contraction and epithelialization progressed faster in the first 2 weeks of repair, possibly as a result of the healthier wound bed granulation tissue. Indeed, wound tissue quality exceeded that of wounds treated conventionally. Microvessels were also occluded significantly more often in wounds dressed with the silicone gel,[45] presumably creating biochemical changes similar to those described by Reno et al. (2003).[43] The proposed best use for this dressing appears to be during the repair and remodeling phases of healing.

Semi-Occlusive Synthetic Dressings (SCSDs)

Fabric Synthetic Dressings (FSDs)

FSDs are commercially available in many forms: petrolatum-impregnated gauze (NU Gauze sponges®, Vaseline Petrolatum Gauze®, Xerofoam®, Jelonet®), petrolatum emulsion dressing (Adaptic®), oil emulsion knitted fabric (Curity®), rayon/polyethylene fabric (Release®), petrolatum-impregnated gauze with 3% bismuth tribromophenate (Adaptic plus Xerofoam®), absorbent adhesive film (Mitraflex®), and perforated polyester film filled with compressed cotton (Telfa®). Newer/advanced SCSDs are also commercially available as a polyurethane sheet or foam. The latter will be covered later in this chapter.

A study evaluating the effects of four SCSDs on the healing of experimentally created full-thickness wounds in dogs found that wounds dressed with petrolatum-containing dressings (PCD) showed more contraction for the first 7 days than did wounds dressed with cotton non-adherent film (CNF) or rayon/polyethylene (RP) dressings.[46] However, by days 14 and 21 there was little difference in the amount of contraction of any of the wounds. At 7, 14, and 21 days, the PCD wounds showed less epithelialization than did wounds dressed with CNF or RP. The commercial petrolatum emulsion dressing (Adaptic®) allowed the best absorption of exudate. Lee (1987) recommended that PCD be used early, in wounds free of necrotic tissue, with newly formed granulation tissue that is still producing exudate.[46] Furthermore, CNF and RP dressings should be used when healthy granulation tissue has formed and epithelialization is beginning (Figure 3.7).

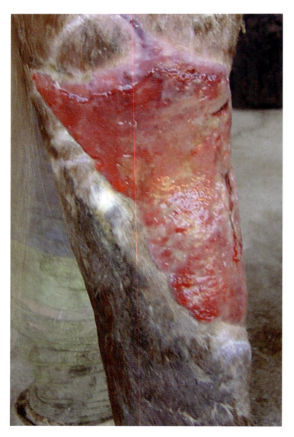

Figure 3.7. Example of a wound that would benefit from the application of a semi-occlusive dressing.

A study evaluating the effects of two semi-occlusive dressings (Telfa® and Mitraflex®), a biologic dressing (equine amnion), and an occlusive dressing (Biodres®) on the healing of experimentally created full-thickness skin wounds on the distal limb in horses found that wounds dressed with Biodres® showed an increased need to trim exuberant granulation tissue, excess exudate, and prolonged wound healing by greater than 2 times that shown by the control (Telfa®) (Figures 3.5 and 3.6).[31] Wounds dressed with amnion required the least trimming of the granulation tissue, and those dressed with Telfa® healed the fastest. A study performed in humans to evaluate the effects of a semi-occlusive dressing (SOD), a semi-permeable silicone membrane (SSM), and an HC dressing on split-thickness skin donor site healing found that wounds dressed with the SOD healed in 10.5 days compared to 15.5 days for the SSM and 19 days for the HC.[6]

Polyurethane Semi-Occlusive (PUS) Dressings

PUS dressings are available as a sheet (e.g., Op-Site®, Tegaderm®, Bioclusive®) or foam (e.g., Hydrosorb®, Hydrosorb®, Sof-Foam®). The film PUS dressings are transparent, waterproof, semipermeable to vapor, oxygen-permeable, adhesive to dry skin, and non-adhesive to the wound, and have an analgesic affect.[47] These dressing are designed to allow excess fluid to be lost by water vapor transmission through the membrane but prevent dehydration of the wound, thus providing an environment for moist wound healing. If the volume of exudate produced exceeds the water vapor transmission rate, the dressing becomes plugged and fluid will accumulate underneath the dressing, making it less effective.[2] The dressing should be changed when this occurs. The wound is also protected against secondary infection by the bacterial impermeability of the film to such organisms as *Pseudomonas, Staphylococcus,* and *Escherichia coli.*[2]

Although these dressings are considered non-adherent, one product (Op-site®) has a tendency to strip newly formed epidermis from the surface of a healing wound when removed.[48] A study performed in pigs comparing Opsite® dressed and gauze dressed full-thickness wounds found that Opsite® created a moist healing environment and there was acceleration into and through the inflammatory and proliferative phases of healing.[32] Although the proposed best use for the sheet dressings in horses is during the repair phase, their unique characteristics allow them to be used during the entire healing period of a clean wound.

PUS foam sponges come as sheet dressings, in situ formed foams, and adhesive foams (e.g., Tielle® hydropolymer adhesive). They are highly conforming, vapor-permeable, absorptive, and easy to apply, and they provide an effective barrier against bacterial penetration.[49] Moisture is absorbed into the dressing, thus decreasing tissue maceration while providing a moist healing environment. These dressings are easily removed without disturbing the healing tissue. The proposed best use for the sponge is the early inflammatory phase of wound healing, when there is considerable exudate in the wound. Under these circumstances the bandage should be changed daily or as indicated according to the amount of fluid produced by the wound. Because of PUSs' semi-occlusive nature it is hypothesized that they may also be effective during the repair phase of healing, much like what is seen with other semi-occlusive dressings. An alternative use of the sponge is to deliver liquid medication or wetting agents to the wound by saturating the sponge prior to placing it on the wound. The same sponge, however, cannot be used for both absorption and medication delivery.[50]

The in situ polymeric foams were developed to dress/fill wounds possessing large cavities. The foam dressings have been found to be clinically superior to packing the wound cavity with ribbon gauze.[1] To our knowledge, in situ foam dressings are not being used routinely in equine practice at the time of this writing.

Antimicrobial Dressings

Infection and bacterial colonization remain very important factors capable of delaying wound healing. Since the widespread use of systemic and topical antibiotics has resulted in increasing numbers of resistant bacterial strains (e.g., methicillin-resistant *Staphylococcus aureus [MRSA]* and Vancomycin-resistant *Enterococcus faecalis* and *pseudomonas aeruginosa)*, it has been suggested that the judicious use of antimicrobial dressings, notably those containing certain antiseptics, can be valuable tools in infection control and in promoting healing.[51]

Iodine-Containing Dressings (ICDs)

A cross-linked polymerized dextran cadexomer ICD (Iodosord®) is available as a sheet, powder, or ointment. When it becomes hydrated within the moist environment of the wound to which it is applied, elemental iodine is released to exert an antibacterial effect and to interact with macrophages to produce tumor necrosis factor-alpha and interleukin-6 which can indirectly influence wound healing.[51] The perceived best use is for contaminated wounds early in the inflammatory phase of repair.

A slow release cadexomer iodine dressing (Iodoflex®) is also available. This particular dressing is designed to ensure adequate local levels of active iodine for at least a 48-hour period.[51] It appears that the slow release of cadexomer iodine in this product does not slow wound healing.[52]

PI-containing dressings are available as a powder (PRN® Wound Dressing) or a hydrogel (Biozide®). Both products have 1% available PI and a broad antimicrobial spectrum, and they are fungicidal and best used during the inflammatory phase, particularly in heavily contaminated wounds. The perceived best use for these iodine-containing dressings is for contaminated wounds early in the inflammatory phase out to the repair phase.

A relatively new bioxygenating hydrogel dressing (Oxyzyme™) that delivers both iodine (~0.04% w/w) and oxygen to the wound's surface was found in an in vitro study to have broad-spectrum antimicrobial activity, encompassing antibiotic-resistant organisms, anaerobes, and yeasts.[53] The technology allowing delivery of both oxygen and iodine from this dressing involves a bi-layered construction with an oxidase enzyme in the top layer and an iodide in the deeper layer. The oxidase enzyme reacts with oxygen in the air to generate hydrogen peroxide, which converts iodide to molecular iodine, which instantly converts hydrogen peroxide into dissolved oxygen; both are then delivered to the surface of the wound. Case studies in humans found the dressing to be effective in the treatment of venous leg ulcers.[54] Studies in humans indicate that Oxyzyme™ may be an effective stimulant for healing in recalcitrant wounds.[54]

This dressing is perceived to be of limited value in wound treatment in horses because it is recommended that it be applied without a secondary dressing to secure it.

In summary, no objective studies attesting to the effects of any of these products on wound healing in horses were available at the time of this writing. That said, one study has documented no delay in healing of horse wounds treated with 10% PI ointment compared to another antimicrobial dressing.[55]

Antimicrobial Gauze Dressing (AMGD)

AMGD (Kerlix®) contains polyhexamethylene biguanide, which has a wide range of antimicrobial activities but is more biocompatible to tissues than its close relative, chlorhexidine.[56] Kerlix® has been shown to resist bacterial colonization within the dressing and to reduce bacterial penetration toward the wound site.[57] The dressing comes packaged as a sponge or roll and the material can be applied wet or dry, as described for plain mesh gauze. The proposed best use for this dressing is during the inflammatory phase of healing in wounds with a high concentration of bacteria and in those in which there is an open synovial cavity (Figures 3.8a,b). This is also an excellent dressing for packing deep contaminated wounds associated with the body or upper limbs (Figures 3.9a,b). This approach facilitates wound debridement, drainage, and the reduction of bacterial numbers. The packing is pre-moistened with sterile salt solution, packed in the wound, and kept in place with loosely "bow tied" large-diameter sutures. The packing is changed daily with less gauze being used subsequently to pack the wound.

Poultice Pad

A poultice pad (Animalintex®) is made of a non-woven cotton pad with plastic backing. According to the manufacturer, the dressing contains boric acid (mild antiseptic) and Tragacanth (poultice). Animalintex® can be applied "wetted," (either hot or cold) or dry. The proposed best use of the product is to apply it dry or wet-hot for infected hoof wounds (e.g., abscesses, dirty wounds, etc.) but it can be used as a poultice for other regions of the body. It may be used wet-cold for sprains and strains and should be applied as a dry dressing over open clean wounds.

Silver-Impregnated Dressings (SIDs)

A range of SIDs (e.g., Silverlon®, Acticoat®, Actisorb® Silver 220, Biopatch®, Silvercel®, Aquacel Silver®, Acticoat®, PolyMem®, Urgotul SSD®) are commercially available (Table 3.1), but comparative data on their antimicrobial efficacies and effects on wound healing are limited. The silver that is released over time in variable concentrations from the dressing kills bacteria.

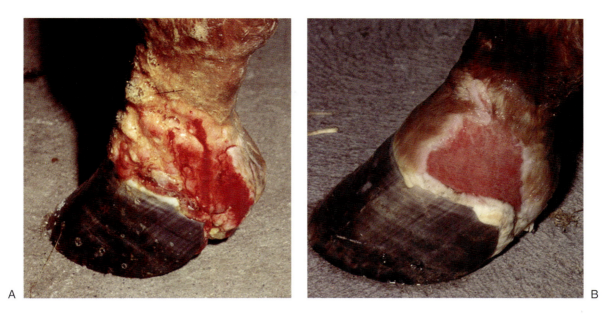

Figure 3.8. (A) Wound on the lateral aspect of the pastern region, entering the distal interphalangeal (coffin) joint. Kerlix® AMD was used to dress this wound. (B) Wound at the time of patient discharge, 8 days later. The coffin joint was closed and a healthy bed of granulation tissue is present. A semi-occlusive dressing was selected for the remainder of the healing period.

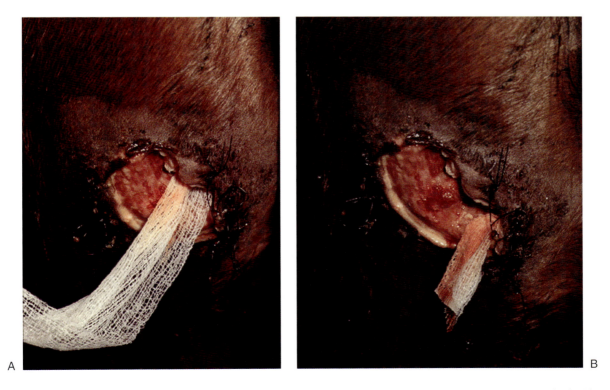

Figure 3.9. Example of a large, undermined, contaminated wound on the cranial surface of the pectoral region, packed with moistened Kerlix® AMD gauze. (A) The wound is being packed with the gauze. (B) Packing the wound is complete; the gauze is attached to the skin with one large suture tied in a bow. Reprinted from Clinical Techniques in Equine Practice, 3, Stashak TS, Update on wound dressings, pp. 148–163, Copyright (2004), with permission from Elsevier.

A non-comparative in vitro experiment found Silverlon® dressing to be antifungal and effective in killing five equine pathogens in vitro.[58] Another in vitro experiment, using a broth method, tested the antimicrobial effects of five commercially available SIDs against nine burn wound pathogens and found that the spectrum and rapidity of action ranged widely for different dressings.[59] Acticoat® and Contreet® dressings exerted broad spectrum bactericidal activities against both Gram-positive and -negative bacteria while the other dressings demonstrated a narrower range of bactericidal activities. For methicillin-sensitive and -resistant *Staphylococcus aureus* (MRSA) Acticoat® and Contreet® exerted maximal bactericidal activity within the shortest period of time. Aquacel Silver® and PolyMem® dressings exhibited little reduction in MRSA, whereas with Urgotul SSD®, an increase in MRSA growth was observed at 24 hours. Although all five of the SIDs were bactericidal on coliform species, Contreet® achieved the most rapid killing. PolyMem® and Urgotul SSD® were less satisfactory, because re-growth of bacteria was observed within 24 hours.

A comparative study of the cytotoxicity of these latter five SIDs in monolayer cell, tissue explant, and animal models found Acticoat®, Aquacel Silver®, and Contreet® were likely to produce the most significant cytotoxic effects on both cultured keratinocytes and fibroblasts, while PolyMem® and Urgotul SSD® demonstrated the least cytotoxicity.[60] The cytotoxicity correlated with the silver released from the dressings and measured silver concentrations in culture medium. In the tissue explant model, in which epidermal cell proliferation was evaluated, all silver dressings resulted in a significant delay of epithelialization. In a mouse excisional wound model, Acticoat® and Contreet® elicited strong inhibition of wound epithelialization on post-wounding day 7.

While SIDs are generally considered to be useful for control of bacterial infections (as well as against fungi and viruses), key issues remain, including the relative efficacy of different SIDs for wound uses and the existence of silver-resistant microbes. The perceived best use for these dressings is during the inflammatory phase out to the beginning of the repair phase of wound healing.

Activated Charcoal Dressings (ACDs)

ACDs are commercially available (Activate®, Actisorb®, CarboFlex™, Lyofoam®). Most are packaged as a multilayered, non-woven, non-adherent material. The proposed advantages of these dressings are maintaining a moist wound environment for autolytic debridement, effective bacterial absorption, and reduction of wound odor.[61] It has been suggested that they prevent the formation of exuberant granulation tissue in horses[62], although no controlled study has documented this effect. An in vitro study found that Activate® placed in a suspension of bacteria (10^6/ml) resulted in a 3–5 log reduction in bacterial numbers compared to <1 log reduction achieved by the un-carbonized cloth control,[61] presumably via absorption. The reported best use of these dressings is for heavily infected wounds during the inflammatory phase out to the repair phase of healing. Good healing has been observed by the first author in a limited number of cases through the repair phase.

Antibiotic-Impregnated Collagen Sponges (AICS)

AICS have been used extensively in human orthopedic and soft tissue surgery for some time.[63] One such product, Collatamp G®, is made from denatured type I bovine collagen impregnated with gentamicin. Each 10 cm × 10 cm sponge contains 280 mg of collagen and 130 mg of gentamicin. This registered medical device has a hemostatic effect and reportedly is effective in the treatment and prevention of infection.[64] The hemostatic effect relies on adhesion and aggregation of platelets and certain bridge proteins such as fibronectin to the collagen. The dressing facilitates the prevention and treatment of infection by releasing gentamicin from the collagen matrix, initially by passive diffusion then by breakdown of the collagen by wound macrophages. Reportedly high levels of gentamicin are achieved at the implantation site while serum levels remain below toxic levels.[63]

A study comparing the level of gentamicin released in wound exudate after treatment with AICS or gentamicin-impregnated polymethylmethacrylate (PMMA) beads found that on day 1 the concentration of gentamicin in AICS-treated wounds was 15 times greater than in the PMMA-treated wounds and the concentration of gentamicin remained 2 times higher on the third day for the AICS-treated group.[65] In a clinical study in eight horses presenting with synovial sepsis, seven of the eight horses responded favorably to implantation of the AICS sponge into the infected site.[64] Collagen dressings have also been impregnated with amikacin.[66]

Biologic Dressings

Biologic dressings are developed from natural products produced by the body. They reportedly promote wound contraction and epithelialization by retarding the formation of exuberant granulation tissue, and for this reason are considered bioactive. These dressings also induce a mild inflammatory response, which is believed to be beneficial to wound healing.[67] Examples of these dressings are as follows.

Equine Amnion (EA)

EA has been described as possessing most of the qualities of an ideal dressing.[68] Despite its occlusive nature, it did not result in exuberant granulation tissue formation or more rapid healing in the distal limb wounds of horses when compared to a synthetic semi-occlusive control dressing (Telfa®) (Figure 3.6).[31] A study comparing EA, a live yeast cell derivative, and a non-adherent control dressing on second intention healing of distal limb wounds in horses found less exuberant granulation tissue formation, significantly greater epithelialization rates, and significantly reduced number of days to complete healing for EA covered wounds.[68] Another study in ponies found that amnion-enhanced epithelialization and accelerated wound closure in pinch-grafted wounds compared to wounds bandaged with a non-adherent wound dressing.[69]

The proposed best use for this dressing is to suppress the formation of exuberant granulation tissue and accelerate epithelialization in distal limb wounds. Although EA can be used in an acute clean wound for the entire healing period, it is probably best used after a healthy bed of granulation tissue develops or after trimming exuberant granulation tissue. EA is also indicated for accelerating healing of pinch-grafted wounds. In all cases, use of the dressing can be continued until healing is complete. Bandages can be placed over the dressing but is not required. Unbandaged EA is held in place by attaching it to skin with super glue (Figure 3.10).

Allogeneic EA is procured and stored according to Goodrich's recommendations.[69] EA should be harvested within the first 2 hours. The thin, transparent EA is separated from its umbilical attachments and from the

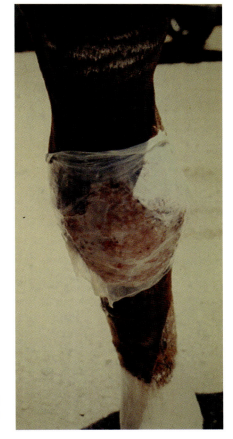

Figure 3.10. Example of a large wound over the left hock with an amnion dressing in place. The dressing was secured to the skin, at its proximal limits, with super glue. No further bandaging was required.

chorionic portion of the placenta, after which the latter two are discarded. Gross contaminants are removed from the EA with water irrigation. Areas in which contaminants cannot be removed should be debrided. Following cleansing, the EA is placed on a sterile impervious drape and cut into 5 cm × 5 cm segments. Segments are washed in a 0.05% solution of chlorhexidine diacetate (1 : 40 dilution of the 2% concentrate) and rinsed in tap water. They are then placed in plastic containers containing 0.05% chlorhexidine diacetate solution and refrigerated at 4°C until use. Amnion can be stored for 3 to 6 months prior to use. If longer storage is required, the EA dressings can be frozen in sterile specimen cups. The frozen dressings should be transferred to a refrigerator 24 hours prior to use to ensure full thawing.

Equine Peritoneum (EP)

EP consists of squamous epithelium overlying a thin layer of connective tissue that is rich in collagen. It has been theorized that when applied as an allogeneic dressing, peritoneum would enhance healing of wounds on the distal extremities of horses. However, one study in horses found no significant differences in healing between peritoneum-dressed wounds of the distal extremities and other wounds dressed with either a biologic dressing or a control non-biologic dressing.[70]

Split-Thickness Allogeneic Skin (STS)

STS is believed to accelerate second intention healing. One study, however, found that wounds dressed with split-thickness allogeneic skin did not heal faster than similar wounds dressed with peritoneum, an acellular matrix, or a synthetic dressing.[70]

Omentum (O)

O, which has a rich blood supply, has been used in dogs and cats to treat chronic non-healing wounds and to support healing of full-thickness skin mesh grafts.[71] The O is tunneled through the abdominal wall and retains its blood supply. Although this technique seems appealing, the use of O in horses appears to be limited due to the O's short attachment fixing it to the stomach.

Collagen Dressings (CDs)

CDs that are made into gels (Collasate®), porous and nonporous membranes, particles (Collamend™), freeze-dried oxidized regenerated cellulose (Promogran®), powder (HyCure®), and porous collagen sponges (Skin Temp®) reportedly enhance wound healing in humans and laboratory animals. Studies evaluating bovine porous and nonporous collagen membranes or gel dressings in horses found no benefit of this dressing over semi-occlusive dressed controls.[72,73] Another study in horses found that porous Skin Temp®-dressed wounds had more frequent scab formation than did control wounds dressed with non-adherent gauze.[73] The fact that scabs formed indicated that the wound surface became dehydrated and therefore the dressing was not acting in an occlusive or semi-occlusive manner. A study found that clean contaminated wounds in dogs dressed with hydrolyzed bovine collagen had a significantly increased rate of epithelialization compared to those dressed with a semi-occlusive non-adherent control dressing.[74]

Promogran® freeze-dried matrix was designed to modify the chronic wound environment by decreasing the activity of key matrix metalloproteinases (MMPs) in the wound fluid.[75] In the presence of wound exudate the dressing absorbs liquid, forming a soft, conformable, biodegradable gel that physically binds and inactivates MMPs. The gel also binds naturally occurring growth factors within the wound and protects them from degradation by proteinases. These growth factors are then released back into the wound in an active form as the gel is slowly broken down.[38]

Collagen sponges impregnated with gentamicin have been used for many years in human soft tissue and orthopedic surgery.[63] For more information, see gentamicin-impregnated collagen sponges under Antibiotic-impregnated Collagen Sponges, above.

Extracellular Matrix (ECM)

A significant body of work has been conducted over the past decade showing that porcine origin acellular ECM scaffolds facilitate constructive, tissue-specific replacement of diverse tissue structures.[76] The ECM scaffolds have been shown to exert a profound angiogenic effect, and although there is immune recognition, it occurs without rejection. ECM apparently has the capability of recruiting marrow-derived stem cells to migrate into the acellular scaffold, resulting in constructive remodeling of the severely damaged or missing tissue.[77] The healed, remodeled tissue is associated with differentiated cell and tissue types including functional arteries and veins, innervated smooth muscle, cartilage, and specialized epithelial structures.[78] Additionally, minimal scar tissue is found in the healed wounds.

Two porcine ECM scaffolds are available to veterinarians: porcine urinary bladder basement membrane (PUBBM) (ACell Vet®) and porcine small intestinal submucosa (PSIS) (Vet BioSISt®). Both products are considered to be biologic devices. A recent study determined that Vet BioSISt® offered no apparent advantage over a non-biological dressing for the treatment of small, granulating wounds on the distal limbs of horses.[70] This said, ECM scaffolds are not intended for applications in which natural healing results in normal or near normal tissue structure and function.[79] ACell Vet® has been on the market for a shorter period and has not been evaluated extensively. The perceived best use for the PUBBM is in large avulsion injuries of the distal extremity (Figure 3.4) (For more information, see The Extracellular Matrix as a Biologic Scaffold for Wound Healing in Veterinary Medicine later in this chapter).

Recently, a synthetic ECM (EquitrX™) became available. According to the company, EquitrX™ is a chemically modified GAG including hyaluronan (HA) suspended in an ECM to fabricate films, sponges, and injectable HGs. The dressing is biocompatible, noninflammatory, and biodegradable at controlled rates and is nonimmunogenic. The product can be used alone or in combination with growth factors, drugs, or autologous cells. The company boasts accelerated scar-free healing in the skin of horses and dogs. A preliminary trial in eight horses with experimentally created distal limb wounds found that wounds treated with Equifilm™ (the sheet form of EquitrX™) healed significantly faster than control treated wounds.[80]

Protein-Free Dialysate of Calf Blood (PFD)

PFD is commercially available (Solcoseryl®). An equine study aimed at enhancing the acute inflammatory response during repair of deep wounds found that in the first month of repair, Solcoseryl® provoked a greater inflammatory response, faster wound contraction, and faster formation of granulation tissue.[81] The continued use of Solcoseryl® beyond the first month of healing inhibited repair by causing protracted inflammation and delayed epithelialization. The perceived best use is for deep wounds during the early inflammatory phase; treatment should be discontinued at the first signs of epithelialization.

Platelet-Rich Plasma (PRP)

Platelets are well known for their role in hemostasis, where they help prevent blood loss at sites of vascular injury.[82] Platelets also release growth factors, cytokines, chemokines, and newly synthesized metabolites that promote tissue repair and influence the reactivity of cells involved in angiogenesis and inflammation.[82,83] The fact that platelets secrete these healing promoters indicates that their use could have a positive influence in clinical situations. One strategy is to prepare a platelet concentrate suspended in plasma, also known as platelet-rich plasma (PRP). The PRP contains both a high number of platelets and the full complement of secretory proteins.[84,85] PRP can either be prepared from the patient's blood (autologous source) or obtained commercially as a homologous source. For more information regarding PRP, see Chapter 1, Wound Repair: Problems in the Horse and Innovative Solutions.

Liquid Adhesives

Cyanoacrylates (CAL)

CAL is one of a group of adhesive chemical compounds which have been shown to be hemostatic and bacteriostatic. It is well tolerated by mammalian tissues and has been used as a surface dressing on animals and humans. A study in rats to assess the healing of full-thickness (2.5 cm × 1.5 cm) experimentally created skin wounds found that cyranoacrylate-sprayed wounds showed reduced edema, inflammatory infiltrates, and granulation tissue compared to controls.[86] A study conducted in horses to evaluate the effects of BC (Nexaband®) on experimentally created 7 cm × 4 cm full-thickness skin wounds on the dorsal metacarpus/metatarsus found

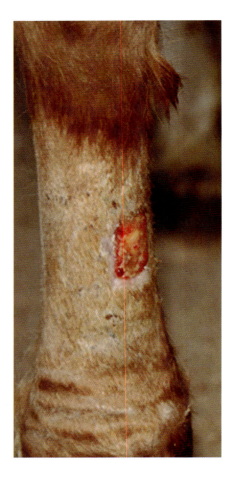

Figure 3.11. Example of a small wound on the medial metacarpal region that would benefit from cyranoacrylate or hydroxyethylated amylopectin dressing.

that healing of the unbandaged BC-treated wounds was equivalent to that of control wounds that were dressed for the entire healing period with an HC. The time required to apply the bandage to control wounds was longer than that to apply BC and both were effective in preventing the formation of exuberant granulation tissue. In this same report, BC was used to treat traumatic wounds to the distal extremities in 10 clinical cases; all wounds healed without the development of exuberant granulation tissue.[87] The proposed best use would be as a protective barrier for small (<10 cm in diameter), clean, limb wounds over the entire healing period.

Hydroxyethylated Amylopectin (HEA)

HEA (Facilatator®), a new patented product, is a polymeric gel which, upon drying over the wound, forms an adhesive barrier. According to the manufacturer the dressing is non-occlusive and water-soluble and can be used in the treatment of many types of wounds. The product is to be thinly applied to the surface of a clean dry wound and re-applied every third day thereafter until healing is complete. The proposed best use is as an effective protective barrier for small, dry, clean wounds of the distal extremities (Figure 3.11).

Conclusion

The selection of a dressing for treatment of wounds destined to heal by second intention or to be treated by delayed closure can be important to the outcome. Different dressings promote healing during different phases of the wound healing process (Box 3.1).

Generally speaking, clean acute wounds are best dressed with an occlusive dressing until a healthy bed of granulation tissue develops. During the transition from inflammation to the formation of granulation tissue, alginate dressings are recommended. Once granulation tissue develops, a semi-occlusive dressing is

---

Box 3.1.

Dressing Selection for Promotion of Healing During Different Phases of Repair

Inflammatory/Cellular Debridement Phase

1. **Occlusive dressings**: Use for clean or contaminated non-infected wounds until healthy granulation tissue forms.
   - Exceptions are Vulketan® and silicone gels, which can be used throughout the entire healing period.
   - Occlusive dressings promote autolytic wound debridement.
2. **Adherent, hydrophilic, and antimicrobial dressings**: Use for heavily contaminated/infected exudative wounds.
   - Discontinue when a healthy bed of granulation tissue is formed.
   - Gauze roll or strips can be used for packing tunneled and undermined wounds; the dressing fills in the dead space and provides drainage.
3. **Alginate dressings**: Use to "kick start" healing in chronic slow/non-healing wounds.
   - Hydrate dressing for dry wounds.
4. **Acemannan-containing dressings**: Use to promote granulation tissue formation in wounds over exposed bone.
   - Discontinue when a healthy bed of granulation tissue is formed.
5. **Protein-free dialysate of calf blood dressings**: Use to promote granulation tissue and contraction in deep wounds.
   - Discontinue at the first signs of epithelialization.
6. **Oxidized regenerated cellulose/collagen**: Use to promote healing in a chronic wound.
   - Inactivates matrix metalloproteinases and binds growth factors, releasing them back into the wound in an active form as the gel is slowly broken down.

Repair Phase

1. **Semi-occlusive dressings**: Use once granulation tissue develops.
   - Sometimes used for the entire healing period in clean, non-infected wounds.
   - Not good for autolytic debridement.
2. **Vulketan® and silicone gels**: Use to promote moist healing.
   - Prevents the formation of exuberant granulation tissue.

All Phases

1. **Vulketan® and silicone gels**: Use to promote moist healing.
   - Suppresses the formation of exuberant granulation tissue and the development of infection in the distal extremities.
2. **Liquid adhesives**: Provide protective barrier for small (<10 cm in diameter), clean limb wounds.
3. **Biologic dressings**: Use to stimulate healing.
   - ECM dressings provide constructive remodeling of clean large avulsive wounds and tendon deficits
   - Some biologic dressings include autologous and homologous platelet-rich plasma gels.

---

recommended. Heavily contaminated or infected wounds are best treated with adherent dressings or hydrophilic or antimicrobial dressings until a healthy bed of granulation tissue develops, at which time a semi-occlusive dressing is selected for the repair phase. Although reports on biologic bioactive dressings are limited, and in some cases conflicting, these represent an important category of dressings that will undoubtedly achieve more use in the future.

References

1. Turner TD: The development of wound management products. In D Krasner, G Rodeheaver, and G Sibbald, editors. *Chronic wound care: a clinical source book for healthcare professionals (3rd edition)* Wayne, PA: HMP communications, 2001, p.293

2. Turner TD: Interactive dressings used in the management of human soft tissue injuries and their potential in veterinary practice. Vet Dermatol 1997;8:235

3. Liptak JM: An overview of the topical management of wounds. Aust Vet J 1997;75:408

4. Stashak TS: Wound dressings: indications and best use, Proc North Am Vet Conf 2007;21:205

5. Alvarez OM, Hefton JM, Eaglstein WH: Grand rounds: healing wounds: occlusion or exposure. Infections in Surgery 1984;3:173

6. Feldman DL, Rogers A, Karpinski HS: A prospective trial comparing Biomembrane, Duoderm and Xerofoam for skin graft donor sites. Surg Gynec Obstet 1991;173:1

7. Stashak TS, Farstvedt E, Othic A: Update on wound dressings: indication and best use. Clin Tech Equine Pract 2004;3:148

8. Blackford JT, Latimer FG, Wan PY: Clinical use of wet-to-dry bandages to debride extremity lacerations in horses. Am Assoc Equine Pract 1995;41:52

9. Pain R, Sneddon JC, Cochrane CA: An in vitro study of the effectiveness of different dressings for debriding fibrin in blood clots from horses. Vet Record 2006;159:712

10. Lim FK, Smith MJ, McTavish J, et al: Normal saline wound dressing—is it really normal. Br J Plastic Surg 2000;53:42

11. Campbell BG: Current concepts and materials in wound bandaging. Proc North Am Vet Conf 2004;18:1217

12. Swaim SF, Gillette RL: An update on wound medications and dressings. Compend Contin Educ 1998;20:1133

13. McFadden EA: Multidex gel for use in wound care. J Pediatr Nurs 1997;12:125

14. Rodeheaver R, Stashak TS: Evaluation of calcium alginate as a wound dressing in horses. In progress

15. Segal HC, Hunt BJ, Bilding K: Effects of alginate and non-alginate wound dressings on blood coagulation and platelet activation. J Biomater Appl 1998;12:249

16. Thomas A, Harding KG, Moore K: Alginates from wound dressings activate human macrophages to secrete tumor necrosis factor-alpha. Biomaterials 2000;21:797

17. Gustafson S: Personal communication 2007

18. Cockbill SME, Turner TD: Management of veterinary wounds. Vet Record 1995;136:362

19. Fanucci D, Seese J: Multi-faceted use of calcium alginates. Ostomy Wound Manage 1991;37:16

20. Tizard I, Busbee D, Maxwell B, et al: Effects of Acemannan, a complex carbohydrate, on wound healing in young and aged rats. Wounds 1994;6:201

21. Bradley DM: The effects of topically-applied Acemannan on the healing of wounds with exposed bone. PhD thesis, Auburn University, 1998

22. Swaim S: Personal communication 2007

23. Okamoto Y, Shibazaki K, Minami S: Evaluation of chitin and chitosan on open wound healing in dogs. J Vet Sci 1995;57:851

24. Jones V, Harding K: Moist wound healing. In D Krasner, G Rodeheaver and G Sibbald editors. *Chronic wound care: a clinical source book for healthcare professionals (3rd edition)* Wayne, PA: HMP communications, 2001, p.245

25. Dolynchuk KN: Debridement. In D Krasner, G Rodeheaver and G Sibbald, editors. *Chronic wound care: a clinical source book for healthcare professionals (3rd edition)* Wayne, PA: HMP communications, 2001, p.385

26. Katz MH, Alvarez AF, Kirsner RS, et al: Human wound fluid from acute wounds simulates fibroblast and endothelial cell growth. J Am Acad Dermatol 1991;25:1054

27. Kunimoto BT: Growth factors in wound healing. In D Krasner, G Rodeheaver and G Sibbald, editors. *Chronic wound care: a clinical source book for healthcare professionals (3rd edition)* Wayne, PA: HMP communications, 2001, p.391

28. Jones V, Harding K: Moist wound healing. In D Krasner, G Rodeheaver and G Sibbald, editors. *Chronic wound care: a clinical source book for healthcare professionals (3rd edition)* Wayne, PA: HMP communications, 2001, p.245

29. Blackford JT, Wan PY, Latimer FG, et al: Treatment of distal extremity lacerations using a flexible hydroactive occlusive dressing. Proc Am Assoc Equine Pract 1993;39:215

30. Morgan PW, Binnington AG, Miller CW, et al: The effects of occlusive and semi-occlusive dressings on the healing of acute full-thickness wounds on the forelimbs of dogs. Vet Surgery 1994;23:494

31. Howard RD, Stashak TS, Baxter GM: Evaluation of occlusive dressings for management of full thickness wounds on distal limbs of horses. Am J Vet Res 1993;54:50

32. Dyson M, Young S, Pendle CL, et al: Comparison of the effects of moist and dry conditions on dermal repair. J Invest Dermatol 1988;91:434

33. Federal Registration. 1999;64:53972–9

34. Flanagan M: The efficacy of hydrogel in the treatment of wounds with non-viable tissue. J Wound Care 1995;6:264

35. Kirker KR, Luo Y, Nielson JH, et al: Glycosaminoglycan hydrogel films as bio-interactive dressings for wound healing. Biomaterials 2002;23:3661

36. Dart AJ, Cries L, Jeffcott LB, et al: Effects of 25% propylene glycol hydrogel (Solugel) on second intention wound healing in horses. Vet Surg 2002;31:309

37. Agren MS: An amorphous hydrogel enhances epithelialization of wounds. Acta Dermatol Venereol 1998;8:119
38. Theoret C: What's new and innovative in wound management: problems and solutions. Proc Am Assoc Equine Pract 2006;52:265
39. Engelen M, Besche B, Lefay MP, et al: Effects of ketanserin on hypergranulation tissue formation, infection, and healing of equine lower limb wounds. Can Vet J 2004;45:144
40. Ovington L, Peirce B: Wound dressings: form, function, feasibility, and fact. In D Krasner, G Rodeheaver and G Sibbald, editors. *Chronic wound care: a clinical source book for healthcare professionals (3rd edition)* Wayne, PA: HMP communications, 2001, p.311
41. Eaglstein WH: Experiences with biosynthetic dressings. J Am Acad Dermatol 1985;12:434
42. Grange-Pruiner A, Couilliet D, Guillaume JC: Allergic contact dermatitis to the Comfeel hydrocolloid dressing. Ann Dermatol Venereol 2002;129:725
43. Reno F, Sabbatini M, Lombardi F, et al: In vitro mechanical compression induces apoptosis and regulates cytokines release in hypertrophic scars. Wound Repair Regen 2003;11:331
44. Ricketts CH, Martin L, Faria DT, et al: Cytokine mRNA changes during the treatment of hypertrophic scars with silicone and non-silicone gel dressings. Dermatol Surg 1996;22:955
45. Ducharme-Desjarlais M, Lepault É, Céleste C, Theoret CL: Determination of the effect of a silicone dressing (CicaCare®) on second intention healing of full-thickness wounds of the distal limb of horses. Am J Vet Res 2005;66:1133
46. Lee AH, Swaim SF, McGuire JA, et al: Effects of nonadherent dressing materials on the healing of open wounds in dogs. J Am Vet Med Assoc 1987;190:416
47. Eaglstein WH: Effect of occlusive dressings on wound healing. Clin Dermatol 1984;2:107
48. Alvarez OM, Mertz BA, Eaglstein WH: The effects of occlusive dressings on collagen synthesis and re-epithelialization in superficial wounds. J Surg Res 1983;35:142
49. Carter K: Hydropolymer dressings in the management of wound exudates. Br J Community Nursing (Suppl 9) 2003;8:10
50. Swaim SF: Advances in wound healing in small animal practice: current status and lines of development. Vet Dermatol 1997;8:249
51. Moore K, Thomas A, Harding KG: Iodine released from the wound dressing Iodosorb modulates the secretion of cytokines by human macrophages responding to bacterial lipopolysaccharide. Int J Biochem Cell Biol 1997;29:163
52. Mertz PM, Oliveria-Gandia MF, Davis SC: The evaluation of cadexomer iodine wound dressing on methicillin resistant *Staphylococcus aureus* (MRSA) in acute wounds. Dermatol Surg 1999;25:89
53. Thorn RM, Greenman J, Austin A: An in vitro study of antimicrobial activity and efficacy of iodine-generating hydrogel dressings. Wound Care 2006;15:305
54. Ivins N, Simmonds W, Turner A, et al: The use of an oxygenating hydrogel dressing in VLU. Wounds UK 2007;3:1
55. Berry DB, Sullins KE: Effects of topical application of antimicrobials and bandaging on healing and granulation tissue formation in wounds of the distal aspect of the limbs in horses. Am J Vet Res 2003;64:88
56. Angelique MR, Rodeheaver GT: Effectiveness of a new antimicrobial gauze dressing as a bacteria barrier (pamphlet) Kendall, Wound care research and development, Mansfield, MA, 2001
57. Lee WR, Tobias KM, Bemis DA, et al: In vitro efficacy of a polyhexamethylene biguanide–impregnated gauze dressing against bacteria found in veterinary patients. Vet Surg 2004;33:404
58. Adams AP, Santschi EM, Mellencamp MA: Antibacterial properties of a silver-coated nylon wound dressing. Vet Surg 1999;28:219
59. Ip M, Lui SL, Poon V, et al: Antimicrobial activities of silver dressings: an in vitro comparison. J Med Microbl 2006;55:59
60. Burd A, Kwok CH, Hung SC, et al: A comparative study of the cytotoxicity of silver-based dressings in monolayer cell, tissue explant, and animal models. Wound Repair Regen 2007;15:94
61. Frost MR, Jackson SW, Stevens PJ: Adsorption of bacteria onto activated charcoal cloth: an effect of potential importance in the treatment of infected wounds. Microbias Letters 1980;13:135
62. Knottenbelt DC: Healing "problem wounds" in the horse. Comments contained in a letter 2002
63. Stemberger A, Grimm H, Bader F, et al: Local treatment of bone and soft tissue infections with collagen gentamicin sponge. Eur J Surg 1997;578:17
64. Summerhays GES: Treatment of traumatically induced synovial sepsis in horses with gentamicin-impregnated collagen sponges. Vet Rec 2000;147:184
65. Letsch R, Rosenthal E, Joka T: A comparative study of two local antibiotic carriers in the treatment of osteomyelits of long bones. In A Stemberger, editor. *Collagen as a drug carrier. Some applications in surgery (1st edition).* London: Franklin Scientific Projects, 1991, p.109
66. Grzybowski J, Kolodziez W, Trafny EA, et al: A new anti-infective collagen dressing containing antibiotics. J Biomed Res 1997;36:163
67. Hunt TK: Basic principles of wound healing. J Trauma Supplement 1990;30:122

68. Bigbie RB, Schumacher J, Swaim SF, et al: Effects of amnion and live yeast cell derivative on second intention healing in horses. Am J Vet Res 1991;52:1376

69. Goodrich LR, Moll DH, Crisman MV, et al: Comparison of equine amnion and a non-adherent wound dressing material for bandaging pinch-grafted wounds in ponies. Am J Vet Res 2000;61:326

70. Gomez JH, Schumacher J, Lauten SD, et al: Effects of 3 biologic dressings of healing of cutaneous wounds on the limbs of horses. Can J Vet Res 2004;68:49

71. Smith BA, Hosgood G, Hedlund CS: Omental pedicle used to manage a large dorsal wound in a dog. J Small Animal Pract 1995;36:267

72. Bertone A, Sullins KE, Stashak TS, et al: Effect of wound location and the use of topical collagen gel on exuberant granulation tissue formation and wound healing in the horse and pony. Am J Vet Res 1985;46:1438

73. Yvorchuk-St.Jean K, Gaughan E: Evaluation of a porous bovine collagen membrane bandage for management of wounds in horses. Am J Vet Res 1995;56:1663

74. Swaim SF, Gillette RL, Sartin EA: Effects of a hydrolyzed collagen dressing on the healing of open wounds in dogs. Abstr, Scott-Ritchey Research Center, 2003

75. Cullen B, Smith R, McCulloch E, et al: Mechanism of action of PROMOGRAN, a protease modulating matrix, for the treatment of diabetic foot ulcers. Wound Repair Regen 2002;10:16

76. Badylak SF, Lantz GC, Coffey AC, et al: Small intestinal submucosa as a large diameter vascular graft in the dog. J Surg Res 1989;47:74

77. Badylak SF, Park K, Peppas N, et al: Marrow-derived cells populate scaffolds composed of xenogeneic extracellular matrix. Exp Hematol 2001;29:1310

78. Cook JL, Tomlinson JL, Kreeger JM, et al: Induction of meniscal regeneration in dogs using a novel biomaterial. Am J Sports Med 1999;27:65

79. Badylak SF: Extracellular matrix as a scaffold for tissue engineering in veterinary medicine: applications to soft tissue healing. Clin Tech Equine Pract 2004;3:172

80. Mann BK, Scott JA, Rees R, et al: Enhanced wound healing in horses and dogs using crosslinked hyaluronic acid-based films. Poster presented at the Society for Biomaterials Annual Meeting, Chicago, IL, April 2007

81. Wilmink JM, Stolk PW, van Weeren PR, et al: The effectiveness of haemodialystae Solcoseryl® for second intention wound healing in horses and ponies. J Vet Med A Physiol Pathol Clin Med 2000;47:311

82. Anitua E, Andia I, Ardanza B, et al: Autologous platelets as a source of proteins for healing and tissue regeneration. Thromb Haemost 2004;91:4

83. Pietrzak WS, Eppley BL: Platelet rich plasma: biology and new technology. J Craniofac Surg 2005;16:1043

84. Marx RD: Platelet-rich plasma (PRP): what is PRP and what is not PRP. Implant Dentistry 2001;10:225

85. Carter CA, Jolly DG, Worden CE, et al: Platelet rich plasma gel promotes differentiation and regeneration during equine wound healing. Exp Mol Pathol 2003;74:244

86. Bhaskar SN, Cutright DE: Healing of skin wounds with butyl cyanoacrylate. J Dent Res 1969;48:294

87. Blackford J, Shires M, Goble D, et al: The use of n-butyl cyranoacrylate in the treatment of open leg wounds in the horse. Proc Am Assoc Equine Pract 1986;32:349

3.2 Topical Wound Treatments and Wound Care Products

Ellis Farstvedt, DVM, MS, Diplomate ACVS, and Ted S. Stashak, DVM, MS, Diplomate ACVS

Introduction

The equine practitioner can choose from a myriad of topical wound care products. Importantly, much of the data available on these products has been obtained from their use in species other than the horse or through in vitro experiments. The practitioner should be aware that favorable results obtained through these research trials have not been reproduced reliably when tested in vivo on wounds in horses.

The physiological aim of topical wound treatment is to remove foreign debris and/or reduce bacterial contamination in a manner exerting minimal impact on the cellular activities required for healing to progress.

Wound location and depth, degree of contamination, and duration since injury should direct the clinician's choice of product. The frequency of use as well as a change of product should depend on the stage of healing and the clinical response to treatment.

The intent of this section is to provide the clinician with a workable knowledge of common topical wound care products currently in use.

Wound Cleansers

An ideal wound cleansing agent combines antiseptic and cleansing properties while minimizing cytotoxicity. These products are typically used during the inflammatory phase of healing to remove foreign material, decrease bacterial load, and rid the wound of necrotic tissue. Interestingly, there is no data on the use of these products in wounds destined to be closed by suturing.

Commercial Soaps

Commercial soaps have been used in the initial preparation of heavily contaminated wounds to remove large amounts of foreign material. Although these products are good skin cleansers, they can be harmful to the healing wound. The following products were tested in vitro on human fibroblasts and keratinocytes: (1) Dial liquid antibacterial soap, (2) Dove moisturizing body wash, and (3) Ivory liquid-gel.[1] In this trial, Dove and Ivory required a 1:100,000 dilution to render them non-toxic to fibroblasts while Dove moisturizing body wash required a 1:10,000 dilution to become non-toxic.[1] When tested on keratinocytes, all three products required a 1:1,000 dilution to become non-toxic.[1] Given this alarming information, the clinician should avoid using commercial soap products for cleansing a wound.

Commercial Wound Cleansers

The cleansing activity of many commercial wound cleansers depends upon a surfactant that breaks the bonds between foreign bodies and the wound surface.[2] Unfortunately, most ionic surfactants and many nonionic surfactants have been shown to be toxic to cells, delay wound healing, and inhibit local defenses against infection.[3]

Constant-Clens™ was found to be the most biocompatible with human fibroblasts, red blood cells, and white blood cells in vitro when compared to Shur-Clens®, SAF-Clens™, Cara-Klenz™ and Ultra-Klenz™.[2] More recent data has shown that Shur-Clens®, SAF-Clens™, and saline were non-toxic to human fibroblasts in vitro (Constant-Clens™ was not included in this trial).[1] When tested on human keratinocytes, Shur-Clens™, Techni-Care™, and Biolex™ were found to be non-toxic.[1]

Equine Vet™ is a relatively new wound cleansing product. One formula contains acemannan, a wound healing stimulant, considered the active component of aloe vera.[4] The product is non-irritating and contains a surface modifier. The adjustable spray nozzle delivers a fluid stream of approximately 12 PSI at a distance of 15 cm. Although this product anecdotally appears to be an effective wound cleansing agent with minimal cytotoxic effects, no studies have compared it to other products. The healing properties of aloe vera and acemannan are discussed later in this chapter.

Vetricyn™(V) is a new cleansing solution that is the veterinary formulation of Dermacyn™(D), produced by using Microcyn® technology. V and D are super-oxidized water products created through electrolysis, resulting in a blend of reactive chlorine and oxygen species. The toxicity and corrosiveness of super-oxidized solutions result from the acidity/alkalinity and high levels of free available chlorine (FAC > 100 ppm). Microcyn technology creates a solution that has a neutral pH with a low FAC (<80 ppm) and is stable for more than 1 year.[5] Toxicity analyses performed in vitro on mouse fibroblasts and in vivo on full-thickness wound beds in rats showed no evidence of cell lysis or histopathologic changes.[6] D has also been reported to stabilize mast cells leading to control of Type I hypersensitivity reactions, suggesting that it is anti-allergenic.[7] (Figure 3.12).

Bactericidal, fungicidal, and sporocidal trials performed in accordance to Environmental Protection Agency (EPA) guidelines have shown that growth of the following organisms is totally inhibited by D: *Mycobacterium bovis* (5 minutes), *Pseudomonas aeruginosa* (10 minutes), *Staphylococcus aureus* (10 minutes), *Salmonella choleraesuis* (10 minutes), methicillin-resistant *S. aureus* (10 minutes), vancomycin-resistant *Enterococcus faecalis* (15 minutes), *Trychophyton mentagrophytes* (10 minutes), and *Bacillus atrophaeus* (15 minutes).[6]

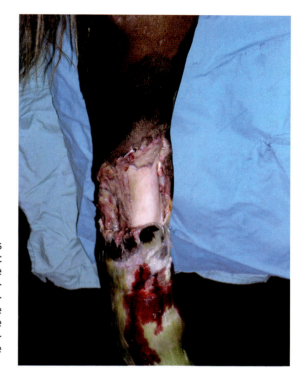

Figure 3.12. Example of a degloving wound to the metatarsus (2 to 3 days duration) that would benefit from irrigation with one of the non-toxic wound cleansers containing a surfactant (e.g., Constant-Clens™ or Equine Vet™). The surfactant would liquefy the exudate contaminated with bacteria (biofilm) at the edges of this wound. This should be followed by irrigation of the wound with an antimicrobial (e.g., Vetricyn™, povidone iodine [0.1% to 0.2%], or chlorhexidine [0.5%]) delivered at an oblique angle with a pressure of ~15 PSI. For more information regarding techniques for wound lavage, see Management Practices That Influence Wound Infection and Healing in Chapter 2.

When compared to 10% povidone iodine (PI) solution in a clinical trial of diabetic foot ulcers, it was found that D significantly decreased the number of positive microbial cultures, had an odds ratio of 3:4 for a successful outcome relative to PI, and significantly decreased healing times.[5] However, the concentration of PI used in this trial is far above the 0.1% to 0.2% solution recommended in the treatment of equine wounds. The authors are not aware of any equine-specific research involving V; however, reports of using D on human wounds is promising. The proposed best use for this product is during the inflammatory out to the repair phase of healing.

Derma-Clens® (DC) is an acidic wound cleansing ointment that contains benzoic, malic, and salicylic acids. According to the manufacturer, the low pH discourages bacterial and fungal growth in wounds. To the authors' knowledge there are currently no scientific reports that evaluate DC's effect on wound healing. Considering the low pH of Derma-Clens®, the authors recommend the use of cleansing solutions approaching a neutral pH. To this effect, a wide range in pH is found among commercial wound cleansing products (Table 3.2). In general, it is believed that products with a lower pH tend to be most cytotoxic. Dermal cleansers, wound/dermal cleansers, and wound antiseptic cleansers containing benzethonium chloride, a synthetic quaternary ammonium compound, tend to have a lower pH and therefore are considered more cytotoxic. See Table 3.3 for more information regarding commercial wound cleansers.

Commercial Fluids

Once the wound is clean, commercially available isotonic fluids are recommended for wound lavage. Saline (0.9% sodium chloride), Normosol-R, and lactated Ringer's solution (LRS) are examples of acceptable isotonic (Figure 3.13). When tested in vitro on human fibroblasts, 0.9% sodium chloride was found to be non-toxic; however, a 1:10 dilution was required to render it non-toxic to human keratinocytes.[1]

Tap Water

Tap water is an acceptable fluid choice for wound irrigation/cleansing. However, the hypotonicity of tap water will encourage cell swelling which can cause significant cell destruction with prolonged use.[8] It is recommended, in most cases, that irrigation with tap water cease at the first sign of granulation tissue formation in the wound bed.

Table 3.2. Commercial wound cleansers.

Wound cleanser	pH	Company
Constant-Clens	7.34	Covidien Animal Health/Kendall, Dublin, OH
Shur-Clens	7.26	Convatec, Princeton, NJ
SAF-Clens	6.7	Convatec, Princeton, NJ
Cara-Klenz wound and skin cleanser	5.62	Carrington Laboratories, Inc., Irving, TX
Ultra-Klenz	7.37	Carrington Laboratories, Inc., Irving, TX
Techni Care	6.5–7.8	Care-Tech Laboratories, Inc., St. Louis, MO
Biolex	5.5	Bard Medical Division, Covington, GA
Ultra-Klenz antiseptic cleanser	7.37	Carrington Laboratories, Inc., Irving, TX
Equine Vet acemannan wound cleanser	5.62	Carrington Laboratories, Inc., Irving, TX
Equine Vet antimicrobial wound cleanser	7.27	Carrington Laboratories, Inc., Irving, TX
Vetericyn	Neutral pH	Oculus Innovative Sciences, Petaluma, CA
Derma-Clens	2.8–3.6	Pfizer Animal Health www.pfizerah.com

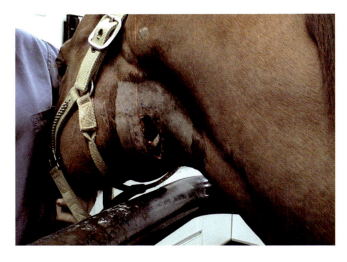

Figure 3.13. This clean, non-infected, 5-day-old wound involving the throat latch region (head is to the left; linguofacial vein is seen in the bottom one-third of the wound) is at the beginning of the repair phase of healing. Sterile saline solution can be used to irrigate the wound at this time. A stent bandage has been used to minimize environmental contamination. For more information regarding methods of stent bandaging, see Chapter 16.

Antiseptics

Povidone Iodine

Povidone iodine (PI) solution (10%) has a broad range of antimicrobial activity that lasts for 4 to 6 hours following application. Solutions diluted to 0.1% to 0.2% (10–20 ml/1,000 ml) are recommended to minimize cytotoxicity and increase the availability of free iodine for its antimicrobial action. At this concentration the PI solution kills bacteria within 15 seconds and there is no known bacterial resistance to the product. On the other hand, PI at a concentration of 5% has been shown to inhibit white blood cell migration, resulting in increased wound infection compared to irrigation with 1% PI or saline.[9]

PI (1%) solution used for irrigation of abdominal incisions after closure of the peritoneum was shown to be significantly superior to saline in reducing post surgical wound infection.[9] PI (0.5%) powder sprayed in contaminated incision wound beds following gastrointestinal surgery significantly reduced infection rates to 9.9% compared to 24.4% for non-sprayed control wounds.[10] Bacterial contamination (confirmed by cultures) at the time of surgery was associated with 52% infection rates in control groups, whereas the infection rate was reduced to 11% in the PI-treated group.[10] Irrigation with 1% PI does not appear to affect gain of tensile strength in healing wounds.[11] PI is inactivated by organic material and blood; serum has been shown to inactivate PI within 2 minutes of contact.[12]

PI ointment (10%) is available for topical wound treatment. In an ex vivo rat model, 10% PI ointment had a negative effect on microcirculation.[13] When applied to human autografts and epidermal sheets, 10% PI ointment caused severe, detrimental effects on tissue histopathology.[14] However, an in vivo wound trial in horses did not find a delay in wound healing when using 10% PI ointment.[15]

Hyperthyroidism, thyrotoxicosis, and hypothyroidism have been reported in humans subjected to repeated contact with PI.[16,17,18] The symptoms, are transient, and most disappear upon discontinuing use of the compound. When PI is combined with a surfactant to form a detergent, it was found to be harmful to wound tissues and to potentiate infection.[19] Dermal hypersensitivity can occur with the use of PI in humans and small animals; however, this reaction is not usually observed in the horse.

The proposed best use of PI solution is for irrigation of a contaminated wound at 0.1% to 0.2% dilution (Figures 3.12 and 3.14).

Chlorhexidine Diacetate

Chlorhexidine diacetate (CHD) solution (2%) has a wide antimicrobial spectrum and prolonged residual effect due to its ability to bind protein in the *stratum corneum*. Advantages of CHD over PI are its residual antibacterial capacity and continued activity in the presence of blood, pus, and organic debris, with less systemic absorption. A potential drawbacks are that *Proteus* and *Pseudomonas* have developed or possess an inherent resistance to this product and it has no effect against fungi or Candida.[20] Contact with the cornea must be avoided because ocular toxicity occurs upon direct contact. There appears to be a narrow margin of dilution safety.

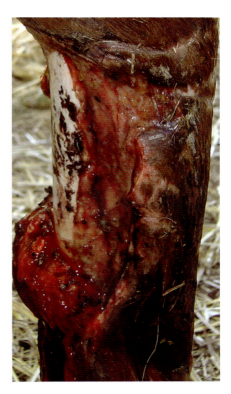

Figure 3.14. Example of a severely contaminated degloving wound of the metatarsus that would benefit from irrigation with either PI (0.1% to 0.2% dilution) or CHD (0.05% dilution) delivered to the wound surface at 10–15 PSI. Courtesy Dr. C. Rogers.

Historically, in vitro cytotoxicity studies have been unreliable as predictors of in vivo wound activity. An in vivo controlled trial using full-thickness wounds in dogs irrigated daily using low pressure lavage with various preparations of 0.05% CHD revealed no significant difference in the percent of wound contraction, epithelialization, or healing compared to controls irrigated with either sterile water or LRS titrated to pH 7.4.[21] The only significant difference found in this study was that of in vitro bacterial testing in which all CHD solutions had a 100% kill rate.[21]

In another in vivo study involving full-thickness wounds in dogs, CHD (0.05%, 0.5%, and 1%) was found to be superior to PI (0.1%, 0.25%, and 0.5%) in reducing wound tissue bacterial load at 48 hours.[22] When comparing in vivo wound healing in dogs using 0.5% CHD solution versus 1% PI, the authors concluded that wound irrigation with CHD favored more rapid healing and contraction over that seen with PI or saline.[23] This study also confirmed that cytotoxicity in vitro is not an adequate model for the study of antiseptic effects on wound healing.[23] Currently a 0.05% solution (1:40 dilution = 25 ml of CHD to 975 ml of solution) is recommended for wound lavage. Concentrations > 0.05% CHD have been shown to delay wound healing (Figure 3.14).[24]

Chlorhexidine ointment is supplied as 1% chlorhexidine acetate (CHA). This concentration of CHA has been shown to delay wound healing, as mentioned above. The authors are unaware of any clinical studies examining this ointment formulation. Chlorhexidine gluconate is typically the compound that is present in soap products (e.g., Hibiclens) and is widely used as a skin disinfectant. Chlorhexidine gluconate (0.05%) has been shown to be toxic to human keratinocytes and fibroblasts.[25] The effects of chlorhexidine gluconate on horse tissues have yet to be examined.

Hydrogen Peroxide

Hydrogen peroxide (HP) (3%) is an effective sporocide, but has a narrow antimicrobial spectrum. Stock solutions of 3% have been shown to be cytotoxic to fibroblasts and result in thrombosis of microvasculature.[26] The toxicity of HP to fibroblasts exceeds its anti-bacterial potency; therefore, it is unsuitable as a wound cleansing solution.[27] Nonetheless, HP appears to be an effective chemical debriding agent.[2]

Dakin's Solution

The use of Dakin's solution (DS) (sodium hypochlorite) was first described by Alexis Carrel during World War I for the treatment of open wounds.[28] DS has a broad antimicrobial spectrum. It has been shown to be more effective than PI and CHD in killing *Staphylococcus aureus*.[29] The bactericidal effect is from the release of chlorine and oxygen. DS was shown to be cytotoxic to fibroblasts in vitro at concentrations of 0.025% and has a narrow margin of dilution safety.[30,31] The clinical indication for DS is to aid in removal of necrotic tissue; therefore, it should never be used on a clean wound.[3] Although DS should not be used routinely as a topical disinfectant, when used for debridement it should be diluted to one-quarter strength (0.125%).[32]

In a pinch, dilute 5% sodium hypochlorite with tap water to achieve a 0.025% solution. In a study evaluating field water from five different sources to dilute sodium hypochlorite, no bacterial growth was found from any of the sources.[33]

Acetic Acid

Acetic Acid (AA) can be used as an antimicrobial agent in wound cleansing. AA (0.25%) requires a 1:10 dilution (0.025%) to be made non-toxic to human fibroblasts and keratinocytes in vitro.[1] AA is typically prepared as a 0.5% or 0.25% solution, which is effective against *Pseudomonas* organisms.[27] Toxicity against fibroblasts and retardation of wound epithelialization outweigh the benefits of AA's bactericidal activity,[27] suggesting that AA is not suitable for wound care.

Acid Replacement Solution-1050

The use of acid replacement solution (ARS)-1050 (Banixx™ Wound and Hoof Care) was recently reported for the treatment of hoof and skin infections and for open wounds in the horse.[34] Tri-hydrated hydronium is the active ingredient in this solution. Concentrated ARS was diluted with water (20 ml to 1,000 ml of water) to achieve a pH of 1.5, and the resultant solution was placed in a spray bottle for topical use. In the case of a foot abscess or an extensive limb wound, the solution was used to saturate gauze pads or sheet cotton dressing before they were applied, while body wounds were sprayed. In either case the solution was re-applied daily until the infection resolved or the wound healed. The observed debridement and antimicrobial effects were attributed to the solution's acidic pH. The perceived best use for this product is for chemical debridement of a chronic infected wound during the inflammatory phase of wound healing.

See Table 3.3 for additional details about antiseptics.

Topical Antibiotics

Topical antibiotics are most effective when applied within 3 hours of wounding.[26] However, if the wound is completely debrided, thus creating a new wound, topical antibiotics can be applied within 3 hours of debridement and are considered effective.

Triple Antibiotic Ointment

Triple antibiotic (TA) ointment (bacitracin, polymixin B, and neomycin) has a wide antimicrobial spectrum but is ineffective against *Pseudomonas aeruginosa*.[27] The zinc component of bacitracin has been shown to stimulate epithelialization (increasing it by 25%), but can retard wound contraction. These antimicrobials are poorly absorbed; therefore, toxicity is rare. In the authors' experience, TA has been effective in preventing postoperative infection in wounds treated with island grafts (Figure 3.15).

Silver Sulfadiazine

Silver sulfadiazine (SS) has a wide antimicrobial spectrum including *Pseudomonas* spp. and fungi. It has been shown in some studies to increase epithelialization by 28%, while in others it slowed epithelialization and may have increased wound fragility.[35] Muller (2003) reported that the combination of aloe vera with SS reverses the inhibitory effects observed when using SS alone.[36] Berry (2003) did not observe in horses the increased rate

Table 3.3. Antiseptics.

Product	Active agent	Best use	Source
Betadine solution	Povidone iodine	Contaminated or infected wound lavage (dilute to 0.1%)	The Purdue Frederick Company Stamford, CT
Nolvasan solution	Chlorhexidine diacetate	Contaminated or infected wound lavage (dilute to 0.05%)	Fort Dodge Laboratories, Inc. Fort Dodge, IA
Hydrogen peroxide	Hydrogen peroxide	Chemical debridement (not recommended for routine use)	Household hydrogen peroxide
Modified Dakin's solution	Sodium hypochlorite	Contaminated or infected wound (dilute to 0.025%); chemical debridement	Household bleach
Vinegar	Acetic acid	Infected wounds (not recommended for routine use); chemical debridement	Household vinegar
Banixx™ Wound and Hoof Care	Tri-hydriated hydronium (ARS-1050)	Infected wounds (20 ml to 1 L water)	Sherborne Corp. Pinehurst, NC

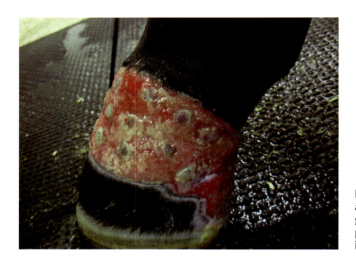

Figure 3.15. This wound is in the repair phase of healing. Triple antibiotic ointment was applied to the wound following punch grafting to prevent infection. Following grafting, the limb was placed in a short limb cast for 2 weeks. This picture was taken immediately after the cast removal.

of epithelialization or decreased rate of wound contraction reported in other species when SS was applied topically.[15] In this particular equine trial there was no significant difference in the rate of wound healing in relation to the topical treatment (1% SS cream, 1% slow release SS matrix, 10% PI ointment), provided exuberant granulation tissue was managed by sharp excision.[15] The authors concluded that a topical slow-release SS product should be used without a bandage if protection of deep structures, reduction of edema, or mechanical stabilization are not necessary because bandaging appeared to favor the development of exuberant granulation tissue in this model,[15] as reported previously by others.[37,38]

Nitrofurazone Ointment

Nitrofurazone ointment (NFO) has a good antimicrobial spectrum against Gram-positive and Gram-negative organisms, but has little effect against *Pseudomonas* spp. It has been shown to decrease epithelialization in laboratory animals and humans by some 24% and it delays wound contraction in horses.[26] The antibiotic Furacin, rather than the vehicle base, is incriminated for the delay in wound healing. NFO (0.02%) has also been shown to be toxic to cultured human keratinocytes and fibroblasts.[25] Although there is a plethora of information surrounding the carcinogenic potential of nitrofurazone, and it is recognized by the state of California as a cancer-causing substance, it is not listed as a carcinogen by the Occupational Safety and Health Association (OSHA).[39]

Gentamicin Sulfate

Gentamicin sulfate (GS) has a narrow antimicrobial spectrum, but it may be applied to wounds infected with Gram-negative bacteria, particularly *Pseudomonas aeruginosa*. In a canine study comparing the rate of healing of full-thickness skin defects treated topically with either a 0.1% GS solution or a 0.1% oil-in-water cream base, it was found that treatment with the 0.1% oil-in-water cream base slowed wound contraction and epithelialization.[27]

Cefazolin

Cefazolin (C) is an effective antimicrobial against Gram-positive and some Gram-negative organisms. When it is applied to a wound at a dose of 20 mg/kg, the concentration in the wound fluid remains above the MIC for a longer period than that observed when the same dose is administered systemically. The powder form provides a prolonged elevated tissue concentration compared to the solution. Therefore, C may be effective in treating established infections. C is also safe to use intrathecally and/or for regional limb perfusion. See chapters 9 and 10 for more information regarding these uses of C.

See Table 3.4 for additional details about topical antibiotics.

Table 3.4. Topical antibiotics.

Product	Active ingredient(s)	Best use	Source
Triple antibiotic (e.g., Neosporin)	Bacitracin zinc, Polymyxin B sulfate, Neomycin sulfate	All phases of wound healing; broad spectrum antimicrobial.	Pfizer Consumer Healthcare Morris Plains, NJ
Silvadine cream	1% silver sulfadiazine	Inflammatory to repair phases.	Monarch Pharmaceuticals, Inc. Bristol, TN
Fura-Zone ointment	0.2% Nitrofurazone	Inflammatory and debridement phases (slows epithelial growth and wound contraction)	Neogen Corp. Lexington, KY
Gentacin	Gentamicin sulfate	Infected wound as indicated by wound culture	
Cefazolin	Cefazolin sodium	Infected wound as indicated by wound culture	

Aerosol Sprays

Furazolidone

Furazolidone (F) aerosol powder is an antibacterial and antiprotozoal agent that is used in people for the treatment of cholera, *Giardia lamblia*, and bacterial diarrhea. Controlled trials using F topically on wounds are lacking in horses. One clinical report on nonhuman primates reported using F on fight-inflicted lacerations in which 74% of the outcomes were rated good to excellent.[40] In this report, *Staphylococcus, Bacillis, Streptococcus*, and *Pseudomonas* were shown to be sensitive to F.[40] *Staphylococcus aureus* isolated from wounds and abscesses on camels has been shown to be sensitive to F, while *Nocardia spp.* and *Aeromonas liquefaciens* isolates were resistant.[41] F is also thought to have some carcinogenic effects, although this data is not uniformly accepted. The proposed best use of this product is for minor abrasions.

Alu-Spray®

Alu-Spray® (AS) is indicated to create a physical barrier for protection of the wound from the surrounding environment. According to the manufacturer, it does not come off with hot or cold water but can be washed off with soap and water. The physical barrier can protect wounds from flies and gnats, common in the environment of horses. The perceived best use is for surgical sites that are not bandaged and for minor lacerations for open wound healing (Figure 3.16).

Cut-Heal®

Cut-Heal® (CH) contains fish oil, raw linseed oil, turpentine, balsam of fir, and sulfuric acid. According to material safety data sheets, sulfuric acid (also called battery acid) and turpentine are recognized as skin irritants. This product is commonly applied to wounds of horses by horse owners; however, the authors do not recommend its use.

Blu-Kote®

Blu-Kote® (BK) contains sodium propionate, gentian violet, and acriflavine (see Gentian Violet). Although not the authors' first choice, the perceived best use is for minor abrasions.

Table 3.5 contains additional details about aerosol sprays.

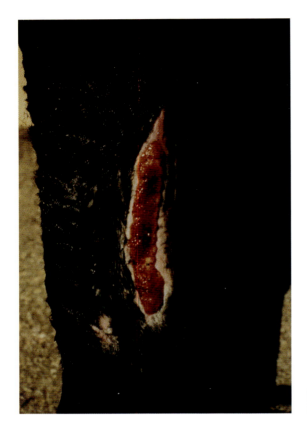

Figure 3.16. An example of a wound that could be treated effectively with Alu-Spray®.

Table 3.5. Aerosol sprays.

Product	Active agent	Best use	Source
Furazolidone® aerosol powder	4% Furazolidone	Minor abrasions	Veterinary Products Laboratory Phoenix, AZ
Alu-Spray®	Aluminum powder (40 mg/gram)	Surgical sites that are not bandaged; minor lacerations for open wound healing	Neogen Corporation Lexington, KY
Cut-Heal®	Sulfuric acid, turpentine	Not recommended	Cut-Heal Animal Care Products Cedar Hill, TX
Blu-Kote®	Gentian violet	Minor abrasions	HW Naylor Co. Morris, NY

Topical Herbal Therapies

Herbal preparations are only one component of alternative medicine, which encompasses a wide variety of approaches. There are a large number of herbal therapies and combinations of therapies for wound care. These preparations usually comprise small amounts of the plant combined with a delivery vehicle (e.g., ointment). The authors have attempted to produce, from the scientific literature, a list of those herbs readily available. Due to the scarcity of rigorous scientific evaluation of herbal therapies, however, this list is undoubtedly incomplete. Very few of these therapies have been tested in the horse for effectiveness and/or toxicity. The authors highly recommend further study by those interested in using herbal remedies. Table 3.6 provides an abbreviated list of available products, as well as their ingredients.

Table 3.6. Topical herbal products with reported wound healing properties.

Product	Ingredients	Best use	Contact information
Bag Balm™	Lanolin, petrolatum, 8-Hydroxyquinoline sulfate	Maturation phase	Dairy Association Co, Inc. Lyndonville, VT www.bagbalm.com
Espree™ 3 in 1 Wound Cream	Aloe vera, yeast extract, herbs, eucalyptus, bitrix	Repair phase	Espree Animal Products, Inc. Grapevine, TX www.espree.com
Pavia™ Natural Wound Care Cream	Lanolin, bee's wax, propylene glycol, DI water, vegetable oil, propolis tincture, comfrey extract	Repair phase	Pavia Sales Group, Inc. Plymouth, MN www.paviasalesgroup.com
Tea-Pro™ Wound Spray	Tea tree oil, comfrey, myrrh, aloe vera, goldenseal	Repair phase	Healing Tree Products Inc. McMinnville, OR www.healing-tree.com

Aloe Vera

Aloe Vera (AV) is reported to stimulate wound healing; possess antibacterial, antifungal, and antiviral properties; act as an immune stimulant; have anti-inflammatory effects; and stimulate collagen production.[4,42] Acemannan, the active ingredient in AV, is derived from the clear gel of the AV plant leaf.[4] AV extract gel with allantoin (Carrasyn®) was shown experimentally to increase epithelialization and the rate of wound healing in open footpad wounds of dogs assessed at 7 days.[43] In contrast, a controlled clinical trial of second intention healing in women showed that AV gel (Carrington Dermal wound gel) caused a significant delay in wound healing.[44] When acemannan was isolated and purified from the AV gel to form a water-soluble product, it was shown to significantly accelerate healing in experimentally created wounds in rats.[4] The proposed reasons for these effects are acemannan's potent macrophage-activating property and its ability to bind growth factors, causing a prolonged stimulating effect on fibroplasia. For more information on the effects of acemannan on wound healing, see the first section of Chapter 3.

AV is reported to be effective against *Pseudomonas aeruginosa*.[45] Clinical investigations have demonstrated the anti-inflammatory effect of AV gel in vitro when tested on human colorectal mucosa. The results showed reduced production of reactive oxygen metabolites and prostaglandin E_2, but failed to show an effect on thromboxane B_2 production.[46] Further evidence of anti-inflammatory effects were demonstrated in an in vivo rat burn wound model when AV significantly reduced the degree of leukocyte adhesion and concentrations of tumor necrosis factor-α and interleukin-6 at the wound site.[47] Its efficacy in horse wounds has not yet been investigated.

Comfrey (Symphytum officinale)

Comfrey (*Symphytum officinale*) (CO) is a natural poultice that reportedly draws exudate and waste products away from the wound.[48] Although scientific literature is lacking to support or refute this claim, there is evidence that CO does have antimicrobial and antifungal properties. Staphylococcal, streptococcal, yeast, coliform, *Pseudomonas*, and some fungal organisms have been killed in as little as 10–30 minutes when put in contact with

CO extract.[49] Karavaev (2001) demonstrated a strong antifungal activity when CO was applied to wheat seedlings.[50]

Eucalyptus (Eucalyptus spp.)

Antibacterial properties of Eucalyptus (EU) against *Pseudomonas aeruginosa* have been reported in human burn patients.[51] There are also a few reports in the veterinary literature that support the use of EU in wound care.[52,53,54] Most products described in these reports contained numerous ingredients and the trial control/design are questionable. Perhaps the best use of EU in wound care is to treat and/or prevent myiasis.[55]

Goldenseal (Hydrastis canadensis)

To the authors' knowledge there are currently no scientific reports available that address the use of goldenseal (G) for wound healing. G has been used for the treatment of athlete's foot and minor skin abrasions in people. Antibacterial properties associated with the constituents of GS have been reported.[56] G is an ingredient of Tea-Pro Wound Spray see (see Table 3.6).

Matihorse (Piper angustifolium)

Matihorse (MA) is a topical wound medicant that is formulated from extracts of *Piper angustifolium*. Products from this plant have been used as a diuretic and an aphrodisiac and for the treatment of gastrointestinal ulcers. The undersurface of the leaf is prepared for topical treatment of minor wounds and lesions caused by leech and to apply following tooth extraction.[57] Camphor and camphene were found, by gas chromatography–mass spectrometry, to be the major constituents of this plant. The isolated oils exhibited bacteriostatic activity toward *Pseudomonas* and *E. coli* as well as some fungistatic activity.[58] The proposed best use of this compound is during the inflammatory phase of wound healing.

Propolis

Propolis (P) is a compound used by bees to protect their hives from bacterial and viral infections. P is made of resinous compounds and balsams (55%), beeswax (30%), aromatic oils (10%), and bee pollen (5%).[59] P also contains various flavonoids, amino acids, B vitamins, and antibiotic substances.[59] When applied topically, P exhibits a significant antimicrobial activity against Gram-positive bacteria and yeasts, but not against Gram-negative bacteria.[60] A synergistic effect between P extract and various antibiotics against *Staphylococcus aureus* has been identified.[61] A marked synergistic effect was demonstrated with streptomycin, while moderate synergy exists with penicillin G, doxycycline, cloxacillin, chloramphenicol, cefradine, and polymixin B.[61] Ampicillin failed to produce a similar synergistic effect in this study.[61]

P is also attributed to have anti-inflammatory properties. In a cisplatin-induced nephrotoxicity rat model, P demonstrated a free-oxygen radical scavenging ability;[62] it was hypothesized that P's anti-oxidative capacity comes from its ability to donate hydrogen atoms in vitro[63] and/or from the activity of the flavonoids.[64] The proposed best use for P is during the inflammatory phase of wound healing.

Tea Tree Oil (Melaleuca alternifolia)

Anecdotally, tea tree oil (TTO) products are nonirritating, increase fibroplasia without causing the formation of exuberant granulation tissue, encourage rapid healing, and are effective in controlling bacterial/fungal infections.[48] The antifungal and antibacterial characteristics of TTO have been well documented.[65,66,67] Takarada (2004) reported that at a concentration of 0.2% TTO had little damaging effect on cultured human umbilical vein endothelial cells.[67] This data suggests that TTO is minimally cytotoxic at a low concentration. To the authors' knowledge there is no scientific literature documenting the effects of TTO on wound healing in horses. The proposed best use of TTO is during the inflammatory through repair phases of wound healing (Figure 3.17).

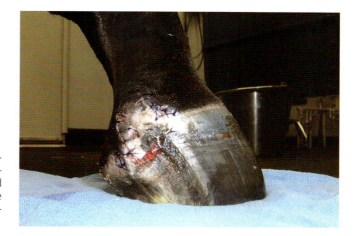

Figure 3.17. Example of a surgical wound in the acute inflammatory stage of wound healing following reduction of a proximally displaced coronary band. The distal portion of this wound is in the repair phase, indicated by the granulation tissue present. This wound was being treated topically with an ointment containing tea tree oil and triple antibiotic.

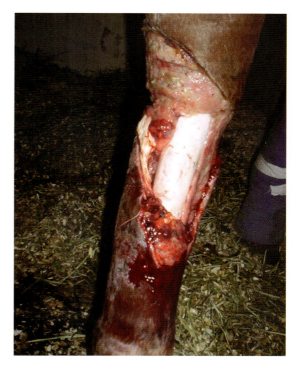

Figure 3.18. Example of a degloving wound that is in the early phase of repair, which may benefit from treatment with a live yeast cell derivative until granulation tissue fills the wound. Debridement of the bone with a rasp or drilling holes in the bone would also stimulate granulation tissue to form on its surface. For more information regarding methods to stimulate granulation tissue to form on bone stripped of periosteum, see Degloving Injuries in Chapter 8. Immobilization of the limb with a bandage cast or bandage cast splint would afford this wound the best opportunity to heal. For more information on these techniques, see Chapter 16.

Other Topical Agents

Live Yeast Cell Derivative

Live yeast cell derivative (LYCD) (Preparation H™) is a water-soluble extract of yeast reported to stimulate angiogenesis, epithelialization, and collagen formation.[29] It has been associated with improved wound healing in dogs.[29] However, in horses it prolonged wound healing by delaying wound contraction and resulted in excessive granulation tissue formation.[68] The perceived best use of LYCD is during the early part of the repair phase and then discontinued after the wound has granulated (Figure 3.18).

Honey

Honey (H) has many potentially useful properties, including broad-spectrum antimicrobial activity, pro- and anti-inflammatory actions, and stimulation of new tissue growth.[69] Although the exact mechanism of H's bacterial inhibition is unknown, possibilities include osmotic activity, low pH, viscosity, and production of hydrogen peroxide.[70] H from Australia and New Zealand (*Leptospermum spp*) have been identified as possessing enhanced antimicrobial activity.[71] H made from the Manuka bush (*Leptospernum scoparium*) have superior antimicrobial activity when compared to artificial H.[72]

H's antimicrobial effects have been demonstrated in vitro against 18 strains of methicillin-resistant *Staphylococcus aureus*, 7 strains of vancomycin-sensitive enterococci, and 20 strains of vancomycin-resistant enterococci.[72] The latter study concluded that inhibition of bacterial growth was not solely dependent upon osmolality.[72] Bang, et al. 2003, described the antibacterial effect of H as a result of hydrogen peroxide production by glucose oxidase in the wound.[73] The concentrations of hydrogen peroxide produced in this study were very low; therefore, cytotoxicity is considered minimal. Further studies have shown that H contains inhibine, an enzyme from bee pharyngeal glands, which breaks down into hydrogen peroxide and glucolactone/gluconic acid; these compounds act as a mild disinfectant and mild antimicrobial, respectively.

H also provides antioxidants which protect wound tissues from the damage imparted by free-oxygen radicals released from inflammatory cells.[74] Finally, H-treated wounds show little neutrophilic infiltration but experience a chemoattractant effect for tissue macrophages and marked proliferation of angioblasts and fibroblasts.[30] H has been shown to enhance granulation tissue formation and epithelialization, possibly via stimulatory activity on tissue macrophages.[75] In particular, it has recently been shown that the stimulatory effect of honey on wound healing may in part be related to up-regulation of inflammatory cytokines (TNF-α, IL-1β, IL-6) within monocytes.[76]

Kingsley (2001) concluded from a series of case studies that not all of the expected benefits of using H for wound treatment are achieved in clinical practice.[69] A review of randomized controlled trials involving the use of H in superficial burns and wounds concluded that the overall design of these studies was poor, such that confidence in the use of H for superficial wounds and burns is low despite the biological rationale for its use.[77] The proposed best use for H is during the inflammatory to early repair phases of wound healing.

Lanolin

Lanolin (L) has been used for centuries as a skin softener and moisturizer. In a controlled clinical trial evaluating partial-thickness wounds in piglets, it was found that lanolin cream alone significantly enhanced the rate of epithelialization and increased dermal thickness when compared to lanolin-human epidermal growth factor cream or gauze controls.[78] The proposed best use for L is for abrasions and during the maturation phase of wound healing (Figure 3.19).

Phenytoin

Phenytoin (PT) was originally introduced in 1937 as an anti-seizure medication; since that time there has been interest in its use as an adjunct to wound care.[79] Intramuscular and topical PT treatment for wounds has been shown to shorten healing time in a rabbit model evaluating superficial and deep wounds.[80] This study also found that topical use of PT resulted in better wound tensile strength when compared to systemic treatment.[80] In a controlled human clinical trial, PT-treated skin ulcers healed in 73% of cases compared to saline-dressed (control) skin ulcers at 28.5%.[79] Although PT had beneficial effects in these trials, the effects of PT on horse wounds remains unknown.

Gallium Nitrate

Gallium nitrate (GN) has been shown to increase the expression of type I collagen and fibronectin in human fibroblasts, proteins which are structural components of the wound matrix.[81] GN also suppresses matrix metalloproteinase (MMP) activity and accelerates in vitro keratinocyte motility.[81] At the time of this writing no information was available regarding GN's efficacy when used clinically.

Gentian Violet

Gentian violet (GV) is often applied topically in a 1% aqueous solution or included in aerosol products (e.g., Blu-Kote). It has been proposed to be an effective wound repair stimulant, though conclusive evidence has yet

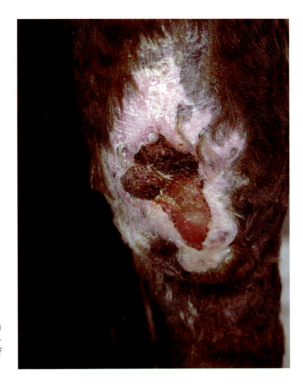

Figure 3.19. This chronic nonhealing wound on the dorsal hock region may benefit from treatment with lanolin and bandaging. Besides softening and moisturizing the wound, lanolin may stimulate the rate of epithelialization.

to be established. Several potential side effects must be considered before it is determined whether or not this agent should even be used. In one study, 3 human patients developed a necrotic, painful, and slowly healing skin reaction after topical application of 1% GV in aqueous solution.[82] GV is also noted to have a tissue-irritating effect that discolors and masks the true color of the skin, necessitating caution when using this agent because tissue color may be skewed.[83]

GV in low concentrations inhibits the formation of granulation tissue in cellulose sponges implanted subcutaneously for 10 days in rats.[83] One application of GV to incised skin wounds before suturing retarded the gain of tensile strength in wounds for more than 3 weeks.[83] It also caused marked vascular proliferation, indicating tissue damage as assessed by microangiography.[83] Finally, granulation tissue slices exposed to GV have a decreased capacity to consume oxygen, incorporate proline into collagen and noncollagenous proteins, and synthesize RNA.[83] Several studies have revealed that GV is a carcinogenic agent when used on open wounds and on mucous membranes.[84,85] In conclusion, GV is not recommended for wound care.

Recombinant Vasoactive Protein

Recombinant vasoactive protein (RVP) is a protein originally isolated and purified from insect saliva. This compound was evaluated for wound healing because it is known to increase blood flow. In a controlled clinical trial using surgical wounds in dogs it was found that intradermal or subcutaneous injection of RVP significantly increased wound breaking strength on day 5.[86] The rate of open wound healing was significantly enhanced at day 21 in dogs treated with RVP intradermally at the time of wounding.[86] The proposed best use of RVP is during the repair phase of wound healing.

Scarlet Oil

Although scarlet oil (SO) has been used in the treatment of horse wounds for many years, there have been no controlled studies evaluating its effectiveness. The ingredients in SO are mineral oil, isopropyl alcohol (30%), methyl salicylate, benzyl alcohol (3%), pine oil, eucalyptus oil, parachlorometaxylenol, and biebrich scarlet red.[87] Pine oil is commonly used as an antiseptic in household cleaning agents. The use of eucalyptus (EU) has been described previously in this chapter. SO can cause a painful contact dermatitis in some horses, causing objection to continued treatment. Most veterinarians use this agent to stimulate granulation tissue formation in large, upper body wounds. There is no data to prove that it is of any benefit and therefore the authors do not recommend its use.

Aminoplex

Aminoplex (AP) contains amino acids, trace minerals, peptides, electrolytes, and nucleosides. The purported properties of AP include the ability to reverse cell damage, increase cellular glucose and oxygen uptake, enhance collagen synthesis, and accelerate epithelialization.[88] In a controlled human clinical trial using AP following CO_2 laser resurfacing, patients that received AP therapy had decreased post-operative pain, healed faster, and had less swelling than that observed in a more traditional laser recovery program.[89] AP spray is available through biO$_2$ Cosmeceuticals, Inc. No data is available documenting its use in the horse.

Sugardine

Sugardine (SD) is made by adding PI solution to granular sugar until a workable paste consistency is reached. This hypertonic agent acts by osmotic action to draw exudate from the wound. SD is commonly used to treat sub-solar abscesses in the horse. When using SD one must keep in mind the information provided under PI in this chapter. For more information on the use of hypertonic wound products, see the first section of this chapter.

Zn7™ Equine Wound Care Formula

Zn7™ (ZE) is a wound cream composed of deionized water, zinc gluconate, carboxymethylcellulose, taurine, L-lysine, methylparaben, and propylparaben.[90] According to the company, it provides substantial anti-pruritic, anti-microbial, and wound healing benefits. The majority of the literature surrounding zinc gluconate is associated with its use in lozenges to treat the common cold in people.[91] Zinc gluconate has been shown in vitro to stimulate a select group of integrins that affect cellular mobility in the early phases of wound healing.[92]

Controversy exists as to whether zinc aids in wound healing; however, it is well known that zinc-deficient animals suffer impaired healing that is reversed with appropriate mineral supplementation.[93] When zinc oxide was applied to full-thickness wounds in pigs, researchers found that insulin-like growth factor-1 mRNA was significantly increased on days 3 and 4 post wounding.[94] This finding could be a mechanism whereby zinc enhances wound healing. Zinc oxide was also found to significantly increase epithelialization of partial-thickness skin wounds in pigs when compared to treatment with zinc sulfate, indicating that the mode of delivery is probably critical to achieve the beneficial effects of zinc.[95] No data is available documenting its use in the horse. The proposed best use of ZE is during the early repair phase of wound healing.

Tripeptide-Copper Complex

Tripeptide-Copper Complex (TCC) is available as a topical or injectable medicant. Reportedly the product promotes angiogenesis, epithelialization, and collagen deposition, and enhances wound contraction.[96] The topical form has been shown to enhance open wound healing in dogs while the injectable form stimulates type I collagen deposition in healing footpad wounds in dogs.[96] TCC has also been shown to enhance healing of chronic, ischemic wounds. To our knowledge TCC is not commonly used in equine practice. The proposed best use for TCC is during the repair phase of wound healing.

Vitamin E

Vitamin E (E) is the major lipid-soluble antioxidant in the skin; however, the effects of exogenous E on surgical wounds is inconclusive.[97] Parenteral supplementation of E in rats has been shown to significantly increase epithelial thickness, fibroblast proliferation, and angiogenesis of tympanic membrane perforations.[98] A double-blinded clinical trial to evaluate the effects of E on the cosmetic appearance of scars in humans found that E had no effect but led to a high incidence of contact dermatitis.[99] E is commonly used during the maturation phase of wound healing in horses, but clinical trials that examine its effects are lacking.

Wound Debridement Agents

Acute open wounds rapidly develop a proteineous surface coagulum that often encompasses surface contaminants and bacteria; as such it prevents contact of topical and systemic antibiotics. Additionally, bacterial proliferation produces a biofilm and exudate resulting in a similar type of coagulum.[100]

Proteolytic enzymes (proteinases) applied topically or secreted by maggots degrade (liquefy) the biofilm and surface coagulum, thus exposing bacteria to topical and systemic antibiotics. These proteinases also remove exudate and necrotic tissue from a wound bed. This is important because excessive exudate not only blocks the effects of topically applied medicants but also breaks down extracellular matrix material and blocks the effects of growth factors.[101] Necrotic tissue, besides acting as a culture medium for bacteria, creates a low oxygen tension and elaborates humoral factors which impair the polymorphonuclear cell's bactericidal functions (Figure 3.20).

The use of wound debriding agents should be considered when surgical debridement is contraindicated because it may cause injury (e.g., a wound adjacent to neurovascular structures) or may result in the removal of tissue needed for reconstruction of the wound at a later time. Additionally, papain/urea-based and collagenase preparations have been shown to stimulate angiogenesis and granulation tissue formation and accelerate epithelialization; thus, they are believed to be effective in stimulating healing of a chronic wound.[102,103] Debriding preparations presently available should be used with caution because bacteremia has been reported in human patients following proteolytic enzymatic debridement.[104] While the authors did not postulate as to the cause of bacteremia, they conjectured that the enzymes dissolved the biofilm, freeing the entrapped bacteria to invade the exposed capillaries. A review of the more common proteolytic enzyme preparations in use today follows.

Papain/Urea-Based Proteinase

Papain/urea-based proteinase (PUBP) is a proteolytic enzymatic combination that has been widely used in humans and to a limited degree in animals.[105] Papain breaks down any protein-containing cysteine residues. This makes papain nonselective because most proteins, including beneficial growth factors, contain cysteine residues. Collagen contains no cysteine residues and is thus unaffected by papain.[106]

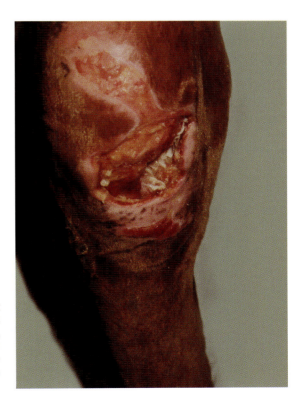

Figure 3.20. Example of an open wound to the plantar hock region that developed a proteineous surface coagulum which often encompasses surface contaminants and bacteria. As such, it prevents contact of topical and systemic antibiotics. Bacterial proliferation also produces a biofilm and exudate resulting in a similar type of coagulum. A topical debridement agent (e.g., collagenase) could be used on this wound at this time.

Urea's role in this combination is to facilitate the proteolytic action of papain by reducing disulfide bridges to expose cysteine residues.[107] The combination of papain and urea is estimated to be twice as effective in protein digestion as papain alone.[108] Importantly, hydrogen peroxide, silver sulfadiazine, gentamicin solution or cream, as well as alcohol-based products can block the effect of PUBP preparations and therefore should not be used simultaneously.

Advantages to PUBP are an effective broad pH range (3–12) and debridement achieved more rapidly than with other products on the market. Disadvantages are their non-selective action and creation of a prominent painful inflammatory response when applied to wounds. Chlorophyllin has been added to PUBP in an effort to remedy this situation and has shown promise.[101,107]

In experimental wounds in animals, the papain/urea combination has been shown to be very effective for debridement.[109] However, in experimental animal and human burns, these preparations may behave too aggressively, both in terms of affecting viable tissue and in causing pain.[110]

Collagenase

The commercially available preparation of collagenase (CG) is derived from bacteria (*Clostridium histolyticum*). CG is a water-soluble proteinase that specifically breaks down collagen.[103] CG is reported to be most effective in a pH range of 6–8. CG can hydrolyze native collagen and thereby facilitate rapid debridement and healing of chronic wounds.[111] The mechanism of CG's action is to degrade collagen and convert it to gelatin, upon which less specific enzymes can act. However, until CG cleaves collagen, no other enzyme is capable of breaking it down. CG acts selectively on nonviable collagen. It appears that CG cleaves the undenatured collagen molecules at the boundary of the necrotic tissue, thus freeing up the necrotic tissue from the wound.[112] Recently CG was shown to have the highest proteolytic activity and the greatest likelihood of achieving a clean wound compared to other non-surgical approaches to wound debridement.[113]

CG has been found to be remarkably gentle on viable cells. The addition of CG derived from *Clostridium histolyticum* to keratinocyte cultures was shown to enhance their proliferation and migration up to 10-fold.[103] It appears that CG can stimulate the formation of granulation tissue and accelerate epithelialization via enhanced migration of epithelial cells under the surface clot.[101]

Elase®

Elase® (EL) -containing fibrinolysin-deoxyribonuclease has been used to treat everything from monilial vulvovaginitis to chronic leg ulcers and burn wounds. EL was examined as a possible enzymatic agent to aid in antimicrobial treatment of contaminated wounds. However, topical application of the active enzymes in EL to contaminated wounds prior to antibiotic treatment did not alter the incidence of infection.[114]

EL powder has been evaluated in patients with chronic leg ulcers prior to autologous skin grafts, in whom it had a significant effect on debridement and enhanced granulation tissue formation, compared to saline controls.[115] Despite EL's many apparent benefits, it has also been reported to facilitate and extend the necrotic process in some cases.[116]

Granulex®

Granulex® (G) is an aerosolized spray that contains trypsin (TR), Peru balsam, and castor oil.[117] TR functions to liquefy fibrin and debride necrotic tissue from ulcerated areas without harming healthy tissue.[118] TR directly hydrolyzes a large number of non-specific naturally occurring proteins. It was hypothesized that T applied topically to a contaminated wound would augment the activity of a concurrently applied antibiotic. However, application of 1 mg of TR to a wound prior to application of topical antibiotic was found to be ineffective in potentiating antibiotic activity.[114]

Peru balsam contains cinnamic and benzoic acids, believed to act as irritants, resulting in enhanced blood flow by local stimulation of the capillary bed.[119] It may also act as a mild antiseptic.[119] Castor oil is a local protective agent that may promote epithelialization.[119] In one case report, G was used to promote tissue healing of a necrotic ulcer of the oral mucosa. After 48 hours of spray treatments, the area had granulated and the site of the eschar had become more normal in appearance.[119] A prospective clinical trial in human patients suffering from decubital ulcers treated with G revealed a faster healing rate than those with no direct medication of the ulcer.[120] Aspiration of G spray is an important consideration if it is sprayed on or around the face because it is oil-based and may cause respiratory irritation.[119]

Meat Tenderizer

Users of meat tenderizer (MT) profess to its debridement activity when applied to open wounds. Bromelain, from pineapple stems, and papain, from papaya, are the two most common meat tenderizers. Bromelain comprises a group of proteolytic enzymes among other substances. Scientific studies on the use of MTs in wound care is lacking; however, there is some information available on the base ingredients (see PUPB, above). Most literature focuses on MTs' use for providing analgesia following jellyfish stings. In all cases, however, MT was found to be ineffective as an analgesic.[121]

Maggot Therapy

See Wound Repair: Problems in the Horse and Innovative Solutions in Chapter 1 for information on this subject.

Topical Fly Repellents

Although many fly repellants are available on the market, few are marketed specifically for use with wounds. Citronella oil, cedar oil, and eucalyptus oil have been used to repel insects and are contained in some products. Pyrethrins are a class of insecticides that are also added to some products. The authors are unaware of any scientific study that examines the use of these compounds on or near wounds.

Avon Skin So Soft (SSS) is a common ingredient of many home remedy fly repellents. SSS Bug Guard and bath oil were shown to repel insects for approximately 10 minutes in a clinical trial.[122] See Table 3.7 for more information on topical fly repellents.

Table 3.7. Topical fly repellents.

Product	Insect repellent ingredients	Contact information
SWAT®	Pyrethrins	Farnam Co., Inc. Phoenix, AZ www.farnam.com
Tri-Care™ 3-way Wound Treatment	Pyrethrins	Farnam Co., Inc.
Flys-Off ® Ointment	Citronella oil	Farnam Co. Inc.
Scram! Fly Repellent Ointment	Citronella oil, eucalyptus oil	Myhorseandme.com Caliente, CA http://store.myhorsenme.com
Espree 3 in 1 Wound Cream	Citronella oil, cedar oil	Espree Animal Products, Inc. Grapevine, TX www.espree.com

Conclusion

This chapter has attempted to provide the clinician with a summary of the existing scientific data on commonly encountered wound care products. Many more products are commercially available, making it very difficult to decide which to use and when. Clinicians are constantly inundated with anecdotal evidence supporting different topical products, of which many have some scientific merit. The authors encourage clinicians to make an educated decision regarding the topical products they apply to wounds.

References

1. Wilson J, Mills J, Prather D, Dimitrijevich S: A toxicity index of skin and wound cleansers used on in vitro fibroblasts and keratinocytes. Adv Skin Wound Care 2005;18:373
2. Rodeheaver GT: Wound cleansing, wound irrigation, wound disinfection. In D Krasner, G Rodeheaver and G Sibbald, editors. *Chronic wound care: a clinical source book for healthcare professionals (3rd edition)*. Wayne, PA: HMP Communications, 2001, p.369
3. Edlich RF, Schmolka IR, Prusak MP, et al: The molecular basis for toxicity of surfactants in surgical wounds. 1. EO:PO block polymers. J Surg Res 1973;14:277
4. Tizard I, Busbee D, Maxwell B, Kemp MC: Effects of acemannan, a complex carbohydrate, on wound healing in young and aged rats. Wounds 1994;6:201
5. Paola L, Brocco E, Senesi A, et al: Super-oxidized solution (SOS) therapy for infected diabetic foot ulcers. Wounds 2006;18:262
6. Gutierrez A: The science behind stable, super-oxidized water. Wounds 2006;Supplement:7
7. Medina-Tamayo J, Sanchez-Miranda E, Balleza-Tapia H, et al: Super-oxidized solution inhibits IgE-antigen–induced degranulation and cytokine release in mast cells. Int Immunopharmacol 2007;7:1013
8. Knottenbelt D: Basic wound management. In D Knottenbelt, editor. *Handbook of equine wound management (1st edition)*. Edinburgh: Elsevier Science Limited, 2003, p.39
9. Viljanto J: Disinfection of surgical wounds without inhibition of normal wound healing. Arch Surg 1980;115:253
10. Grey JG, Lee JR: The effect of topical povidone iodine on wound infection following abdominal surgery. Br J Surg 1981;68:310
11. Mulliken, JB, Nancey A, Healey B, et al: Povidone-iodine and tensile strength of wounds in rats. J Trauma 1980;20:323
12. Hugo WH, Newton JM: The antibacterial activity of a complex of iodine and a non-ionic surface active agent. J Pharm Pharmacol 1964;16:189
13. Peter FW, Li-Peuser H, Vogt PN, et al: The effect of wound ointments on tissue microcirculation and leukocyte behaviour. Clin Exp Dermatol 2002;27:51
14. Duc Q, Breetveld M, Middlekoop E, et al: A cytotoxic analysis of antiseptic medication on skin substitutes and autograft. Br J Dermatol 2007;157:33
15. Berry DB, Sullins KE: Effects of topical application of antimicrobials and bandaging on healing and granulation tissue formation in wounds of the distal aspect of the limbs in horses. Am J Vet Res 2003;64:88
16. Rath T, Meissl G: Induction of hyperthyroidism in burn patients treated topically with povidone-iodine. Burns Incl Therm Inj 1988;14:320
17. Shetty KR, Duthie EH Jr.: Thyrotoxicosis induced by topical iodine application. Arch Intern Med 1990;150:2400
18. Nobukuni K, Hayakawa N, Namba R, et al: The influence of long-term treatment with povidone-iodine on thyroid function. Dermatol 1997;2:69
19. Rodeheaver G, Bellamy W, Kody M, et al: Bacterial activity and toxicity of iodine-containing solutions in wounds. Arch Surg 1982;117:181
20. Prince HN, Nonemaker WS, Norgard RC: Drug resistance studies with topical antiseptics. J Pharm Sci 1978;67:1629
21. Lozier S, Pope E, Berg J: Effects of four preparations of 0.05% chlorhexidine diacetate on wound healing in dogs. Vet Surg 1992;21:107
22. Amber EI, Henderson RA, Swaim SF, et al: A comparison of antimicrobial efficacy and tissue reaction of four antiseptics on canine wounds. Vet Surg 1983;12:63
23. Sanchez IR, Swaim SF, Nusbaum KE, et al: Effects of chlorhexidine diacetate and povidone-iodine on wound healing in dogs. Vet Surg 1988;17:291
24. Lee AH, Swaim SF, McGuire JA, et al: Effects of chlorhexidine diacetate, povidone iodine and polyhydroxydine on wound healing in dogs. J Am Anim Hosp Assoc 1988;24:77
25. Boyce S, Warden G, Holder I: Cytotoxicity testing of topical antimicrobial agents on human keratinocytes and fibroblasts for cultured skin grafts. J Burn Care Rehabil 1995;16:97
26. Stashak TS: Selected factors that affect wound healing. In T Stashak, editor. *Equine wound management (1st edition)*. Philadelphia: Lea and Febiger, 1991, p.19

27. Swaim SF: Topical wound medications: A review. J Am Vet Med Assoc 1987;190:1588
28. Carrel A, Dehelly G: *The treatment of infected wounds*. New York, NY: Hoeber, 1917
29. Lozier SM: Topical wound therapy. In J Harari, editor. *Surgical complications and wound healing in the small animal practice*. Philadelphia: WB Saunders Co, 1993, p.63
30. Liptak JM: An overview of the topical management of wounds. Aust Vet J 1997;75:408
31. Lineaweaver W, Howard R, Soucy D, et al: Cellular and bacterial toxicities of topical antimicrobials. Arch Surg 1985;120:267
32. Lemarie RJ, Hosgood G: Antiseptics and disinfectants in small animal practice. Compend Contin Educ 1995;17:1339
33. Cyr S, Hensley D, Benedetti G, et al: Treatment of field water with sodium hypochlorite for surgical irrigation. J Trauma-Injury Crit Care 2004;57:231
34. Bello TR, Allen TM: The use of ARS-1050 in wound care of horses. J Equine Vet Sci 2005;25:303
35. Southwood LL, Baxter GM: Instrument sterilization, skin preparation, and wound management. Vet Clin N Am Equine Pract 1996;12:173
36. Muller MJ, Hollyoak MA, Moaveni S, et al: Retardation of wound healing by silver sulfadiazine is reversed by aloe vera and nystatin. Burns 2003;29:834
37. Barber SM: Second intention wound healing in the horse: the effect of bandages and topical corticosteroids. Proc Am Assoc Equine Pract 1990;35:107
38. Theoret CL, Barber SM, Moyana TN, Gordon JR: Expression of transforming growth factor β1, β3 and basic fibroblast growth factor in full-thickness skin wounds of equine limbs and thorax. Vet Surg 2001;30:269
39. http://www.sciencelab.com/xMSDS-Nitrofurazone-9926271, 2007
40. Greer WE: Furazolidone aerosol powder in the treatment of wounds in nonhuman primates. Southwestern Vet 1971;25:45
41. Qureshi S: In vitro evaluation of efficacy of some antibiotics against *S. aureus* and other bacterial microflora isolated from skin wounds and abscesses in camel. J Camel Pract Res 2004;11:67
42. Rund C: Alternative topical therapies for wound care. In D Krasner, G Rodeheaver and G Sibbald, editors. *Chronic wound care: a clinical source book for healthcare professionals (3rd edition)*. Wayne: HMP Communications, 2001, p.329
43. Swaim S, Vaughn D, Kincaid S, et al: Effects of locally injected medications on healing of pad wounds in dogs. Am J Vet Res 1996;57:394
44. Schmidt JM, Greenspoon JS: Aloe vera dermal wound gel is associated with a delay in wound healing. Obstet Gynecol 1991;78:115
45. Cera LM, Heggers JP, Robson MC, et al: The therapeutic efficacy of aloe vera cream in thermal injuries: two reports. J Am Anim Hosp Assoc 1980;16:768
46. Langmead L, Makins RJ, Ramptom DS: Anti-inflammatory effects of aloe vera gel in human colorectal mucosa in vitro. Aliment Pharmacol Ther 2004;19:521
47. Duansak D, Somboonwong J, Patumraj S: Effects of aloe vera on leukocyte adhesion and TNF-alpha and IL-6 levels in burn wound rats. Clin Hemorheol Microcirc 2003;29:239
48. Witherspoon E: Healing Tree® Products Healing Tree Products, Inc., McMinnville, Oregon (pamphlet and personal comm.) 2004
49. Heckman RA: The bactericidal properties of comfrey (*Symphytum officinale*) herbal extracts. Department of Zoology, Brigham Young University, Pavia Sales Group, Inc., Plymouth, MN (pamphlet) 2004
50. Karavaev VA, Solntsev MK, Iurina TP: Antifungal activity of aqueous extracts from the leaf of cow parsnip and comfrey. Izv Akad Nauk Ser Biol 2001;4:435
51. Al-Saimary IE, Bakr SS, Jaffar T, et al: Effects of some plant extracts and antibiotics on Pseudomonas aeruginosa isolated from various burn cases. Saudi Med J 2002;23:802
52. Agrawal AK: Therapeutic efficacy of an herbal gel for skin affections in dogs. Ind Vet J 1997;74:417
53. Bhagwat V, Mitra SK, Suryanarayana T: Therapeutic efficacy of a herbal formulation "Scavon" on the wound healing in cattle. Ind Vet J 2000;77:636
54. Bansod KV: Efficacy of topicure on wounds in canines. Ind Vet J 2003;80:1300
55. Pearse BHG, Peucker SKJ: Comparison of a liquid and a powder insecticidal dressing to aid healing and prevent fly strike of mulesing wounds in lambs. Aust Vet J 1991;68:163
56. Hwang BW, Roberts SK, Chadwick LR, et al: Antimicrobial constituents from Goldenseal (the rhizomes of Hydrastix Canadensis) against selected oral pathogens. Planta Medica 2003;69:623
57. www.botanical.com, 2007
58. Tirillini B, Valsquez ER, Pellegrino R: Chemical composition and antimicrobial activity of essential oil of Piper augustifolium. Planta Med 1996;62:372
59. Pavia J: Pavia Natural Wound Care Cream. Pavia Sales Group, Inc. Minnetonka, MN. 2004 (pamphlet and personal comm)

60. Stepanovic S, Antic N, Dakic I, et al: In vitro antimicrobial activity of propolis and synergism between propolis and antimicrobial drugs. Microbiol Res 2003;158:353

61. Krol W, Scheller S, Shani J et al: Synergistic effect of propolis and antibiotics on the growth of *staphylococcus aureus.* Arzneimittelforschung 1993;43:607

62. Ozen S, Akyol O, Iraz M: Role of caffeic acid phenethyl ester, an active component of propolos, against cisplatin-induced nephrotoxocity in rats. J Appl Toxicol 2004;24:27

63. Scheller S, Wilczok T, Imielski S, et al: Free radical scavenging by ethanol extract of propolis. Int J Radiat Biol 1990;57:461

64. Krol W, Czuba Z, Scheller S, et al: Anti-oxidant property of ethanolic extract of propolis (EEP) as evaluated by inhibiting the chemiluminescence oxidation of luminal. Biochem Int 1990;21:593

65. Hammer KA, Carson CF, Riley TV: Antifungal activity of the components of *Melaleuca alternifolia* (tea tree) oil. J Appl Microbiol 2003;95:853

66. Olivia B, Piccirilli E, Ceddia T, et al: Antimycotic activity of *Melaleuca alternifolia* essential oil and its major components. Letters Appl Microbiol 2003;37:185

67. Takarada K, Kimizuka R, Takahashi N, et al: A comparison of the antibacterial efficacies of essential oils against oral pathogens. Oral Microbiol Immunol 2004;19:61

68. Bigbie RB, Schumacher J, Swaim SF: Effects of amnion and live yeast cell derivative on second-intention healing in horses. Am J Vet Res 1991;52:1376

69. Kingsley A: The use of honey on the treatment of infected wounds: case studies. Brit J Nurs 2001;10:22S(abs)

70. Mathews KA, Binnington AG: Wound management using honey. Compend Contin Educ 2002;24:53

71. Lusby PE, Coombes A, Wilkinson JM: Honey: a potent agent for wound healing? J Wound Ostomy Continence Nurs 2002;29:273

72. Cooper RA, Molan PC, Harding KG: The sensitivity to honey of Gram-positive cocci of clinical significance isolated from wounds. J Appl Microbiol 2002;93:857

73. Bang LM, Buntting C, Molan P: The effect on dilution on the rate of hydrogen peroxide production in honey and its implication for wound healing. J Altern Complement Med 2003;9:267

74. Frankel S, Robinson GE, Berenbaum MR: Antioxidant capacity and correlated characteristics of 14 unifloral honeys. J Apic Res 1998;37:27

75. Molan PC: The role of honey in the management of wounds. J Wound Care 1999;8:415

76. Tonks AJ, Cooper RA, Jones KP, et al: Honey stimulates inflammatory cytokine production from monocytes. Cytokine 2003;21:242

77. Moore OA, Campbell F, Seers K: Systematic review of the use of honey as a wound dressing. BMC Complement Altern Med 2001; 1:Epub (http://www.biomedcentral.com/1472-6882/1/2)

78. Chvapil M, Gaines JA, Gilman T: Lanolin and epidermal growth factor in healing of partial thickness pig wounds. J Burn Care Rehabil 1988;9:279

79. Pendse AK, Sharma A, Sodani A et al: Topical phenytoin in wound healing. Int J Dermatol 1993;32:214

80. Dehghani S, Abrishami A: Effect of phenytoin on wound healing in rabbits. Indian J Vet Surg 1993;14:10

81. Goncalves J, Wasif N, Esposito D, et al: Gallium nitrate accelerates partial thickness wound repair and alters keratinocyte integrin expression to favor a motile phenotype. J Surg Res 2002;103:134

82. Bjornberg A, Mobacken H: Necrotic skin reactions caused by 1 percent gentian violet and brilliant green. Acta Derm Venerol 1972;52:55

83. Mobacken H, Zederfeldt B: Influence of a cationic triphenylmethan dye on granulation tissue growth in vivo: An experimental study in rats. Acta Derm Venerol 1973;53:161

84. Dealy C: *The care of wounds (1st edition).* Oxford: Blackwell Scientific Publications, 1994, p.11

85. Ryan TJ: Wound healing and current dermatologic dressings. Clin Derm 1990;8:21

86. Cupp MS, Swaim SF, Amalsadvala T, et al: Use of a recombinant vasoactive protein (rSVEP) to enhance healing of surgically-created wounds. Wounds 2004;16:85

87. First Priority, Inc., Elgin, IL. 2004 (personal comm.)

88. biO$_2$ Cosmeceuticals: Amino-Plex®. Beverly Hills, CA.2004 (pamphlet)

89. McGuire MF, Hayman S: Enhanced healing after CO$_2$ laser resurfacing: A controlled clinical study. biO$_2$ Cosmeceuticals, Beverly Hills, CA.2004 (pamphlet)

90. Addison Biological Laboratory, Inc.: http://addisonlabs.com/Zn7EquineWoundCare.htm, 2004

91. Turner RB, Cetnarowski WE: Effect of treatment with zinc gluconate or zinc acetate on experimental and natural colds. Clin Infect Dis 2000;31:1202

92. Tenaud I, Sainte-Marie I, Jumbou O, et al: In vitro modulation of keratinocyte wound healing integrins by zinc, copper, and manganese. Br J Dermatol 1999;140:26

93. Ruberg RL: Role of nutrition in wound healing. Surg Clin North Am 1984;64:705

94. Tarnow P, Agren M, Steenfos H, et al: Topical zinc oxide treatment increases endogenous gene expression of insulin-like growth factor-1 in granulation tissue from porcine wounds. Scand J Plast Reconstr Surg Hand Surg 1994;28:255

95. Agren MS, Chvapil M, Franzen L: Enhancement of re-epithelialization with topical zinc oxide in porcine partial-thickness wounds. J Surg Res 1991;50:101
96. Swaim SF: What's new in wound management? Proc N Am Vet Conf; Small Animal 2003;17:117
97. MacKay D, Miller AL: Nutritional support for wound healing. Altern Med Rev 2003;8:359
98. Susaman N, Yalcin S, Ilhan N, et al: The effect of vitamin E on histopathologic healing and lipid peroxidation levels in experimentally induced traumatic tympanic membrane perforations. Kulak Burun Borgaz Ihtis Derg 2003;10:3(abs)
99. Baumann LS, Spencer J: The effects of topical vitamin E on the cosmetic appearance of scars. Dermatol Surg 1999;25:311
100. Wilson DA: Principles of early wound management. Vet Clin North Am; Equine Pract 2005;21:45
101. Falanga V: Wound bed preparation and the role of enzymes: A case for multiple actions of therapeutic agents. Wounds 2002;14:47
102. Raffetto JD, Mendez MV, Marien BJ: Changes in cellular motility and cytoskeletal actin in fibroblasts from patients with chronic venous insufficiency and neonatal fibroblasts in the presence of chronic wound fluids. J Vasc Surg 2001;33:233
103. Herman I: Stimulation of human keratinocyte migration and proliferation in vitro: Insights into the cellular responses to injury and wound healing. Wounds 1996;8:33
104. Hummel RP, Kautz PD, MacMillan BG, et al: The continuing problem of sepsis following enzymatic debridement of burns. J Trauma 1974;14:572
105. Berger MM: Enzyme debriding preparations. Ostomy Wound Manage 1993;39:61
106. Smith B: Expression and regulation of the collagen family in skin. In V Falanga, editor. *Cutaneous wound healing (1st edition)*. London: Martin Dunitz Publishers, 2001, p.57
107. Miller JM, Howard F: The interaction of papain, urea and water-soluble chlorophyll in proteolytic ointment for infected wounds. Surg 1958;43:939
108. Silverstein P, Ruzicka FJ, Jeimkamp GM: In-vitro evaluations of enzymatic debridement of burn eschar. Surg 1973;73:15
109. Hebda PA, Flynn KJ, Dohar JE: Evaluation of efficacy of enzymatic debriding agents for the removal of necrotic tissue and promotion of healing in porcine skin wounds. Wounds 1998;10:83
110. Curtis R, Blache C, Johnston K: Accuzyme papain-urea-based ointment versus collagenase Santyl ointment in the treatment of partial thickness burn wounds. Proc Am Burn Assoc 1999
111. Boxer AM, Gottesman N, Bernstein H, Mandl I: Debridement of dermal ulcers and decubiti with collagenase. Geriatrics 1969;24:75
112. Howes EL: Early investigations of the treatment of third degree burns with collagenases. In M Ines, editor. *Collagenase (1st edition)*. New York: Gordon and Breach Science Publishers, 1972, p.123
113. Mosher BA, Cuddigan J, Thomas DR: Outcomes of 4 methods of debridement using a decision analysis methodology. Adv Wound Care 1999;12:81
114. Rodeheaver G, Marsh D, Edgerton MT, Edlich RF: Proteolytic enzymes as adjuncts to antimicrobial prophylaxis of contaminated wounds. Am J Surg 1975;129:537
115. Westerhof W, Jansen FC, de Wit FS, Cormane RH: Controlled double-blind trial of fibrinolysin-desoxyribonuclease (Elase) solution in patients with chronic leg ulcers who are treated before autologous skin grafting. J Am Acad Dermatol 1987;17:32
116. Chapple JS: Elase and wound debridement. N Z Med J 1984;97:701
117. http://www.drugs.com/mtm/granulex.html, 2007
118. Reynolds JEF: Marindale L the extra pharmacopoeia. Pharmaceutical Press 1980;315(659)
119. Noble TA, Carr DS, Gonzales MF: Use of a trypsin, Peru balsam, and castor oil spray on the oral mucosa: case report and review of the literature. Pharmacother 1989;9:386
120. Yucel VE, Basmajian JV: Decubitus ulcers: healing effect of an enzymatic spray. Arch Phys Med Rehabil 1974;55:517
121. Thomas CS, Scott SA, Galanis DJ, et al: Box jellyfish (Carybdea alata) in Waikiki. The analgesic effect of sting-aid, Adolph's meat tenderizer and fresh water on their stings: a double-blinded, randomized, placebo-controlled clinical trial. Hawaii Med J 2001;60:205
122. Fradin MS, Day JF: Comparative efficacy of insect repellents against mosquito bites. N Engl J Med 2002;347:13

3.3 The Extracellular Matrix as a Biologic Scaffold for Wound Healing in Veterinary Medicine

Stephen F. Badylak, DVM, PhD, MD; Cooper Williams, DVM; and Julie Myers-Irvin, PhD

Introduction

An extraordinary amount of research has been devoted to the treatment of acute and chronic (non-healing) wounds in both human and veterinary medicine. In spite of significant advances in stem cell biology, cytokine and growth factor biology, and off-the-shelf wound care products—including wound dressings—there has been little notable change in the outcome of animals suffering from large wounds involving soft tissue.

Tissue engineering/regenerative medicine has introduced many novel therapeutic options for wound care including the use of tissue-engineered skin, biologic scaffolds, bioactive cytokines, and cell-based therapies, but these are not widely recognized in veterinary medicine. This section will focus upon the use of biologic scaffolds derived from the extracellular matrix (ECM) as a potential therapeutic option for the treatment of both acute and chronic soft tissue injuries in veterinary medicine.

The ECM is by definition nature's ideal biologic scaffold material. The ECM is custom designed and manufactured by the resident cells of each tissue and organ and is in a state of dynamic equilibrium with its surrounding microenvironment.[1] The structural and functional molecules which compose the ECM provide the means whereby adjacent cells communicate with each other and with the external environment.[2-4] The ECM is biocompatible because it is produced by host cells. The ECM also provides a supportive medium or conduit for blood vessels, nerves, and lymphatics, and for the diffusion of nutrients from the blood to surrounding cells. In other words, the ECM possesses all of the characteristics of the ideal tissue-engineered scaffold or biomaterial. Perhaps more pertinent to the context of this section, the ECM provides many of the critical modulators of the host response to injury.

Composition of the Extracellular Matrix

The ECM represents a mixture of structural and functional molecules organized in a tissue-specific 3-dimensional architecture. The major components of the ECM include collagen, fibronectin, laminin, glycosaminoglycans, and growth factors.

Collagen is the most abundant protein within the mammalian ECM and accounts for greater than 90% of its dry weight.[5] More than 20 distinct types of collagen have been identified, each with a unique biologic function. Type I collagen is the major structural protein present in tissues and is ubiquitous within both the animal and plant kingdoms. Type I collagen is abundant in tendinous and ligamentous structures and provides the necessary strength to accommodate the uniaxial and multiaxial mechanical loading to which these tissues are commonly subjected. These same tissues provide a convenient source of collagen for many medical device applications. Bovine type I collagen is harvested from Achilles tendon and is perhaps the most commonly used xenogeneic ECM component intended for therapeutic applications.

Other collagen types exist in the ECM of most tissues but typically in much lower quantities. These alternative collagen types provide distinct mechanical and physical properties to the ECM and simultaneously contribute to the population of ligands that interact with the resident cell populations. Each type of collagen is, of course, the result of specific gene expression patterns as cells differentiate and tissues and organs develop and spatially organize.[5,6] In nature, collagen is intimately associated with glycosylated proteins, growth factors, and other structural proteins such as elastin and laminin to provide unique tissue properties.[6] Each of these molecules exist within most of the ECM sources that are used as scaffolds for the constructive remodeling of tissues, but their concentration and distribution differ depending upon the tissue of origin of the ECM[7] (Figures 3.21a–c).

Fibronectin is second only to collagen in quantity within the ECM. Fibronectin, with a molecular mass of 250,000, is a dimeric molecule that exists both in soluble and insoluble/tissue isoforms and possesses ligands for adhesion of many cell types.[8–11] The ECM of submucosal structures, basement membranes, and interstitial tissues all contain abundant fibronectin.[8–10] The cell-friendly characteristics of this protein have made it an attractive substrate for in-vitro cell culture and for use as a coating for synthetic scaffold materials to promote host biocompatibility. Fibronectin is rich in the Arg-Gly-Asp (RGD) subunit; a tripeptide that is important in cell adhesion via the $\alpha 5\beta 1$ integrin.[6] Fibronectin is found at an early stage within the ECM of developing embryos and is critical for normal biologic development, especially that of vascular structures. Fibronectin was the first "structural" molecule shown to have a functional motif.

Laminin is a complex adhesion protein found in the ECM, especially within basement membrane ECMs.[10] This protein plays an important role in early embryonic development and is perhaps the best studied of the ECM proteins found within embryonic bodies.[12] This trimeric cross-linked polypeptide exists in numerous forms that depend upon the particular mixture of peptide chains (e.g., $\alpha 1$, $\beta 1$, $\gamma 1$).[13,14]

The prominent role of laminin in the formation and maintenance of vascular structures is particularly noteworthy when considering the ECM as a scaffold for tissue reconstruction.[15,16] The crucial role of the $\alpha 1$ integrin chain in mediating hematopoietic stem cell interactions with fibronectin and laminin has been firmly established.[15,16] Loss of the $\alpha 1$ integrin receptors in mice results in intrapartum mortality. This protein appears to be among the first and most critical ECM factors in the process of cell and tissue differentiation. The specific role of laminin when ECM is used as a scaffold for tissue and organ reconstruction in adults is unclear, but its importance in developmental biology suggests that this molecule is essential for self assembly of cell populations and for organized tissue development as opposed to scar tissue formation.

The ECM contains a mixture of glycosaminoglycans (GAGs) depending upon the tissue location of the ECM in the host, the age of the host, and the microenvironment. The GAGs bind growth factors and cytokines, promote water retention, and contribute to the gel properties of the ECM. The heparin-binding properties of numerous cell surface receptors and of many growth factors (e.g., fibroblast growth factor [FGF] family, vascular endothelial cell growth factor [VEGF]) make the heparin-rich GAGs important components of naturally occurring substrates for cell growth. The GAGs present in ECM include chondroitin sulfates A and B, heparin, heparan sulfate, and hyaluronan.[17,18]

Hyaluronan has been most extensively investigated as a scaffold for tissue reconstruction and as a carrier for selected cell populations in therapeutic tissue engineering applications. The concentration of hyaluronan within ECM is highest in fetal and newborn tissues and therefore tends to be associated with desirable healing properties. The specific role, if any, of this GAG upon progenitor cell proliferation and differentiation during adult wound healing is unknown.

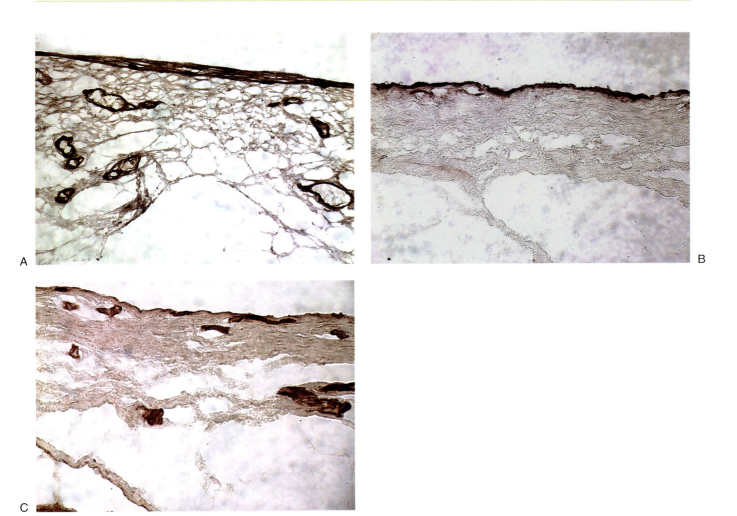

Figure 3.21. Immunoperoxidase staining shows the presence of (A) collagen IV, (B) collagen VII, and (C) laminin in the urinary bladder matrix (UBM) (×40). Collagen IV and laminin, but not collagen VII, are present in other ECM scaffolds such as SIS but their distribution and quantity are different from that in UBM.

The list of molecules of which the ECM is composed represents the "who's who" of materials from which wound care products have been manufactured. However, the amount and organization of these molecules relative to native ECM is markedly different. The complex 3-dimensional organization of the structural and functional molecules of which the ECM is composed has not been fully characterized. Therefore, synthesis of this biomaterial in the laboratory is not possible. However, individual components of the ECM such as collagen, laminin, fibronectin, and hyaluronan can be isolated, harvested, and used both in vitro and in vivo to facilitate cell growth, cell differentiation, and wound healing.

Various forms of intact ECM have been used as biologic scaffolds to promote the constructive remodeling of tissues and organs.[19–26] The term "constructive remodeling" refers to the process of scaffold degradation, cellular infiltration, and vascularization, and the differentiation and 3-dimensional organization and self-assembly of site-appropriate tissues. Commercial products composed of ECM include AlloDerm™ (Lifecell, Branchburg, NJ), Integra™ (Integra Neurosciences, Plainsboro, NJ), Apligraf® (Organogenesis Inc., Canton, MA), Oasis® (Cook Biotech, West Lafayette, IN), ACell Vet™ (ACell Vet™ Inc., Jessup, MD), and Vet BioSist (Global Vet Products, New Buffalo, MI) (Figure 3.22).

All except ACell Vet™ and Vet BioSist are intended solely for human use and therefore the cost has been prohibitive for most veterinary applications. These ECM scaffolds have been harvested from the small intestine, skin, and urinary bladder, among other tissues. Two of the most widely studied ECM scaffolds for veterinary

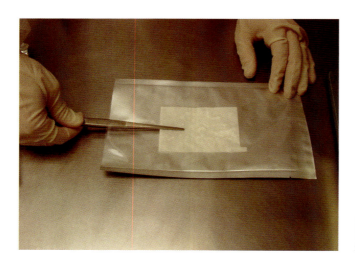

Figure 3.22. ACell Vet™ is composed of urinary bladder matrix (UBM). This figure shows a sample of the hydrated form of the single layer of ACell Vet™.

medicine applications are derived from the tunica propria and basement membrane of the porcine urinary bladder (UBM)[27–30] and small intestinal submucosa (SIS).[31–46] The composition, macrostructure and microstructure, biomechanical properties, in vivo degradation rate, cell:matrix interactions, and ability to support constructive remodeling in a variety of preclinical studies have been exhaustively investigated in a number of species for these two ECM materials.[32,47–53] It should be noted, however, that very little of this information is in the mainstream veterinary literature.

Xenogeneic, porcine-derived UBM and SIS will be used as prototype ECM scaffold materials for the present discussion but the comments and principles most likely apply to all ECM materials that are thoroughly decellularized, sterilized, and not modified by chemical crosslinking agents or other processing methods that produce unnatural protein cross-links.

The Bioinductive Properties of Extracellular Matrix Scaffolds

The mechanisms whereby scaffolds composed of naturally occurring ECM facilitate the constructive remodeling of tissues are only partially understood. It is clear that the bioinductive properties of these scaffolds play a very important role in tissue remodeling. The biomechanical properties and the ability to support host cell attachment through collagen, fibronectin, and laminin ligands are not sufficient to explain the constructive remodeling events that are observed following in vivo implantation of ECM scaffolds.

Angiogenesis, abundant host cell infiltration, mitogenesis, as well as deposition and organization of new host ECM are common events occurring during the remodeling of ECM scaffolds such as UBM and SIS. Component growth factors such as VEGF, basic FGF, and transforming growth factor beta (TGF-β) are released during scaffold degradation and exert their biologic effects as they are uncoupled from their binding proteins and are activated.[45,54–58] These growth factors survive tissue processing and sterilization[57,59] and promote angiogenesis, mitogenesis, and cellular differentiation during the tissue remodeling phase of the wound healing process. Growth factors that can be found in the ECM include VEGF, epidermal growth factor (EGF), FGF, stromal-derived growth factor (SDF-1), platelet-derived growth factor (PDGF), hepatocyte growth factor (HGF), keratinocyte growth factor (KGF), TGF-β, and others.[60–62]

Significant research effort is being placed on the use of biologic wound dressings that incorporate growth factors or antibiotics into the base material. Controlled release of various growth factors or antibiotics from such dressings is considered to be a desirable property. Examples of controlled release wound dressings include gelatin sponges or bilayer devices loaded with either free EGF or EGF encapsulated in microspheres[63] and gelatin sponges loaded with FGF-filled microspheres.[64]

While such dressings may demonstrate enhancement of a selected aspect of wound healing (e.g., angiogenesis), effective wound healing requires a complex mixture of growth factors rather than the activity of a single factor. The therapeutic use of isolated growth factors as adjuncts to wound healing can be difficult to optimize because of the inability to control the release pharmacokinetics at the target site. Growth factors are usually bound to matrix molecules as inactive precursors and then released in their active form when needed. Growth factors also work in concert with other growth factors in vivo. Therefore, isolating and applying purified forms of individual growth factors to a wound site in vivo often causes unexpected and disappointing results.[65]

ECM scaffolds are rapidly degraded in vivo by enzymatic and cellular processes. Release of the ECM constituent molecules, including the various growth factors, occurs during the degradation process. When utilized for topical applications, the ECM is typically degraded within 7 to 10 days. When utilized to repair injuries within the body, complete ECM degradation takes approximately 60–75 days.

It has recently been shown that degradation products of the parent molecules that constitute the ECM mediate a series of remodeling events. Cryptic peptides created by the degradation process initiate and sustain the recruitment of circulating, bone-marrow derived stem cells that actively participate in long-term tissue remodeling.[66,67] Antimicrobial peptides that protect the remodeling site from potential pathogens are also generated during ECM degradation.[30,39,68,69] Peptides that modulate angiogenesis and the recruitment of endothelial cells are recruited to facilitate the development of a rich blood supply to the remodeling tissue for as long as 6 to 8 weeks following ECM scaffold implantation.[70] Because of these events, sustained bioinductive properties are a hallmark of ECM scaffolds that are susceptible to in vivo degradation; i.e., not chemically crosslinked. In summary, the use of an ECM scaffold to support wound healing alters the default mechanisms of wound healing which include chronic inflammation, migration of fibroblasts, and eventual scar tissue formation.

The Antimicrobial Activity of Extracellular Matrix Scaffolds

Control of bacterial infection following injury is critical for successful tissue repair. Naturally occurring antimicrobial peptides are widespread among the animal and plant kingdoms. More than 500 such peptides have been reported.[71] It has been shown that ECM scaffolds derived from porcine SIS and UBM possess antibacterial activity against both Gram-positive and Gram-negative bacteria[30,68] (Figure 3.23). Interestingly, antibacterial activity from ECM scaffolds is only associated with degradation products of the ECM[68] and not with intact ECM.[72]

Clinical and preclinical studies have demonstrated that ECM scaffolds are resistant to bacterial infections, even in clinical applications at a high risk for bacterial infection, such as traumatic wounds and wounds with

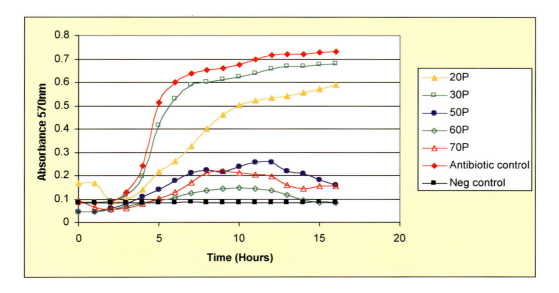

Figure 3.23. Effect of ammonium sulfate fractions of UBM-ECM digests on *S. aureus* growth. The antibacterial effects of ECM degradation products were examined. The biologic scaffold was digested with acid at high temperatures, fractionated sequentially by ammonium sulfate precipitation (20 P = 20% ammonium sulfate precipitate, etc.), and tested for antibacterial activity in a standardized in vitro assay. Ammonium sulfate fractions of the digested ECM demonstrated varying antibacterial activities against *S. aureus*.

gastrointestinal contamination.[39,73–77] In one preclinical study, dogs were subjected to infrarenal aorta replacement with either a synthetic graft or SIS. The grafts were deliberately contaminated with a pathogenic strain of 10^8 S. aureus at the time of surgery. Half of the dogs treated with synthetic grafts had positive bacterial cultures at the time of necropsy and all of the dogs in this group showed clinical evidence of persistent infection after 30 days. In contrast, all of the dogs implanted with SIS had negative bacterial cultures and the histological appearance of constructive remodeling and were free of any clinical signs of inflammation after 30 days.[39]

The short-term antimicrobial effects of ECM degradation products may protect against clinical infection long enough to allow the host inflammatory cell response and humoral immune response to become activated. The antimicrobial effects will persist as long as there is active ECM scaffold degradation taking place. This period of time will vary from several days to several weeks depending upon factors such as blood supply, size of the wound, and general state of health of the animal.[30]

The described studies demonstrate the role and importance of ECM degradation products in numerous biologic activities that promote constructive tissue remodeling. The knowledgeable and prudent use of ECM scaffolds provides the opportunity to change the wound repair process from one of inflammation and scarring to one of constructive tissue remodeling.

Host Tissue Response to Xenogeneic Extracellular Matrix

The use of xenogeneic ECM as a biologic scaffold should logically raise questions regarding the host (recipient) immune response. Many ECM scaffolds are of porcine origin, including UBM and SIS, but bovine tissue such as TissueMend® (TEI Biosciences, Boston, MA) and allogeneic human tissue (e.g., AlloDerm®, Lifecell, Inc., Branchburg, NJ) are also represented among the group of ECM biomaterials that are available for the treatment of acute and chronic wounds. Non-autologous biologic materials have been used for many years in humans without evidence of adverse immunologic outcomes. For example, porcine heart valves for valve replacement and porcine skin for the temporary treatment of burn victims have widely been accepted as safe products for human use.

Few controlled studies have evaluated and characterized the host immune response to non-autologous ECM scaffold materials. One such material, however, xenogeneic SIS-ECM, has been studied in depth. It has been shown[78] that SIS-ECM contains small amounts of the galactosyl 1,3 galactose epitope (i.e., gal-epitope),[78] but its presence does not result in complement activation or cell-mediated rejection following implantation.[79] van Seventer evaluated the T-cell response to SIS and found that human helper T-cell activation and differentiation are suppressed when these cells are cultured in vitro in the presence of processed SIS material.[80]

When examining the effects of ECM implantation on systemic immunity in mouse models, the tissue cytokine and serum humoral response to SIS were shown to be consistent with a Th-2 type immune response (accommodation) in contrast to the expected Th-1 (cell mediated rejection) type of response.[81] Repeat exposure to xenogeneic ECM failed to cause sensitization or a Th-1 type response in a mouse model. Recipients of SIS-ECM scaffolds recognize the material as "non-self" and produce antibodies, but these antibodies appear to be limited to the non-complement fixing Th-2 profile, a finding consistent with their ability to induce constructive remodeling and avoid a classic tissue rejection response. It is unknown whether the simple absence of the cellular component provides for this favorable immunologic response or whether there is an immune modulatory component of the ECM that directs this response. In summary, the host immune response in animal models shows the xenogeneic scaffold approach to be safe. In fact, the Th-2 type immune response may even be required for the constructive remodeling outcome.

The method of preparation of the ECM scaffold material can greatly affect the host response. The response to unmodified (i.e., not chemically cross-linked) ECM such as Restore™ (DePuy, Warsaw, IN) or ACell Vet™ (ACell, Jessup, MD) promotes rapid degradation of the scaffold along with deposition of new host matrix and tissue repair with minimal scar tissue.[82] Some ECM materials are crosslinked by chemicals such as glutaraldehyde, carbodiimide, isocyanate, or photo-oxidizing agents to modify their mechanical, immunogenic, or physical properties. However, such cross-linking promotes a foreign body response with fibrous tissue formation, chronic inflammation, and inhibition of cellular infiltration and scaffold degradation.[82]

A recent study utilized a rodent model of body wall repair to compare the host response to five commercially available ECM scaffolds. Autologous tissue was used as a control scaffold.[26] Marked differences were shown in the amount and temporal appearance of inflammatory cells, the morphologic structural integrity of the devices over time, and the type of host tissue that either replaced or surrounded the ECM-derived devices. It was clear

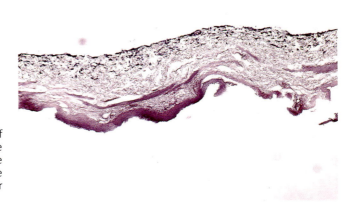

Figure 3.24. Fibroblasts growing on the abluminal surface of UBM. The spindle-shaped cells grow on the surface and invade into the underlying layers. When cultured on the opposite surface of UBM where a basement membrane is present, the cells do not invade the scaffold but rather form a confluent layer on the surface.

that manipulation of the native ECM by chemical cross-linking methods provoked a chronic inflammatory response and fibrous connective tissue deposition when compared with the host response to ECM scaffolds that were minimally manipulated. On the other hand, powder forms and gel forms of ECM scaffolds such as UBM that are suitable for injection have been produced without loss of bioactivity. The scaffold processing method, host of origin, and tissue of origin are important determinants in the host tissue response and subsequent clinical outcome.

Other factors which may have an important role in the host response to ECM scaffolds include the processes used to decellularize, disinfect, and terminally sterilize these devices. While these procedures are necessary for clinical use, they can alter the protein structures within the ECM and their ability to interact with host cells.[56] It has been shown that disinfection with peracetic acid (PAA) and terminal sterilization with gamma irradiation does not affect cell adhesion to scaffold derived from porcine bladder or small intestine and that proteins involved in cell attachment, such as fibronectin and collagen type IV, retain their ability to interact with cells.[56,83,84] Moreover, these processes do not affect the integrity of the basement membrane of ECM scaffolds such as UBM (ACell, Jessup, MD). The presence of an intact basement membrane in biologic scaffolds can aid and direct the growth of selected cell populations[85] (Figure 3.24). Decellularization can be accomplished by a number of methods. Most methods will leave remnants of cellular material, which may or may not be visible upon histologic examination, but these remnants do not appear to contribute to an adverse host response.

There is a great need for a better understanding of the relationship between the classic indicators of inflammation such as cellular infiltration, hyperemia, and tissue swelling and the same processes that are involved in constructive remodeling of tissue. Necessary and critical components of constructive ECM scaffold remodeling include cellular infiltration, deposition of new ECM in response to mechanical stimuli, self-assembly of various cell populations, and re-establishment of an interface between remodeling tissue and adjacent normal tissue. If biologic scaffold materials such as UBM and SIS are intended to modify the default mechanisms and patterns of wound healing toward more constructive tissue remodeling, then a re-examination of the spatial and temporal events that characterize similarities and differences between these two processes is warranted.

Recently, the role of mononuclear macrophages in the host response to implanted biologic scaffold materials was investigated.[86] These studies suggest that macrophages differentiate toward a phenotype that is associated with either cytotoxic inflammation or constructive remodeling.[87,88] The factors that influence the pro-inflammatory (M1) versus anti-inflammatory (M2) polarization profile of a mononuclear macrophage population are largely unknown. It appears, however, that ECM scaffold materials that are resistant to degradation (e.g., CuffPatch™) elicit a pro-inflammatory (M1) type of response whereas the anti-inflammatory (M2) macrophage phenotype predominates with native ECM scaffold materials that are readily degraded (e.g., Restore™).

Environmental Factors That Affect Tissue Reconstruction

The macro and microenvironment in which ECM scaffold remodeling occurs plays a large role in the eventual outcome. Proliferation and differentiation of the cells are strongly influenced by factors such as pH, oxygen tension, and importantly, mechanical loading. Cells destined to be of connective tissue phenotype such as fibroblasts and muscle cells depend upon and respond to mechanical loading. Protection from loading with casting and splinting can actually inhibit a constructive wound healing response for load-bearing musculotendinous tissue. The adage of "use it or lose it" is very applicable in an ECM mediated wound healing environment. Progressive loading with active assisted rehabilitation typically results in self-assembly of the participating cell population into organized, strong, and site-appropriate connective tissue rather than simple scar tissue.

Similarly, exposure of an epithelial cell surface to air promotes keratinization, whereas exposure of the same surface to fluid promotes the development of a single layer of cells.[89,90] Sheer stresses are known to affect cell orientation and phenotype. In summary, the microenvironment clearly affects the course of remodeling. Translation of this principle to the wound care setting is important. The type of dressing (wet versus dry), duration of a wound covering, and use of adjuvant treatments that affect pH, O_2 tension, and nutrient diffusion all play important roles in the remodeling of ECM scaffolds used for wound care.

Clinical Applications for Extracellular Matrix Scaffold Materials in Veterinary Medicine

Mammalian wound healing can differ significantly in the time course and degree of scar tissue formation from one individual to the next and from one species to another. Optimal wound healing in a non-infected, clean wound in most species results in a satisfactory outcome. It is difficult, if not impossible, to improve upon Mother Nature's optimal wound healing process. Therefore, results of studies that compare various scaffold materials and other wound healing interventions in uncomplicated wounds frequently yield no obvious differences.[91,92] Stated differently, there is no need for the use of ECM scaffolds in non-complicated wounds in which minimal scarring is expected. However, in sites of potential complications such as active movement around a joint and open wounds exposed to the environment and at risk for infection, and in areas where excessive scar tissue formation is a common sequelae, the use of ECM scaffolds can have dramatic positive effects. In addition, damage or injury to load-bearing structures such as ligaments or tendons frequently require external support during the time in which there is gradual replacement of the injured tissue by the host, followed by a period of rehabilitation and return of strength. The use of ECM technology as a reinforcement for such musculotendinous injuries has excellent potential in veterinary medicine.

Injuries to the superficial digital flexor tendon and/or suspensory ligaments are common and can become problematic if left untreated or if treated inappropriately. The placement of an ECM scaffold, with its inductive properties of cell recruitment, angiogenesis, and antimicrobial activity, provides a potentially valuable adjunct to conventional therapy (Figure 3.25).

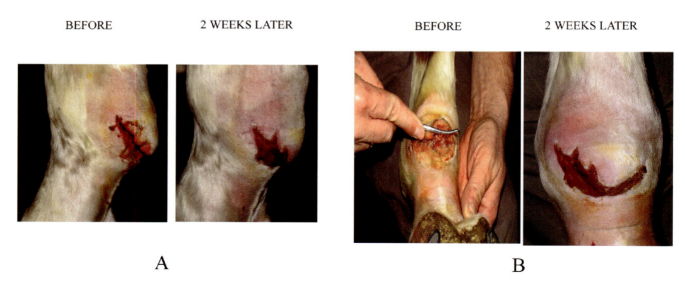

BEFORE   2 WEEKS LATER   BEFORE   2 WEEKS LATER

A   B

Figure 3.25. Contaminated wound of the left hind fetlock, which dehisced 5 days after primary closure. The wound was treated with UBM ACell Vet™ Scaffold. The photos show the wound (A) at the time of dehiscence and (B) 2 weeks post-treatment with UBM.

Injectable forms of ECM (e.g., a particulate suspension), can be placed in selected areas by injection or other minimally invasive approaches. The presence of such an inductive scaffold not only can accelerate wound healing, but in fact the tissue reconstruction process is optimized when rapid return of function (loading) is encouraged. Percutaneous injection of particulate ECM has been used for injuries involving the deep digital flexor tendon, inferior check ligament, sesamoidean ligaments, collateral ligaments, patellar ligaments, gastrocnemius tendon, and other musculotendinous structures that otherwise prove difficult to treat. In such cases, 0.2 g (dry weight) of ECM powder suspended in 3 ml of sterile saline has proven sufficient to induce a constructive remodeling response. Ultrasound guidance of the injection to ensure appropriate placement of the bioscaffold increases the likelihood of success. Serial ultrasound examinations can be used to determine when re-treatment is necessary.

Dissecting septic tendonitis, a potentially devastating complication of soft tissue injury, has been shown to respond very well to the presence of a lyophilized form of ACell Vet™ (Figure 3.26). The antimicrobial properties of the ECM degradation products, combined with the aggressive angiogenesis that occurs as part of the tissue response, clearly play roles in this type of injury.

When placed in a soft tissue defect that undergoes significant load bearing, multilaminate sheets of ECM scaffold may be required (Figure 3.27). In such cases, the presence of ECM can facilitate re-attachment of the superficial digital flexor tendon to the calcaneal tuberosity.

Wound healing in sites where there are large defects or loss of tissue can be improved with the use of appropriate ECM scaffolds. In such cases, default wound healing would typically result in excessive scar tissue formation, contracture, and loss of function. The provision of an inductive scaffold that supports cellular infiltration, neo-vascularization, and organization of differentiated connective tissues can result in functional tissue that, although not perfectly normal, is a significant improvement over default wound healing (Figure 3.28).

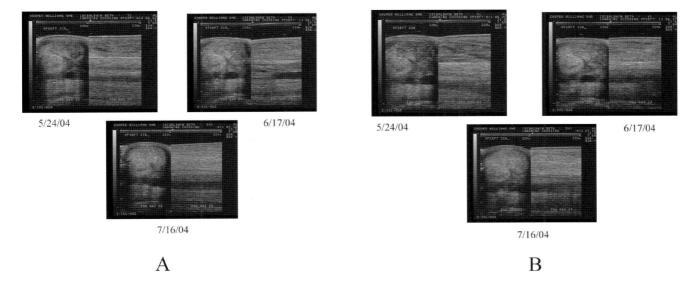

5/24/04   6/17/04   5/24/04   6/17/04

7/16/04   7/16/04

A   B

Figure 3.26. These sonograms were taken of a severe dissecting septic tendonitis of the right front superficial digital flexor tendon. The involved tissue was treated with lyophilized ACell Vet™ via ultrasound-guided injection. There was progressive healing over three tendon zones before treatment. (A) Represents sonographic findings in zone 2b and (B) represents zone 3a. The three images in each figure represent the appearance before treatment, 1 month following treatment, and 2 months following treatment. This horse returned to partial work within 3 months and full work within 6 months following treatment.

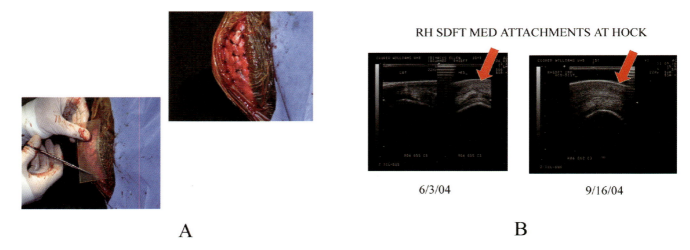

6/3/04   9/16/04

A   B

Figure 3.27. (A) Intraoperative photographs of a right hind superficial flexor tendon whose medial attachments are torn away from the calcaneal tuberosity. The area of tendon attachment is being repaired with a multiple layer ACell Vet™ Scaffold. (B) The sonograms show the torn attachments before (left) and 3 months (right) after the repair.

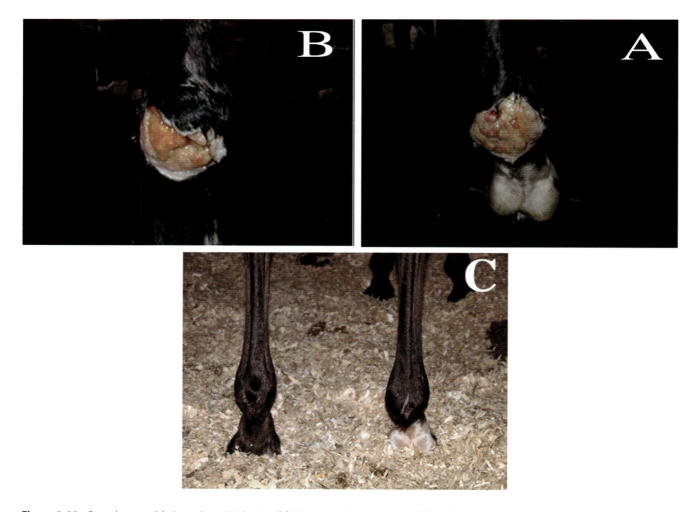

Figure 3.28. Race horse with "run down" injuries. (A) Right hindleg injury and (B) left hindleg injury. The injuries to this racehorse healed three times with scar formation, followed by repeated breakdown within 4 days of wound closure. (C) After treatment with UBM (ACell Vet™) scaffolds, the wounds closed within 2 weeks followed by complete healing within 3 months. This horse won two of its next three races.

Conclusion

The use of ECM as a biologic scaffold for wound healing is in its infancy. Unlike traditional approaches to wound healing that attempt to modulate individual events such as angiogenesis, inflammation, or scar tissue formation, the therapeutic use of ECM scaffolds is an attempt to redirect the host wound healing response to a constructive tissue remodeling response. The appropriate use of ECM scaffolds sends signals to the host that indicate a need for tissue development/reconstruction rather than response to injury.

Many of the processes of tissue development and the tissue response to injury are similar. Angiogenesis, cell recruitment, and deposition of new tissue are events common to both processes. However, the degree of angiogenesis, types of cells recruited, and spatial and temporal reorganization of tissues differ markedly between these two processes. Mother Nature has invested a complex mixture of signals within the ECM that modulate cell recruitment, cell proliferation and differentiation, and tissue assembly. Environmental factors that affect the process of tissue reconstruction such as mechanical forces, pH, and state of hydration, among others, can have a marked effect upon the end result.

An understanding of the biology of ECM mediated wound healing is essential to achieve optimal results for the use of this potentially valuable therapeutic modality in veterinary medicine.

References

1. Bissell MJ, Aggeler J: Dynamic reciprocity: how do extracellular matrix and hormones direct gene expression? Prog Clin Biol Res 987;249:251
2. Kleinman HK, Philp D, Hoffman MP: Role of the extracellular matrix in morphogenesis. Curr Opin Biotechnol 2003;14:526
3. Rosso F, Giordano A, Barbarisi M, et al: From cell-ECM interactions to tissue engineering. J Cell Physiol 2004;199:174
4. Brown E, Dejana E: Cell-to-cell contact and extracellular matrix editorial overview: Cell-cell and cell-matrix interactions—running, jumping, standing still. Cur Opin Cell Biol 2003;15:1
5. van der Rest M, Garrone R: The collagen family of proteins. FASEB J 1992;5:2814
6. Yurchenco P, Birk D, Mecham R: *Extracellular matrix assembly and structure.* San Diego: Academic Press, 1994, p.214
7. Brown B, Lindberg K, Reing J, et al: The basement membrane component of biologic scaffolds derived from extracellular matrix. Tissue Eng 2006;12:519
8. McPherson T, Badylak SF: Characterization of fibronectin derived from porcine small intestinal submucosa. Tissue Eng 1998;4:75
9. Miyamoto S, Katz BZ, Lafrenie RM, et al: Fibronectin and integrins in cell adhesion, signaling, and morphogenesis. Ann N Y Acad Sci 1998;857:119
10. Schwarzbauer JE: Basement membranes: putting up the barriers. Curr Biol 1999;9:R242
11. Schwarzbauer JE: Fibronectin: from gene to protein. Curr Opin Cell Biol 1991;3:786
12. Li S, Harrison D, Carbonetto S, et al: Matrix assembly, regulation, and survival functions of laminin and its receptors in embryonic stem cell differentiation. J Cell Biol 2002;157:1279
13. Timpl R: Macromolecular organization of basement membranes. Curr Opin Cell Biol 1996;8:618
14. Timpl R, Brown JC: Supramolecular assembly of basement membranes. Bioessays 1996;18:123
15. Ponce ML, Nomizu M, Delgado MC, et al: Identification of endothelial cell binding sites on the laminin gamma 1 chain. Circ Res 1999;84:688
16. Werb Z, Vu TH, Rinkenberger JL, et al: Matrix-degrading proteases and angiogenesis during development and tumor formation. Apmis 1999;107:11
17. Entwistle J, Zhang S, Yang B, et al: Characterization of the murine gene encoding the hyaluronan receptor RHAMM. Gene 1995;163:233
18. Hodde JP, Badylak SF, Brightman AO, et al: Glycosaminoglycan content of small intestinal submucosa: A bioscaffold for tissue replacement. Tissue Eng 1996;2:209
19. Chagraoui J, Lepage-Noll A, Anjo A, et al: Fetal liver stroma consists of cells in epithelial-to-mesenchymal transition. Blood 2003;101:2973
20. Dahms SE, Piechota HJ, Dahiya R, et al: Composition and biomechanical properties of the bladder acellular matrix graft: comparative analysis in rat, pig and human. Br J Urol 1998;82:411
21. Huang M, Khor E, Lim LY: Uptake and cytotoxicity of chitosan molecules and nanoparticles: effects of molecular weight and degree of deacetylation. Pharm Res 2004;21:344
22. Meyer T: Extracellular matrix proteins in the porcine pancreas: a structural analysis for directed pancreatic islet isolation. Transpl Proc 1998;30:354
23. Robinson K, Matheny R: Myocardial tissue replacement with extracellular matrix scaffolds. J Am Coll Cardiol 2003;41(Suppl.2):514

24. Schenke-Layland K, Vasilevski O, Opitz F, et al: Impact of decellularization of xenogeneic tissue on extracellular matrix integrity for tissue engineering of heart valves. J Struct Biol 2003;143:201

25. Sutherland RS, Baskin LS, Hayward SW, et al: Regeneration of bladder urothelium, smooth muscle, blood vessels and nerves into an acellular tissue matrix. J Urol 1996;156:571

26. Valentin J, Badylak J, McCabe G, et al: Extracellular matrix bioscaffolds for orthopaedic applications: a comparative histologic study. J Bone Joint Surg Am 2006;88:2673

27. Kochupura PV, Azeloglu EU, Kelly DJ, et al: Tissue-engineered myocardial patch derived from extracellular matrix provides regional mechanical function. Circulation 2005;112(Suppl.9):I144

28. Wood JD, Simmons-Byrd A, Spievack AR, et al: Use of a particulate extracellular matrix bioscaffold for treatment of acquired urinary incontinence in dogs. J Am Vet Med Assoc 2005;226:1095

29. Nieponice A, Gilbert T, Badylak SF: Reinforcement of esophageal anastomoses with an extracellular matrix scaffold in a canine model. Ann Thor Surg 2006;82:2050

30. Brennan E, Reing J, Chew D, et al: Antibacterial activity within degradation products of biologic scaffolds composed of extracellular matrix. Tissue Eng 2006;12:2949

31. Abraham GA, Murray J, Billiar K, et al: Evaluation of the porcine intestinal collagen layer as a biomaterial. J Biomed Mater Res 2000;51:442

32. Alpert S, Cheng E, Kaplan W, et al: Bladder neck fistula after the complete primary repair of exostrophy: a multi-institutional experience. J Urol 2005;174(4 Pt 2):1687

33. Jones S, Vasavada S, Abdelmalak J, et al: Sling may hasten return of continence after radical prostatectomy. J Urol 2005;65:1163

34. Le Visage C, Okawa A, Kadakia L, et al: Intervertebral disc regeneration using small intestinal submucosa as a bioscaffold. Comput Methods Biomech Biomed Engin 2005;Suppl.1:177

35. Tian X, Xue W, Pang X, et al: Effect of small intestinal submucosa on islet recovery and function in vitro culture. Hepatobiliary Pancreat Dis Int 2005;4:524

36. Ueno T, Pickett LC, de la Fuente SG, et al: Clinical application of porcine small intestinal submucosa in the management of infected or potentially contaminated abdominal defects. J Gastrointest Surg 2004;8:109

37. Badylak S, Kokini K, Tullius B, et al: Strength over time of a resorbable bioscaffold for body wall repair in a dog model. J Surg Res 2001;99:282

38. Badylak S, Meurling S, Chen M, et al: Resorbable bioscaffold for esophageal repair in a dog model. J Pediatr Surg 2000;35:1097

39. Badylak SF, Coffey AC, Lantz GC, et al: Comparison of the resistance to infection of intestinal submucosa arterial autografts versus polytetrafluoroethylene arterial prostheses in a dog model. J Vasc Surg 1994;19:465

40. Badylak SF, Lantz GC, Coffey A, et al: Small intestinal submucosa as a large diameter vascular graft in the dog. J Surg Res 1989;47:74

41. Herbert ST, Badylak SF, Geddes LA, et al: Elastic modulus of prepared canine jejunum, a new vascular graft material. Ann Biomed Eng 1993;21:727

42. Hiles MC, Badylak SF, Geddes LA, et al: Porosity of porcine small-intestinal submucosa for use as a vascular graft. J Biomed Mater Res 1993;27:139

43. Hiles MC, Badylak SF, Lantz GC, et al: Mechanical properties of xenogeneic small-intestinal submucosa when used as an aortic graft in the dog. J Biomed Mat Res 1995;29:883

44. Lantz GC, Badylak SF, Hiles MC, et al: Treatment of reperfusion injury in dogs with experimentally induced gastric dilatation-volvulus. Am J Vet Res 1992;53:1594

45. Voytik-Harbin SL, Brightman AO, Kraine MR, et al: Identification of extractable growth factors from small intestinal submucosa. J Cell Biochem 1997;67:478

46. Freytes D, Tullius R, Badylak S: The effect of storage upon material properties of lyophilized porcine extracellular matrix derived from the urinary bladder. J Biomed Mat Res:b—Applied Biomat 2006;78:327

47. De Ugarte D, Choi E, Weitzbuch H, et al: Mucosal regeneration of a duodenal defect using small intestine submucosa. Am Surg 2004;70:49

48. Helton W, Fisichella PM, Berger R, et al: Short-term outcomes with small intestinal submucosa for ventral abdominal hernia. Arch Surg 2005;140:549

49. Jones J, Rackley RR, Berglund R, et al: Porcine small intestinal submucosa as a percutaneous mid-urethral sling: 2-year results. Br J Urol Int 2005;96:103

50. Misseri R, Cain M, Casale A, et al: Small intestinal submucosa bladder neck slings for incontinence associated with neuropathic bladder. J Urol 2005;174(4 Pt 2):1680

51. Pu LL: Small intestinal submucosa (Surgisis) as a bioactive prosthetic material for repair of abdominal wall fascial defect. Plast Reconstr Surg 2005;115:2127

52. Shell DHT, Croce MA, Cagiannos C, et al: Comparison of small-intestinal submucosa and expanded polytetrafluoroethylene as a vascular conduit in the presence of gram-positive contamination. Ann Surg 2005;241:995

53. Smith A, Walsh R, Henderson J: Novel bile duct repair for bleeding biliary anastomotic varices: case report and literature review. J Gastroint Surg 2005;9:832

54. Hodde J, Record R, Tullius B, et al: Fibronectin peptides mediate HMEC adhesion to porcine-derived extracellular matrix. Biomat 2002;23:1841

55. Hodde JP, Record RD, Liang HA, et al: Vascular endothelial growth factor in porcine-derived extracellular matrix. Endothelium 2001;8:11

56. Hodde JP, Record RD, Tullius RS, et al: Retention of endothelial cell adherence to porcine-derived extracellular matrix after disinfection and sterilization. Tissue Eng 2002;8:225

57. McDevitt CA, Wildey GM, Cutrone RM: Transforming growth factor-beta1 in a sterilized tissue derived from the pig small intestine submucosa. J Biomed Mater Res 2003;67A:637

58. Hodde J, Hiles M: Bioactive FGF-2 in sterilized extracellular matrix. Wounds 2001;13:195

59. Hodde JP, Ernst DM, Hiles MC: An investigation of the long-term bioactivity of endogenous growth factor in OASIS Wound Matrix. J Wound Care 2005;14:23

60. Bonewald LF: Regulation and regulatory activities of transforming growth factor beta. Crit Rev Eukaryotic Gene Expres 1999;9:33

61. Kagami S, Kondo S, Loster K, et al: Collagen type I modulates the platelet-derived growth factor (PDGF) regulation of the growth and expression of beta1 integrins by rat mesangial cells. Biochem Biophys Res Commun 1998;252:728

62. Roberts R, Gallagher J, Spooncer E, et al: Heparan sulphate bound growth factors: a mechanism for stromal cell mediated haemopoiesis. Nature 1988;332:376

63. Ulubayram K, Nur Cakar A, Korkusuz P, et al: EGF containing gelatin-based wound dressings. Biomat 2001;22:1345

64. Huang S, Deng T, Wu H, et al: Wound dressings containing bFGF-impregnated microspheres. J Microencapsul 2006;23:277

65. Badylak SF: Extracellular matrix as a scaffold for tissue engineering in veterinary medicine: applications to soft tissue healing. Clin Tech Equine Pract 2004;3:173

66. Zantop T, Gilbert, TW, Yoder MC, et al: Extracellular matrix scaffolds attract bone marrow derived cells in a mouse model of Achilles tendon reconstruction. J Orthop Res 2006;24:1299

67. Badylak S, Park K, McCabe G, et al: Marrow-derived cells populate scaffolds composed of xenogeneic extracellular matrix. Exp Hematol 2001;29:1310

68. Sarikaya A, Record R, Wu CC, et al: Antimicrobial activity associated with extracellular matrices. Tissue Eng 2002;8:63

69. Badylak SF, Wu CC, Bible M, et al: Host protection against deliberate bacterial contamination of an extracellular matrix bioscaffold versus Dacron mesh in a dog model of orthopedic soft tissue repair. J Biomed Mater Res 2003;67B:648

70. Li F, Li W, Johnson SA, et al: Low–molecular-weight peptides derived from extracellular matrix as chemoattractants for primary endothelial cells. Endothelium 2004;11:199

71. Zasloff M: Antimicrobial peptides of multicellular organisms. Nature 2002;415:389

72. Holtom PD, Shinar Z, Benna J, et al: Porcine small intestine submucosa does not show antimicrobial properties. Clin Orthop Relat Res 2004;427:18

73. Jernigan TW, Croce MA, Cagiannos C, et al: Small intestinal submucosa for vascular reconstruction in the presence of gastrointestinal contamination. Ann Surg 2004;239:733

74. Kim BS, Baez CE, Atala A: Biomaterials for tissue engineering. World J Urol 2000;18:2

75. Mantovani F, Trinchieri A, Castelnuovo C, et al: Reconstructive urethroplasty using porcine acellular matrix. Eur Urol 2003;44:600

76. Ruiz CE, Iemura M, Medie S, et al: Transcatheter placement of a low-profile biodegradable pulmonary valve made of small intestinal submucosa: a long-term study in a swine model. J Thorac Cardiovasc Surg 2005;130:477

77. Kim MS, Hong KD, Shin HW, et al: Preparation of porcine small intestinal submucosa sponge and their application as a wound dressing in full-thickness skin defect of rat. Int J Biol Macromol 2005;36:54

78. McPherson TB, Liang H, Record RD, et al: Galalpha (1,3) Gal epitope in porcine small intestinal submucosa. Tissue Eng 2000;6:233

79. Raeder RH, Badylak SF, Sheehan C, et al: Natural anti-galactose alpha1,3 galactose antibodies delay, but do not prevent the acceptance of extracellular matrix xenografts. Transplant Immunol 2002;10:15

80. Palmer EM, Beilfuss BA, Nagai T, et al: Human helper T cell activation and differentiation is suppressed by porcine small intestinal submucosa. Tissue Eng 2002;8:893

81. Allman AJ, McPherson TB, Merrill LC, et al: The Th2-restricted immune response to xenogeneic small intestinal submucosa does not influence systemic protective immunity to viral and bacterial pathogens. Tissue Eng 2002;8:53

82. Badylak SF: The extracellular matrix as a scaffold for tissue reconstruction. Semin Cell Dev Biol 2002;13:377

83. Hodde J, Janis A, Ernst D, et al: Effects of sterilization on an extracellular matrix scaffold: part I. Composition and matrix architecture. J Mater Sci: Mater Med 2007;18:537

84. Hodde J, Janis A, Hiles M: Effects of sterilization on an extracellular matrix scaffold: part II. Bioactivity and matrix interaction. J Mater Sci: Mater Med 2007;18:545

85. Brown B, Lindberg K, Reing J, et al: The basement membrane component of biologic scaffolds derived from extracellular matrix. Tissue Eng 2006;12:519
86. Badylak S, Valentin J, Ravindra A, et al: Macrophage phenotype as a determinant of biologic scaffold remodeling. Tissue Eng, in press
87. Mantovani A, Sica A, Sozzani S, et al: The chemokine system in diverse forms of macrophage activation and polarization. TRENDS Immunol 2004;25:677
88. Mantovani A, Sica A, Locati M: Macrophage polarization comes of age. Immun 2005;23:344
89. Knowles N, Miyashita Y, Usui M, et al: A model for studying keratinocyte attachment morphology at the interface between skin and percutaneous devices. J Biomed Mater Res 2005;74:482
90. Zeltinger J, Holbrook K: A model system for long-term serum-free suspension organ culture of human fetal tissues: experiments on digits and skin from multiple body regions. Cell Tissue Res 1997;290:51
91. Winkler JT, Swaim SF, Sartin EA, et al: The effect of porcine-derived small intestinal submucosa product on wounds with exposed bone in dogs. Vet Surg 2002;31:541
92. Gomez JH, Schumacher J, Lauten SD, et al: Effects of 3 biologic dressings on healing of cutaneous wounds on the limbs of horses. Can J Vet Res 2004;68:49

4 Approaches to Wound Closure

4.1 Selection of Approaches to Wound Closure

Ted S. Stashak, DVM, MS, Diplomate ACVS

Introduction

The therapeutic goal in the case of any wound should be to return the horse to normal function as soon a possible while achieving a cosmetic outcome. Many interdependent factors must be considered when selecting a treatment approach: time elapsed since injury; location, depth, and configuration of the wound; degree of contamination, severity and nature of the trauma; and status of the blood supply to the wound, as well as the patient's condition. Other factors to consider include cost, patient temperament, and intended use of the horse. Rigid guidelines dictating whether a wound should be sutured are inadvisable; such a decision should be made only after objective information has been obtained from an evaluation of both the patient and the wound.

This said, whenever possible, wounds should be managed by primary closure (closed within several hours following injury). The "golden period" relates to the time that it takes multiplying bacteria in a wound to reach infective levels, considered to be $>10^5$ organisms per gram of tissue in a sutured wound.[1] This may take longer in very clean, minimally contaminated wounds and it may be shorter in heavily contaminated, contused wounds. Primary closure is considered ideal for fresh, minimally contaminated wounds of the extremities (not involving vital structures), wounds of the head region, flap wounds with a good blood supply, and wounds of the upper body when an improved cosmetic result is desired. Wounds caused by contact with sharp objects are often closed primarily (Figure 4.1).

Delayed primary closure is defined as that carried out before the development of granulation tissue, which usually occurs 4 to 5 days following injury. Delayed secondary closure (secondary closure) most typically refers to wound apposition after observable formation of granulation tissue, usually >5 days following injury. While it has been suggested that both delayed primary and delayed secondary closure be referred to simply as delayed closure, they will be considered as distinct since granulation tissue may be visible in horses by 3 days post injury.[2] Delayed primary closure is often selected for acute wounds (<6–8 hours duration) that are moderately contaminated, contused, and swollen (Figure 4.2). Many wounds that penetrate synovial structures are handled this way, although some wounds <6–8 hours old may be closed primarily following the treatment approaches outlined in Chapter 9.

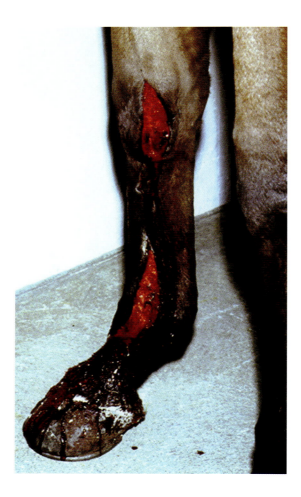

Figure 4.1. Example of acute wounds of <4 hours duration that could be managed by primary closure. The injuries occurred when the horse reared and subsequently fell on the farrier's tool box; a hoof knife was the cause. The lacerations were overlying the carpal and fetlock joints and may have involved the tendon sheaths and bursae. Joint involvement was evaluated by placing a needle into each joint space, in a site remote to the wounds, and then injecting sterile fluid under pressure. Tendon sheath and bursa involvement could be ruled out by digital palpation. None of the synovial cavities were breached by these injuries.

Delayed secondary closure is often selected for more chronic wounds that are infected or have a compromised blood supply (Figure 4.3). The wound is closed following the development of a healthy bed of granulation tissue. An exception to this is the "degloving" type of injury which usually involves the metacarpus/metatarsus (Figure 2.4). These wounds should be sutured as early as possible, ideally within 4 days, to reduce the risk of bone sequestrum formation, tendon degeneration, and potentially uncontrolled infection.[3] Management of degloving wounds will be discussed under the section of delayed primary closure in this chapter and is reviewed in more detail in the first two sections of Chapter 8.

Second intention healing (granulation tissue formation, wound contraction, and epithelialization) is selected for large wounds over highly mobile regions (e.g., pectoral, axilla, groin and gluteal, etc.) (Figure 4.4). Skin grafting is useful in cases in which the tissue deficit exceeds the capability of wound contraction and epithelialization. Reconstructive surgery and scar tissue revision can be used to obtain a better cosmetic and functional end result in a wound that is already healed.[4] In many cases, wound closure is unachievable due to the surrounding soft tissue damage, size of the wound, or loss of skin (Figure 4.5). For information regarding the management of such wounds, see Degloving Injuries in Chapter 8.

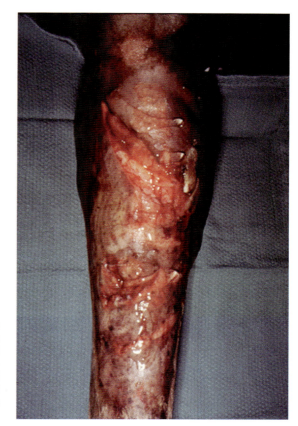

Figure 4.2. Example of wounds of <4 hours duration that could be managed by delayed primary closure. The lacerations resulted from this horse kicking the inside of a horse trailer. Note the limb swelling and edema associated with these wounds. Following wound cleansing, examination, and debridement, the limb was immobilized in a bandage cast splint in preparation for possible closure within the next 2 days. The blunt nature of the trauma made it inadvisable to suture these wounds primarily.

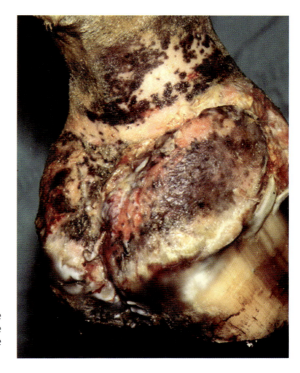

Figure 4.3. Heel bulb laceration of several days duration that could be managed by delayed secondary closure. The cause was barbed wire. The horse was 4/5 lame in the affected limb and the wound was exudative and swollen, indicating infection.

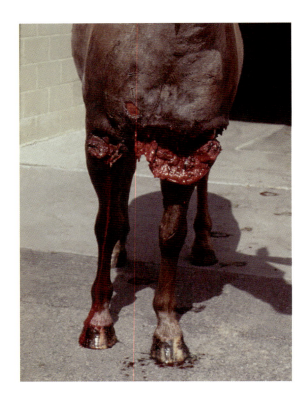

Figure 4.4. Example of large wounds (~24 hours duration) involving the upper cranial antebrachium and pectoral region that can be managed by second intention healing without loss of function. These lacerations resulted from the horse running through several barbed wire fences.

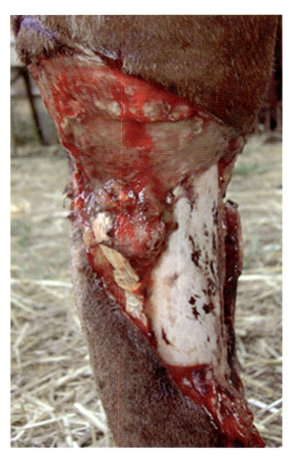

Figure 4.5. Large avulsive contaminated wound of the proximal metatarsal region that will have to be managed by second intention healing.

Preparation of the Wound for Closure

Appropriate preparation of the wound prior to closure is critical to the final outcome. Some horses will require sedation and/or tranquilization prior to wound preparation, though phenothiazine tranquilizers should be avoided in horses suffering hemorrhagic shock. Local anesthesia can be accomplished by regional, perineural, or intralesional (direct) infiltration of an anesthetic agent. Direct infiltration of the wound is acceptable following cleansing. With the wound protected by means of sterile moist gauze sponges, a wide area of hair around the wound is then clipped and the wound edges are shaved with a recessed head razor. Dampening the hair with water or coating it lightly with K-Y water-soluble jelly will prevent the hair from falling into the wound. The clipped area is scrubbed at least 3 times with antiseptic soap (e.g., povidone-iodine or chlorhexidine); between scrubs, the area is rinsed with a sterile isotonic salt solution.

Although time-honored, firm scrubbing of the wound with gauze sponges and saline may not be as beneficial in decreasing infection in a contaminated wound as was once thought. Trauma to the wound surface apparently offsets the benefits of removing contaminants and bacteria.[5] On the other hand, the mechanical effect of lavaging (irrigating) the wound under pressure is important to remove adherent contaminants and bacteria. To be effective, irrigation solutions should be delivered by fluid jet and impact the wound at an oblique angle with at least 7 PSI.[6] However, since pressures of 10–15 PSI have been shown to remove approximately 80% of the microorganisms from the wound surface,[7] the author prefers using these higher pressures. Addition of a diluted antiseptic solution[8] or antibiotic(s) to the irrigation solution enhances its ability to prevent wound infection.[9–11] Povidone-iodine (0.1% to 0.2% [10–20 ml/L sterile salt solution]) or chlorhexidine (0.05% [1:40 = 25 ml of the 2% concentrate diluted with 975 ml of sterile isotonic crystalloid]) have proven effective[12–14] and are preferred by the author, though greater concentrations of these antiseptics are cytotoxic and may increase the incidence of infection.[7] While addition of antibiotics such as 0.5% neomycin, 0.5% kanamycin, and 0.1% gentamicin to the irrigation solution has been recommended, the author sees no real advantage to their use over antiseptics unless culture and sensitivity results justify it.

The effect of the timing of wound irrigation is also important. Early irrigation appears to improve the ability to remove bacteria from the surface of the wound. An experimental study using goat wounds contaminated with a fixed number of bacteria found that irrigation with 6 L saline solution delivered by a Stryker inter-pulse irrigation system™ resulted in ~70%, ~52%, and ~37% reduction in bacterial counts from the pre-irrigation levels at 3, 6, and 12 hours, respectively.[15] The reason that earlier irrigation resulted in greater bacterial removal was believed to be that bacterial adhesion begins about 3 hours, followed by the establishment of a biofilm as early as 5 hours, after inoculation, with maturation of the biofilm by 10 hours.[16] Even though the effects of wound debridement were not considered in this study it nevertheless provides key information regarding the importance of early irrigation.

The amount of fluid required to adequately cleanse/irrigate the wound will vary with the size of the wound and the degree of contamination. Minimally, the gross contaminants within the wound should be eliminated. Lavage should be discontinued before the tissues take on a "water-logged" appearance and become discolored by a gray hue.

After the wound has been thoroughly cleansed and is free of devitalized tissue and debris, it can be explored either by digital palpation or with a sterile instrument. Sterile gloves, rinsed free of talcum powder, should be worn to palpate the wound's depth. A sterile instrument to probe a penetrating tract can be helpful in identifying a foreign body or determining whether bone has been contacted by the injury. If the location of the probe in relation to synovial structures is questionable, a radiograph should be taken (Figure 2.13a).

If suspicion persists, contrast material can be injected into the tract and a second radiograph taken (Figure 2.13b). This can be accomplished by inserting a Foley catheter into the wound, inflating the balloon tip, and injecting contrast dye. Moreover, synovial fluid may be identified by stringing it between the thumb and forefinger. In such cases a fluid sample may be submitted for cytologic examination.

Finally, if there remains a doubt about whether a synovial cavity has been penetrated, sterile fluid can be injected under pressure into the joint, taking care to insert the needle at a site far removed from the wound (Figure 2.15).[17] In the event of synovial capsule penetration, injected fluid will be seen in the wound bed. In this case the needle is left in place to flush the synovial cavity with a sterile isotonic salt solution. For more information on the management of wounds involving synovial structures, see Chapter 9.

A management plan is designed following wound examination. In the event of primary closure, one must decide whether it can be done in the standing sedated horse or if general anesthesia is required. In either case, perioperative antibiotics are most often indicated and the tetanus immunization updated. If a synovial structure has been penetrated, combination therapy with broad-spectrum antimicrobials is recommended. When primary closure is used, the wound is prepared immediately for suture. If the horse has to be transported, topical, water-soluble antibiotics are placed in the wound and a sterile, non-adherent dressing is applied followed by sterile bandaging. Nonsteroidal anti-inflammatory drugs can be administered at this time if necessary (excessive swelling, lameness, etc.). The aim of this chapter is to review the various approaches for wound closure and discuss indications. For more detailed information regarding preparation of the wound for closure, see Chapter 2.

Primary Closure

Whenever possible, immediate closure of a traumatic wound is desirable because it has several advantages over other techniques. Primary closure reduces the chances of further wound contamination and infection; it apposes the wound edges in their normal anatomic position and thus reduces healing time and scarring; it usually requires less aftercare (e.g., wound irrigation, debridement, and bandaging) and consequently reduces expenses; and it enables an earlier return to function.

Successful primary closure relies on several important features including an adequate blood supply to the wounded tissues and a bacterial inoculum (bioburden) $<10^5$ microorganisms per gram of tissue. Although there are laser Doppler instruments that can measure cutaneous blood flow to the wound (e.g., Periflux™, models 4000–5000, Perimed Inc., North Royalton, OH [www.perimed.com]; SIM LD12™, Moor Instruments Ltd., Devon, UK [www.moor.co.uk]), assessment of an adequate blood supply is largely accomplished by clinical examination of the wound and a knowledge of the vascular supply to the affected region (e.g., distal extremities have a limited blood supply compared to the head).

On the other hand, accurate clinical assessment of the bacterial inoculum in the wound, before and after cleansing, may be difficult. Several procedures can provide a more accurate assessment of the bacterial burden (bioburden). Gram-stained smears provide important information about the identity of the bacteria present in the wound. The presence of *beta-hemolytic streptococci,* for example, is associated with wound infection and dehiscence despite comparatively low inoculums, in relation to the production of cytotoxins and enzymes that depolymerize connective tissue components and enhance microbial invasion.[18,19] Smears prepared from wound biopsies are superior to surface swabs,[19] and samples should be taken following irrigation and wound debridement to provide a measure of the efficacy of wound decontamination.[20]

Quantitative procedures can be used to estimate the wound bioburden, which may direct decisions on wound closure.[21,22] Wound biopsy, the current gold standard, relies on weighing the biopsy specimen after which it is homogenized and the number of organisms determined by serial dilution cultures of the homogenate.[23] Unfortunately, this test, because it only samples a small part of the wound, lacks sensitivity for detecting all bacterial pathogens and has poor reproducibility in quantifying total bacterial burden.[20] Moreover, it is time-consuming. As a result, it is rarely used in routine clinical practice in humans and horses. A modified rapid slide technique offers results in 30 minutes and is convenient for intraoperative assessment of wounds being considered for closure.[22] A single organism on the slide indicates a bioburden $>10^5$ organisms per gram of tissue, making closure ill-advised. The reproducibility of this technique has not been extensively studied; therefore, it cannot be recommended at this time. The special equipment and personnel required for these quantitative procedures typically limit their use to referral and institutional practices. For more information regarding the detrimental effects of the bacterial bioburden on wound healing, see Chapter 2.

Once primary closure has been selected, the wound must be prepared properly, as outlined previously in this chapter and in more detail in Chapter 2. Debridement of the entire wound should be performed following proper cleansing and exploration. This is best done systematically, beginning with the removal of a thin margin of skin, when indicated, then with tissue within the wound from one margin, advancing across the wound and finishing at the other margin (Figure 4.6). Excisional layered debridement is most effective for removing contaminants and bacteria from within the superficial layers of the wound.[3,24] In some wounds complete excisional debridement is impossible; simple or piecemeal debridement of all abnormal tissue, performed in a systematic fashion, may suffice for these (Figure 2.21).

Whenever possible, sharp excision of the wound edges and its surfaces is best. Scraping the wound with a scalpel is ineffective and traumatizes the wound, making it more susceptible to infection. Care should be taken to avoid penetrating and transecting vital structures. Once debridement is complete, the wound is irrigated with a dilute antiseptic sterile salt solution. Surgical gloves are changed, the wound is re-draped, the instruments

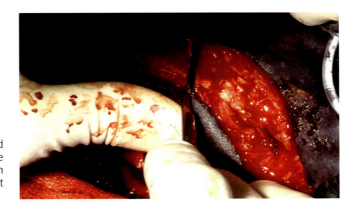

Figure 4.6. Same wound as in Figure 4.1. Excisional layered debridement is being used to eliminate contaminants and the bioburden, thus creating a new wound. Note that a thin margin of skin is being excised at the wound edge. Layered debridement of the deeper tissues within the wound followed.

used for debridement are discarded, and new ones are used for suturing and placement of a drain if needed. For more information on preparation of the wound for closure the reader, see Chapter 2.

Although the use of antibiotics topically applied to or injected directly into the wound just prior to closure is controversial, this practice is generally thought to decrease infection rates.[11,25,26] The author recommends this approach for wounds with marginal blood supply that require prompt closure (e.g., degloving injury). In these cases only water-soluble nonirritating antibiotics should be used.

The least number of sutures to effectively appose wound tissues under minimal tension should be used.[27,28] Sutures should be placed in deeper tissue only to appose prominent fascial layers, retinaculae, and joint capsules, as well as transected flexor tendons or ligaments. Although synthetic absorbable sutures create minimal inflammatory response, they nonetheless represent a foreign body within the tissues, which may prolong the inflammatory phase of healing and make the wound more susceptible to infection.[27,28] For more information regarding suture patterns and materials, see Selection of Suture Materials, Suture Patterns, and Drains for Wound Closure later in this chapter.

Tension suturing patterns can be employed to reduce the tension on the primary suture line.[29] Widely placed vertical mattress sutures with or without support such as buttons, gauze, or rubber tubing are quite effective for this purpose (Figures 4.28a–c, 4.29, and 4.30). While tension sutures with supports are mostly used in regions that can't be effectively bandaged (e.g., upper body and neck regions), they should not be placed under pressure bandages or casts because this can induce skin necrosis (Figure 4.30). Tension sutures should be removed in 4 to 10 days, depending on the amount of tension generated upon closure. Staggered removal over several days is advisable when excessive tension was present at closure. Tension sutures employed to aid in wound stabilization (e.g., wounds over the cranial surface of the stifle) are left in place for at least 7 to 10 days. For more information regarding methods of reducing skin tension upon closure, see Selection of Suture Materials, Suture Patterns, and Drains for Wound Closure later in this chapter.

Drains are used when considerable dead space will remain after suture closure (Figures 4.7a,b). However, these must be maintained in a sterile environment. Drainage can be directed into a sterile bandage in the case of wounds on the extremities, while fluid can flow into a sterile stent bandage that is sutured over the wound to cover the drain in the case of upper body wounds. Drains should be sutured proximally, traverse the wound adjacent to but not directly underneath the sutured skin edges, and exit through an incision created adjacent or distal to the distal limit of the wound (Figure 4.7b). The drain should also be sutured at the point of exit (Figure 4.36). This method of placement reduces the risk of retrograde infection directly involving the suture line. Drains are usually left in place for 24–48 hours but may remain longer if drainage persists. For more information regarding wound drains, see Selection of Suture Materials, Suture Patterns, and Drains for Wound Closure later in this chapter.

If treated appropriately (as outlined in chapter 9), acute synovial wounds (<6–8 hours) only contaminate the synovial structure without causing a true infection.[3,30] Primary wound closure should be considered in these cases. If doubt exists, it is probably best to leave the wound to heal by second intention; alternatively, delayed primary closure of the wound may be performed after 2 to 4 days.[3,30] Delaying closure permits a greater time to re-sterilize the synovial cavity following the administration of appropriate broad-spectrum antimicrobials (systemic and intrasynovial) prior to wound edge apposition.

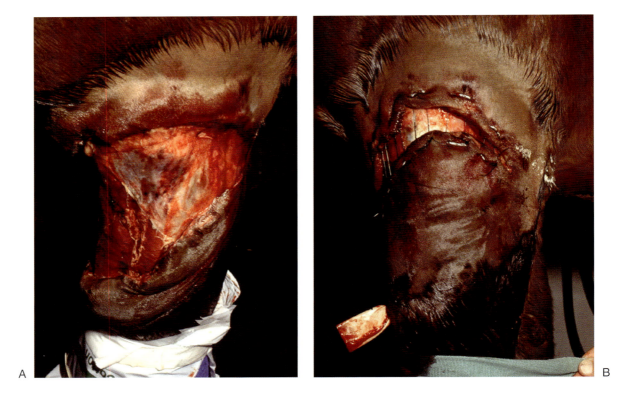

Figure 4.7. Example of a wound in which a drain should be used. (A) An acute wound of <4 hours duration involving the proximal antebrachium. Note the skin flap at the distal extent of the wound which has become displaced distad. Suturing the skin flap into its normal position will create a sizeable dead space underneath the skin flap. (B) The wound could not be completely closed because of increased skin tension. Note that the Penrose drain is exiting the undermined skin flap at its distal most limits. The drain was fixed in place by sutures attaching it to the skin, proximally and distally. The drain exit site was covered with sterile bandages.

Although delaying repair for a few days will likely hinder closure of the wound as a result of granulation tissue formation and skin retraction, this can usually be accomplished by removal (debulking) of the granulation tissue, limited undermining of the skin edges, and use of skin tension suturing techniques. It is typically unnecessary to close small puncture type wounds involving a synovial cavity, but larger wounds in high motion regions should be closed to minimize wound healing complications.

The final decision to close a wound breaching a synovial cavity is often based on the clinical examination (lameness, drainage, swelling, etc.) and laboratory findings (synovial WBC count and total protein concentration). See Chapter 9 for more information regarding the examination and the clinical and laboratory findings associated with penetrating wounds to synovial cavities.

Some wounds cannot be completely closed due to the excess tension required to bring the wound edges in contact. In these, partial closure is acceptable (Figure 4.7). If the sutured wound edges are not too far apart a cosmetic result can be achieved, particularly when this approach is used for upper limb and body wounds (Figures 4.8a,b).

A retrospective study documenting the effects of primary closure in 217 horses and 41 ponies with similar wounds (60% of which were located on the lower limb) found primary closure was significantly more often successful in ponies (41%) compared to horses (26%). This difference was most apparent in the limbs, where 37% of the wounds in ponies healed by primary intention compared to 21% in the horses. Sequestra were formed significantly more often in horses. The reasons for these differences may relate to the ponies' superior inflammatory response following injury, which may result in a better local defense against wound infection.[31] See Chapter 8 for more information regarding the management and complications associated with distal limb injuries.

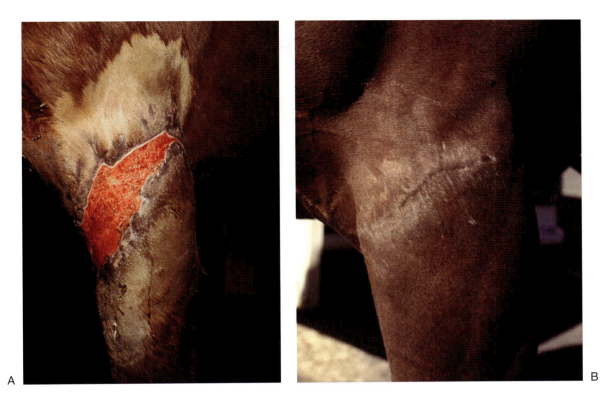

Figure 4.8. Same horse as in Figure 4.7. (A) The wound, 3 weeks following partial closure. The drain was removed within 48 hours and the skin sutures were removed 2 weeks post-operatively. (B) The wound ~3 months post surgery. Note the good cosmetic outcome.

Delayed Closure

The ability of delayed closure to reduce wound infection in contaminated wounds is well established.[32–35] Successful delayed closure is reported in 80% to 95% of wounds considered likely to become infected with immediate closure.[36,37] Research also indicates that healing and gain in tensile strength are not significantly deferred by delayed closure.[38]

Delayed Primary Closure

Delayed primary closure is suturing a wound prior to the formation of granulation tissue, usually within 4 days of injury. The type of wound amenable to this approach has already been reviewed in the introduction. While a shorter delay (<4 days) has been suggested,[32] a study of contaminated skin wounds in guinea pigs revealed gross infection in 73% of wounds closed after 24 hours, in 33% of wounds closed after 48 and 72 hours, and in 3% of wounds closed after 96 hours (4 days).[39] Another study using an infective dose of *Staphylococcus aureus* to contaminate experimental wounds showed that delayed closure performed at 24, 48, and 72 hours resulted in 76%, 22%, and 30% infection rates, respectively, while wounds closed at 4 days developed infection at a rate similar to that of control, non-infected wounds.[40] While these studies provided important information on the wound's normal defense mechanisms against infection, they did not consider the effects of antibiotics, administered systemically or topically, of wound debridement, or irrigation on infection rates. In the author's experience many wounds can be managed by delayed primary closure in <4 days following injury (Figure 4.9).

Prior to suture closure, the wound should be maintained in a sterile bandage and evaluated at bandage changes performed either daily or on alternate days. Antibiotics and non-steroidal anti-inflammatory drugs are usually administered during this period. Assessment of the wound's readiness for closure is based on several

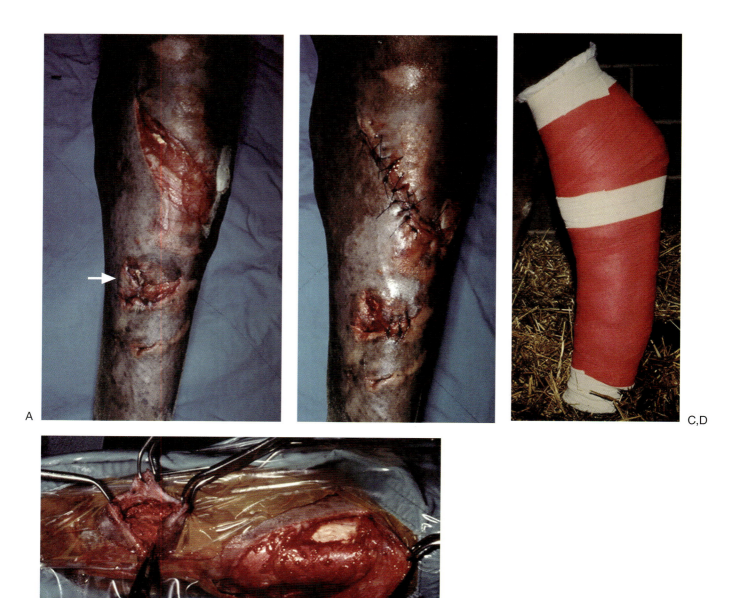

Figure 4.9. Same horse as in Figure 4.2. (A) Appearance of the wounds 24 hours after cleansing and debridement and following limb immobilization in a bandage cast splint. Note the reduction in limb swelling and wound edema compared to that seen at presentation in Figure 4.2. This proximal (upper) wound appeared clean, healthy, and ready for closure. Conversely, the tissue in the intermediate wound, particularly on the lateral side (arrow), appeared bruised and was not ready for closure. The most distal wound was very superficial and therefore not a concern. (B) The proximal wound (right) has been debrided and irrigated in preparation for wound closure. Note the exposed fibular tarsal bone (upper right) following debridement with a hip arthroplasty rasp. The intermediate wound is being prepared for debridement. (C) The proximal wound (top) after suturing; good apposition was achieved. Note that partial closure of the intermediate wound was used in this case; the bruised tissues on the lateral side were left open to heal by second intention. The most distal wound (bottom) was not sutured. (D) The limb was immobilized in a bandage cast splint for 2 weeks and sutures were removed 2 weeks postoperatively. The horse was dismissed to the care of a veterinarian. Six-month follow-up by phone confirmed that this horse was back in performance (jumping) and that a cosmetic outcome had been achieved.

factors: its appearance, the presence or absence of swelling, and the nature of the wound fluid. Wounds that appear clean and healthy with minimal swelling and only clear, serous, non-odiferous fluid are ready for closure (Figure 4.9a). Although bacteria in the wound bed can be quantified via wound biopsy, swab, or rapid slide techniques, the author generally relies on clinical observations.

The wound should be prepared with further clipping, shaving, and antiseptic preparation. Although some feel it is unnecessary, the author prefers to debride the wound again following the steps previously outlined (Figure 4.9b). The wound is then apposed with sutures following the same principles described for primary closure (Figure 4.9c and 4.9d). The selection of bandaging or casting will be considered under a separate section later in this chapter.

A special consideration, as previously mentioned, is the "degloving" injury, which usually involves the metacarpal or metatarsal region. The periosteum is often stripped off a portion of the bone and the paratendon may be missing from the tendons (Figure 2.4). Bone sequestration or tendon degeneration and uncontrollable infection may develop if blood supply to the avascular tissues is not rapidly restored in an effort to support the healing process. Because bone stripped of its periosteum and tendons missing their paratendon represent a relatively avascular surface, they won't readily support the formation of granulation tissue and consequently are very susceptible to infection. If delayed primary closure is selected to manage these cases, any present loose skin should be held in place with a few sutures to temporarily provide a covering for the exposed bone and/or tendon until the wound is ready for closure (Figure 2.5). This effort will reduce desiccation of underlying structures. Thorough debridement of the devitalized tissue should precede the delayed primary closure. A bandage splint or cast will often be required to support the wound after closure.

Delayed Secondary Closure

Delayed secondary closure, carried out after the formation of granulation tissue, is relegated to chronic, severely contaminated, or infected wounds. Heel bulb lacerations frequently fall into this category (Figure 4.3). At the time of suture closure the wound is handled in a manner similar to that described for primary closure and delayed primary closure. The exception is that any excessive granulation tissue is excised (removed) to allow apposition of the skin edges (Figures 4.10a–d). In cases in which considerable dead space remains, a drain may be employed to prevent the accumulation of serum within the wound. A bandage or cast is required to protect the wound (Figure 4.9d). For information regarding the use and application of bandages and casts, see Chapter 16.

While no such data exist for equine patients, retrospective analysis of 48 human patients suffering from sternal wound infections following coronary bypass surgery and that were treated by muscle flap closure found 17 of 22 patients (77%) undergoing closure 4 days or less after sternal debridement and irrigation suffered serious wound complications (re-infected requiring treatment >1 month). No major wound complications occurred in 25 patients undergoing delayed closure 5 days or more after sternal debridement and irrigation.[41] After 5 days the granulation tissue typically appeared healthy, exudate was minimal, and the patients were not exhibiting signs of either local or systemic infection. It is this author's opinion that it likely took 5 days for the body's natural defenses to clear the wound of infection and for healthy granulation tissue to develop.

Second Intention Healing

Second intention healing relies on wound contraction and epithelialization to close and resurface the wound. This approach is selected in cases with significant tissue loss and in wounds of the upper limbs, body, and neck (Figures 4.4 and 4.5). These wounds, though left open, are prepared with the same care as described for primary closure and delayed primary closure with the exception that wounds of the upper forearm and upper hind leg are left uncovered (Figure 4.4). These uncovered wounds should be cleansed daily at first to remove the accumulated exudate. The skin below the wound should be cleansed and then smeared with petrolatum jelly (Vaseline) to prevent serum scalds. If the wound is located in the proximal extremities of the limb, the limb distal to the wound should be bandaged to reduce swelling. Once a healthy bed of granulation tissue has formed, the frequency of cleansing is reduced and antibiotic therapy, if initiated, is discontinued unless skin grafting is contemplated. If a skin flap is present or the wound is gaping, a few strategically placed sutures may help support the wound, though it is important to avoid trapping deep-seated contaminants when so doing.

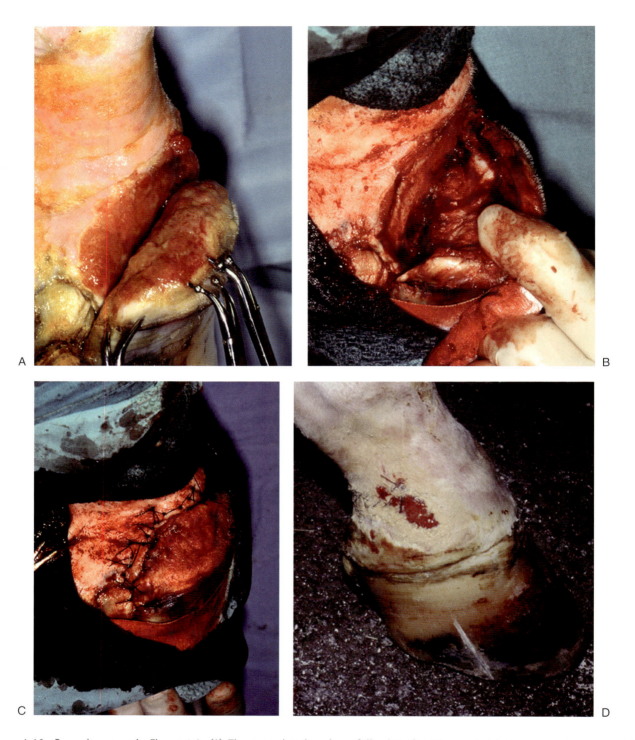

Figure 4.10. Same horse as in Figure 4.3. (A) The wound 5 days later following cleansing and debridement and antimicrobial therapy. Note the healthy bed of granulation tissue. This wound is ready for delayed secondary closure. (B) The wound following excision of granulation tissue. The lateral ungual cartilage (cartilage of the distal phalanx) was damaged and therefore debrided (white tissue proximal to the gloved digit). (C) The partially sutured wound. The coronary band has been apposed at the heel bulb but the skin at the dorsal limits of the wound (just to the right of the last suture) could not be apposed due to a tissue deficit (missing skin). A foot pastern cast was applied after surgery and left in place for 2 weeks. (D) The wound 2 weeks following cast removal. The sutured wound healed and the area of tissue deficit (granulating wound) will heal by second intention under a bandage. The coronary band healed primarily, obviating the development of a hoof wall defect.

When the upper limb (just above the hock or carpus) is injured and second intention healing has been selected, the wound should be supported with bandages and cleansed frequently until granulation tissue forms.

Wounds of the distal limb (carpus or tarsus and below) suffering large tissue deficits present a special problem with the formation of exuberant granulation tissue. Studies show that horses have the ability to form granulation tissue very rapidly when compared to laboratory animals.[42] Other factors that may contribute to the formation of exuberant granulation tissue include increased movement, lack of soft tissue covering, excessive contamination, and reduced blood supply to the distal extremities. Importantly, treatment should be aimed at prevention of the formation of exuberant granulation tissue. For more information regarding the development and treatment of exuberant granulation tissue, see chapters 1 and 8.

Wounds of the upper extremities (proximal antebrachium and proximal crus), body, and neck regions heal effectively by second intention. Usually a good functional and cosmetic end result is achieved (Figures 4.11a,b). Conversely, large full-thickness wounds involving the distal extremity heal very slowly, and ultimately are covered by a thin layer of new epithelium overlying a bed of scar tissue. Typically, the epithelial covering is easily damaged and lacks or develops sparse adnexa (hair follicles, sebaceous and sweat glands) (Figures 4.12 and 8.9b). In these, skin grafting is recommended to improve the appearance and strength of the scar tissue. For more information regarding skin grafting, see chapter 11.

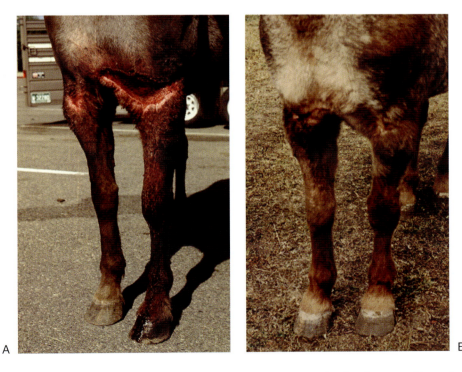

A   B

Figure 4.11. Same horse as in Figure 4.4. (a) The wound 2.5 months post injury is healing by second intention. No treatment was being administered at this time. (b) The wound 4 months post injury had almost completely healed and the horse had resumed its intended function.

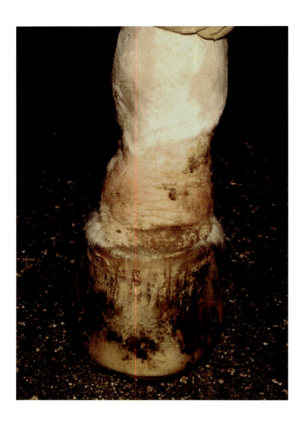

Figure 4.12. This horse sustained an extensive full-thickness skin wound to the pastern region 2 years earlier, which healed by second intention. Note the hairless zone in the pastern region representing scar tissue epithelium.

Selection of Wound Supports

Proper support of the wound is important to the outcome. Following the application of an appropriate dressing (see chapter 3 for information regarding wound dressings), a bandage is often applied to wounds involving the extremities. The bandage protects the wound from further contamination, reduces edema and movement of the affected part, and absorbs secretions from open wounds. Bandages also limit the loss of CO_2 from the wound surface, lowering its pH and shifting the oxygen hemoglobin dissociation curve, which renders oxygen more available for healing. The lower pH also inhibits bacterial growth.

While the techniques of bandaging vary, closed wounds are generally covered with a non-adherent dressing followed by application of conforming gauze (e.g., Kling gauze™, Johnson and Johnson, New Brunswick, NJ). If pressure is required, elastic adhesive bandage (e.g., Elasticon™, Pitman-Moore Inc., NJ) is applied, followed by further bandaging with cotton. If bandage pressure is not critical, several layers of cotton are applied and held in place with conforming gauze. An elastic, self-adherent bandage (e.g., Vet Wrap™, 3M Animal Care Products, St. Paul, MN) is applied as a final covering (tertiary layer).

If limb immobilization is important, a polyvinyl chloride splint can be incorporated into the bandage, or cast application can be selected. A cast is recommended following suture apposition of a laceration to the coronary band, heel bulb, and dorsal surface of the fetlock, and for many degloving injuries as well as for a laceration to tendons and or ligaments. A cast is also recommended following repair of a deep laceration that is oriented perpendicular or oblique to the long axis of a limb because movement of the fetlock and/or the carpus or hock can greatly influence the tension on this type of wound.[43] Moreover, movement of sutured tissue layers deep to the skin (e.g., paratendon) can be independent of that of the sutured skin, creating a shearing force which can lead to dehiscence if these wounds are not stabilized with a splint or cast (Figure 2.3b). Generally, wounds that are sutured under tension should be stabilized with bandage splints or casts to provide the best end result.

Sutured wounds of the upper limb, body, and neck regions can be protected with either a stent or a tie-over bandage. See Chapter 3 for a more complete discussion of wound dressings and Chapter 16 for further discussion of bandaging and casting techniques.

Conclusion

Wound closure should only be performed when all injured tissues are ready to be sutured. Closure prior to this time is premature and invites infection, wound dehiscence, and all related consequences.[44] The best functional and cosmetic end result can be achieved by following the principles of wound preparation and selecting the appropriate options for wound closure. This should benefit the horse and the pleasing end result will be recognized by most clients.

References

1. Noyes H, Chi N, Linah L, et al: Delayed topical antimicrobials as adjuncts to systemic antibiotic therapy of war wounds: bacteriologic studies. Mil Med 1967;132:461
2. Caron JP: Management of superficial wounds. In Jorge Auer, ed. *Equine surgery (1st edition)*. Philadelphia: WB Saunders, 1992, p.232
3. Stashak TS: Wound infection: contributing factors and selected techniques for prevention. Proc Am Assoc Equine Pract 2006;52:270
4. Stashak TS: Reconstructive surgery in the horse. J Am Vet Med Assoc 1977;170:143
5. Edlich RF, Madden JE, Prusak M, et al: Studies in the management of the contaminated wound. VI. The therapeutic value of gentle scrubbing prolonging the limited period of effectiveness of antibiotics in contaminated wounds. Am J Surg 1971;121:668
6. Madden J, Edlich RF, Schauerhamer R, et al: Application of principles of fluid dynamics to surgical wound irrigation. Curr Topic Surg Res 1971;3:85
7. Rodeheaver GT: Wound cleansing, wound irrigation, wound disinfection. In: Diane Krasner, George Rodeheaver, and Gary Sibbald, eds. *Chronic wound care (3rd edition)*. Wayne PA: HMP Communications, 2001, p.389
8. Bhandari M, Anthony D, Schemitsch EH: The efficacy of low-pressure lavage with different irrigating solutions to remove adherent bacteria from bone. J Bone Joint Surg 2001;83:412
9. Cutright DE, Bhaskar SN, Gross A, et al: Effect of vancomycin, streptomycin and tetracycline pulsating jet lavage on contaminated wounds. Military Med 1971;136:810
10. Singleton AO, Julian J: An experimental evaluation of methods used to prevent infection in wounds which have been contaminated with feces. Ann Surg 1960;151:912
11. Lindsey D, Nava C, Marti M. Effectiveness of penicillin irrigation in control of infection in sutured lacerations. J Trauma 1982;22:186
12. Sanchez IR, Swaim SF, Nusbaum KE, et al. Effects of chlorhexidine diacetate and povidone iodine on wound healing in dogs. Vet Surg 1988;17:291
13. Amber EI, Henderson RA, Swaim SF, et al: A comparison of antimicrobial efficacy and tissue reaction of four antiseptics on canine wounds. Vet Surg 1983;12:63
14. Berkelman RL, Holland BW, Anderson RL: Increased bactericidal activity of dilute preparations of povidone-iodine solution. J Clin Microbiol 1982;15:635
15. Owens BD, Wenke JC: Early wound irrigation improves the ability to remove bacteria. J Bone Joint Surg Am 2007;89:1723
16. Gristina AG, Naylor PT, Myrvik QN: Mechanisms of musculoskeletal sepsis. Orthop Clin 1991;22:363
17. Stashak TS: Current concepts in wound management in horses: parts I–III. Proc N Am Vet Conf 2003;17:231
18. Robson MC, Heggars JP: Quantitative bacteriology and inflammatory mediators in soft tissue. In T Hunt, R Heppenstall. Pines E and Roveeds D, eds. *Soft and hard tissue repair. biological and clinical aspects (1st edition)*. New York: Prager, 1984, p.483
19. Robson MC, Duke WF, Krizek TJ: Rapid bacterial screening in the treatment of civilian wounds. J Surg Res 1973;14:426
20. Dow D: Infection in chronic wound care. In Diane Krasner, George Rodeheaver, and Gary Sibbald, eds. *Chronic wound care (3rd edition)*. Wayne PA: HMP Communications, 2001, p.343
21. Cooney WP, Fitzgerald RH, Dobyns JH, et al: Quantitative wound cultures in upper extremity trauma. J Trauma 1982;22:112
22. Hackett RP, Dimock BA, Bentinck-Smith J: Quantitative bacteriology of the experimentally incised skin wound in the horse. Equine Vet J 1983;15:37
23. Edlich RF, Rodeheaver GT, Thacker JG, et al: Management of soft tissue injury. Clin Plast Surg 1977;4:191
24. Hackett RP: Management of traumatic wounds. Proc Am Assoc Equine Pract 1978;24:363
25. Lord JW: Intraoperative antibiotic wound irrigation. Surg Gyn Obstet 1983;157:357
26. Stone HH, Hester TR: Topical antibiotic and delayed primary closure in the management of contaminated surgical incisions. J Surg Res 1972;12:70

27. Stashak TS, Yturraspe DJ: Consideration for selection of suture material. J Vet Surg 1978;7:48

28. DeHoll D, Rodeheaver GT, Edgerton MT, et al: Potentiation of infection by suture closure of dead space. Am J Surg 1974;127:716

29. Stashak TS: Suture patterns used for wound closure in veterinary surgery. Proc Am Assoc Equine Pract 1978;24:383

30. Baxter GM: Treatment of wounds involving synovial structures. Clin Tech Equine Pract 2004;3:204

31. Wilmink JM, van Herten J, van Weeren PR, et al: Retrospective study of primary intention healing and sequestrum formation in horses compared to ponies under clinical circumstances. Equine Vet J 2002;34:270

32. Bernard HR, Cole WR: Wound infections following potentially contaminated operations: Effect of delayed primary closure of the skin and subcutaneous tissue. J Am Med Assoc 1963;184:118

33. Hackett RP: Delayed wound closure. A review and report of use of the technique on three equine limb wounds. Vet Surg 1983;12:48

34. Baxter GM, Doran RE, Moore JN: Management of lower leg wounds with delayed closure in horses. Proc Am Assoc Equine Pract 1986;32:341

35. Baxter GM: Wound healing and delayed wound closure in the lower limb of the horse. Equine Pract 1988;10:23

36. Verrier ED, Bossart KJ, Heer FW: Reduction of infection rates in abdominal incisions by a delayed closure technique. Am J Surg 1979;138:22

37. Robson MC, Heggers JP: Delayed wound closures based on bacterial counts. J Surg Oncol 1970;2:379

38. Fogdestam I: Biomechanical study of healing rat skin incisions after delayed primary closure. Surg Gynecol Obstet 1981;153:191

39. Edlich RF, Rogers W, Kasper G, et al: Studies in the management of the contaminated wound: I. Optimal time for closure of contaminated open wounds: II. Comparison resistance to infection of open and closed wounds during healing. Am J Surg 1969;117:323

40. Heaton LD, Rosgay H, Fisher GW, et al: Military surgical practices of the United States Army in Vietnam. Proc Current Probl Surg, 1966, p.19

41. Lindsey JT: A retrospective analysis of 48 infected sternal wound closures: delayed closure decreases wound complications. Plast Reconst Surg 2002;109:1882

42. Chvapil M, Pfister T, Escalada S, et al: Dynamics of the healing of skin wounds in the horse as compared to the rat. Exp Mol Pathol 1979;30:349.

43. Stashak TS: Plastic and Reconstructive Surgery. In Paul Jennings, ed. *Textbook of large animal surgery, (1st edition)*, vol 1, Philadelphia: WB Saunders, 1984, p.277

44. Brown PW: The prevention of infection in open wounds. Clin Orthop 1973;96:42

4.2 Selection of Suture Materials, Suture Patterns, and Drains for Wound Closure

Christophe Céleste, DrVet, MS, Diplomate ECVS, Diplomate ACVS, and Ted S. Stashak, DVM, MS, Diplomate ACVS

Introduction

Sutures serve important functions in wound repair, namely, blood vessel ligation or holding tissues in apposition as they heal. Equine veterinarians have a broad range of suture materials from which to choose. Knowledge of the advantages and disadvantages of each suture material, assessment of wound location and condition, as well as familiarity with the healing rate of the particular tissue involved will allow the surgeon to make an appropriate selection of suture material.

Although this selection is important, more vital is the surgical technique used to close the wound. Satisfactory results will be best achieved if the surgeon uses the appropriate suture material and pattern for wound closure. The proper application of a wound drain is very important in facilitating elimination of dead space by evacuating existing fluid and gas accumulations.

The aim of this chapter is to review the various suture materials and patterns used for wound closure and to discuss the proper use of wound drains.

[A]Syneture, United States Surgical Corp. and Davis and Geck™, Norwalk, CT.
[B]Ethicon, Inc., Johnson and Johnson Company, Sommerville, NJ.

Suture Material

Ideal Material

The ideal suture material should:

- Retain adequate tensile strength until its purpose is achieved, then be absorbed without inducing postoperative complications
- Have first-throw holding strength and good knot security
- Stimulate minimal tissue reaction to avoid creating a situation favorable to bacterial growth
- Be non-electrolytic, non-capillary, non-allergenic, non-carcinogenic, non-corrosive, and non-toxic
- Be inexpensive, readily available, and easily sterilized without alteration of its properties
- Be easy to handle and comfortable to use.

The ideal suture material does not presently exist; however, many of the available suture materials boast excellent properties.[1,2,3,4]

Classification

Suture materials are classified as absorbable or nonabsorbable, natural or synthetic, and monofilament or multifilament. Absorbable sutures undergo degradation and loss of tensile strength within 60 days, either by enzymatic degradation and subsequent hydrolysis or by hydrolysis alone (e.g., polyglycolic acid Dexon[TMA]). Non-absorbable sutures retain tensile strength for longer than 60 days (e.g., polypropylene Prolene[TMB]). Some examples of natural sutures are surgical gut (catgut) and collagen, and some examples of synthetic sutures are poliglecaprone 25 (Monocryl[TMB]) and stainless steel. Refer to Table 4.1 for more details about absorbable and nonabsorbable synthetic and natural materials.

Sutures constructed of one filament are referred to as monofilament (e.g., polydioxanone PDS II[TMB]), while those constructed of multiple filaments that are either braided or twisted together are referred to as multifilament (e.g., polyglactin 910 Vicryl[TMB]). It is widely accepted that synthetic absorbable and non-absorbable suture materials are superior to the natural suture materials and thus should be favored. The most important characteristics of commonly used absorbable and non-absorbable, natural and synthetic, and monofilament and multifilament suture materials are summarized in Tables 4.2a and 4.2b.

Selection

The goal of suturing is to provide secure partial or complete wound closure while minimizing morbidity. Knowledge of the advantages and disadvantages of each type of suture material as well as assessment of location and condition of the wound and knowledge of the healing rate of the type of tissue involved allows the surgeon to make an appropriate selection of suture material.

Certain principles should be considered in selecting the appropriate suture material:

- Sutures should be at least as strong as the normal tissue through which they are placed.[3] During the first days of healing, the strength of the sutured wound depends almost entirely on the suture material. As examples, skin and fascia are among the strongest tissues, requiring larger diameter and stronger sutures to hold them together, while the stomach, small intestine, and urinary bladder are much weaker tissues and require smaller diameter sutures with less structural strength.[5]
- The relative rates at which a suture material loses tensile strength and the wound gains strength should concord for optimal wound healing.[3] Visceral wounds heal rapidly and attain maximal strength in 14–21 days, such that absorbable suture materials are adequate for these tissues. On the other hand, fascia heals slowly, attaining only 50% of maximal strength at day 50.[4] Therefore, rapidly absorbed suture materials are contraindicated, whereas non-absorbable suture materials, or the more slowly absorbable synthetic suture materials, are the most appropriate choices for fascia closure. Skin also heals slowly such that a non-absorbable suture material should thus be selected for its closure.

Table 4.1. Available implant forms as suture material.

Material	Natural vs. synthetic	Absorbable vs. non-absorbable	Forms available
Collagen	Natural	Absorbable	Surgical suture, hemostatic sponge (ULTRAFOAM Collagen Sponge[a])
Poliglecaprone	Synthetic	Absorbable	Surgical suture (MONOCRYL Suture[b])
Polyamide	Synthetic	Non-absorbable	Surgical suture (Ethlilon Nylon Suture[b], Nurolon Braided Nylon Suture[b], MONOSOFT[c], NYLON[d], SUPRAMID[e])
Polybutester	Synthetic	Non-absorbable	Surgical suture (Novafil[c])
Polydioxanone	Synthetic	Absorbable	Surgical suture (PDS II Suture[b]), surgical pins (OrthoSorb Resorbable pins[f])
Polyester	Synthetic	Non-absorbable	Surgical suture (Coated Ethibond Eecel Polyester Suture[b], Mersilene Polyester Fiber Suture[b], Polyester[d])
Polyglactin	Synthetic	Absorbable	Surgical suture (Coated Vicryl Suture[b], Coated Vicryl Rapid Suture[b], Coated Vicryl plus Antibacterial Suture[b]), surgical staples (Premium polysorb[c])
Polyglycolic acid	Synthetic	Absorbable	Surgical suture (Dexon[c]), surgical staples (Insorb 20 Absorbable Staple[g])
Polypropylene	Synthetic	Non-absorbable	Surgical suture (Prolene Polypropylene Suture[b], Polypropylene[d])
Silk	Natural	Non-absorbable	Surgical suture (Perma-Hand Silk Suture[b], silk[dh])
Stainless steel	Synthetic	Non-absorbable	Surgical suture (Surgical Stainless Steel Suture[b]), surgical staples (Appose ULC[c])
Surgical gut	Natural	Absorbable	Surgical suture (Plain Gut[dh], Care Express Ethicon Absorbable Suture–Chromic Gut[b], Chromic Gut[dh])

Adapted from Blackford[4]
[a] Davol, Inc., Cranston, RI
[b] Ethicon, Inc., Johnson and Johnson Company, Somerville, NJ
[c] Syneture, United States Surgical Corp. and Davis and Geck™, Norwalk, CT
[d] Schering-Plough, Union, NJ
[e] S. Jackson, Inc., Alexandria, VA
[f] Johnson and Johnson Gateway, LLC, Piscataway, NJ
[g] Incisive Surgical, Inc., Plymouth, MN
[h] C.P. Medical, Portland, OR

- If the suture biologically alters the process of wound healing, these changes must be considered in selecting a suture material.[3] Most suture materials act as a foreign material and can potentiate the development of wound infection when used in excess (too much suture, too large a diameter, or too many knots).[1,6] The number of bacteria needed to produce an active infection is reduced by a factor of 10–10,000 in the presence of foreign material. Even the least reactive suture acts as foreign material and impairs the ability of the wound to resist infection; therefore, the use of suture material should always be minimized, especially in contaminated wounds.[1,3] Technically, the smallest-diameter synthetic absorbable monofilament suture material should be used,[7] and held only by surgical knots (square or surgeon's; the former is preferred).[6]

In cases in which primary closure is not possible, because of massive tissue loss, excessive bacterial contamination, or undue tension on wound edges after closure, delayed primary or secondary closure should be considered as an alternative.[2] For information regarding sutures recommended for specific tissues, refer to Table 4.3.

Table 4.2a. Characteristics of the most commonly used absorbable suture materials.

Suture type	Raw material	Properties		Advantages and uses	Disadvantages
		Absorption	Tensile strength		
Polydioxanone (monofilament) (PDS II Suture[a])	Polymer of polydioxanone	Absorbed by hydrolysis in 180–190 days	Loss of 26% of tensile strength after 14 days, 42% after 28 days, and 86% after 56 days. Tensile strength half-life: 6 weeks.	Good knot security. Minimal tissue drag. Strength before implantation exceeds that of nylon and polypropylene. Minimal foreign body reaction.	Poor handling characteristics (stiffness and memory).
Polyglyconate (monofilament) (MAXON Suture[b])	Copolymer of glycolic acid and trimethylene	Absorbed by hydrolysis starting at day 60 and complete by day 180.	Retains tensile strength for more than 21 days. Breaking strength half-life: 28 days.	Good handling characteristics. Best effective post-implantation strength of all absorbable materials. 3 times stronger than VICRYL™ at day 21 of wound healing. Best knot security of all absorbable materials. Superior to nylon and polybutester for tendon repair.	
Poliglecaprone 25 (monofilament) (MONOCRYL Suture[a])	Copolymer of caprolactone and glycolide	Absorbed by hydrolysis in 90 to 120 days.	Loses tensile strength by 50% at day 7, 75% at day 14 and 100% at day 21.	Excellent knot security. One of the strongest absorbable materials initially. Good handling characteristics (decreased flexibility, minimal memory). Used for tissues that heal rapidly. Minimal tissue reaction.	Rapid loss of tensile strength. Should not be used in cases of delayed healing.
Surgical catgut (monofilament)—plain	Submucosa of ovine intestine or serosa of bovine intestine.	Absorbed quickly by phagocytosis.	Retains tensile strength for less than 14 days.	Rarely used.	Induces inflammatory reaction. Rapid loss of tensile strength.
Surgical catgut (monofilament)—chromic	Similar to plain. Treated with chromium salt, which increases bonding, improves tensile strength, minimizes tissue reaction.	Absorbed by phagocytosis more slowly owing to added chromium salt (90+ days).	Retains tensile strength for 14 to 28 days.	Good handling characteristics. Used for tissues that heal rapidly. May be used in contaminated wound.	Inflammatory reaction leads to fibrosis.
Polyglycolic acid (braided multifilament) (DEXON[b])	Polymer of glycolic acid.	Absorbed by hydrolysis in 100 to 120 days. Hydrolysis more rapid in alkaline environment. Degradation products have some antibacterial effects.	Loses tensile strength by 33% within 7 days of implantation, and by 80% within 14 days.	Wide variety of uses in clean and contaminated wounds (binds bacteria, however). Superior tensile strength when compared to surgical gut. Good handling characteristics.	Prematurely absorbed in urine. Tends to drag through tissues, cut friable tissue, and have poor knot security (good tightening of each throw is mandatory).

Table 4.2a. *Continued*

Suture type	Raw material	Properties		Advantages and uses	Disadvantages
		Absorption	**Tensile strength**		
Polyglactin 910 (braided multifilament) (some coated forms) (VICRYL Suture[a])	Copolymer of glycolic acid and lactic acid. Coated with calcium stearate (ratio 9:1)	Absorbed by hydrolysis over a period of 100–120 days.	Retains tensile strength for 14 to 21 days.	Coated form: easier to handle, less tissue drag, minimal tissue reaction, stable in contaminated wounds, higher tensile and knot strength, excellent size-to-strength ratio. Stable in alkaline urine.	Non-coated forms have significantly higher tissue drag.

Adapted from Blackford;[4,33] Toombs[12]
[a] Ethicon, Inc., Johnson and Johnson Company, Somerville, NJ
[b] Syneture, United States Surgical Corp. and Davis and Geck™, Norwalk, CT

Table 4.2b. Characteristics of the most commonly used non-absorbable suture materials.

Suture type	Raw material	Properties: absorption, tensile strength	Advantages and uses	Disadvantages
Polypropylene (monofilament) (PROLENE Suture[a])	Polyolfin plastic	Biologically inert. Retains strength with no reduction after implantation.	Higher knot security than all monofilament non-metallic synthetic suture materials. The least thrombogenic suture (vascular surgery). The least likely to convert a contaminated wound to an infected one. Stable in contaminated wound environment. Best suture available for skin.	Lower tensile strength than all monofilament non-metallic synthetic suture materials. Medium handling characteristics (slippage).
Polybutester (monofilament) (NOVAFIL[b])	Copolymer of polybutylene, polyglycol, and polytetramethylene terephtalates	Biologically inert. Retains strength after implantation.	Strong, with good handling characteristics and knot security. High degree of elastic stretch under low loads (good for wounds where swelling is anticipated). Non-reactive in tissues. Provides prolonged support for slow-healing tissues.	Marginal knot quality unless force is applied to the material, causing fibers to interlock.
Silk (twisted or braided multifilament) (SILK[acd])	Raw silk, spun by silkworm. Sometimes coated with oil, wax or silicone.	Loses 80% of tensile strength within 8 days. May be absorbed or persist for several years.	Excellent handling characteristics and knot security. Inexpensive. Ophthalmology.	Rapid loss of tensile strength. Coating reduces knot security. Incites tissue reaction. May potentiate infection. Capillarity.

Table 4.2b. *Continued*

Suture type	Raw material	Properties: absorption, tensile strength	Advantages and uses	Disadvantages
Surgical stainless steel (monofilament or twisted multifilament)[a]	Alloy of iron, chromium, nickel, and molybdenum	Biologically inert. Retains strength after implantation.	Noncapillary as a monofilament. Greatest tensile strength of all sutures. Maintains strength when implanted. Good for tissues that heal slowly or are infected. Minimal tissue reaction except at the suture ends.	Poor handling characteristics. Inflexible ends can generate inflammation and tissue necrosis, leading to localized skin infection. Tends to cut tissue. Cannot withstand repeated bending without breaking. Multifilament wire tends to fragment and migrate, leading to sinus formation.
Polymerized caprolactam (monofilament / multifilament) (SUPRAMID[e], BRAUNAMID[f])	Polyamide polymer	Retains no tensile strength after 6 months.	Superior tensile strength compared with nylon. Best use is for skin. Should not be buried because it absorbs up to 10% of its weight in fluid.	Poor handling characteristics. Heat sterilization required before use. Elicits moderate to severe tissue reaction, swelling, and sinus tract formation.
Nylon (ETHILON[a])				
Monofilament	Polyamide polyester	Biologically inert. Loses about 30% of its original tensile strength within 2 years.	Incidence of infection very low, even in contaminated wound (similar to stainless steel). Degradation products have antibacterial properties.	Poor handling characteristics and knot security (slippage). Not recommended for use within a serous or synovial cavity. The buried sharp ends may cause frictional irritation.
Multifilament		Biologically inert. Retains no tensile strength after 6 months in tissue.	Degradation products have antibacterial properties.	
Polyester fiber (braided multifilament) (MERSILENE[a], Coated ETHIBOND[a])	Synthetic material made from chemicals such as polyethylene terephthalate. Coating: polybutylate, teflon, and silicone.	High initial tensile strength with little or no loss after implantation.	One of the strongest non-metallic suture materials available. Good handling characteristics improved by coating. Provides prolonged support for slow-healing tissues. Non-wicking.	Poor handling characteristics. Non-coated form has a high coefficient of friction. Coating reduces friction and knot security. Causes the most tissue reaction of the synthetic non-absorbable suture materials. Should not be used in contaminated wound (persistent local infection, excessive tissue reaction, and sinus tract formation).

Adapted from Blackford;[4,33] Toombs[12]
[a] Ethicon, Inc., Johnson and Johnson Company, Somerville, NJ
[b] Syneture, United States Surgical Corp. and Davis and Geck™, Norwalk, CT
[c] Schering-Plough, Union, NJ
[d] C.P. Medical, Portland, OR
[e] S. Jackson, Inc., Alexandria, VA
[f] Jorgensen Laboratories, Inc., Loveland, CO

Table 4.3. Guideline for suture material selection in equine wound management.

Tissue type	Suture size (USP)	Suture type
Skin—appositional suture	2-0–0	Non-absorbable monofilament (polypropylene, nylon, polybutester)
Skin–tension suture	0–2	Non-absorbable monofilament (polypropylene, nylon)
Subcutis	3-0–2-0	Absorbable monofilament (poliglecaprone 25, glycomer 631) or multifilament (polyglactin 910, polyglycolic acid)
Fascia	0–3	Slow absorbable monofilament (polyglyconate, polydioxanone) or multifilament (polyglactin 910)
Muscle	2-0–2	Absorbable monofilament (polyglyconate, polydioxanone) or multifilament (polyglactin 910)
Tendon	2	Slow absorbable monofilament (polydioxanone, polyglyconate)
Vessel (ligatures)	3-0–0	Absorbable monofilament (poliglecaprone 25) or multifilament (polyglycolic acid, polyglactin 910)
Vessel (sutures)	6-0–5-0	Non-absorbable monofilament (polypropylene, nylon)
Nerve	10-0–7-0	Non-absorbable monofilament (polypropylene, nylon) or multifilament (silk)
Eye—eyelid	6-0–4-0	Non-absorbable monofilament (nylon) or multifilament (silk)
Eye—sclera	8-0–6-0	Non-absorbable monofilament (nylon)
Eye—conjunctiva and cornea	9-0–7-0	Absorbable monofilament (e.g., polydioxanone) or multifilament (polyglactin 910, polyglycolic acid)

Adapted from Boothe,[3] Blackford,[4,33] MacKay,[34] Miller,[35] Millichamp,[36,37] Nasisse[38]

Size and Tension

Selecting inappropriately large suture material and exerting undue tension on it is not recommended. Use of unsuitably large suture material results in excessive tissue reaction and unnecessary foreign material in the wound, which alter the tissue's architecture and ability to resist infection.[1,3] Excessive tension leads to tissue necrosis by interfering with local blood supply (ischemia) and increasing edema to the wound and surrounding tissues,[8,9,10,11] which favor wound dehiscence.

Certain principles underlie the selection of appropriate suture material size and tension: (1) The injured tissue's ability to hold suture bears a greater influence on the strength of a repair than does the tensile strength of the suture material itself.[12,13] (2) Use of oversized suture material weakens the wound repair and should thus be avoided. (3) The suture's functions are to appose accurately and to hold together the wound edges, while minimally interfering with the blood supply.[4,8,14] (4) For a wound under mild to moderate tension, increasing the number of sutures apposing the primary suture line[2,4] and/or using tension sutures is wiser than increasing the size of the chosen suture material.

If suturing alone cannot reduce the tension to an optimal level, other tension-relieving techniques, such as undermining, tension release incisions, mesh expansion, plasties (V-to-Y, Z, W), or flaps should be used before closure in an effort to mobilize the wound edges.[2,11,14] Refer to Chapter 5 for more information regarding the mobilization of skin to reduce tension.

While guidelines for suture material selection (type and size) in large animal surgery have not yet been officially established, Table 4.3 reflects the authors' preferences for wound management in the horse.

Surgical Needles

Some important factors should be considered when selecting a surgical needle: needle characteristics, suture material size, wound configuration, and tissue characteristics[3] are foremost. Surgical needles are manufactured from stainless steel (an alloy of iron, chromium, nickel, and molybdenum) and are available as eyed needles or swaged needles. Eyed needles, in which the suture material has to be threaded, are more traumatic to tissues during suture placement because of the bigger diameter of the eye and because a double strand of suture material is pulled through the tissues while suturing. Eyed needles are reusable, so they are less expensive. However, they are less efficient because they become dull with reuse, which can exacerbate tissue trauma. Swaged needles (eyeless needles) are less traumatic to tissues because the suture material is directly attached to their ends and only one strand of suture material is pulled through the tissues, which makes them easier to handle. Swaged needles are always sharp because they are nonreusable.

Surgical needles vary in size, shape, and type of needle point. The needle should be long enough to penetrate both sides of the incision in one bite. Its diameter should be the smallest that allows tissue penetration without buckling or bending; in view of limiting tissue trauma a length-to-diameter ratio <8:1 is recommended.[15] The common needle shapes are straight, half-curved, and parts of a circle (1/4, 1/2, 3/8, and 5/8) (Figure 4.13).

Tissue type as well as wound depth, size, and accessibility to suturing are factors which guide the selection of needle shape.[3] Straight needles are usually used on or near the surface of the body. Half and 5/8 curved needles are convenient for both superficial and deep wounds. In most situations, the 3/8 needle is preferred because it is easier to handle within tissues.

The shape of the surgical needle point and body determine its ability to penetrate tissue and should be considered prior to surgical needle selection (Figure 4.14). Non-cutting (taper-point) needles have a sharp point and cylindrical body and are generally used for soft tissues such as viscera, fat, and muscles, with minimal risk of injury to adjacent structures.

Cutting needles are designed to penetrate much denser tissues such as fascia or skin. Several types of cutting surgical needles are available: (1) conventional curved cutting needle, with the cutting edge along the concave surface, (2) reverse curved cutting needle, with the cutting edge along the convex surface to avoid cutting out of the tissues when the needle passes through them, and (3) tapered cutting needle, which combines a round shaft with a reverse cutting point that is useful in delicate yet dense tissue (e.g., fascia, periosteum, tendon).[15,16]

When choosing a surgical needle, the following requirements should be met: (1) the hole made by the needle should be just large enough to permit the passage of suture material; (2) the sutured tissue should not be weakened by needle passage; (3) microorganisms, foreign bodies, chemicals, or other substances should not be introduced into the wound by the needle passage; (4) the design and diameter of the needle should minimize tissue damage and needle breakage; and (5) the needle should have the appropriate design to permit rapid, accurate, and precise suturing.[16]

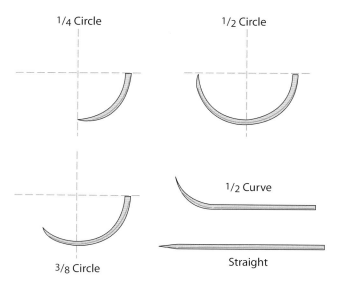

Figure 4.13. Various surgical suture needle shapes.

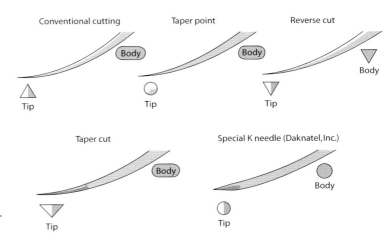

Figure 4.14. Various point and body designs of surgical suture needles.

Suture Techniques

Accurate apposition of the wound edges with minimal interference to the blood supply enhances wound healing. The technique and pattern of suture material placement, the number of sutures, and the suture line support are also critical to optimal wound outcome.

Suture Placement

It is generally recommended that sutures be placed at a distance from the wound edge equal to the thickness of the wound edge itself. However, factors such as tension on the wound edges as well as thickness and stiffness of the wound must also be considered. Because inflammation and collagen lysis occurring during early wound healing weaken the suture-holding power of a wound, sutures should be placed at a distance greater than 0.5 cm from the wound edge for improved security.[17] Neo-epithelium lacks holding power; therefore, sutures should be placed well back from the wound edge to ensure optimal holding strength when repair is to be achieved by delayed closure.

When suturing a vertical incision, it is best to start from the end most distant to the surgeon and proceed toward the closest end. When suturing a horizontal incision, it is best to place sutures from right to left if right-handed, and from left to right if left-handed.[2]

Recommendations regarding the number of sutures required to close a wound also have been made.[17,18] In human surgery, placing interrupted sutures 0.5 cm apart ensures good tissue apposition, minimal tension on individual sutures, and maximum wound holding strength.[17] Placing interrupted sutures closer together may result, in some instances, in delayed healing secondary to excessive tissue reaction and unwarranted interference to the blood supply of the wound edges.[2] A good rule of thumb is to place sutures in sufficient numbers to provide good apposition of wound edges (Figure 4.15). Spacing between sutures can be increased in thick-skinned regions and regions where incisions or lacerations are parallel to the skin tension lines. The opposite is true in thin-skinned regions and regions where incisions or lacerations are perpendicular to the skin tension lines.[2]

Suture Knots

Sutures are most commonly tied in square knots because these are among the most secure. When the first throw of a square knot does not accurately appose the wound edges, it can be modified into a surgeon's knot (Figure 4.16a,b). However, the surgeon's knot places more suture material within the wound, thus potentiating the development of wound infection; therefore, it should be used only when needed. The surgeon's knot is contraindicated when using chromic catgut. Indeed, the increased friction provoked by the double throws weakens the suture by fraying the material at the knot.[4]

Knot-tying techniques and characteristics of suture materials' influence on knot and suture line security are summarized in Table 4.4.

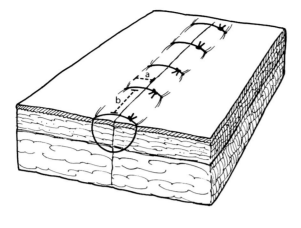

Figure 4.15. Simple interrupted sutures. Knots should be offset so they do not rest upon the apposed skin margins. Sutures should be placed close enough to prevent gaping. a = distance from the wound edge where the suture should be placed to ensure optimal holding strength (>0.5 cm). b = minimal distance between two consecutive sutures (±0.5 cm).

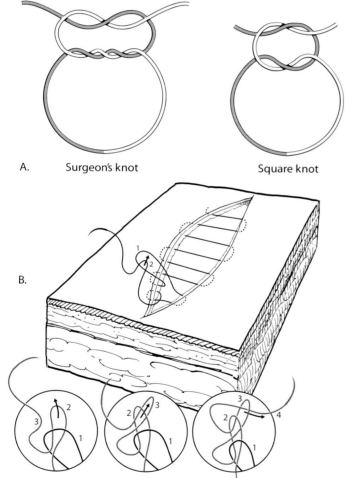

A.   Surgeon's knot   Square knot

B.

Figure 4.16. Surgical knots: (A) Left, surgeon's; right, square. (B) Chain-stitch.

Three knot-tying techniques exist: one-handed, two-handed, and instruments ties. These techniques are discussed in depth elsewhere in the literature (Ethicon Knot-Tying Manual, available free online) and therefore will not be addressed here.

Absorbable sutures, when placed in subcutaneous or intradermal tissues, frequently have their knots buried (Figures 4.16b and 4.17). If a large knot remains immediately below or within the skin, it may cause excessive pressure resulting in local skin necrosis, suture extrusion, wound infection, and a poor cosmetic result. For

Table 4.4. Minimal number of throws required (including the first) for a secure square knot in interrupted suture patterns and continuous suture patterns.

Suture type	Interrupted suture pattern	Beginning continuous suture pattern	Ending continuous suture pattern
Polydioxanone abs, mono	4	4	7
Catgut abs, multi	3	4	5–6
Polyclycolic acid abs, multi	3	3	5–6
Polyglactin 910 abs, multi	3	3	5–6
Polypropylene Non-abs, mono	3	3	5–6
Nylon Non-abs, multi/mono	4	4	6–7

Adapted from Rosin[39]
abs = absorbable
non-abs = nonabsorbable
mono = monofilament
multi = multifilament

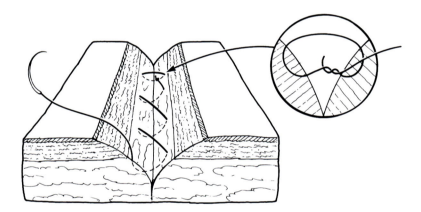

Figure 4.17. Suture placement for a subcutaneous continuous or running suture pattern. The initial knot is buried in the subcutaneous tissues.

subcutaneous closure, the knot is buried by introducing the needle first deep within the subcutaneous tissues, passing the suture toward the dermis, and exiting just below the dermis. The suture crosses the incision line, and then the needle is re-introduced in the subcutaneous tissues just below the dermis and recovered deep in the subcutaneous tissues (Figure 4.17). The technique to bury the knot in an intradermal suture pattern is similar, except the suture material passes through the dermis and the knot is tied just beneath the dermis in the subcutaneous tissues. The chain stitch knot can be used to secure the intradermal suture pattern (Figure 4.16b).

The volume of suture material and symmetry of buried knots within the wound are critical determinants of suture extrusion. Indeed, additional useless throws should be avoided (see Table 4.4) and buried knots must always be symmetrical and positioned perpendicular to the linear wound incision to prevent suture extrusion.[19]

Suture Patterns

A wide variety of suture patterns have been described for use in animals. They have been categorized according to the following criteria: (1) anatomical areas in which they are placed; (2) tendency to promote apposition, eversion, or inversion of tissues; (3) ability to overcome tension forces that may disrupt accurate approximation of tissues; and (4) placement in a continuous or an interrupted fashion.[12]

Suture patterns are usually divided into four groups:

1. Appositional (Figures 4.18, 4.19, 4.20a,b, 4.21a-c, 4.22, 4.23a,b, 4.24, 4.25, 4.26, 4.27)
2. Inverting
3. Everting (Figures 4.21a and 4.23a)
4. Tension sutures (Figures 4.28a-c, 4.29, 4.30, 4.31, 4.32).

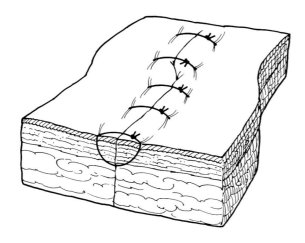

Figure 4.18. Simple interrupted sutures. The independent nature of each suture allows for mobility and use in irregularly shaped areas.

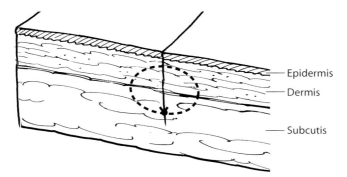

Epidermis

Dermis

Subcutis

Figure 4.19. Interrupted intradermal suture.

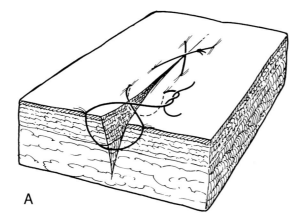

A

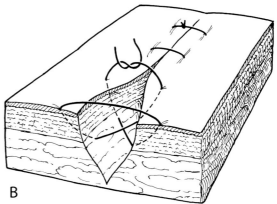

B

Figure 4.20. (A) A cruciate mattress suture pattern. (B) An inverted cruciate mattress suture pattern.

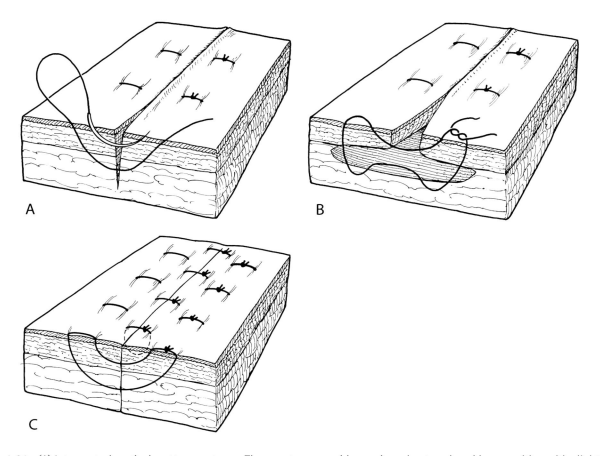

Figure 4.21. (A) Interrupted vertical mattress sutures. These sutures provide precise edge-to-edge skin apposition with slight eversion after they are tied. They also minimally compromise skin vasculature. (B) Interrupted vertical mattress suture used to decrease dead space. (C) Alternating vertical mattress and simple interrupted sutures to prevent skin inversion. Note: There is no biomechanical advantage over simple interrupted sutures when placed as described. The alternating vertical mattress suture pattern can, however, be placed widely to reduce tension on the primary suture line or associated with rubber "stents" or buttons (see Figures 4.28 and 4.30).

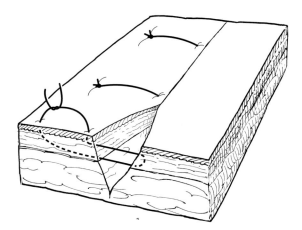

Figure 4.22. The Allgöwer corium vertical mattress suture pattern. This minimally traumatic suture pattern provides good apposition of skin margins with minimal or no eversion of the skin edges.

205

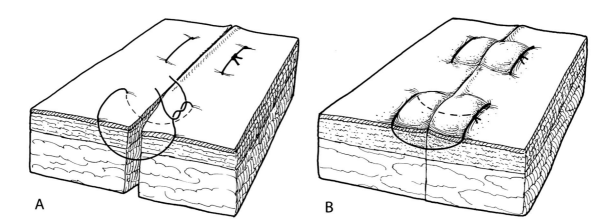

Figure 4.23. (A) Horizontal mattress sutures. Slight eversion and some gaping of the wound edges occur after they are tied. (B) If the sutures are tied too tightly or if tissues swell excessively after placement, reduction of the skin blood supply occurs (elevated tissue and dashed lines within the suture pattern) and can impair wound healing.

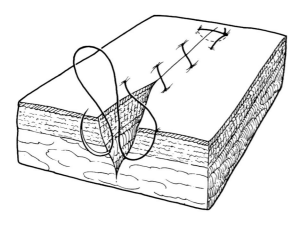

Figure 4.24. Suture placement through all skin layers in a simple continuous suture pattern.

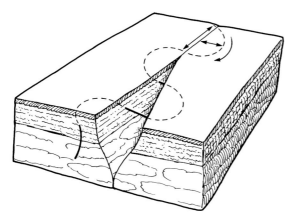

Figure 4.25. Continuous intradermal suture. The suture should pass through the dermis perpendicular to the long axis of the wound. Suture bites in the dermis should be of equivalent depth. Spacing between bites should also be regular.

Inverting sutures are rarely used in wound management; therefore, they will not be discussed in this chapter. (Refer to Blackford 2006a[4] or Toombs 2003[12] for more detail.)

In wounds with no tissue loss, an appositional suture pattern provides superior approximation of wound edges leading to secure anatomic closure and good cosmetic results. Wounds with large defects or tissue loss are much more difficult to close without creating tension on the suture line. Use of tension sutures allows the

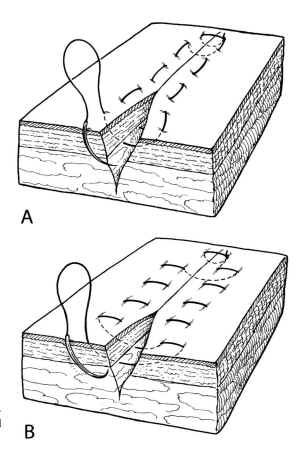

Figure 4.26. Continuous mattress suture pattern that creates slight eversion of the sutured skin edges. (A) Horizontal mattress. (B) Vertical mattress.

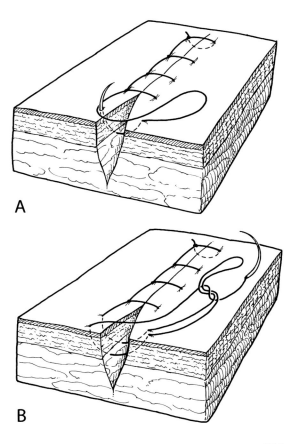

Figure 4.27. Continuous locking or Ford interlocking suture. (A) Passage of the suture. (B) Tying the suture after completion.

redistribution of tension across the wound edges, minimizing tissue strangulation and necrosis. Everting sutures are sometimes useful for skin closure because skin edges tend to invert during healing.

Interrupted Versus Continuous Suture Patterns

The choice of an interrupted versus a continuous suture pattern is somewhat contentious because each presents advantages and disadvantages. The major advantages of interrupted suture patterns (Figure 4.15) are their ability to precisely control tension at each point along the wound, the possibility of adjustments for good alignment of wound edges in irregularly shaped lacerations (Figure 4.18), and the minimal interference of the suture pattern with the skin's blood supply when properly applied.[2,14] Simple interrupted sutures also have been shown to increase the gain in skin tensile strength compared to a simple continuous suture out to 21 days.[20] Disadvantages of interrupted suture patterns include increased surgery time (to tie multiple knots and cut the suture ends), increased volume of foreign material left in the wound, especially when sutures are buried, as well as poor suture material economy.[12]

In contrast, continuous suture patterns are quickly placed, use less suture material, and minimize the number of knots, reducing both the operating time and the amount of foreign material left within the wound (Figures 4.24, 4.25, 4.26, 4.27).[12] They also form a more airtight or watertight seal.[21] On the downside, it is not possible to vary the tension on the suture line to the same degree as with an interrupted suture pattern, and knot failure or suture material breakage can have a disastrous effect on the closure. It is thus imperative that strands of suture used in continuous patterns be handled carefully and that knots' throws be applied correctly and tied securely.

Recent studies either recommend the incorporation of the chain-stitch knot as the termination knot for continuous intradermal pattern for a better security of suture line[22] (Figure 4.16b) or demonstrate that in selected cases, the "pulley knot-free" continuous intradermal pattern is as secure as the buried-knot continuous intradermal pattern to close a skin incision.[23] Moreover, because of their design, simple continuous suture patterns tend to compromise the microvascular supply to wound edges.[20] If this occurs, the resulting edema can unduly prolong the inflammatory phase of wound healing, thus delaying the wound's gain in tensile strength. The Ford interlocking suture pattern (Figure 4.27) represents a compromise between interrupted and continuous suture patterns.

Inverting Versus Everting Suture Patterns

Depending on the wound's anatomical location, the ability of a suture pattern to invert or evert tissues may or may not be sought. Inversion is often desirable only for closure of hollow viscera to prevent leakage; however, excessive inversion will reduce luminal diameter. Slight eversion to counter the tendency of wound edges to invert during healing is mandatory to proper healing of the skin. Consequently, slight skin eversion results in the most cosmetic outcome following suture removal (Figures 4.21a, 4.23a, 4.26).[2]

Continuous Intradermal Patterns

A continuous intradermal pattern provides secure skin closure and better cosmetic results and precludes suture removal following healing of the skin edge. Care must be taken to avoid including the epidermis in the closure because of the potential for the formation of suture fistulas (Figure 4.25). Refer to Table 4.5 for the general features, advantages versus disadvantages, and common uses of appositional and everting sutures.

Tension Sutures

Large wounds are difficult to close without creating tension on the suture line. Some suture patterns offer mechanical advantages over others, by requiring less force to achieve wound closure.[24] While clinical experience suggests that equine wounds can be closed with a reasonable amount of tension,[14] when the forces required on individual appositional sutures increase to the point where cutting out of sutures and compromise to the blood supply threaten to occur, tension sutures should be used. They draw the wound edges together with minimal risk of vascular damage, tissue necrosis, or wound dehiscence (Figures 4.28a-c, 4.29, 4.30, 4.31).

Table 4.5. Appositional suture patterns for wound management.

Suture type	Advantages	Disadvantages	Common uses
Simple interrupted (Figures 4.15 and 4.18)	Easily applied. Precise suture tension possible. Minimally alters the skin architecture. Provides secure, anatomic closure. Concurrent closure of skin, subcutis, and underlying fascia may reduce dead space. Minimal alteration in blood supply.	Requires increased time for placement. Excessive tension causes inversion of skin margins.	Skin, subcutis, fascia, blood vessels, nerves.
Interrupted intradermal or subcuticular (Figure 4.19)	Similar to SI (upside down SI suture placed in dermis and subcutis).	Requires increased time for placement compared to the SI and continuous suture pattern.	Intradermal skin closure. Rarely used.
Interrupted cruciate or cross mattress (Figures 4.20a,b)	Easiest of all mattress sutures to apply; more rapidly applied than SI. No alteration of blood supply, even when placed under tension. Provides stronger closure than SI. Resists tension. Prevents eversion of wound edges at fascia level.	Excessive tension causes inversion of skin margins. Skin margins tend to gap between sutures.	Fascia, occasionally skin.
Interrupted vertical mattress (Figures 4.21a,b,c)	Provides precise wound edge-to-edge apposition with slight eversion when tied. Minimal alteration in skin blood supply. A single layer can be used for concurrent closure of skin and subcutis to eliminate dead space.	Takes longer to apply and creates slightly more inflammation because the suture is passed through tissue 4 times.	Skin, subcutis, fascia. Can be alternated with SI sutures to prevent inversion and gaping.
Allgöwer corium vertical mattress (Figure 4.22)	Minimal trauma (through dermis only). Perfect alignment of skin margins without inversion and with minimal or no eversion. Cosmetically superior closure.	May have less holding strength than a traditional vertical mattress.	Skin.
Interrupted horizontal mattress (Figures 4.23a,b)	Appositional to everting suture, depending on suture tension and whether suture penetrates tissue full- or split-thickness. Less suture material than IVM.	Tends to reduce skin blood supply. Potential for tissue strangulation (can be reduced with stents). Excessive scar formation when used alone because of skin eversion and gaping.	Skin, subcutis, fascia, muscle, tendon.
Simple continuous (Figure 4.24)	Saves time. Promotes suture economy. Provides good apposition of wound edges or skin margins. Provides airtight or watertight seal.	Good only for layers under low tension. Provides less strength than SI. Wound tensile strength gain is delayed compared to SI sutures. Excessive tension causes puckering and strangulation of skin.	Skin, subcutis, fascia, blood vessels.
Continuous intradermal or subcuticular (Figure 4.25)	Similar to II (modified horizontal mattress suture). Saves time. Promotes suture economy.	Provides less strength than skin closure.	Intradermal skin closure.

Table 4.5. *Continued*

Suture type	Advantages	Disadvantages	Common uses
Continuous mattress; horizontal (Figure 4.26a) and vertical (Figure 4.26b)	Horizontal: appositional to everting suture, depending on suture tension. Facilitates rapid closure. Vertical: minimal alteration in blood supply; precise edge-to-edge skin contact.	Horizontal: can cause skin eversion/gaping. Vertical: difficult to apply; rarely used.	Skin, subcutis, fascia.
Continuous lock or Ford interlocking (Figure 4.27)	Similar to SC. Provides greater security than SC if broken.	Similar to SC. Requires large amount of suture. Time consuming to apply. May cause pressure necrosis and become buried when placed under tension.	Skin.

Adapted from Bailey,[14] Blackford,[4] Toombs,[12] Stashak[2]
IHM = interrupted horizontal mattress
II = interrupted intradermal
IVM = interrupted vertical mattress
SC = simple continuous
SI = simple interrupted

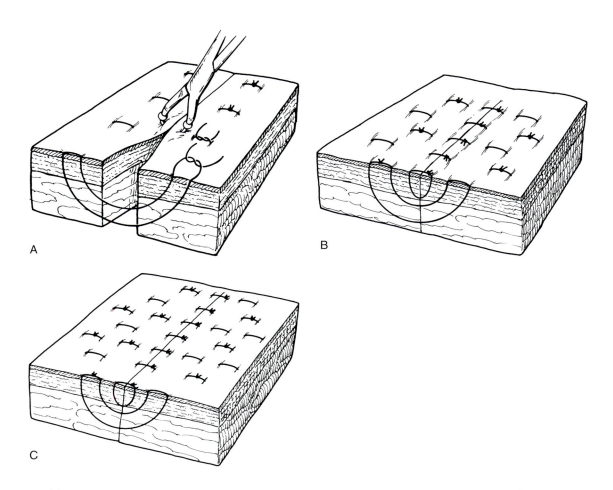

Figure 4.28. (A) Vertical mattress sutures are preplaced and the skin edges apposed with towel clamps. (B) Two rows of vertical mattress sutures are used to reduce the tension at the site of primary closure. (C) Three rows of vertical mattress sutures are used to reduce the tension at the site of primary closure. Both (B) and (C) placement of interrupted vertical mattress sutures are in an "echelon" pattern.

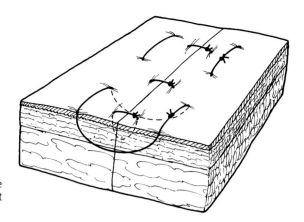

Figure 4.29. Widely placed interrupted horizontal mattress and simple interrupted sutures reduce tension on the primary repair site and prevent eversion of the skin edges.

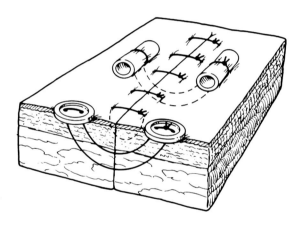

Figure 4.30. Quilled or stented tension sutures augmented by supports (rubber stents or buttons).

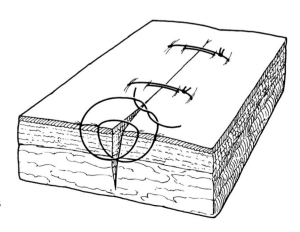

Figure 4.31. A far-near near-far suture pattern. The far component reduces tension while the near component holds the tissue edges in apposition.

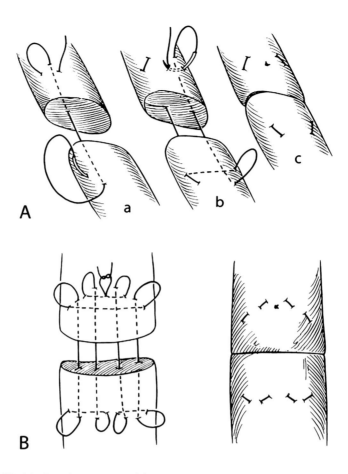

Figure 4.32. (A) Single modified locking loop suture. (B) Double modified locking loop suture pattern.

Tension sutures, placed well away from the wound edges to prevent strangulation, can be used either alone (Figure 4.31) or in combination with appositional suture patterns (Figures 4.28a-c, 4.29, 4.30). Tension sutures are usually preplaced first. Skin edges are then apposed with the aid of towel clamps and preplaced tension sutures are tied. Finally, the suture line is closed with an appositional suture pattern (Figures 4.28b,c, 4.29, 4.30).[2]

Additional support in the form of buttons, rubber tubing, and/or gauze either placed under the tension sutures or incorporated into them before they are tied (Figure 4.30) will reduce the risk of cutting out of sutures. This technique is referred to as a quilled or stented suture and is best used in regions with good soft tissue support (neck and trunk)[2] where pressure bandages cannot be applied. If bandages or a cast are applied, areas of necrosis corresponding to the surface area of these additional supports usually develop. When managing a wound under a bandage or cast, it is recommended to place several rows of tension sutures without supports rather than use buttons, rubber tubing, or gauze as suture supports. Tension suture patterns for tendon and nerve apposition are needed in some instances (Figures 4.32, 4.33, 4.34). Refer to Table 4.6 for the general features, advantages versus disadvantages, and common uses of tension sutures.

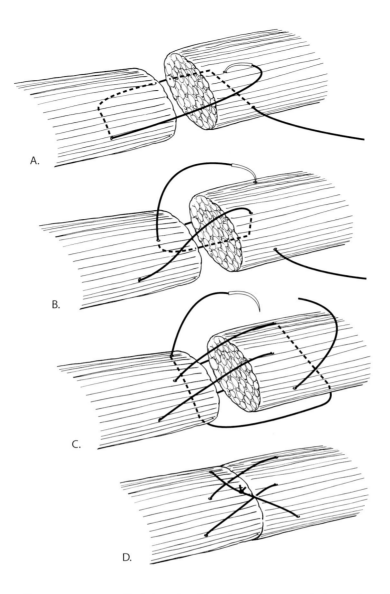

Figure 4.33. The Three-loop pulley suture pattern. Each loop is oriented 120 degrees relative to the others. (A) The first loop is in a near-far suture pattern, (B) the second loop is equidistant from the transected ends of the tendon and (C and D) the third loop is placed in a far-near pattern.

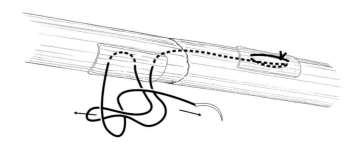

Figure 4.34. Intraneural pattern.

Table 4.6. Tension suture patterns for wound management.

Suture pattern	Advantages	Disadvantages	Common uses
Interrupted vertical mattress (Figures 4.28a,b,c)	Minimal alteration in cutaneous blood supply. Adding more, widely placed rows of IVM suture reduces the tension on the appositional primary suture line. Stronger than IHM in tissues under tension.	Occasionally, suture will cut out when placed under excessive tension.	Undermined skin under tension. Used with supports (bandage, buttons, stents).
Interrupted horizontal mattress (Figure 4.29)	Placed widely, IHM suture reduces the tension on the appositional primary suture line. Less suture material than IVM.	Tends to compromise skin blood supply. Does not reduce tension as effectively as IVM. Potential for tissue strangulation (can be reduced with stents).	Skin, subcutis, fascia, muscle, tendon. Supports are added to reduce cutting out of sutures in regions that cannot be bandaged.
Quilled or stented (Figure 4.30)	Similar to IVM (variation of IVM that loops over a stent on either side of the incision). Very effective in reducing tension on the appositional primary suture line. Everting mainly. Can also be a variation of the IHM.	Skin necrosis underneath the quilled/stented sutures can occur if too much suture tension exists.	Combined with appositional suture for skin in areas of extreme tension where bandage cannot be applied.
Near and far (or far and near) (Figure 4.31)	Combines a tension suture (the far portion) and an appositional suture (the near portion). Higher tensile strength than either an SI or a mattress pattern. Provides necessary tension for wound edge approximation without applying tension to the wound edge itself.	Excessive tightening can cause inversion. Leaves a large amount of suture material in the wound.	Skin, subcutis, fascia.
Locking loop (Figure 4.32)	Provides good apposition compared with other tendon sutures, with equal holding strength.	May compromise intrathecal blood supply.	Tendon.
Three-loop pulley (Figure 4.33)	Has slightly higher tension strength compared to the LL. Minimal alteration in the blood supply.	More suture is exposed compared to the LL.	Tendon.
Intraneural (Figure 4.34)	Centrally placed neurorrhaphy suture anchored externally with silicone buttons.	N/A	Nerve.

Adapted from Bailey,[14] Blackford,[4] Toombs,[12] Stashak[2]
IHM = interrupted horizontal mattress
IVM = interrupted vertical mattress
LL = locking loop
SI = simple interrupted

Walking Sutures

Walking sutures are buried sutures that: (1) move skin progressively toward the center of the wound or the opposite wound margin, (2) distribute tension, and (3) obliterate subcutaneous dead space and so prevent the formation of serum pockets (Figure 4.35).[4] They are not commonly used in equine wound management because increasing the number of buried sutures increases the tissue reaction and foreign body response, thus making the wound more susceptible to infection.

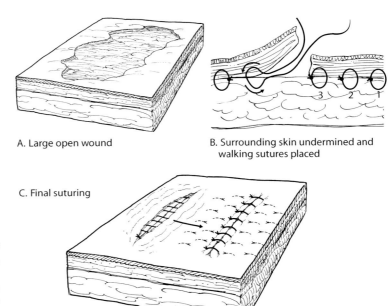

A. Large open wound

B. Surrounding skin undermined and walking sutures placed

C. Final suturing

Figure 4.35. Walking sutures. Skin around the initial wound is undermined. Using absorbable suture material, the first bite is taken deep within the dermis (without penetrating the epidermis). The second bite is taken in the underlying fascia toward the center of the wound or the opposite wound margin. Tying the suture advances the skin flap in the chosen direction. Walking sutures are placed on both sides of the wound until the skin margins are close enough to allow closure with an appositional suture pattern placed without tension.

Staples

In wound management, surgical staples are mainly used for rapid skin closure. Surgical staples made of absorbable or non-absorbable materials are now available. Both are associated with a lower risk of wound infection than conventional suture materials.[25] Absorbable surgical staples induce a less severe inflammatory response in the early stages of skin healing than do other methods of wound closure, including non-absorbable staples,[26] leading to better cosmetic results.[25,26] Although their application is rapid, absorbable or non-absorbable surgical staples are not as strong as sutures; therefore, they should not be used when skin is under tension unless it is also supported by tension sutures.

Support for Suture Lines

Supplying adequate support for the suture line can determine the wound's success or failure in healing. In many instances, bandages (regular, pressure, or stent) may be used to support a suture line, immobilize surrounding skin and adjacent joints, minimize edema formation, and obliterate dead space.[18] In all cases, a subtle balance should be sought between providing adequate support to the suture line and interfering with regional cutaneous blood supply,[14] the critical occluding pressure of skin arterioles being as low as 30 mm Hg. Careful monitoring is therefore very important in such cases.

Drains

Indications for Use

Drains are implants designed to channel unwanted debris, fluids, tissues, or gas out of a body cavity or away from a wound on a temporary basis. They serve a number of important functions such that proper use of drains usually speeds up the healing process. These implants are not benign, however, and inappropriate use may result in delayed healing and complications including retrograde bacterial migration, tissue inflammation, drain entrapment or loss, and hemorrhage.

Established indications for drain implantation are those of facilitating elimination of dead space and evacuating existing fluid and gas accumulations. The prophylactic use of drains to prevent the anticipated formation of fluid or gas collections remains debatable.[27,28]

Ideal Material

The ideal drain material should:

- Efficiently channel the unwanted fluids or gas out of body cavities or away from wounds
- Be sterile, non-reactive, non-allergenic, non-carcinogenic, and pyrogen-free, not corrosive or toxic
- Be soft and compliant
- Stimulate minimal tissue reaction to avoid creating a situation favorable to bacterial contamination and growth
- Be inexpensive, readily available in different sizes, and easily sterilized without alteration of its properties
- Be easy to handle and comfortable to users and patients
- Be radio opaque to be retrieved easily if it disappears inside a wound or a body cavity.

The ideal drain material does not presently exist; however, many available drain materials do boast excellent properties.

Principles of Drain Usage

Drains are implants designed to facilitate the healing process; they are not a substitute for proper wound management and surgical technique and therefore cannot compensate for inadequate wound cleansing, debridement, and lavage.[27] Drains are also foreign bodies which increase the wound's susceptibility to infection and can cause some mechanical injury to tissue. Consequently, they should not be placed in the immediate vicinity of delicate tissues (blood vessels and nerves) or lie directly under or exit from a suture line.[2,27,29,30]

The most frequent complication associated with drain use is retrograde contamination of the wound by environmental multiresistant bacteria. To minimize this risk, drains should be applied under aseptic conditions. The sterile environment should then be maintained by covering the wound and drain exit site with a sterile absorptive dressing that is changed frequently. The amount of drainage and its consistency dictate the frequency with which bandages need to be changed (passive drains) or vacuum containers emptied (active drains). The sterile absorptive dressing is held in place using standard bandaging techniques for the extremities and a stent or tie-over bandage can be used in the upper body. If bandaging of an upper body wound is impractical because of its location or if it is too large and more than one drain is used, then the exit site(s) for the drain(s) should be cleansed at least twice daily with an antiseptic soap, followed by rinsing with a dilute antiseptic solution after which an antiseptic ointment is applied to the drain exit site(s).

Classification of Drains

Passive Drains

Passive drains can be either soft latex (Penrose drain) or a more rigid tube of red rubber, polypropylene, or silicone. Passive drains usually rely to a large extent on gravity and capillary action to evacuate fluid and gas away from the wound. They should exit the wound or dead space below its most distal or ventral aspect and be long enough to avoid disappearing into the wound in response to the horse's movements. The proximal or dorsal end of the drain should be buried into the proximal or dorsal aspect of the wound to avert descending bacterial infection and be secured with a single penetrating suture tied on the outside of the intact skin adjacent to the wound (Figure 4.36). An exception should be made when placing drains in wounds in the axillary or inguinal regions. In these cases, exiting the proximal or dorsal end of the drain through a more proximal or dorsal skin incision will prevent subcutaneous air entrapment as the horse moves.

Another exception may be made when a drain is placed in a wound in the ventral throat latch region or in the cranial ventral two thirds of the neck; having cranial and caudal drain exit sites may facilitate drainage of these wounds no matter the position of the head and neck (extension, flexion, or neutral).

Exiting the distal or ventral end of the drain through a single stab incision in a dependent position near the wound is strongly recommended (Figure 4.37). This latter end should be secured with individual sutures to prevent its retreat into the wound. These sutures should be easily distinguishable to avoid premature removal of sutures securing an incision when the drain is removed. Refer to Table 4.7 for more details about passive drains commonly used in equine wound management.

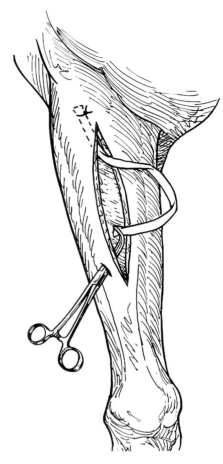

Figure 4.36. Proper placement of a Penrose drain to facilitate passive drainage. The proximal end of the drain is buried within the proximal aspect of the wound and is secured with a single penetrating suture tied on the outside of intact skin adjacent to the wound. The distal end exits the wound below its most distal aspect through a single stab incision in a dependent position near the wound. The wound is subsequently closed.

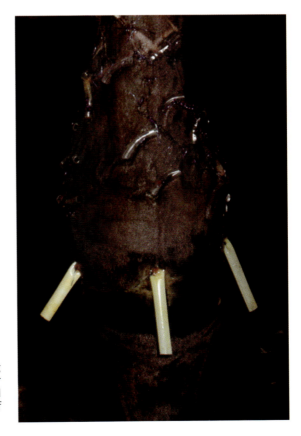

Figure 4.37. Traumatic carpal wound with multiple Penrose drains exiting the wound distally through stab incisions in a dependent position near the wound. The drains were removed within 5 days and the wound healed by primary intention under a full limb cast. Courtesy of the University of Montreal.

Table 4.7. Characteristics of the most commonly used passive drains.

Type	Raw material	Mechanism of action	Advantages and uses	Disadvantages
Gauze drains[a]	Fine mesh gauze.	Drainage occurs by gravity and capillary action.	Economical. May be soaked with antibiotics or antiseptics or made from commercially available antimicrobial dressing material (Kerlix® Antimicrobial Dressing[b]) May be applied as packing in profusely bleeding cavities or in abscesses. Adherence of surrounding tissues and fibrin clots to the gauze exerts a debriding action.	Greater foreign body reaction, increasing inflammation and potential for infection. Prolonged use can result in a fibrous tract. Wicking effect facilitates ascending infection. Should not be used in the abdominal or thoracic cavities.
Penrose drains[d]	Soft and pliable latex.	Drainage occurs mostly extraluminally by gravity and capillary action (hollow tube). **WARNING:** Fenestration weakens the drain and reduces the surface area of drainage, which decreases its efficacy.	Economical. Easily sterilized. Readily available in various sizes. Little foreign body reaction. Radio-opaque. Many applications: in contaminated wounds not completely debrided, in fluid-filled dead spaces, underneath skin grafts, in second-intention healing, in synovial cavities left open for lavage.	Kink easily. Cannot be used in abdominal or thoracic cavity. Cannot be used with suction. May facilitate ascending infection. Some contain zinc diethyldithiocarbamate, a vulcanizing accelerator, which has been shown to be toxic.
Silicone Penrose drains[c]	Soft and pliable nonreactive silicone.	As regular Penrose drain.	As regular Penrose drain. Less irritating. Latex-free for sensitive patients. Contains radiodense markers.	As regular Penrose drain.
Sheet drains	Waved sheet of red rubber. Smooth surface.	Drainage occurs by gravity and capillary action.	Relative stiffness: there is a gap between the two layers of drain, which resists obstruction when folded. Can be cut to size.	Increased foreign body reaction. Impurities can support bacterial growth.
Stiff tubular drains	Red rubber. Smooth surface.	Drainage occurs by gravity and capillary action.	Relative stiffness: rarely compressed or occluded. Suction can be applied.	Increased foreign body reaction. Impurities can support bacterial growth. Easily obstructed by debris.
Soft tubular drains (Flexi-Drain[c]), J-VAC Drain[a])	Soft and pliable nonreactive silicone.	Drainage occurs by gravity and capillary action. Drainage is increased when tubes are joined together.	Contains radiodense markers. Can be split longitudinally to size. Suction can be applied.	Easily obstructed by debris.

Adapted from Auer,[29] Blackford[4]
[a] Ethicon, Johnson and Johnson Company, Inc., New Brunswick, NJ
[b] Tyco Healthcare Kendall, Mansfield, MA
[c] Benson Medical Industries, Inc., Toronto, ON
[d] Sherwood Medical, St. Louis, MO

Not all latex drains are created equal. For example, latex drains that are vulcanized using zinc dithiocarbamates (e.g., Perry latex Penrose drains, Ansell Perry Inc., Massillon, OH) to improve the aging behavior and thermal resistance of the product have been shown to induce severe local and systemic toxicity in mice.[31]

Active Drains

Active drains create an artificial gradient for fluid and gas evacuation by applying negative pressure to the wound, sometimes against gravity. Refer to Table 4.8 for details about active drains commonly used in equine wound management.

Open suction using sump drains is infrequently employed in equine wound management. Briefly, sump drains are double-lumen tubes with a large outflow lumen and smaller inflow lumen. Venting occurs when air enters the drainage area through the small inflow lumen. Air breaks the vacuum, forcing air and fluid into the larger outflow lumen. Certain types of sump drains have a third lumen which is used to irrigate the wound while maintaining suction via the other lumen.

Table 4.8. Characteristics of the most commonly used drains in closed active drainage.

Type	Material	Material description	Mechanism of action	Advantages and uses	Disadvantages
Redon drain[a]	Polyvinylchloride (PVC)	Round multifenestrated tube at its distal end with nonfenestrated extension. Length of the multifenestrated part: 14 cm. Total length of drain: 50–80 cm. Diameter: 3–6 mm.	Active or passive drainage intraluminally.	Can be used as a closed or open drainage system. Excellent for evacuation of fluids from body cavities. Available in different diameters.	Attaching the suction device may be difficult, depending on the wound location. Fibrin can plug/clog the drain. This can be prevented by flushing the tube with full-strength sterile heparin prior to implantation.
Jackson-Pratt drain[b]	Silastic, Teflon	Flat multifenestrated drain at its distal end with nonfenestrated plastic extension.	Active or passive drainage intraluminally.	Can be used as a closed or open drainage system. Excellent for evacuation of fluids from body cavities. Less reactive (can be left in place for longer period of time).	Attaching the suction device may be difficult, depending on the wound location.
Black drain[c]	Silicone	Flat or round drains with four channels along the sides with a solid core center connected to an extension tubing. Available either 3/4 fluted or full fluted, with or without a trocar.	Active or passive drainage intraluminally.	Available in a wide variety of sizes. Greater tissue contact area than regular perforated drains. Offers multiple drainage routes to resist clogging. Minimal tissue irritation = greater patient comfort. Removal may be less traumatic to surrounding tissues.	Relatively voluminous, making it hard to fix it to the horse's body and limbs. Suction possible only when skin suture is tight. Single use only.

Adapted from Auer[29]
[a] Zimmer, Inc., Dover, OH
[b] Nelaton, Ruesch, Belp, Switzerland
[c] Ethicon, Johnson and Johnson Company, Inc., New Brunswick, NJ

Closed suction is very useful to evacuate fluid and collapse dead space within large cavities in horses. Closed suction drains are frequently used in the management of infected synovial cavities and large, deep wounds or to evacuate the pleural space.[29] They usually consist of a multifenestrated drain with a nonfenestrated extension (drain tube) which is connected to a drain reservoir. Most multifenestrated drains are made of polyvinylchloride (Redon drain) or silicone/silastic (Black drain, Jackson-Pratt drain).

Suction can be either continuous or intermittent. Continuous suction is usually more efficient, preventing drain occlusion and reducing the amount of time that the drain is in place.[23] Several portable commercial continuous-suction devices are available and consist of a bellows-type drain reservoir (Figures 4.38 and 4.39) that is compressed, attached to the drain tube, then released. The 80 mm Hg of negative pressure generated by these units is sufficient to evacuate fluid and collapse dead space but does not damage tissues.[32]

Homemade active drains (Figures 4.40 and 4.41) can also be constructed by connecting the external end of a drain tube through a three-way stopcock to a syringe (e.g., 60 ml) acting as a drain reservoir. The plunger of the syringe is withdrawn to achieve the desired negative pressure. It is usually held in that position to maintain the negative pressure by introducing a large needle or a small pin across the plunger through a predrilled hole. The three-way stopcock allows interruption of the suction action prior to removing the syringe for emptying.[27,29] It is extremely important that the drain reservoir not become disconnected from the drain tube inadvertently, which would cause a rapid loss of negative pressure and introduce environmental bacteria into the wound.

Multifenestrated drains are positioned into the wound or body cavity and secured to the skin at the level of the drain tube. Drain tubes can be sutured to the skin using a variety of suture patterns. The "Chinese finger trap" suture pattern and the "double clove hitch" are the patterns most frequently used (Figure 4.42). Drain reservoirs are usually secured to the skin at a remote site and protected with bandages. Drain reservoirs should be monitored frequently to ensure that adequate negative pressure is present, particularly in the first 24 hours following insertion, when fluid withdrawal is maximal. Anticipated volume of drainage should dictate in part the size of the reservoir. A larger reservoir is preferable in most cases.

Closed suction systems reduce saturation of bandages with wound fluid and help prevent contamination by environmental bacteria. Furthermore, they significantly decrease the likelihood of ascending infection

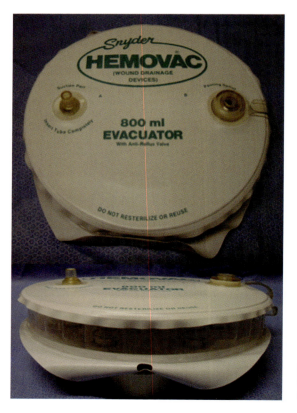

Figure 4.38. Snyder Hemovac wound drainage device, 800 ml. Bellows-type drain reservoir, used as active drainage system. Courtesy of the University of Montreal.

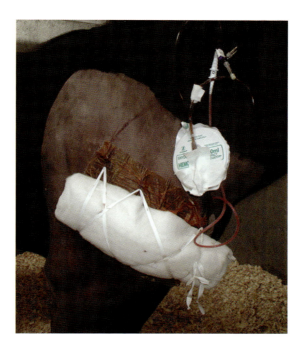

Figure 4.39. Active drainage system (Jackson-Pratt drain connected to a bellows-type Snyder Hemovac reservoir) used in the management of septic arthritis (shoulder joint). Courtesy of Dr. F. David.

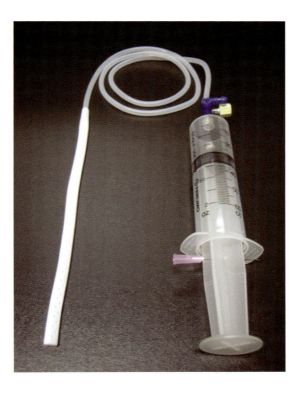

Figure 4.40. Homemade active drain constructed by connecting one end of a tube to a Jackson-Pratt drain and the other end to a three-way stopcock. The stopcock is attached to a 60 ml syringe which acts as a drain reservoir. The plunger of the syringe is withdrawn to achieve the desired negative pressure and held in that position by introducing a large needle through the syringe handle. Courtesy of the University of Montreal.

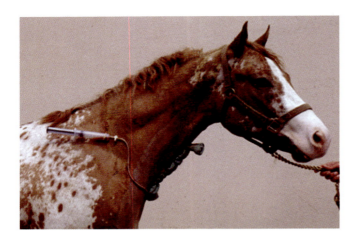

Figure 4.41. Homemade active drain used in the management of a case of interbody cervical fusion.

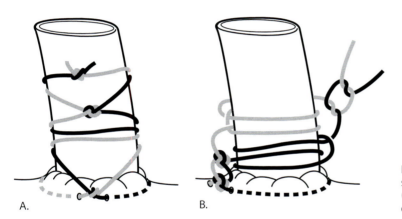

A.   B.

Figure 4.42. Suture patterns commonly used to secure a suction drain to the body or limb. (A) "Chinese finger trap" suture pattern. (B) "Double clove hitch" pattern.

attributed to passive drains. A special closed suction system has been used successfully to promote granulation tissue production in avulsion wounds with bone exposure both in humans and horses (vacuum-assisted closure). For more details, see New and Innovative Approaches to Wound Closure later in this chapter.

Drain Removal

All drains can incite a foreign body reaction and induce the production of secretions. Therefore, they should be removed in an aseptic manner as soon as possible.

The duration of drain placement varies according to the situation. A good indication for drain removal is a significant decrease in the drainage volume and a change in its characteristics, from a purulent or serosanguineous to a serous, non-odoriferous, non-turbid fluid. As a rule, the average time for maintaining a drain within a wound is 2 to 4 days (inflammatory phase of wound repair), but there are exceptions to this rule: (1) When drains are placed in small cavities to evacuate capillary bleeding, they can usually be removed within 24 hours; (2) When drains are placed to treat bacterial infections, they are usually maintained for 48 to 72 hours; (3) When drains are placed into large body cavities to promote the union of local tissues, they may be necessary for 1 week or more.[27,29] Upon removal, the drain should be carefully examined to verify its integrity. If a portion of the drain is accidentally left in the wound, wound drainage will persist until the fragment has been removed completely.

Conclusion

Sutures and drains serve important functions in wound repair; proper use usually speeds up healing and allows for a better cosmetic and functional outcome. A broad range of suture and drain materials is now available. Knowledge of the advantages and disadvantages of each material, assessment of wound location and condition, as well as familiarity with the healing rate of the tissues involved dictate the appropriate selection. Although this choice is important, more vital is the fundamental approach to managing the wound. Indeed, sutures and drains are not a substitute for proper wound management. They cannot compensate for cleansing, debridement, and lavage. Inappropriate use may result in delayed healing and the development of major complications including increased susceptibility to infection, which could lead to death.

References

1. Stashak TS, Yturraspe DJ: Consideration for the selection of suture materials. Vet Surg 1978;7:48
2. Stashak TS, Yturraspe DJ: Selection of suture materials and suture patterns for wound closure. In Ted Stashak, ed. *Equine wound management (1st edition)*. Philadelphia: Lea and Febiger, 1991, p.52
3. Boothe HW: Suture materials, tissue adhesives, staplers, and ligating clips. In Doug Slatter, ed. *Textbook of small animal surgery (7th edition)*. Philadelphia: WB Saunders, 2003, volume 1, p.235
4. Blackford LW, Blackford JT: Suture Materials and Patterns. In Jorge Auer and John Stick, eds. *Equine surgery (3rd edition)*. Philadelphia: Saunders Elsevier, 2006, p.187
5. Van Winckle W Jr, Hastings JC: Considerations in the choice of suture material for various tissues. Surg Gynecol Obstet 1972;135:113
6. Hendrickson DA: Management of superficial wounds. In Jorge Auer and John Stick, eds. *Equine surgery (3rd edition)*. Philadelphia: Saunders Elsevier, 2006, p.288
7. Van Rijssel EJ, Brand R, Admiraal C, et al: Tissue reaction and surgical knots: the effect of suture size, knot configuration, and knot volume. Obstet Gynecol 1989;74:64
8. Stashak TS: Suture patterns used for wound closure in veterinary surgery. Proc Am Assoc of Equine Pract 1978;24:383
9. Moy LS: Management of acute wounds. Dermatol Clinics 1993;11:759
10. Trostle SS, Wilson DG, Stone WC, et al: A study of the biomechanical properties of the adult equine linea alba: relationship of tissue bite size and suture material to breaking strength. Vet Surg 1994;23:435
11. Hendrickson D, Virgin J: Factors that affect equine wound repair. Vet Clin N Am Equine Pract, Wound Management 2005;21:33
12. Toombs JP, Clarke KM: Basic operative techniques. In Doug Slatter. ed. *Textbook of small animal surgery (7th edition)*. Philadelphia: WB Saunders, 2003, p.199
13. Fierheller EE, Wilson DG: An in vitro biomechanical comparison of the breaking strength and stiffness of polydioxanone (sizes 2,7) and polyglactin (sizes 3,6) in the equine linea alba. Vet Surg 2005;34:18
14. Bailey JV: Principles of Reconstructive and plastic surgery. In Jorge Auer and John Stick, eds. *Equine surgery (3rd edition)*. Philadelphia: Saunders Elsevier, 2006, p.255
15. Heath MM: Needle selection in veterinary surgery. Anim Health Tech 1983;4:45
16. Trier WC: Considerations in the choice of surgical needles. Surg Gynecol Obstet 1979;149:84
17. Forrester JC: Suture materials and their uses. Nurses Mirror 1975;140:48
18. Swaim SF: Management and reconstruction in the dog and cat. In Steven Swaim, ed. *Surgery of traumatized skin (1st edition)*. Philadelphia: WB Saunders, 1980, p.165
19. Drake DB, Rodeheaver PF, Edlich RF, et al: Experimental studies in swine for measurement of suture extrusion. J Long Term Eff Med Implants 2004;14:251
20. Speer DP: The influence of suture technique on early wound healing. J Surg Res 1979;27:385
21. Knecht CD: Fundamental techniques in veterinary surgery. In Charles Knecht, Algernon Allen, David Williams and Jerry Johnson, eds. *Fundamental techniques in veterinary surgery (3rd edition)*. Philadelphia: WB Saunders, 1987, p.205
22. Richey ML, Roe SC: Assessment of knot security in continuous intradermal wound closures. J Surg Res 2005;123:284
23. Gillespie BW, Martinez SA, Smith LV, et al: Comparison of the tensile strength between two intradermal suture patterns: buried-knot and "pulley knot-free" techniques in the dog. Proc Am Coll Vet Surg 2006;152:17
24. Austin BR, Henderson RA: Buried tension sutures: Force-tension comparisons of pulley, double butterfly, mattress, and simple interrupted suture patterns. Vet Surg 2006;35:43
25. Pineros-Fernandez A, Salopek LS, Rodeheaver PF, et al: A revolutionary advance in skin closure compared to current methods. J Long Term Eff Med Implants 2006;16:19
26. Fick JL, Novo RE, Kirchhof N: Comparison of gross and histologic tissue responses of skin incisions closed by use of absorbable subcuticular staples, cutaneous metal staples, and polyglactin 910 suture in pigs. Am J Vet Res 2005;66:1975

27. Miller CW: Bandages and drains. In Doug Slatter, ed. *Textbook of small animal surgery (7th edition)*, 2 volumes. Philadelphia: WB Saunders, 2003, p.244

28. Roush KJ: The use and misuse of drains in surgical practice. Prob in Vet Med 1990;2:482

29. Auer JA: Drains, bandages, and external coaptation. In Jorge Auer and John Stick, eds. *Equine surgery (3rd edition)*. Philadelphia: Saunders Elsevier, 2006, p.203

30. Baines SJ: Surgical drains. In David Fowler and John M. Williams, eds. *Manual of canine and feline wound management and reconstruction (1st edition)*. London: Br Small Anim Vet Assoc, 1999, p.44

31. Nicolaysen PH, Klink KJ, Shriver E, et al: Local and systemic toxicity in mice following subcutaneous implantation of latex Penrose drains. J Toxicol Cutan Ocul Toxicol 2004;23:233

32. Hampel NL, Johnson RG: Principles of surgical drains and drainage. J Am Animal Hosp Assoc 1985;21:21

33. Blackford JT, Blackford LW, Disegi J, et al: Biomaterials, surgical implants and instruments. In Jorge Auer and John Stick, eds. *Equine surgery (3rd edition)*. Philadelphia: Saunders Elsevier, 2006, p.96

34. MacKay RJ: Peripheral nerve injury. In Jorge Auer and John Stick, eds. *Equine surgery (3rd edition)*. Philadelphia: Saunders Elsevier, 2006, p.684

35. Miller TR: Eyelids. In Jorge Auer and John Stick, eds. *Equine surgery (3rd edition)*. Philadelphia: Saunders Elsevier, 2006, p.702

36. Millichamp NJ: Conjunctiva. In Jorge Auer and John Stick, eds. *Equine surgery (3rd edition)*. Philadelphia: Saunders Elsevier, 2006, p.716

37. Millichamp NJ: Principles of ophthalmic surgery. In Jorge Auer and John Stick, eds. *Equine surgery (3rd edition)*. Philadelphia: Saunders Elsevier, 2006, p.693

38. Nasisse MP, Jamieson VE, Brooks DE: Cornea and sclera. In Jorge Auer and John Stick, eds. *Equine surgery (3rd edition)*. Philadelphia: Saunders Elsevier, 2006, p.731

39. Rosin E, Robinson GM: Knot security of suture materials. Vet Surg 1998;18:269

4.3 New and Innovative Approaches to Wound Closure

David A. Wilson, DVM, MS, Diplomate ACVS

Introduction

The current method of closing wounds and surgical incisions with sutures dates back thousands of years. Based on skeletal remains and the presence of eyed needles, wound closure with needle and suture is thought to have occurred as long ago as 50,000 to 30,000 B.C.[1] In 1862, an Egyptologist named Edwin Smith discovered the first reference to sutures in several papyri dated ~1600 B.C. for the treatment of a gashed shoulder: "thou shouldst draw together for him the gash with two strips of linen."[1] The oldest physical evidence of preserved suture is that found in a mummy dated ~1100 B.C.[2]

The material used for suture has changed through the years but the principles of wound closure were not altered significantly until the last century. The advent of antimicrobial-impregnated sutures, barbed sutures, suture anchors, tissue adhesives, skin expanders, tissue fusion, and vacuum-assisted closure (VAC) has promised to change the way we close wounds and surgical incisions. These innovative products hold the potential to close wounds located in areas that challenge conventional methods or to provide a more stable closure with fewer complications and a superior cosmetic outcome.

The purpose of this chapter is to describe the new and future developments in wound closure. Some of these methods may never become commercially available, but reviewing the current literature may stimulate the inquisitive mind to think of other potential methods of closure.

Suture Innovations

Antimicrobial-impregnated Sutures

While sutures have been used for thousands of years to close wounds and incisions, this practice has not been problem-free. Because sutures act as a foreign body, considerable inflammation as well as infection can develop around the suture material. Synthetic monofilament sutures have significantly decreased but have not eliminated adverse tissue reactions to sutures. In the 1980s, techniques were developed to impregnate suture material with antibiotics.[3,4]

More recently, two triclosan antibiotic-impregnated sutures have been commercialized.[5,6] The basic suture materials are polyglactin 910 (Vicryl Plus, Ethicon, Inc., New Brunswick, NJ) and poliglecaprone 25 (Monocryl Plus, Ethicon, Inc., New Brunswick, NJ). A third triclosan antibiotic-impregnated suture material, polydioxanone (PDS Plus, Ethicon, Inc., New Brunswick, NJ), is also available.[7]

Triclosan is a synthetic non-ionic broad-spectrum antimicrobial agent that has been used in personal care products for more than 30 years. Its common uses are in the prevention of oral plaque and as an active ingredient for surgical scrubbing. Triclosan has been shown to have no effect on tissue reaction, healing response, or the absorption profile of Vicryl Plus sutures.[6] Additionally, triclosan-impregnated suture has shown evidence of inhibiting the in vitro growth of wild-type and methicillin-resistant *Staphylococcus aureus* and *Staphylococcus epidermidis*.[5] The development of antimicrobial-impregnated suture will likely improve wound closure options in areas that are at increased risk for infection in the horse, such as contaminated skin wounds and wherever a lumen—such as intestine, bladder, trachea, or esophagus—is closed.

Barbed Sutures

Barbed or self-anchoring sutures, manufactured from polydioxanone monofilament material, have recently been described.[8,9] The sutures consists of axially placed barbed segments on each side of a midpoint at which the barbs change direction (Figure 4.43). Every suture has a curved needle crimped onto each end for tissue insertion. Suturing begins at the midpoint of an incision and the suture is advanced through the tissue in a horizontal curvilinear sinusoidal pattern toward one end of the wound. The other end of the suture is then inserted in a mirror image to the first, extending to the opposite end of the wound/incision. Instead of a knot, a reverse bite is taken to secure each end of the suture. Excess suture is then cut at the dermal layer and discarded (Figure 4.44).

In a clinical trial of 195 women undergoing Cesarean section, barbed sutures made from size 0 polydioxanone monofilament were used for dermal closure.[8] There were no differences in closure time, pain, and cosmesis scores; rates of infection; dehiscence; or other adverse events between the control group using a continuous intradermal subcuticular 3–0 polydioxanone suture-II and the barbed suture group. A study in pigs comparing barbed (size 0 polydioxanone monofilament) to regular knotted sutures (size 2–0 polyglactin 910 multifilament) indicated similar failure forces, operative times, and incision integrity, but fibrosis was increased in the barbed suture closures.[9]

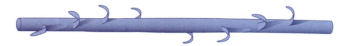

Figure 4.43. Modified self-anchoring suture to increase tissue drag and approximate tissue without the need for suture ligation. Modified from Weld, et al.[9] (Elsevier, Inc.)

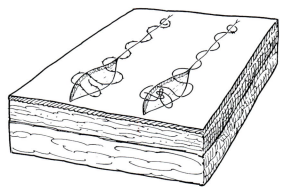

Figure 4.44. Insertion technique of the barbed suture (left) and normal subcutaneous suture pattern. Modified from Murtha, et al.[8] (J.B. Lippincott Co.)

The barbed sutures are not yet commercially available. The prototype sutures present an interesting future option for wound closure. A potential use could certainly be envisioned for laparoscopic or endoscopic procedures and for areas of limited access where suturing and knot tying are problematic.

Suture Anchors

Suture anchors come in a variety of configurations according to their intended purpose. They are mostly used to attach or reattach soft tissues to bone, primarily ligaments, joint capsules, or tendons.[10] A number of applications have been developed including solid organ parenchymal closure,[11] visceral closure and repair of rotator cuff injuries,[12] meniscal tears,[13] and lumbar and ventral hernias.[14,15] Currently, the most common clinical use of suture anchors is to repair rotator cuff injuries in humans.

There is variation in the characteristics of available commercial anchors: screw versus non-screw anchors, pull-out strength, size and shape, method of insertion, bioabsorbability, and radio-opacity of suture anchors.[16–18] Typically, they have a metal end and an "eye" for suture attachment. The metal end may be configured as either a screw or toggle bar for attachment to a particular surface.

In a comparison of pull-out strength to failure of six different metal anchors used in veterinary medicine, screw-type, self-tapping, transcortical tissue anchors (4.7 mm and 4 mm screw-type anchor, 6 mm length, IMEX, Inc., Longview, TX) were superior to Bone Biter (Bone Biter™ #5 suture anchor, Androcles Inc., distributed by Innovative Animal Products, Rochester, MD) and TwinFix (TwinFix™ Ti 5.0 Preloaded Suture Anchor System, Smith & Nephew, Andover, MD) metal anchors. They compared favorably with cortical and cancellous bone screws (3.5 mm cortex screw and 4 mm cancellous screw, each 10 mm length, Synthes, Paoli, PA)[18] (Figure 4.45).

There have been few reports on the use of suture anchors in veterinary medicine. In small animals, their primary use has been in ligament reconstruction.[19–20] In the horse, suture anchors have been reported to facilitate the successful repair of collateral ligament instability of the carpus and the metacarpophalangeal joint of two foals.[21] In this report, Mitek suture anchors (DePuy Mitek, Inc., Johnson and Johnson Co., Raynham, MA) (Figure 4.46) were used to repair a medial collateral ligament in the carpus of a 4-week-old thoroughbred

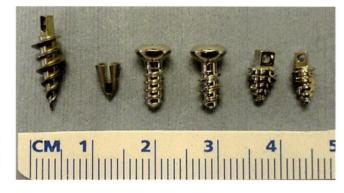

Figure 4.45. Metal anchors tested were (left to right) TwinFix (Smith & Nephew, Andover, MD); BoneBiter (Androcles Inc., Warsaw, IN); Cortical Screw; Cancellous screw; IMEX 4.7; and IMEX 4.0. Reprinted with permission from Robb, et al.[18]

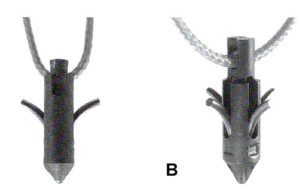

Figure 4.46. (A) Mitek GII suture anchor, (B) Mitek SuperAnchor (DePuy Mitek, Inc., Johnson and Johnson Co., Raynham, MA). Reprinted with permission from Rodgerson, et al.[21]

A   **B**

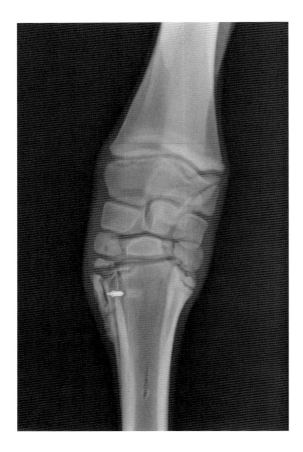

Figure 4.47. Mitek Suture anchor in position to repair a ruptured medial collateral ligament in a 4-week-old thoroughbred filly. Courtesy of Dr. D. Rodgerson.

filly (Figure 4.47) and the fetlock of a 2-week-old miniature horse filly. Larger or multiple suture anchors would be required for most collateral ligament applications in adult horses.

Greater use of suture or tissue anchors will no doubt result from development of new laparoscopic and endoscopic techniques and additional soft tissue applications in adult horses following appropriate biomechanical studies.

Tissue Adhesives

Cyanoacrylates

Cyanoacrylate (CA) adhesives were developed in 1949 and have been used in humans and animals for more than 35 years.[22,23] Initially, the inadequate adhesive properties, low tensile strength, brittleness following curing, and associated tissue inflammation, limited the use of CA adhesives in medical applications. The development of medium chain CAs, primarily butyl-cyanoacrylate and more recently the longer chain octyl-2-cyanoacrylate (2-OCA), have reduced the problems associated with CA use and significantly improved their advantages.

Reported surgeon benefits of the newer forms of CA tissue adhesives include shorter wound closure times, reduced risk of needle stick, and possibly a better cosmetic outcome.[23] Reported patient benefits include improved cosmetic appearance and overall comfort, less concern about getting the suture line wet, easier dressing changes, reduced tension on the wound, fewer hygiene problems, and fewer allergic reactions.[23]

The CAs are reported to be bacteriostatic against Gram-positive organisms[24] and have been used in a variety of medical circumstances. The uses of CAs in wound healing include controlling bleeding and providing an airtight seal following pulmonary biopsy,[25] wound closure,[26,27] dural closure,[28] peripheral nerve repair,[29] cleft palate repair,[30] as a tissue adhesive for solid and hollow organs,[31] repair of corneal perforations and melts,[24,32] and as a drug delivery system.[33]

The reported uses of CAs in the horse include CA spray bandages,[34] as an anchor for IV or nasolacrimal catheters, as a capillary hemostatic,[35] and to seal the nerve ends following neurectomy in an effort to decrease neuroma formation.[36] CAs have also been used in combination with other materials to facilitate closure of wounds and incisions.[37] Examples of combination procedures in the horse include stabilizing grafts to repair acute and chronic hoof injuries,[38,39] attaching split-thickness grafts to graft sites,[40] attaching bovine collagen preparations to granulating wounds,[41] and holding amnion dressings in place (e.g., unbandaged hock wounds).[42]

Incisions or lacerations that may benefit from closure with these adhesives are those that would normally require sutures of size 5–0 or smaller.[26] Therefore, the use of CA adhesives in equine patients is limited at this time, although investigators are finding uses in the horse either alone or in combination with other closure methods. It is anticipated that these combination applications will afford the best future use for these adhesives in the horse.

Fibrin Glue/Sealants

Fibrin sealants are composed primarily of fibrinogen, thrombin, and calcium chloride and are used in a wide range of surgeries, primarily as hemostatic agents but also to assist tissue sealing and wound healing.[43] The final composition of the sealants varies considerably depending on their anticipated use. Higher fibrinogen concentrations boost the clot strength, whereas higher thrombin concentrations enhance the speed of clotting. The addition of factor XIII may increase the tensile strength and stability of the clot, thus improving hemostatic properties. Antifibrinolytic agents such as aprotinin and aminocaproic acid increase the lifespan of the clot. The viscosity of the sealant also varies, depending on the fibrinogen content—the higher the fibrinogen concentration, the more viscous the sealant.

Investigators have evaluated many potential uses for fibrin sealants, including tissue flap repair,[44] closure of sinus membrane perforations,[45] control of air leakage from alveolar sacs,[46] and sealing of gastrointestinal and venous anastomoses.[47,48] Fibrin sealants have also been used in combination with mesh materials for dural repair[49] and corneal ulcer therapy.[50]

Much of the research concerning fibrin sealants has been performed in rodents, dogs, and pigs. Specific evaluations include hemorrhage control,[51] renal vessel anastomosis,[52] skin wound closure,[52,53] closure of pericardium,[54] and sealing of exposed edges of the liver.[55] Hence, there is a good body of knowledge about specific uses of fibrin glues and how they will react in the rodent, dog, and pig. In a study comparing four different ureterotomy closure methods in pigs—fibrin glue, laser welding, Endo-Stitch suture placement (4–0 polyglactin), and free needle suture placement (4–0 polyglactin)—fibrin glue produced better contrast radiographic assessments of closure, flow characteristics, and histology, suggesting that it currently holds the most promise as an alternative or adjunct to laparoscopic suturing.[56]

There have been few reports in the equine veterinary literature concerning the use of fibrin glues.[57,58] One study comparing fibrin glue and sutures to attach split-thickness grafts showed no significant difference in graft survival between glue and sutures.[58]

The future use of fibrin glues in equine procedures is probably limited to those previously described plus ophthalmic, laparoscopic, and endoscopic procedures in which traditional suturing is difficult and a cosmetic outcome is desired. We can also expect that fibrin glues, like cyanoacrylates, will be useful in combination with other materials to provide secure closure. As the use of commercial sealants becomes more prevalent, it is anticipated that the products will improve and subsequently yield consistently better results.

Skin Expanders

Skin is capable of considerable expansion if given enough time and stimulation. Enlarging tumors, hematomas, cellulitis, and advancing pregnancy may all stimulate skin to expand. Therapeutic skin expansion involves the progressive distension of a balloon placed subcutaneously to produce "excess" skin to cover an adjacent skin defect. Indications for the use of skin expansion include repair of defects surrounded by negligible redundant skin, creation of flaps not otherwise possible (such as for the repair of large eyelid defects), and where hair color and texture similar to the surrounding skin is preferred.

Balloon expansion techniques were originally described following partial amputation of a human ear in an effort to expand the skin sufficiently to cover a cartilaginous graft.[59] They have since been used in a variety of situations to treat chronic wounds or large tissue defects, in preparation for breast reconstruction, and to achieve primary closure in the repair of severe clubfoot deformities in children.[60]

The use of skin expanders in horses was first reported in 1989.[61] Compared to that of other species, equine skin on the head and distal limbs is tightly stretched, is strongly adhered to the underlying tissue, and is frequently the limiting factor in the treatment of many distal limb and head wounds. Tissue expanders are placed subcutaneously adjacent to the defect, usually with the patient under general anesthesia, such that excess skin produced by the balloon expansion can be moved to cover the defect (Mentor Tissue Expanders, Mentor Corporation, Santa Barbara, CA) (Figures 4.48, 4.49, 4.50).

The dermis initially thins in response to expansion, but expansion stimulates the epidermis to increase mitotic activity resulting in a net increase in epidermal tissue while a thick, fibrous capsule develops around the tissue expander.[62] A major advantage of using tissue expanders is that the "new" skin is similar in texture,

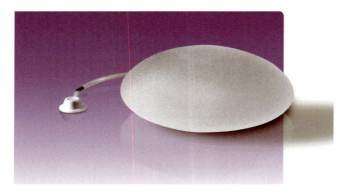

Figure 4.48. Oval tissue expander. Reprinted with permission from Mentor Corporation, Santa Barbara, CA.

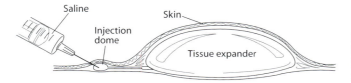

Figure 4.49. Schematic representation of the tissue expander illustrating saline injections into the injection dome to fill the tissue expander. Redrawn with permission from Mentor Corporation Website (Mentor Corporation, Santa Barbara, CA).

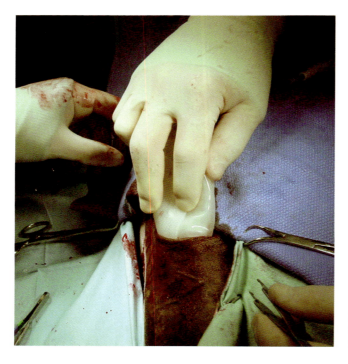

Figure 4.50. Inserting the tissue expander into the subcutaneous space overlying the cranial maxillary sinus in a horse. Courtesy of Dr. J. Kramer.

thickness, and hair color, although the hair may appear sparse because additional follicles are not formed. Furthermore, in contrast to free skin grafts, the blood supply is not disrupted.

At least 10 days are allowed for healing of the implantation site prior to filling the expander. Saline is injected every 4 to 7 days thereafter. In humans, the rate of filling is based on pain upon injection, skin color, and capillary refill time, although these parameters may not be fully adequate. Horses do not predictably demonstrate discomfort upon injection, and skin color and capillary refill time are difficult to assess. Therefore, in the horse, saline is injected until a significant increase in back-pressure within the syringe is noted and the skin over the expander is tight. Once sufficient skin expansion has been achieved, the horse is re-anesthetized, the expander is removed, and the newly-generated skin flap is surgically advanced or rotated over the defect. The skin flaps should be made to maximize the pedicle size and vascular supply, which requires some pre-operative planning.

Complications of the procedure include implant failure such as leakage from the injection portal and subcutaneous rupture of the expander, dehiscence of the suture line, pain upon expansion, seroma formation, widening of scars, infection, exposure of the expanders, and ischemia of the overlying skin caused by overfilling of the expander.

There will likely always be a need for tissue expanders in the horse due to the lack of redundant skin in the distal limb and head regions. Potential future developments include site-specific equine tissue expanders based on the cutaneous blood supply and the required shape of the flap.

Tissue Fusion

Tissue fusion was first described following the use of high-frequency electrocoagulation to create end-to-side portocaval shunts in dogs in 1962.[63] Laser tissue welding was subsequently reported in 1979 for the repair of small incisions in rat blood vessels.[64] The next year a successful microvascular anastomosis using the Nd:YAG laser was reported.[65] Laser tissue bonding relies on localized heating of the skin above the temperature required for collagen denaturation and is believed to result from the intertwining of collagen molecules from the tissue edges as the skin then cools. Initially, application of laser welding was limited because of the large zone of thermal damage produced, relatively low bond strength, and inconsistent results.

Laser tissue welding has the potential for application in situations in which suturing and stapling is difficult, such as microscopic, laparoscopic, and endoscopic procedures. It has been successful in apposing skin and anastomosing nerves, biliary tissue, bowel, and ureters.[56,66]

The ultimate goal of laser tissue welding is to achieve tissue closure that is durable, scarless, and resistant to infection.[66] Many variables governing tissue welding have been investigated. Laser parameters include wavelength, power output, exposure time, focal length, and the use of tissue solder and chromophores that affect the laser-to-tissue interactions. The depth of laser penetration generally increases with decreasing wavelength.[66] For example, an argon laser (wavelength of 488 nm) will have greater penetration than a CO_2 laser (wavelength of 10,600 nm). Additionally, differences between tested tissues, including composition (especially water content), thickness, and pigmentation, also affect the efficiency of energy transmission.[67]

Refinements of the initial procedure are directed at limiting the volume of heated tissue, monitoring and controlling the temperature rise of the surrounding tissue, and producing a higher initial bond strength. Laser tissue welding with naturally-occurring protein solders has been reported to represent an improvement over conventional suture closure because it offers an immediate watertight tissue closure, decreases operative time (especially in microsurgical or laparoscopic applications), reduces trauma, and eliminates foreign body reactions to sutures and clips.[67]

The relative strength and effectiveness of the protein solders depend on their source, concentration, and solubility. The most popular solder material is albumin. The solder is first applied to the tissue to be approximated, and then a laser irradiates the protein solder which bonds the tissue.[68] Albumin used in this way has been shown by electron microscopy to intertwine with the tissue collagen matrix and subsequently fuse with the collagen to effect bonding.[69] Laser-activated protein solders are absorbed within a few days and therefore are unlikely to trigger significant scar formation.

Sources of albumin evaluated include bovine, human, canine, and porcine.[70] Bovine serum albumin (BSA) is either fatty acid–containing or fatty acid–free.[70] The former has been reported to increase the quality of tissue fusion. Bovine serum albumin has been further evaluated in three forms: solid, semi-solid, and liquid, and at least initially, the semi-solid BSA was stronger with better handling characteristics.[71]

Moreover, increasing the BSA concentration from 25% to as high as 68% greatly increased the tensile strength of repair.[69]

While the addition of serum albumin solder has significantly improved laser tissue welding, the use of xenogenic or allogenic serum albumin is reported to carry associated risks of allergic reactions and transmission of disease.[72] Previous methods of serum albumin preparation were time-consuming, which could preclude the use of autogenous serum albumin when needed. A process has recently been developed to produce concentrated autologous plasma protein from unfractionated plasma;[72] initial evaluation has indicated its appropriateness as a biochemically-neutral solder for laser welding. The use of an autologous solder is expected to improve the long-term effects on healing and obviate immunological responses that characterize foreign protein solders.

Tissue solubility is a further variable that appears to affect the quality of fusion. Highly soluble proteins may be diluted in physiological fluids prior to laser tissue welding, which weakens the tensile strength of the repair.[73] Reducing the solubility of the proteins does not seem to affect tissue welding properties. Another potential advantage of the insoluble solder is that it may serve as a delivery system (antibiotics, growth factors, etc.) to aid in healing.

Additional technological advancements include chromophore enhancement and temperature control, which have improved the welding process by augmenting precision, reproducibility, and thus overall tensile strength of the repair.[69–73] A chromophore is any substance that can absorb electromagnetic radiation, such as hemoglobin, melanin, India ink, indocyanine green, fluorescein, carbon black, and gold nanoshells. The chromophores absorb particular wavelengths of the laser light in such a way as to tightly confine energy deposition to the edges of the incision, resulting in a narrower zone of thermal damage. Selection of the appropriate chromophore depends upon the laser unit being used. Lasers with wavelengths within the near infrared (NIR) window (~650–900 nm), where tissue components have minimal absorption, are preferred. Wavelengths of various laser units are: argon = 488 nm, potassium-titanyl-phosphate = 532 nm, continuous-wave diode = 805 nm, Nd:YAG = 1064 nm, and CO_2 = 10,600 nm. Indocyanine green dye is a frequently used chromophore because its absorption peak in aqueous albumin solution is 805 nm, an ideal match in the NIR spectrum with the relatively available and inexpensive diode laser. Cryogens can also be used to minimize peripheral thermal damage. Cryogen cooling applied at the time of laser welding was reported to reduce lateral thermal damage near the tissue surface, increase initial weld strengths, and shorten operative time.[74]

A potential improvement in tissue bonding is reported with a light-based closure method called photochemical tissue bonding (PTB), which does not rely on heating the tissue. PTB involves application of a dye to the walls of the wound followed by laser irradiation. Immediate bonding results from absorption of light energy by the dye, which initiates chemical reactions between proteins on the apposing tissue surfaces to form covalent crosslinks. Two dyes, naphthalimide and Rose Bengal, have been shown to be equal to standard sutures for wound closure in rabbit and pig skin, in terms of cosmetic outcomes and safety.[75]

Tissue welding holds the most potential for laparoscopic and endoscopic procedures in which space constraints make traditional suture closure difficult. As solder protein development, chromophore enhancement, and temperature control variables and their interactions mature, one can expect improved tensile strength, minimal scarring, and quicker procedures. A major advantage of tissue fusion is the rapidity of execution, while disadvantages include the start-up costs and detailed preparation required. Because of the increasing presence of diode lasers in practice, the costs to implement tissue fusion are becoming less significant and the detailed preparation will be simplified as the products become commercially available.

Vacuum-assisted Closure

Vacuum-assisted closure (VAC), the technique of applying sub-atmospheric pressure to wounds, was first reported in 1993.[76] While originally intended for the treatment of chronic wounds, significant progress has made this technique applicable to a variety of wounds including infected surgical wounds, traumatic wounds, pressure ulcers, wounds with exposed bone ± orthopedic implants, diabetic foot ulcers, and venous stasis ulcers.[77]

With the aid of a small electric pump, open cell foam, and an impermeable sheet of adhesive plastic, suction is applied to the wound to remove exudate via fenestrated tubing positioned within the foam. The foam is placed over the wound, which is then covered with the adherent, occlusive dressing, thus effectively converting it into a controlled closed wound environment (Figures 4.51, 4.52, 4.53).

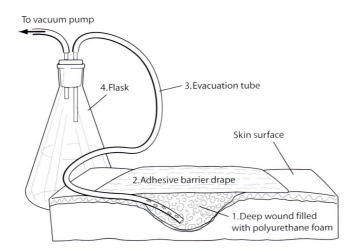

Figure 4.51. Basic components and configuration of the VAC system (1) polyurethane foam filling the wound cavity; (2) adhesive barrier drape sealing the wound; (3) evacuation tube; (4) flask for collecting fluid aspirated from the wound. Redrawn with permission from Gemeinhardt, et al.[83]

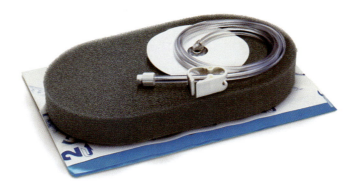

Figure 4.52. Commercial packaging of the disposable components of the VAC system. The evacuation tube has a large foot plate to facilitate free flow of debris from the wound. Reprinted with permission from Kinetic Concepts, Inc. (KCI), San Antonio, TX, http://www.kci1.com.

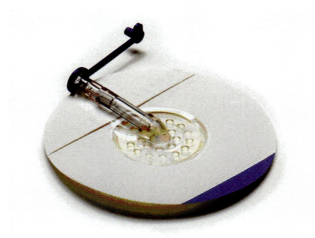

Figure 4.53. Close-up of fenestrated foot plate. Reprinted with permission from Kinetic Concepts, Inc. (KCI), San Antonio, TX, http://www.kci1.com.

The small electric pump applies continuous or intermittent suction to generate sub-atmospheric pressure within the wound, which increases blood flow, decreases interstitial edema, and removes harmful mediators from the wound bed, consequently bestowing the following benefits:

- Centripetal attraction of wound edges favoring increased local blood flow and tissue oxygenation by minimizing the pressure on small vessels
- Diminished wound-associated edema
- Decreased bacterial cell counts
- Removal of inflammatory mediators such as collagenases, stromelysins, and gelatinases that may inhibit wound healing
- Promotion of superior fibroplasia
- Enhancement of angiogenesis
- Lessened need for bandage changes

The VAC device can be applied over any type of tissue or material, including dermis, fat, fascia, tendon, muscle, blood vessels, bone, Gortex grafts, synthetic mesh, and orthopedic implants.[78] The only prerequisites are that the wound be free of necrotic debris and not be ischemic.

Since first described, several refinements have been made to the procedure. The current recommendation for use of VAC in human wounds is an optimum sub-atmospheric pressure of ~125 mm Hg utilizing an alternating pressure cycle of 5 minutes of suction followed by 2 minutes of rest. Cyclical rather than continuous application of sub-atmospheric pressure has been shown to optimize blood flow, increase granulation tissue production, increase the rate of cell division, decrease local tissue edema, and remove excessive fluid and other inhibitory factors from the wound bed.[79,80]

Sub-atmospheric pressure causes a 4-fold increase in blood flow, but the effect lasts only 5 to 7 minutes. Restoring normal pressure for 2 minutes and then resuming the negative pressure ensures that increased blood flow will recur. By alternating 5 minutes on and 2 minutes off, increased blood flow can be maintained indefinitely. This ability of tissue to respond to mechanical stress is attributed to an alteration of the cytoskeleton of wound cells, triggering the release of intracellular messengers which up-regulate cell proliferation.[81,82]

Use of VAC has recently been described in the horse for neck, body, and proximal limb wounds.[83] The methodology is similar to the procedure described above except that a depilatory cream is used to remove the hair around the wound to ensure adhesion of the plastic sheet. Minor technical problems to be resolved in the equine patient include the difficulty of maintaining an airtight seal over the wound, excessive coiling and kinking of the evacuation or extension tubing as the patient moves about the stall, and strategic placement of the vacuum pump out of harm's way yet easily accessible to the caregiver. The case report encourages the use of this technique in difficult equine wounds because of its potential to accelerate healing and simplify wound management once the system is in place.[83]

Equine veterinarians are frequently faced with acute or chronic large open wounds that cannot be easily closed by conventional methods. VAC offers the potential to facilitate the management of these challenging wounds. Distal limb wounds in horses have a relatively poor blood supply compared to upper body and head wounds. The use of VAC to increase blood supply via application of intermittent sub-atmospheric pressure may allow more effective management of wounds in this location.

Conclusion

We are at the cusp of great developments in the world of wound healing. The evolution has been slow, with gradual advancements for thousands of years. In the last 100 years there has been a relative explosion of potential wound closure developments. Many new and innovative methods of closure are currently being evaluated. Many will fail, while others will withstand the rigors of clinical trials and the marketplace and will be added to our armamentarium to provide better wound closure. We hope these new methods will be quick and easy to perform, affordable, more secure, and associated with reduced patient morbidity and scar formation. It will be exciting to follow these future developments.

References

1. MacKenzie D: The history of sutures. Medical History 1973;17:158
2. Black JJ: A stitch in time. 1. The history of sutures. Nursing Times 1982;78:613
3. Smailys AJ, Predikis YY, Vaichyuvenas VA, et al: Processing of surgical material with antibacterial and anticoagulant properties (German author's transl). Zentralbl Chir 1980;105:87
4. Rodeheaver GT, Kurtz LD, Bellamy WT, et al: Biocidal braided sutures. Arch Surg 1983;118:322
5. Rothenburger S, Spangler D, Bhende S, et al: In vitro antimicrobial evaluation of Coated Vicryl Plus Antibacterial Suture (coated polyglactin 910 with triclosan) using zone of inhibition assays. Surg Infect (Larchmt) 2002;3:S79
6. Barbolt TA: Chemistry and safety of triclosan, and its use as an antimicrobial coating on Coated VICRYL* Plus Antibacterial Suture (coated polyglactin 910 suture with triclosan). Surg Infect (Larchmt) 2002;3:S45
7. Brown G: Director, New Technologies Development, Ethicon, Inc., New Brunswick, NJ, personal communication
8. Murtha AP, Kaplan AL, Paglia MJ, et al: Evaluation of a novel technique for wound closure using a barbed suture. Plast Reconstr Surg 2006;117:1769
9. Weld KJ, Ames CD, Hruby G, et al: Evaluation of a novel knotless self-anchoring suture material for urinary tract reconstruction. Urol 2006;67:1133
10. Singer MJ, Pijanowski G, Wiley R, et al: Biomechanical evaluation of a veterinary suture anchor in the canine cadaver pelvis and femur. Vet Comp Orthop Traum 2005;18:31
11. Ames CD, Perrone JM, Frisella AJ, et al: Comparison of holding strength of suture anchors for hepatic and renal parenchyma. J Endourol 2005;19:1221
12. Mazzocca AD, Millett PJ, Guanche CA, et al: Arthroscopic single-row versus double-row suture anchor rotator cuff repair. Am J Sports Med 2005;33:1861
13. Zantop T, Eggers AK, Musahl V, et al: Cyclic testing of flexible all-inside meniscus suture anchors: biomechanical analysis. Am J Sports Med 2005;33:388
14. Carbonell AM, Kercher KW, Sigmon L, et al: A novel technique of lumbar hernia repair using bone anchor fixation. Hernia 2005;9:22
15. Kumar SS: Mesh fixation in laparoscopic repair of ventral hernia: a new method. Surg Innov 2005;12:151
16. Barber FA, Herbert MA, Click JN: Internal fixation strength of suture anchors—update 1997. Arthroscopy 1997;13:355
17. Lee S, Mahar A, Bynum K, et al: Biomechanical comparison of bioabsorbable sutureless screw anchor versus suture anchor fixation for rotator cuff repair. Arthroscopy 2005;21:43
18. Robb JL, Cook JL, Carson W: In vitro evaluation of screws and suture anchors in metaphyseal bone of the canine tibia. Vet Surg 2005;34:499
19. Robinson A: Clinical application of prong-type tissue anchors in small animal surgery. J Sm Anim Pract 2000;41:207
20. Baltzer WI, Schulz KS, Stover SM, et al: Biomechanical analysis of suture anchors and suture materials used for toggle pin stabilization of hip joint luxation in dogs. Am J Vet Res 2001;62:721
21. Rodgerson DH, Spirito MA: Repair of collateral ligament instability in 2 foals by using suture anchors. Can Vet J 2001;42:557
22. Cooper HN, Joyner FB, Sheere NH: Chemistry and performance of cyanoacrylate adhesive. J Soc Plast Surg Engl 1959;1:5
23. Coulthard P, Worthington H, Esposito M, et al. Tissue adhesives for closure of surgical incisions. Cochrane Database of Systematic Reviews 2002, Issue 3. Art. No.: CD004287. DOI: 10.1002/14651858.CD004287.pub2.; http://www.mrw.interscience.wiley.com/cochrane/clsysrev/articles/CD004287/frame.html, April 8, 2007
24. Vote BJ, Elder MJ: Cyanoacrylate glue for corneal perforations: a description of a surgical technique and a review of the literature. Clin Exp Ophth 2000;28:437
25. Esposito C, Damiano R, Settimi A, et al: Experience with the use of tissue adhesives in pediatric endoscopic surgery. Surg Endoscopy 2004;18:290
26. Bruns TB, Worthington JM: Using tissue adhesive for wound repair: a practical guide to Dermabond. Am Family Physician 2000;61:1383
27. Handschel JG, Depprich RA, Dirksen D, et al: A prospective comparison of octyl-2-cyanoacrylate and suture in standardized facial wounds. Int J Oral Maxillofacial Surg 2006;35:318
28. Ozisik PA, Inci S, Soylemezoglu F, et al: Comparative dural closure techniques: a safety study in rats. Surg Neurol 2006;65:42
29. Pineros-Fernandez A, Rodeheaver PF, Rodeheaver GT: Octyl 2-cyanoacrylate for repair of peripheral nerve. Ann Plast Surg 2005;55:188
30. Turkaslan T, Ozcan H, Dayicioglu D, et al: Use of adhesives in cleft palate surgery: a new flap fixation technique. J Craniofacial Surg 2005;16:719
31. Fotiadis C, Leventis I, Adamis S, et al: The use of isobutylcyanoacrylate as a tissue adhesive in abdominal surgery. Acta Chirurgica Belgica 2005;105:392

32. Setlik DE, Seldomridge DL, Adelman RA, et al: The effectiveness of isobutyl cyanoacrylate tissue adhesive for the treatment of corneal perforations. Am J Ophthalmol 2005;140:920

33. Vauthier C, Dubernet C, Fattal E, et al: Poly(alkylcyanoacrylates) as biodegradable materials for biomedical applications. Adv Drug Delivery Rev 2003;55:519

34. Blackford J, Shires M, Goble D, et al: The use of N-butyl cyanoacrylate in the treatment of open leg wounds in the horse. Proc Am Assoc Equine Pract 1986;32:349

35. Pallaoro GA, Long SA, Pallaoro DL, et al: Putting tissue adhesives to work in equine practice. Vet Med 1986;81:823

36. Turner AS, Trotter GW, Powers BE: Evaluation of tissue adhesive to contain axonal regeneration in horses. Vet Surg 1995;24:308

37. Chigira M, Akimoto M: Use of a skin adhesive (octyl-2-cyanoacrylate) and the optimum reinforcing combination for suturing wounds. Scand J Plast Reconstr Surg Hand Surg 2005;39:334

38. Sigafoos R: Polymeric Composite repair for acute and chronic refractory hoof injuries in horses. Proc Am Assoc Equine Pract 1995;41:253

39. Pardoe CH, Wilson AM: In vitro mechanical properties of different equine hoof wall crack fixation techniques. Equine Vet J 1999;31:506

40. Schumacher J: Practical, split-thickness skin grafting of the horse. Am Coll Vet Surg Proceedings 2004, p.137

41. Bello TR: Practical treatment of body and open leg wounds of horses with bovine collagen, biosynthetic wound dressing and cyanoacrylate. J Equine Vet Sci 2002;22:157

42. Stashak TS: Personal communication

43. Albala DM, Lawson JH: Recent clinical and investigational applications of fibrin sealant in selected surgical specialties. J Am Coll Surg 2006;202:685

44. Atalay C, Kockaya EA, Cetin B, et al: The role of fibrin tissue adhesives in flap necrosis in rats. J Invest Surg 2005;18:97

45. Choi BH, Zhu SJ, Jung JH, et al: The use of autologous fibrin glue for closing sinus membrane perforations during sinus lifts. Oral Surg Oral Med Oral Path Oral Rad Endodontics 2006;101:150

46. Kawamura M, Gika M, Izumi Y, et al: The sealing effect of fibrin glue against alveolar air leakage evaluated up to 48 h: comparison between different methods of application. Eur J Cardio-Thoracic Surg 2005;28:39

47. Li Y, Bao Y, Jiang T, et al: Effect of the combination of fibrin glue and growth hormone on incomplete intestinal anastomoses in a rat model of intra-abdominal sepsis. J Surg Res 2006;131:111

48. Uysal AC, Uraloglu M, Orbay H, et al: An alternative method of vein anastomosis with fibrin glue. Ann Plast Surg 2005;54:579

49. Hida K, Yamaguchi S, Seki T, et al: Nonsuture dural repair using polyglycolic acid mesh and fibrin glue: clinical application to spinal surgery. Surg Neurol 2006;65:136

50. Hick S, Demers PE, Brunette I, et al: Amniotic membrane transplantation and fibrin glue in the management of corneal ulcers and perforations: a review of 33 cases. Cornea 2005;24:369

51. Curtin WA, Wang GJ, Goodman NC, et al: Reduction of hemorrhage after knee arthroplasty using cryo-based fibrin sealant. J Arthroplasty 1999;14:481

52. Park W, Kim WH, Lee CH, et al: Comparison of two fibrin glues in anastomoses and skin closure. J Vet Med—Series A 2002;49:385

53. Scardino MS, Swaim SF, Morse BS, et al: Evaluation of fibrin sealants in cutaneous wound closure. J Biomed Mat Res 1999;48:315

54. Moro H, Hayashi J, Ohzeki H, et al: The effect of fibrin glue on inhibition of pericardial adhesions. Jpn J Thorac Cardiovasc Surg 1999;47:79

55. Scotte M, Dujardin F, Amelot A, et al: Experimental measure of the tensile strength of biological sealant–collagen association after hepatectomy in dogs. Eur Surg Res 1996;28:436

56. Wolf SJ Jr, Soble JJ, Nakada SY, et al: Comparison of fibrin glue, laser weld, and mechanical suturing device for the laparoscopic closure of ureterotomy in a porcine model. J Urol 1997;157:1487

57. Vachon AM, McIlwraith CW, Trotter GW, et al: Morphologic study of repair of induced osteochondral defects of the distal portion of the radial carpal bone in horses by use of glued periosteal autografts [corrected—published erratum appears in Am J Vet Res 1991;52:636]. Am J Vet Res 1991;52:317

58. Schumacher J, Ford TS, Brumbaugh GW, et al: Viability of split-thickness skin grafts attached with fibrin glue. Can J Vet Res 1996;60:158

59. Neumann CG: The expansion of an area of skin by progressive distention of a subcutaneous balloon. Plast Reconstr Surg 1957;19:124

60. Rosselli P, Reyes R, Medina A, et al: Use of a soft tissue expander before surgical treatment of clubfoot in children and adolescents. J Ped Orthop 2005;25:353

61. Madison JB, Donawick WJ, Johnston DE, et al: The use of skin expansion to repair cosmetic defects in animals. Vet Surg 1989;18:15

62. Austad Ed, Thomas SB, Pasyk K: Tissue expansion: dividend or loan? Plast Reconstr Surg 1986;78:63

63. Sigel B, Acevedo FJ: Vein anastomosis by electrocoaptive union. Surg Forum 1962;13:291

64. Jain KK, Gorisch W: Repair of small blood vessels with the neodymium-YAG laser: a preliminary report. Surg 1979;85:684

65. Jain KK: Sutureless microvascular anastomosis using a neodymium-YAG laser. J Microsurg 1980;1:436

66. Talmor M, Bleustein CB, Poppas DP: Laser tissue welding: A biotechnological advance for the future. Arch Facial Plast Surg 2001;3:207

67. Bass LS, Treat MR: Laser tissue welding: a comprehensive review of current and future clinical applications. Lasers Surg Med 1995;17:315

68. Lauto A, Poppas DP, Murrell GAC: Solubility study of albumin solders for laser tissue-welding. Lasers Surg Med 1998;23:258

69. McNally KM, Sorg BS, Welch AJ, et al: Photothermal effects of laser tissue soldering. Phys Med Biol 1999;44:983

70. Bleustein CB, Felsen D, Poppas DP: Welding characteristics of different albumin species with and without fatty acids. Lasers Surg Med 2000;27:82

71. Bleustein CB, Walker CN, Felsen D, et al: Semi-solid albumin solder improved mechanical properties for laser tissue welding. Lasers Surg Med 2000;27:140

72. Stewart RB, Bleustein CB, Petratos PB, et al: Concentrated autologous plasma protein: a biochemically neutral solder for tissue welding. Lasers Surg Med 2001;29:336

73. Lauto A, Poppas DP, Murrell GAC: Solubility study of albumin solders for laser tissue-welding. Lasers Surg Med 1998;23:258

74. Fried NM, Walsh JT Jr: Cryogen spray cooling during laser tissue welding. Phys Med Biol 2000;45:753

75. Kamegaya Y, Farinelli WA, Vila Echague AV, et al: Evaluation of photochemical tissue bonding for closure of skin incisions and excisions. Lasers Surg Med 2005;37:264

76. Fleischmann W, Strecker W, Bombelli M, et al: Vacuum sealing as a treatment of soft tissue damage in open fractures. Unfallchirurg 1993;96:488

77. Venturi ML, Attinger CE, Mesbahi AN, et al: Mechanisms and clinical applications of the vacuum-assisted closure (VAC device). Am J Clin Dermatol 2005;6:185

78. DeFranzo AJ, Argenta LC, Marks MW, et al: The use of vacuum-assisted closure therapy for the treatment of lower-extremity wounds with exposed bone. Plast Reconstr Surg 2001;108:1184

79. Morykwas MJ, Argenta LC, Shelton-Brown EI, et al: Vacuum-assisted closure: a new method for wound control and treatment: animal studies and basic foundation. Ann Plast Surg 1997;38:553

80. Saxena V, Hwang CW, Huang S, et al: Vacuum-assisted closure: microdeformations of wounds and cell proliferation. Plast Reconstr Surg 2004;114:1086

81. Urschel JD, Scott PG, Williams HTG: The effect of mechanical stress on soft and hard tissue repair: a review. Br J Plast Surg 1988;41:182

82. Olenius M, Dalsgaard C, Wickman M: Mitotic activity in the expanded human skin. Plast Reconstr Surg 1993;91:213

83. Gemeinhardt KD, Molnar JA: Vacuum-assisted closure for management of a traumatic neck wound in a horse. Equine Vet Ed 2005;17:27

5 Principles and Techniques for Reconstructive Surgery

Ted S. Stashak, DVM, MS, Diplomate ACVS

Introduction

When a full-thickness skin wound, caused either by trauma or excision of a skin lesion, cannot be closed by suturing alone, mobilization of adjacent skin should be considered, particularly if the objective is to achieve the best functional and cosmetic end result.[1–8] A combination of the extent of skin loss and the amount of loose skin surrounding a wound often dictates whether or not the surgeon will be able to successfully close a wound.[9]

This said, some reconstructive surgical techniques (e.g., presuturing, adjustable suture, and tension suturing techniques) allow tension-free closure of many wounds heretofore deemed impossible to close. Skin expansion techniques (e.g., intraoperative tissue expansion and implanted elastomers) allow the surgeon to stretch the skin adjacent to a lesion to be excised, thus reducing the suture tension required for closure. Additional tension relief may be obtained by simply undermining the skin surrounding the wound, making a longitudinal relaxing incision, using a skin mesh expansion technique, or using a V-Y or Z plasty. A combination of tissue debulking (excision of granulation tissue or scar tissue), skin mobilization, and tension relief may be compulsory for cosmetic reconstruction of large, open granulating wounds and reconstruction following excision of large skin lesions (e.g., scar or tumor).

The shape of the wound is also an important consideration. While fusiform-shaped wounds often require only local undermining of the surrounding skin to provide enough tension relief for closure, large rectangular, square, triangular, and circular wounds more typically entail a combination of strategically placed incisions with local undermining to create a skin flap capable of covering the wound. In some cases a transposition flap may be needed to cover circular wounds in tight-skinned regions.

Skin flaps differ from skin grafts in that they retain attachment to their blood supply through a pedicle of skin and subcutaneous tissue. Randomly based flaps derive their blood supply from many small, direct arteries (described later under Cutaneous Blood Supply), whereas axial pattern flaps rely on a single neurovascular trunk for supply to the tissue. Randomly based pedicle flaps are used most commonly in equine surgery.[10] Because a significant relationship between flap width and viable length has been demonstrated in an experiment in ponies, it is recommended to design the pedicle so its base is as broad as possible.[11] Axial pattern flaps, when compared to random pattern flaps, were shown to have superior skin perfusion and a greater ability to maintain a larger percentage of baseline perfusion when submitted to tension.[12] Relatively few axial pattern flaps have been identified in horses compared with dogs, cats, and humans. A type of axial pattern flap referred to as the Estlander flap was used to repair a large chronic lip laceration in a foal.[13] Skin flaps are also classified according to their design (see Table 5.1). Free transfer skin flaps will be discussed later under that heading.

Reconstructive techniques can be used in conjunction with primary closure (the exception is skin expansion using a silicone elastomer) and delayed closure and for closure following tumor excision or scar tissue revision. The advantages of these techniques over open wound management are an overall reduction in healing time, an increased percentage of the wound surface being covered by full-thickness skin, and a more cosmetic outcome with an earlier return to function. When indicated, mobilization of adjacent tissue to cover a skin defect is

Table 5.1. Classification of local skin flaps according to their design.

Flap design	Definition	Best use
Rotation flap		
Unilateral	A semicircular or three-fourths circular flap of skin and subcutaneous tissue that rotates about a pivot point into a defect to be closed.	Triangular defects that have skin available on one side. Limited use in the horse, in the author's experience.
Bilateral	Rotation flaps designed on two sides.	Triangular defects that have skin available on two sides. Limited use in the horse, in the author's experience.
Pedicle advancement flap	Flap of skin that is mobilized by undermining and advancing it into a defect without altering the plane of the pedicle.	Rectangular or square defect.
Single (French flap)	Skin that is available for closure on one side of the defect (e.g., eyelid)	Half H-plasty (Figure 5.33).
Modified single	Skin that is available for closure on one side of the defect.	To cover irregular or unequal angular defects (Figures 5.36, 5.37). To cover triangular-shaped defects (Figures 5.38, 5.39, 5.40). More practical than rotation flaps, in the author's experience.
Two opposing	Skin that is available for closure on two sides of the defect.	H-plasty (Figure 5.32). Use primarily for large defects.
Transposition flap	Usually a rectangular piece of skin and subcutaneous tissue which is rotated on a pivot point to cover an adjacent defect.	To cover defects in tight-skinned regions such as the face. To be most effective, the flap is developed close to the defect so minimal rotation is required (Figure 5.41).

preferable to skin grafting of an open wound because it provides more reliable healing and better cosmetic and functional results.[8]

Before undertaking such reconstructive procedures it is important to discuss the owner's expectations, the potential complications, the expected outcome, and the costs associated with the procedure. This is particularly true when undertaking elective cosmetic procedures where failure to accomplish an esthetic outcome can lead to considerable client dissatisfaction. This said, a successful outcome can be very rewarding professionally and especially pleasing to the client. The aim of this chapter is to review cutaneous reconstructive surgical techniques and describe their clinical applications.

Cutaneous Blood Supply

An understanding of the cutaneous blood supply is crucial to successful reconstructive surgery. While detailed descriptions of the vascular supply to the skin of humans[14,15] and dogs[16,17] have been the basis for significant advancement of cutaneous reconstructive surgery, little information is available for the horse. This said, two types of cutaneous blood supply have been identified in mammals: perforating musculocutaneous vessels and direct cutaneous vessels. Perforating musculocutaneous arteries pass though the body of a muscle to supply the overlying skin. These arteries are larger and sparser in areas where the skin is loose, and smaller and more densely packed in regions where the skin is less mobile.[15] Microangiograms[11] and latex vascular injections[18] demonstrate that horses and ponies, similar to dogs and cats, do not have musculocutaneous arteries.

Direct cutaneous arteries pass through fascial septa between muscles and supply a larger area of skin than do perforating musculocutaneous vessels. They are found in loose-skinned regions, running parallel to the skin surface in close association with the panniculus muscle when present, while in the distal extremities they run beneath and parallel to the dermis in most animals. Smaller vessels branch off these direct cutaneous arteries and in the dog arborize in the dermis, forming three interconnected plexuses: the subcutaneous (deep) plexus, the cutaneous (middle or intermediate) plexus, and the superficial (sub-epidermal or sub-papillary) plexus which together supply the dermis and the adnexa directly and the epidermis by passive diffusion.[19] All three of these vascular plexuses are important to consider when manipulating and/or undermining skin.

Physical and Biomechanical Properties of Skin

Interaction between the skin's structural components, collagen, and elastic fibers, as well as ground substance, provides skin with its natural tension and its viscoelastic properties. Knowledge of these properties allows the surgeon to select the appropriate direction in which to excise a mass or reconstruct a wound that will create the least amount of suture tension upon closure, and the ability to stretch skin to overcome the forces of tension.

Lines of Skin Tension

The normal tension that exists in skin is a result of elastic fibers in the dermis. As such, when the skin is incised its edges retract. Lines of skin tension (Langer's lines) have been referred to as maximal skin tension. However, because skin is anisotropic (lacking similar properties in all directions) and these tension lines can be influenced by movement of an anatomic part, it is probably more accurate to refer to them as relaxed skin tension lines.[20] Incisions made parallel to these lines will gap to a lesser extent and heal with a finer scar than incisions made at right or oblique angles. Incisions made at oblique angles to the lines will take on a curvilinear shape. Incisions made perpendicular to these lines tend to gape widely, are subject to greater tension, and require more sutures to bring them into apposition, and consequently are inclined toward developing a wider scar. Thus, the ideal incision is made parallel to these lines of tension and wounds should be closed in a direction that will avert or minimize skin tension.[21] Tension lines have been well described in humans[22] and dogs[23] but have been investigated only to a limited extent in horses.

Extensibility

Inherent extensibility refers to the skin's normal stretching capacity while an anatomic part is at rest.[24,25] This property allows the surgeon to excise a small fusiform-shaped piece of skin and perform primary closure of the resultant wound. A skin biopsy punch wound model showed that lines of maximal skin extensibility of the equine carpus, upon flexion and extension, run in the same direction as Langer's lines, which is parallel to the limb's long axis.[26] Therefore, the best direction for an incision would be straight and parallel to lines of maximum extensibility.

Pinching the skin to elevate it over the proposed site of excision of a tumor or scar or over a site of proposed reconstruction of a wound can provide a rough estimate of the skin's inherent extensibility.[3,9,24] Maximal skin extensibility should be assessed with the anatomic part in its normal position, at rest, followed by movement of the part (e.g., flexion and extension of the joints of the limb) which can greatly influence extensibility.[4]

Creep

Mechanical creep is the biomechanical property of skin which allows it to stretch, within minutes, beyond the normal limits of extensibility when placed under a constant load.[24] In effect, as the load (stretching force) is applied, intertwined randomly oriented collagen fibers in the dermis straighten longitudinally and become aligned parallel to the stretching force, allowing stress relaxation (discussed later under this heading).[27]

Biological creep, on the other hand, is different from mechanical creep in that the skin does not stretch.[24] Biological creep occurs when a subcutaneous mass (e.g., tumor, chronic exuberant granulation tissue, etc.) enlarges slowly. The skin does not thin, as with mechanical creep, but gradually responds by increasing epidermal mitotic activity and in-growth of blood vessels and cells into the dermis in proportion to the growth of the mass; both of these processes allow more skin to develop.[24,28]

Stress Relaxation

Stress relaxation occurs when a piece of skin is placed under the influence of constant strain. Over time the amount of strain required to maintain elongation decreases and the skin becomes less taut as a result of mechanical creep. This biomechanical property of skin explains why the tension on a suture line decreases within hours after surgery.[9,24] The amount of tension required to successfully achieve stress relaxation in the clinical situation is unknown; however, it is readily acknowledged that excess tension on a suture line can compromise blood flow to the skin edges, resulting in ischemia and dehiscence. Therefore, clinical judgment is needed to make use of this important property of skin.

General Principles of Reconstructive Surgery

Developing a Surgical Plan

Mobilization of adjacent tissue to cover a full-thickness skin defect should be planned. Skin extensibility should be determined while the affected anatomic part is in a normal relaxed position (inherent extensibility) as well as during movement (maximal extensibility) by puckering the skin either over or adjacent to the wound or lesion to be removed (Figures 5.1a–c). In some cases elevating a lesion to be excised with the thumb and forefingers will suffice to evaluate extensibility. Evaluating skin extensibility in a systematic manner will delineate the regions of skin availability for tension relief and mobilization and for skin flap formation.

On limbs, the lines of skin tension and maximum skin extensibility are generally parallel to the long axis.[8,26] Therefore, wounds that are parallel to the limb's long axis are not subjected to the same amount of tension during flexion or extension as are wounds that are oblique or at a right angle to the limb's long axis.[5] Wounds located on the dorsal or palmar/plantar surface that are perpendicular or oblique to the limb's axis typically separate widely during limb flexion and extension (Figure 5.2). Post-operative immobilization of these wounds is usually required. Whenever possible, a lesion should be removed such that the longitudinal axis of excision parallels the long axis of the limb. Skin is then mobilized in a transverse plane (lateral to medial) rather than from proximal to distal, which would subject the wound to greater stress.

Wounds or lesions of the upper limb, trunk, and neck should be manipulated through their full range of motion prior to making a final decision regarding skin extensibility (Figure 5.3a). During surgery the part should be maintained in a position that creates the greatest tension so that the appropriate surgical approach can be selected to close the wound and reduce the risk of post-operative dehiscence (Figure 5.3b). The choice of excision pattern is dictated by available skin and defect configuration. A sterile ruler, sterile marking pen, or sterile

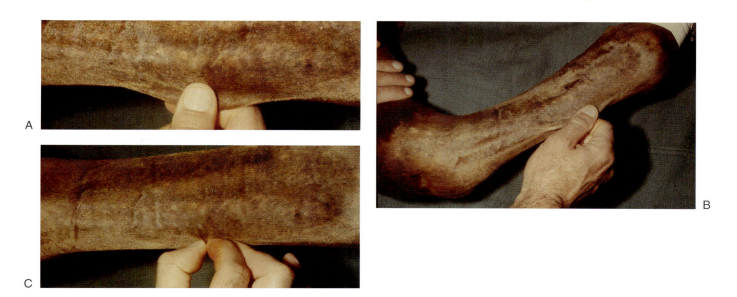

Figure 5.1. Forelimb skin tension lines and maximal extensibility are parallel to the limb's long axis. (A) Forelimb in its normal position at rest. Skin extensibility is evaluated by pinching the skin, parallel to the limb's long axis, over the dorsal mid-metacarpal region. (B) Carpus and fetlock flexed. Skin extensibility and tension remains the same. (C) Carpus and fetlock flexed. Skin extensibility is assessed perpendicular to the limb's long axis over the dorsal mid-metacarpal region. Skin tension has increased markedly and the extensibility has decreased.

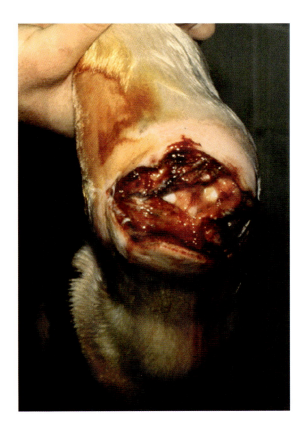

Figure 5.2. Transverse laceration involving the dorsal aspect of the fetlock joint. The wound gapes widely while the joint is flexed, whereas the wound edges were in contact when the fetlock was extended. Courtesy of Dr. G.W. Trotter.

243

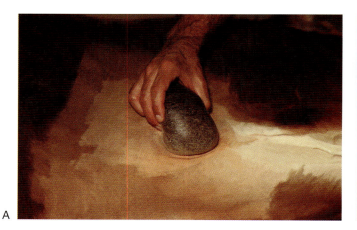
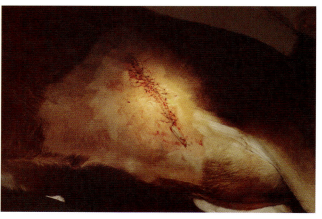

A   B

Figure 5.3. This large solitary melanoma on the right ventral lateral thoracic region in a cow is used to illustrate the value of movement of a part to determine the correct axis for excision and to predict the extent of excision required to remove this lesion. The melanoma was freely movable, somewhat pedunculated, and appeared to be attached by a stalk of skin approximately 10 cm in diameter while the cow was standing. (A) Under general anesthesia in left lateral recumbency, the right limb was extended forward as would occur during walking or when resting in sternal recumbency. The lesion became sessile when the limb was extended. (B) The extent of excision required to remove the melanoma was greater than would have been predicted while the animal was standing. The limb was maintained in extension during surgery to ensure that the appropriate surgical approach, skin mobilization, and suturing techniques to close the wound were selected.

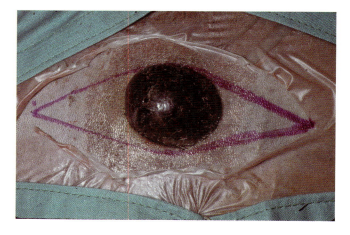

Figure 5.4. Solitary melanoma on the caudal thigh of a horse. A sterile marking pen was used to draw this fusiform pattern on the skin in preparation for excision.

methylene blue applied with a sterilized instrument can be used to draw this pattern on the skin (Figure 5.4). After incision, the skin is mobilized or flaps are created by separating tissues in their natural cleavage planes deep within the subcutaneous tissue.

Tension-reducing Suturing Techniques

Suturing techniques which allow tension free closure of a defect rely on two biomechanical properties of skin: mechanical creep and stress relaxation.

Presuturing

Presuturing is a technique whereby sutures are placed preoperatively to imbricate (elevate) skin over a proposed site of excision or to relieve tension on the wound margin.[24] It is performed by spanning the wound with heavy sutures, placed in an interrupted or mattress Lembert suture pattern, hours before a lesion is to be

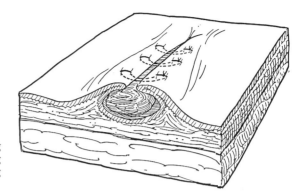

Figure 5.5. Illustration of the presuturing technique. Adapted from Liang MD, Briggs P, Heckler FR, et al: Presuturing—A new technique for closing large skin defects: Clinical and experimental studies. Plast Reconstr Surg 1988;81:694.

excised or a wound is debrided and sutured. It is most applicable to lesions or wounds of the body and proximal region of the limbs, but sometimes may be useful in closing wounds of the distal portion of the limb.

Using heavy, nonabsorbable suture, such as no. 1 or no. 2 polypropylene or nylon, suture bites are placed in the skin perpendicular and 2 cm to 6 cm to either side of the lesion or the wound edge. Tension applied to the sutures elevates and folds skin over the lesion or wound (Figure 5.5). The procedure is performed between 2 and 8 hours before surgery, using sedation and local or regional anesthesia. Placing sutures 24 hours or more in advance of surgery may cause tissue surrounding the wound to become edematous, complicating closure.[24,26–31]

Presuturing experimentally created wounds on pigs showed that closing a presutured wound required 40% less force than that required to close a non-presutured wound.[24] When compared with simply undermining the surrounding skin, presuturing resulted in some tissue gain and an initial decrease in closing tension.[30]

While the original description of this technique suggests that presuturing avoids the potential complications of undermining,[24] the combination of presuturing and undermining (discussed later) may provide additional advantages, because by reducing skin tension, less undermining of adjacent skin will be required to close a defect.[9]

Adjustable Suture Technique

Problems associated with delayed closure of a wound—particularly on the distal aspect of limbs in horses, such as retraction of the wound margins and ineffective wound contraction—can be obviated to a large degree by placing constant tension on the wound margin with an adjustable suture, a technique referred to as augmented wound contraction.[32] To perform this technique, the wound and surrounding tissue are desensitized using local infiltration or regional anesthesia, and a heavy suture is placed intradermally at the wound margin using a continuous horizontal mattress suture pattern. Each end of the suture exits the skin, and by applying tension to these suture ends the skin on one side of the wound is drawn toward that on the opposite side. Each end of the suture is threaded through a button, and after tension has been applied to the margin of the wound by tightening the suture, the ends are anchored to the button using a human umbilical clamp or split-shot (Figure 5.6).

The margins of the wound are pulled closer together by tightening the suture daily. The most rapid decrease in the size of the wound occurs during the first 3 days.[32] Subsequently, skin edges are apposed, if possible, or the wound is left to heal by second intention. The technique can be used not only to augment contraction but also to prevent expansion of an acute wound. A commercially available wound closure system (Canica®, Ogdensburg, NY) uses multiple anchors which are inserted in the skin on opposite sides of the wound. Tension on the wound's edges is created when elastomer bands are affixed to the anchors.

Tension Suturing Techniques

Tension suturing techniques are most often used in conjunction with other skin mobilization techniques (e.g., undermining, which is discussed later). Horizontal or vertical mattress sutures placed well away from the skin edges can be used to decrease tension at the wound margin. The skin edges are then approximated, without tension, usually with simple interrupted sutures or with vertical mattress sutures placed closer to the skin edge. Vertical mattress tension sutures are less apt to interfere with blood supply than are horizontal mattress tension

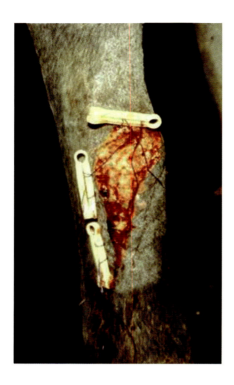

Figure 5.6. Technique of augmented wound contraction used to pull the margins of this wound on a metacarpus closer together. Umbilical clamps anchor the ends of mattress sutures that span the wound. Courtesy of Dr. J. Schumacher.

sutures. Sections of rubber tubing (supports) placed under the loops of the tension sutures will distribute pressure and may prevent interruption of blood flow underlying these sutures (Figure 4.30).

This approach, however, should be reserved for regions that cannot be supported by bandaging (e.g., upper limb, neck, and trunk). If used under a pressure bandage the section of rubber tubing can result in pressure necrosis in the skin underlying these supports. The mattress tension sutures are removed in 5 to 7 days, at which time tension on the approximating sutures should have greatly dissipated. Far-near-near-far sutures serve as both a tension and an approximating suture.[33] The far component relieves tension on the near component, which itself approximates wound margins. Tension on the sutured wound can be relieved by closing the wound with walking sutures. For a complete discussion of tension sutures and suturing techniques, see Chapter 4.

Skin Stretching and Expansion Techniques

As with tension-reducing suturing approaches, skin stretching and expansion techniques rely on the skin's biomechanical properties of mechanical creep and stress relaxation to effect the desired outcome of tension-free closure of a defect.

External Stretching Devices

Externally applied devices designed to pull, thus stretch the skin surrounding a wound or excisional site, are commercially available (e.g., Sure-Closure™, Life Medical Sciences, Princeton, NJ; Wisebands™, IVC Research Center, Tel-Aviv, Israel).[34–36] One such device using adherent skin pads and connecting cables has been described in dogs.[35] Placement of the adherent pads in relation to the skin edge can be adjusted according to the amount of skin needed to cover the wound; thus large areas of skin can be mobilized adjacent and more distant to a surgical or wound site. Tension on the cables is adjusted every 6 to 8 hours, and in most cases enough skin is recruited to allow closure within 48–72 hours. The system can also be left in place for 2 to 4 days following wound closure to offset excessive tension at the suture site. Separation of the pad from the skin during the process of stretching is the most common complication associated with the use of this system.

Another system (Sure-Closure™) attaches the skin to the undersurface of the device using inward-facing hooks that abut against intradermal needles (8 cm long) placed on opposite sides of the wound, and

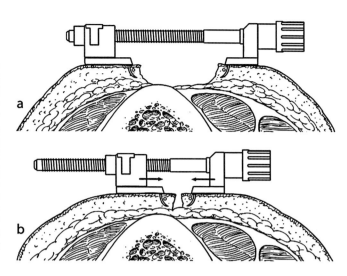

Figure 5.7. Schematic drawing of a skin stretching system (Secure Closure™) being used to stretch skin and the underlying subcutaneous tissue over exposed bone without undermining the skin. (a) Application of the system involves placement of two straight 8 cm long needles in the dermis opposite each other and 0.5 cm from the wound edges (small circles axial to the hooks in the skin contact plate). The skin contact U-shaped arms are secured to the skin by two inward-facing intradermal hooks (two hooks on each U-shaped plate) that after insertion through the skin abut against previously placed intradermal pins. (b) The threaded screw is tightened to increase tension, which is monitored by a tension gauge located on the device, and the wound is brought into apposition and is ready for suturing. Adapted from Hirshowitz B, Lindenbaum E, Har-Shai Y: A skin-stretching device for the harnessing of the viscoelastic properties of skin. Plast Reconstr Surg 1993;92:260.

uses a 7.5 cm long screw-driven tension rod to increase the tension (Figure 5.7).[34] A tension gauge on the device is not engaged when <1 Kg of tension is applied to skin and a safety clutch disengages the device, thus neutralizing tension, when the tension is >2.5 Kg. The advantages to this system are that under sterile technique the device can be applied using local infiltration or regional anaesthesia, undermining of the skin edges is not required, the stretching force on the skin margin is spread over a wide area (8 cm long intradermal needles), incremental traction with periods of tension relaxation can be accomplished, and the skin can be sutured while the device is in place. The disadvantage is that it is difficult to apply tension to a wound that is >7.5 cm wide.

The Wisebands™ skin closure system is composed of a stretching device and a 50 cm long polypropylene band which encircles the skin and underlying tissues (e.g., subcutaneous fat, fascia, and muscle), allowing closure of these more complex wounds.[36] A gauge permits 1 Kg/cm^2 of tension, and greater tension releases the tension. The advantage to this system is that it can be applied to assist the closure of complex wounds, no matter their shape or depth, and it can be applied to most regions of the body. The disadvantages are that it requires general anesthesia for application and the gauge only allows 1 Kg/cm^2 of tension to be applied, which is considerably lower than the maximal safe tension for skin stretching of 3 Kg/cm^2;[34] thus, a longer period is required to close the defect.

These systems rely on the creep and stress-relaxation properties of skin. In general, the greatest gain in skin stretching is achieved within 48–72 hours following application.[35] However, in acute clean wounds, when skin and subcutaneous tissue are normal, stretching can be achieved in a shorter time span (~20–30 minutes).[34] The time required for skin stretching in chronic wounds is often prolonged as a result of edema and fibrosis along the skin margins. Applying tension in cycles, with relaxation periods between loadings, allows for far greater elongation of tissues beyond their intrinsic extensibility capabilities.[34,37,38]

To the author's knowledge the use of these devices has not been reported in the horse. This said, the author believes these systems may hold some promise for wounds of the body, upper limbs, and possibly some involving the head region that do not require pressure bandaging or cast immobilization.

Intraoperative Tissue Expansion

Intraoperative tissue expansion has been advocated as a means of decreasing the incision closure tension. The technique involves rapid expansion of the surrounding skin by attaching towel clamps to the skin edges and applying tension or by inserting an inflatable balloon (e.g., Foley catheter) subcutaneously for several minutes.[39] The original theory postulating that this technique causes mechanical creep, which occurs when normally intertwined collagen fibers straighten and align under the influence of constant force, has been challenged since the histologic changes normally attributed to mechanical creep are lacking.[40] It is likely that the undermining of the surrounding skin required to place an inflatable balloon accounts for the decrease in closing tension on sutures.[41,42]

Silicone Elastomer Expander

A technique that expands the normal tissue adjacent to the defect by stretching it 2- to 3-fold has been described.[43–45] This is accomplished by inserting a silicone elastomer (Tissue Expander™, Cox UpHoff, Costa Mesa, CA) in the subcutaneous tissues adjacent to a cosmetic defect that is to be reconstructed (Figure 5.8a). As a rule of thumb, the elastomer expander's base area should be 2.5 times that of the defect to be closed.[46,47] Attached to the expander by a tube is a self-sealing injection dome which is implanted conveniently nearby yet remote to the silicone expander (Figure 5.8b). After the implant incision has healed (~7–10 days), tissue expansion is accomplished by injecting sterile saline into the injection dome to inflate the expander until the skin becomes taut (Figure 5.8c). The skin over the injection portal is cleansed with alcohol prior to

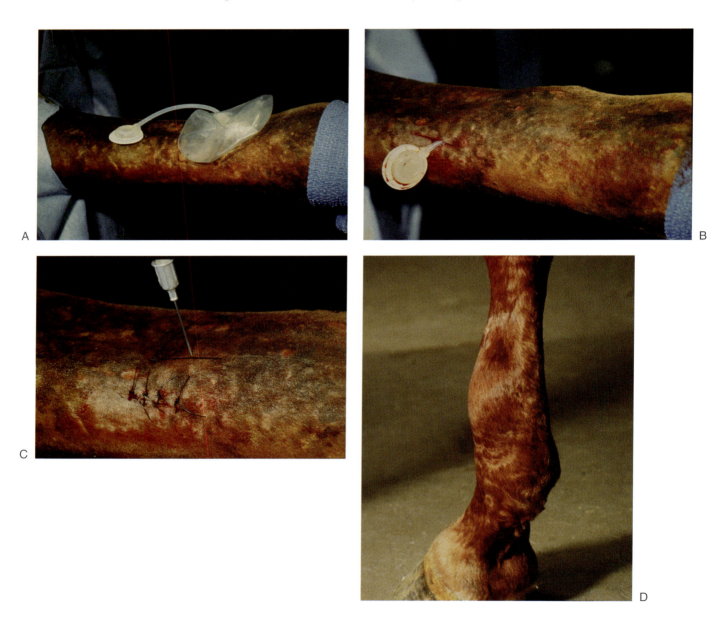

Figure 5.8. (A) A silicone elastomer tissue expander is positioned on the limb at the proposed site of implantation. The clear expander is to the right and the injection dome is to the left. (B) The tissue expander has been inserted in the subcutaneous tissue and the injection portal will be implanted nearby. (C) Sterile saline is being injected into the injection dome to inflate the expander until the skin becomes taut. (D) Note the tissue expansion (swelling) on the lateral surface of the metacarpus. Courtesy of Dr. L. Booth.

administering the injection. Similar injections are carried out at 4-to-7-day intervals until sufficient skin expansion has occurred to permit closure of the wound (Figure 5.8d). Once expansion is sufficient, the expander and injection dome are removed and the expanded skin is undermined and mobilized to cover the defect. Microscopic changes seen in the skin are consistent with mechanical creep.[40]

Generally, the skin can be expanded to 3 times its original surface area; however, slow expansion of the skin is required to prevent ischemic necrosis. The epidermis responds to tissue expansion by an increase in mitotic activity, resulting in a net increase in epidermal tissue. The dermis thins in response to expansion, which is compensated for by a thick fibrous capsule that develops around the expander.[48] The net result of expanded skin plus fibrous capsule is the same thickness as normal unexpanded skin.

The fact that normal skin with the same hair color and texture directly adjacent to the wound can be used to cover the defect makes this technique somewhat attractive, although more experience is required before its full benefit and limitations become known.

Skin Mobilization Procedures to Reduce Tension

Excess tension on a suture line can result in considerable patient discomfort, ischemia of the skin margins, and suture line tear-out with partial or complete wound dehiscence and excessive scarring. These consequences can be ameliorated, to a large extent, by undermining the skin surrounding a lesion, using tension sutures (previously discussed under Tension-reducing Suturing Techniques) or using skin mobilization techniques. These techniques may be used alone or in combination to reduce tension on the suture line.

Undermining Surrounding Skin

Undermining the skin can be used alone or in combination with other tension-relieving techniques (e.g., mesh expansion, skin flaps, etc.) and is a time-honored approach for reducing skin tension on a suture line. It is commonly used in conjunction with suturing techniques that reduce tension on the primary suture line (the sutures that appose skin edges).

Undermining is accomplished by separating the skin and subcutaneous tissue from their underlying attachments to fascia in the extremities; occasionally, the cutaneous muscle is undermined in the neck and body regions where it exists. As with any surgery the tissue should be handled gently and every effort made to protect the blood supply.

Skin can be undermined either by blunt or sharp dissection. Blunt dissection involves opening the blades of a scissor after it has been inserted closed into the desired tissue plane and repeating until the tissue has been adequately undermined. An alternative is to insert the handle of a scalpel and move it in a back-and-forth motion. Blunt dissection has the advantage of minimizing the damage to the cutaneous blood supply and the disadvantages of tearing tissue, creating more trauma, and being of limited use when attempting to undermine chronic fibrotic wounds. The author finds this approach most useful in relatively loose-skinned regions (e.g., neck and some parts of the trunk).

Even though sharp dissection using a scalpel (Figure 5.9) or scissors (Figure 5.10) has the disadvantage of potentially transecting blood vessels, this is of limited concern in the extremities of the horse such that this technique is preferred by the author for these regions. When using a scalpel, one deep, cleanly made incision following the contour of the anatomic part, which separates the attachment of the subcutaneous tissue from the underlying fascia, is preferred to multiple small, shallowly made incisions, which create more tissue trauma and a greater chance of hemorrhage. When using scissors, rather than making multiple small snips to separate the tissue, the author prefers to insert the sharp blades in a half closed position, which, with pressure, converts it to a cutting instrument (Figure 5.10). In the author's opinion multiple snips with a scissor creates more tissue trauma and therefore should be avoided.

The depth at which the skin is undermined depends on the neurovascular anatomy of the region, and therefore it should be reviewed prior to surgery to avoid injury to these structures. On the distal limbs the dissection should be as deep as possible between the subcutaneous tissue and deep fascia.[3,8,21] Skin on the trunk should be elevated below the cutaneous muscles when it is adhered to the dermis; if subcutaneous tissue is present, it is dissected as described for the distal limb. In most cases these planes of tissue are easily identified; an exception is an older scarred wound in which it is difficult to readily identify a tissue plane until dissection has been continued for some distance. In this situation, it is appropriate to either begin with an incision in normal skin

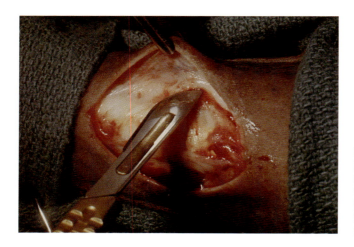

Figure 5.9. Undermining the skin using a scalpel. The scalpel blade is oriented flat against the fascia; it is then used to make a clean incision, following the contour of the anatomic part, which separates the attachment of the subcutaneous tissue from the underlying fascia. One cleanly made incision is preferred to multiple small shallowly made incisions, which create more tissue trauma and a greater chance of hemorrhage.

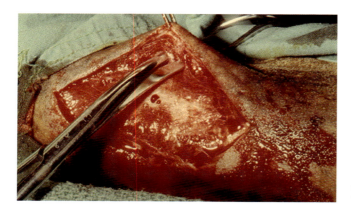

Figure 5.10. A scissor is being inserted with the blades in a half-closed position. This position allows the scissor to be used as a cutting instrument to separate the subcutaneous tissue from its attachments to the underlying fascia.

proximal, distal, lateral, or medial to the wound, or extend the dissection until normal skin is encountered. This will enable the surgeon to identify the proper tissue plane.[3]

The amount of skin that needs to be undermined can be roughly determined by pulling the skin edges together with towel forceps. As a general rule, in fresh wounds a distance equal to the width of the defect itself should be undermined on either side of the wound.[21] Once accomplished, the skin edges are drawn together using towel forceps and the tension is assessed. If the tension appears too great, undermining can be extended half as much again.[9,21] Given the potential for disruption of the cutaneous blood supply when undermining skin, careful judgment is needed. If a question exists, combining undermining with another skin mobilizing procedure (e.g., relaxing incisions, Z or V-Y plasty) should be considered.

The extent to which skin can be undermined without damaging the blood supply and causing necrosis has not been established. In companion animals, it is thought that undermining can be quite extensive without causing necrosis as long as the blood supply remains intact. Clinical experience suggests the same is true for horses.[3,33,49] Used in conjunction with a mesh expansion technique on the limbs of dogs, 360° undermining of the skin was not associated with any major complication.[50]

If hemorrhage appears to be a problem, the surgeon should consider using a drain and a properly applied pressure bandage to avoid the deleterious effects (increasing suture line tension/pressure and providing a medium for bacterial growth) of a hematoma. For more information regarding the use and application of drains, see Chapter 4. For information regarding pressure bandaging, see Chapter 16.

Severing subcutaneous tissue attachments to the underlying fascia allows wound edges to be pulled toward one another and makes use of the elastic properties of skin. The closing tension for a defect varies greatly with the anatomic region involved and is correlated to the amount of loose skin in the area.[41] It appears that the amount of tension relief derived from undermining diminishes as the extent of undermining increases. Thus, it is important to frequently check the amount of tension relief achieved to avoid unnecessary undermining and to prompt the decision for using other methods of tension relief prior to the onset of deleterious effects of undermining (e.g., interruption of the cutaneous blood supply and hematoma formation). In chronic scarred wounds much of the skin's elasticity has been lost such that extensive undermining to achieve the desired end result may be required.

Tissue Debulking

Although not classically considered a tension-relieving procedure, the removal of exuberant granulation tissue or fibrous tissue (debulking) followed by undermining of the adjacent skin will provide considerable tension relief and allow cosmetic reconstruction of many wounds of the distal limb (Figures 5.11a–c). Skin incisions should extend beyond the extremities of the wound into normal tissue so the thickness of the skin can be identified. Using the normal skin thickness as a guide, the skin overlying the granulation or scar tissue (Figure 5.11b) is dissected free until a normal subcutaneous tissue plane is encountered. Once the surrounding skin is free, excessive tissue (granulation or scar) within the wound is excised in an effort to conform the wound bed to the normal underlying tissues. Care must be taken to maintain the blood supply to the undermined skin and to avoid transecting a vital support structure (e.g., tendon) or entering a synovial cavity.

Skin tension is tested following undermining; if more under-mining is needed it should be performed at this time. A Penrose drain placed under the resultant skin flap and brought out through a stab incision distal to the surgical site is used to drain the undermined region. The drain should be secured with sutures at the proximal and distal or dorsal and ventral extents of the undermined tissue. The incision for the distal/ventral exit site for the drain should be separate from the wound edges and the hole should be large enough to allow

A 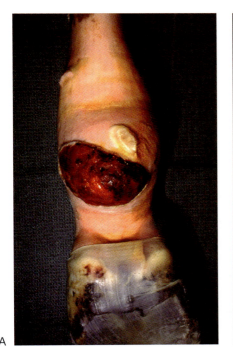 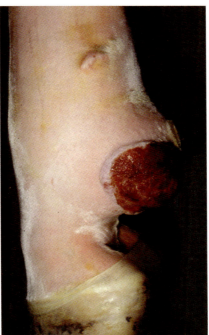 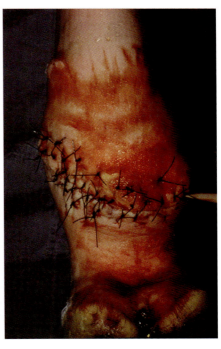 B,C

Figure 5.11. Example of how removal of exuberant granulation tissue (debulking) allows wound closure. (A) Plantar view of a non-healing wound of ~6 months duration. The chronic exuberant granulation was acting as a barrier, which prevented healing (e.g., epithelialization and/or contraction) of this wound. (B) Side view of the same. Note how the skin has attempted to heal over the chronic granulating mass. At this point it is presumed by the author that skin has undergone biologic creep which will allow closure of the wound with little suture tension following excision of the granulation tissue. (C) Following removal of the exuberant tissue, the skin edges were easily apposed with sutures. Because there was considerable dead space for blood to accumulate, a drain was used. A lower limb cast was applied and left in place for 2 weeks. The cast was removed by the referring veterinarian and primary healing was ultimately achieved.

free drainage (Figure 4.36). Additionally, the drain should not reside directly underneath the incision line after closure. If it does, it will hinder the subcutaneous tissue's contribution to the healing process. If required, tension sutures are used to reduce the tension on the primary incision line, after which the skin is closed with inter-rupted nonabsorbable sutures (Figure 5.11c). See Chapter 4 for more information regarding drains and suturing patterns and techniques.

The choice of physical restraint (e.g., bandage versus bandage splinting versus cast) is dictated by lesion location and the amount of tension on the primary suture line. Stent bandages and tie-over bandages are useful in regions that are not amenable to routine bandage or cast applications (Figures 16.13 and 16.14). They protect the wound from external contamination and if secured tightly with sutures reduce the tension on the primary suture line and provide uniform pressure to the surgical site. See Chapter 16 for more information regarding bandaging and casting techniques.

Generally, drains are removed in 1 to 2 days unless drainage persists, in which case they may be left in place longer. Casts are usually removed between 14 and 21 days, depending on the amount of skin mobilization and suture tension required to close the wound. The greater the skin mobilization and suture tension required for wound closure, the longer the cast is left in place. Compress bandages are maintained for 4 to 5 weeks for the best cosmetic end result. Tension sutures and drains are removed at the time of cast removal, whereas tension sutures used under bandages are usually removed after 7 to 10 days, depending upon skin tension.

Longitudinal Relaxing Incisions

Longitudinal relaxing incisions are made adjacent to the wound margin, which can aid in advancing skin to cover the wound.[33] A single incision created parallel to the long axis of the wound is termed a simple relaxing incision. The skin between the relaxing incision and the wound is undermined and advanced toward the wound. The width of the skin between the simple relaxing incision and the wound should be equal to the width of the wound.[32] When the wound is closed by creating only one relaxing incision, the defect created by that incision is generally about the same size as the original wound, whereas making a relaxing incision on either side of the wound results in two smaller wounds. When two relaxing incisions are created, one on either side of the wound, the distance between the original wound and each relaxing incision should equal the width of the original wound.

Wounds created by relaxing incisions heal by second intention, and one large relaxing incision heals more slowly than two smaller relaxing incisions. Creating one or two relaxing incisions to close a wound may be justi-fied if the incision allows closure of a wound that exposes a ligament or tendon. When planning for relaxing incisions, efforts should be made to create the secondary defect over healthy tissue, thereby minimizing the problems associated with second intention healing.

Mesh Expansion

A mesh expansion method, which allows greater mobilization of adjacent skin than can be achieved by undermining alone, has been described.[49] With this method the skin is undermined to free the attachment of the subcutaneous tissue to the underlying fascia after which 10 mm–15 mm long tension-relieving incisions are made parallel to the wound in the undermined skin adjacent to the wound edges (Figure 5.12). As the skin is drawn over the wound, the tension-relieving incisions widen as would occur with a mesh skin graft and the tension required for suture closure is reduced. When the skin is thickened and fibrotic, 15-mm long incisions are recommended. Although these small wounds heal much faster and impart a better cosmetic appearance than do one or two long, relaxing incisions,[32] they do not provide as much skin relaxation as long relaxing incisions.

V-Y Plasty

V-Y plasty provides tension relief when the apex of the V-shaped incision is directed away from the under-mined skin defect to be closed. Once closure of the original defect has been accomplished, closure of the V inci-sion is completed by converting it to a Y, gaining length and relieving tension. In the author's experience, this technique provides very little tension relief for a large defect in the distal limb of horses. The author finds the

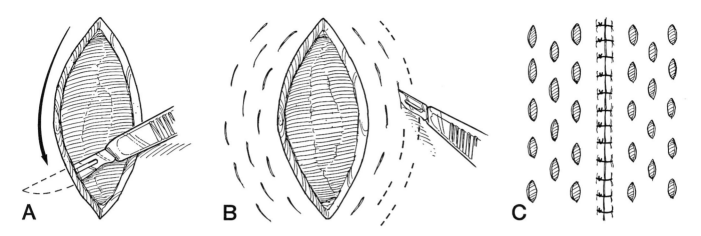

Figure 5.12. Illustration of the mesh expansion method. (A) The skin adjacent to the fusiform defect is being undermined to separate the subcutaneous tissue attachments to the underlying fascia. (B) Strategically placed stab incisions, 10 mm to 15 mm long, are made through the full thickness of the undermined skin. (C) Following apposition of the skin edges with simple interrupted sutures, the stab incisions open in a mesh fashion to reduce tension. Adapted from Bailey JV, Jacobs KA: The mesh expansion method of suturing wounds on the legs of horses. Vet Surg 1983;12:78.

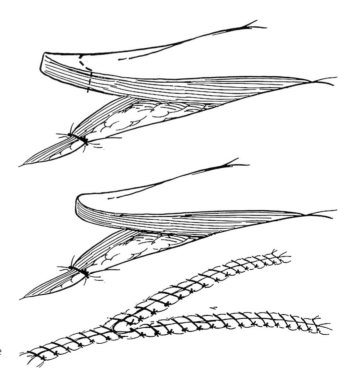

Figure 5.13. Closure of a chevron-shaped skin laceration where the tip of the chevron has been lost.

technique most useful for closure of chevron-shaped lacerations where the tip of the V has been lost (Figure 5.13) and for management of scar tissue contracture associated with the palpebrum (Figure 5.14). A V-Y closure can be used to increase skin tension if needed.

Z Plasty

A Z plasty is composed of a central limb, two arms, and two angles where the two arms join the central limb (Figure 5.15a). The two arms and central limb should be of the same length. While the angles can range

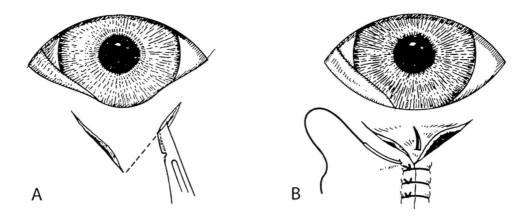

Figure 5.14. V-Y plasty being used to reduce skin tension at the ventral palpebrum. (A) The apex of the V-shaped incision is directed away from the palpebrum and the V is undermined. (B) The apex of the V is advanced toward the palpebrum and the Y-shaped incision is apposed with simple interrupted sutures.

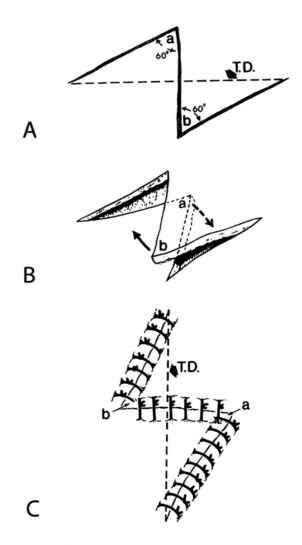

Figure 5.15. Z plasty (A) Line a-b is the central limb. Two arms attach to the central limb at angles of 60°. Transverse diagonal (TD; dotted line) is an imaginary line drawn to connect the ends of the arms. TD is 75% longer than the central limb. The length of the TD will become reoriented vertically after the flaps are undermined and transposed. (B) Undermined skin flaps are being transposed. (C) Simple interrupted sutures appose skin. Note the TD dotted line is oriented vertically and the central limb is now oriented transversally.

from 30° to 90°, in the author's experience 60° for both angles works best in the horse. The Z plasty is developed by making a Z-shaped skin incision which is followed by undermining and then transposing two triangular skin flaps. This results in a change in the orientation of the central limb of the Z and a gain in length (Figure 5.15b).[51] The gain in length achieved by the procedure is in the direction of the original central limb prior to transposition. This may be more easily understood if an imaginary line connecting the ends of the limbs, referred to as the transverse diagonal (TD) measurement, is visualized or drawn (Figure 5.15a). If the angle where the arms join the central limb is 60°, the TD will be 75% longer than the central limb. When the flaps are transposed the TD reorients itself to replace the central limb while the central limb reorients to replace the TD.[21] Although gain in length in the direction of the original central limb is dictated somewhat by the angles of the Z plasty (larger angles give more relaxation), in this author's experience, due to the relatively inelastic properties of equine skin, a gain of only 50% in length can be expected in most instances.

Z plasty can be used to lengthen or excise a contracted (bowstring) scar (Figure 5.16), dilate a scarred stenotic orifice (e.g., stenotic nares; Figure 5.17),[52] and relieve tension associated with closure following fusiform excision (discussed later under cosmetic closure of elongated defects; Figure 5.18).[3,21] In all instances the gain in length or relaxation will be in the direction of the central limb of the Z after the flaps of the Z have been transposed.

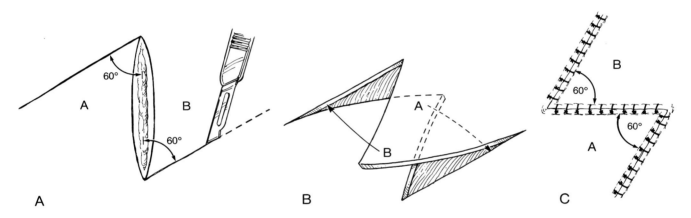

Figure 5.16. A through C illustrates how Z plasty can be used to remove and lengthen a site occupied by a contracted (bowstring) scar.

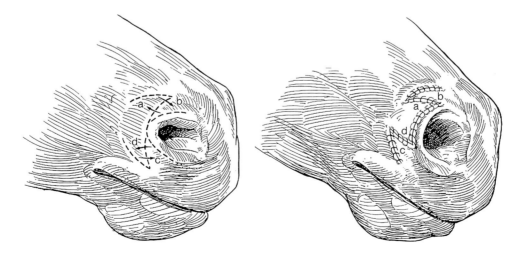

Figure 5.17. Left, a constricted right nostril due to scar formation following injury. Dotted lines indicate the site where two connected Z-plasty incisions will be made. Right, Z plasties complete. The diameter of the nostril is enlarged.

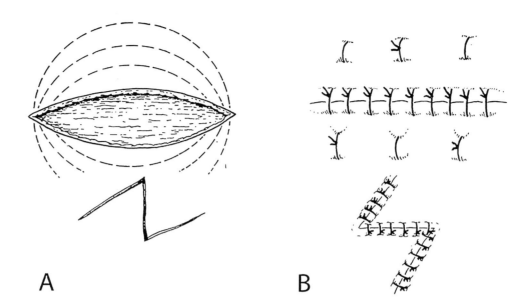

Figure 5.18. Z plasty being used to relieve the skin tension associated with a fusiform defect. (a) The central limb of the Z plasty is centered over the region of greatest tension, which is perpendicular to the long axis of the defect. Dashed lines indicate undermining. (b) Vertical mattress tension sutures are used as support for the closure of the fusiform defect itself, accomplished with simple interrupted sutures. Flaps of the Z plasty were transposed and sutured.

When Z plasty is used to lengthen a bowstring scar, the central limb is oriented in the direction of the scar (Figure 5.16). In this case the scar is most often excised at the site of the central limb, after which the arms are incised followed by undermining and transposition of the flaps. In the case of a scarred stenotic orifice, more than one Z plasty may be required to achieve the desired dilation (relaxation) (Figure 5.17).

In an effort to relax a wound involving the trunk, the surrounding skin should be elevated to determine whether there is sufficient skin in one plane to allow the required relaxation. Because the skin of the distal limb has minimal inherent extensibility, the Z plasty is simply oriented with the central limb in the direction in which relaxation is needed (Figure 5.18). When Z plasty is used to relieve tension associated with fusiform excision of a wound, the undermining should extend from the defect to include the Z plasty.

In all cases, after undermining is complete, the flaps of the Z are transposed and the apices are secured with nonabsorbable sutures placed in a vertical mattress pattern. If Z plasty was used to excise a bowstring scar, the rest of the Z plasty is apposed with simple interrupted sutures. On the other hand, if Z plasty was used to reduce suture tension for closure of a fusiform defect, the defect is sutured before suturing of the Z plasty. In the latter case a drain is often used because considerable dead space is created following undermining of the defect and Z plasty. For more information regarding the indications and use of drains, refer to Chapter 4.

A drawback to the Z plasty, when used to relieve tension associated with closure of a fusiform excision, is that it prolongs surgery considerably and therefore is only used by the author as a last resort. Although it has been reported that the most common complication of Z plasty in the horse is ischemia and necrosis of the tips of the triangular skin flaps,[9] in the author's experience this has not been a problem as long as the angles of the Z plasty are of 60°.

Cosmetic Closure of Various Shaped Defects

Elongated Defects

Elongated wounds may be converted to a fusiform shape (Figure 5.19), and circular or elongated lesions may be removed by a fusiform excision (Figures 5.20a,b). The term fusiform is preferred because the incision ends are tapered, whereas a true ellipse is oval. The shape of the fusiform excision lends itself to a superior cosmetic closure more than an ellipse because it adapts readily to a straight line upon closure (Figure 5.21).

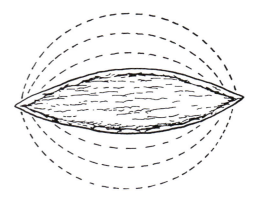

Figure 5.19. Fusiform-shaped defect. The dotted lines represent the required extent of undermining of the skin to allow tension-free closure.

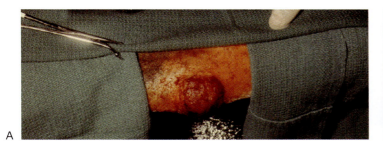

A

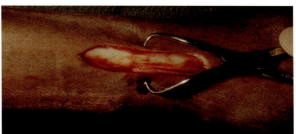

B

Figure 5.20. (a) Circular shaped mass of exuberant granulation tissue on the dorsal surface of the metacarpus. The owners requested reconstructive surgery to improve cosmesis. (b) A fusiform excision was used to remove the mass and facilitate tension-free closure. Towel forceps are used to estimate skin tension and the amount of undermining required to reduce tension for closure.

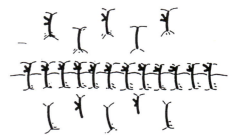

Figure 5.21. Following undermining of the skin as illustrated in Figure 5.19, the fusiform excision is apposed with vertical mattress tension suture to reduce the tension of the simple interrupted sutures that are apposing the skin edges.

The correct axis for removal is determined by lesion shape, its position, tension lines, and skin extensibility. Pre-marking reference points or drawing the fusiform pattern at the site of excision, prior to incising, will reduce the chances of removing excess tissue and improve mirror imagery; as a result a superior cosmetic closure can be anticipated (Figures 5.4, 5.22a–c). In most instances closure will require tension suture support and sometimes an additional tension-relieving procedure (Figures 5.21, 5.22d–f).

Dog ears (bunching of the skin at the end of the incision) may accompany skin closure after fusiform excision. In the design of a fusiform excision, it has been stated that whenever possible the length-to-width ratio should approach 4:1 to prevent this problem.[21] However, lesser ratios have resulted in cosmetic closure following fusiform excision of scar tissue revision in the lower limbs of horses (Figures 5.27a–g, see pages 261–262). When dog ears occur, however, they can be removed in the following manner: when a dog ear develops as a result of one side of the excision being longer than the other, it can be corrected by making a short, right-angle incision at the base of the bunched skin (Figures 5.23 and 5.24). The excess skin that overlaps the wound is excised to permit wound closure (Figure 5.25).

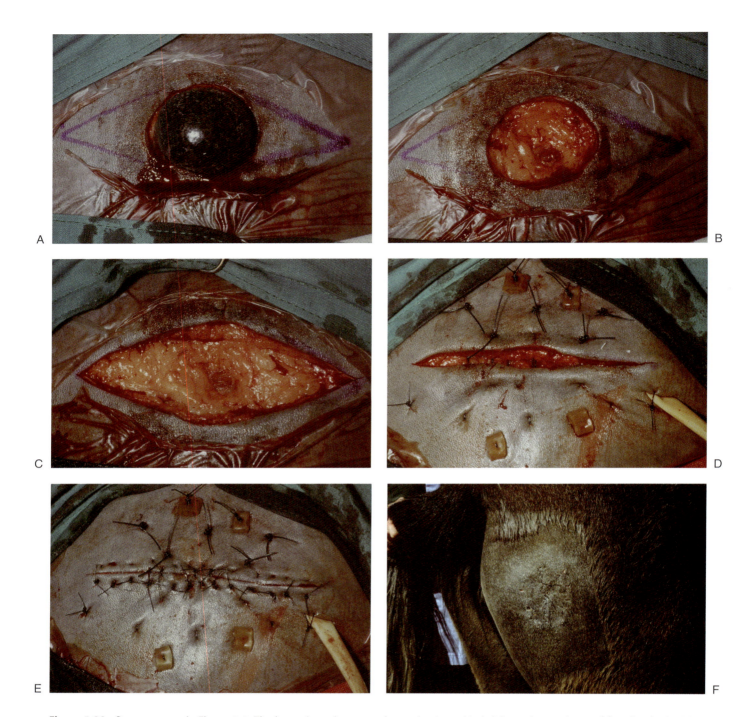

Figure 5.22. Same case as in Figure 5.4. The horse is under general anesthesia and in left lateral recumbency (A) A circular incision is made around the border of the melanoma. (B) The melanoma is completely removed. (C) Fusiform excision is complete and the skin was undermined. (D) Widely placed vertical mattress sutures were used to reduce tension on the primary suture line. Vertical mattress sutures subjected to the greatest tension were supported with soft rubber tubing. A Penrose drain was placed. (E) The skin was apposed with interrupted vertical mattress sutures. (F) The surgical site, in the standing horse, following suture removal 2 weeks post-operatively.

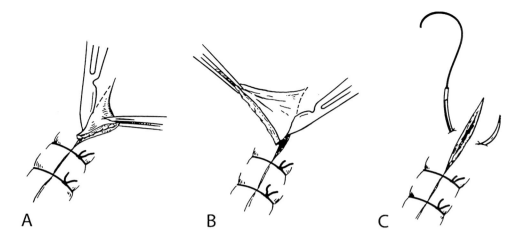

Figure 5.23. Removal of a "dog ear" by making an incision on either side of its base. (A) Scalpel is incising one side of the base of the dog ear. (B) Incision is made in the base on the opposite side of the dog ear. (C) Closure after removal of the dog ear.

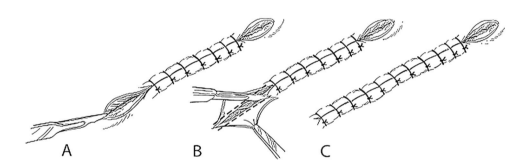

Figure 5.24. Removal of a dog ear by extending the incision through the bunched tissue. (A) Extending the incision through the dog ear. (B) Excision of the two skin triangles. (C) Closure after dog ear removal. Adapted from Swaim SF, Henderson R: Various-shaped wounds. In Stephan Swaim and Ralf Henderson, eds. *Small animal wound management (1st edition)*. Philadelphia: Lea and Febiger, 1990, p.131.

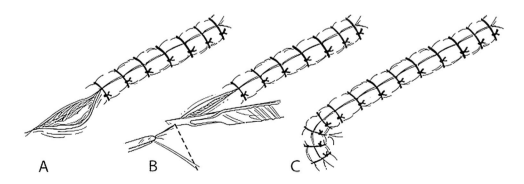

Figure 5.25. Dog ear resulting from one side of the wound being longer than the other. (A) One-sided dog ear. (B) Short, right-angle incision made at the base of the dog ear; the dotted line defines the skin to be excised. (C) Closure after dog ear removal. Adapted from Swaim SF, Henderson R: Various-shaped wounds. In Stephan Swaim and Ralf Henderson, eds. *Small animal wound management (1st edition)*. Philadelphia: Lea and Febiger, 1990, p.131.

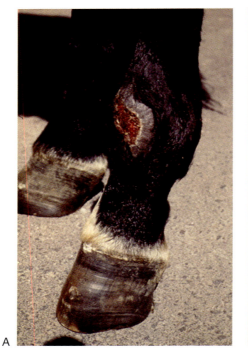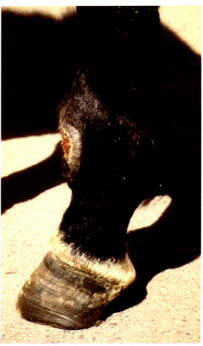

A   B

Figure 5.26. (A) Wound over the dorsal fetlock region, 1 year duration. The wound would crack open and bleed periodically, particularly following forced exercise. (B) Lateral view of the same. Note the swelling deep to the wound and haired skin overlying the fetlock. It is presumed that biologic creep of the skin occurred following slow enlargement of the scar tissue associated with this swelling. Tension-free closure following excision of the underlying scar would be expected.

One of the most rewarding applications of fusiform excision, in the author's experience, is for cosmetic reconstruction of scars on the distal limbs in horses (Figures 5.26a,b). The procedure involves selecting the appropriate axis for the fusiform excision, which must take into account tension lines, maximal skin extensibility, and the skin that will be available following excision of scar tissue. For large scars, the outline for the proposed fusiform excision should be drawn with a sterile marker before the incisions are made (Figure 5.27a). The incision along the pre-marked site is begun proximal or distal to the scar so that the thickness of normal skin is documented and any important anatomic structures (e.g., tendons, joint capsules, etc.) underlying the scar are identified before the scar tissue is removed and undermining begins (Figure 5.27b). Knowing the thickness of normal skin provides the surgeon with a guideline as to how deep to undermine the skin that is adhered to the scar, whereas identifying important structures in advance of removing the scar from the wound bed will minimize the risk of severing a support structure or entering a synovial cavity (Figure 5.27c).

Once the scar tissue has been completely excised the decision is made as to whether the skin should be undermined further to allow its apposition or whether more skin needs to be excised so proper tension on the apposed skin is achieved (Figures 5.27d–f). Closure involves placement of a drain, in most cases, and the use of tension sutures to appose the skin (Figures 5.27g and 5.28). This approach has also been rewarding for the removal of extensive scar tissue deep to the skin (Figures 5.29a–e).

To achieve the most cosmetic end result, most of these cases will require cast immobilization or bandage splinting. For information regarding the techniques for applying a cast or bandage splint see Chapter 16. A good cosmetic end result is usually achieved in the absence of complications (Figures 5.30, 5.31).

Square Defects

Sliding H plasty may be used to repair/reconstruct square or rectangular defects (Figure 5.32). Normally, two flaps are created. However, if skin is available on only three sides of a defect, one-half of the H plasty is used (Figure 5.33).[3,6,21]

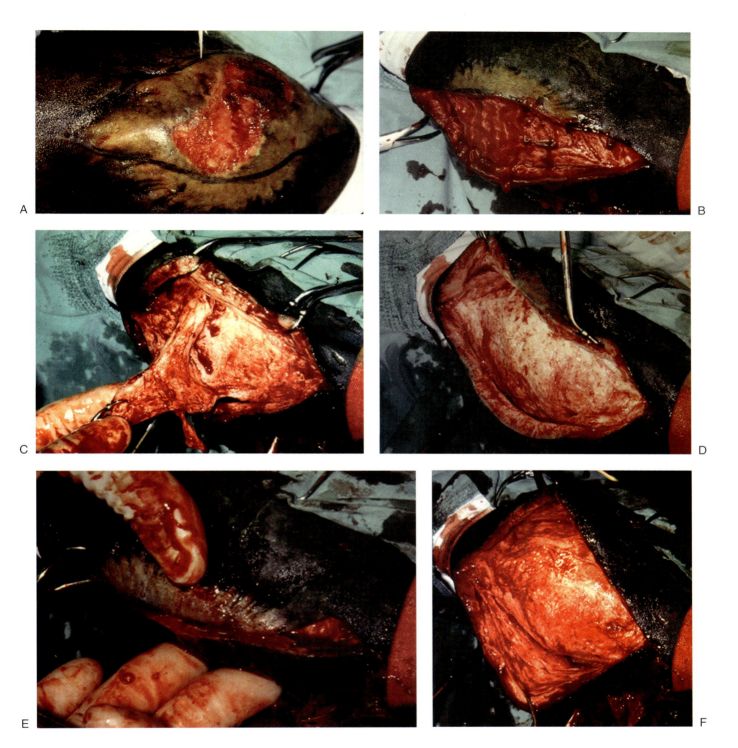

Figure 5.27. Same case as in Figure 5.26. The horse is under general anesthesia and in lateral recumbency. Proximal is to the left. (A) The outline for the proposed fusiform excision was drawn with a sterile marker. Note the un-haired epithelium and centrally located non-healed wound. A major surgical objective was to remove all the non-healed wound. (B) The incision along the pre-marked site is complete. The thickness of normal skin and the extensor tendon in this region were identified prior to removal of the scar in the wound. (C) Scar tissue overlying the extensor tendon is being removed. (D) Scar tissue has been removed and the skin is undermined until normal subcutaneous tissue was encountered. (E) Pushing the undermined skin edges toward each other, using finger pressure, documents excess tension-free skin. Note the non-haired epithelium axial to the thumb; this will be removed prior to suturing. (F) Un-haired epithelium has been excised and the wound bed lavaged in preparation for suturing. (G) (next page) Following closure. Note that the drain exit site is separate from the sutured incision. The drain was sutured at its proximal and distal limits and was placed in the dead space adjacent to the sutured incision. Betadine ointment was applied to the drain exit site after which sterile dressing and conforming gauze were applied in preparation for application of a lower limb cast.

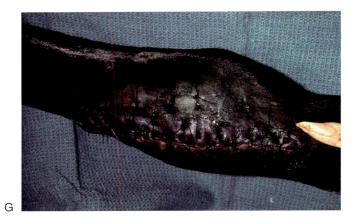

G

Figure 5.27. *Continued*

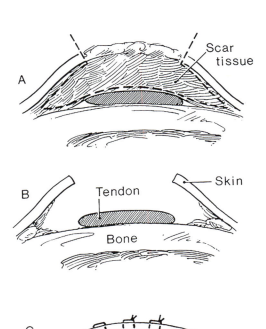

A Scar tissue

B Tendon Skin

Bone

C

Figure 5.28. Technique used in Figure 5.27, illustrated in cross section. (A) Dotted line illustrates excision of the scar tissue overlying the extensor tendon. (B) Following removal of scar tissue and undermining of the skin, sufficient skin is available for tension-free closure. (C) Skin closure complete.

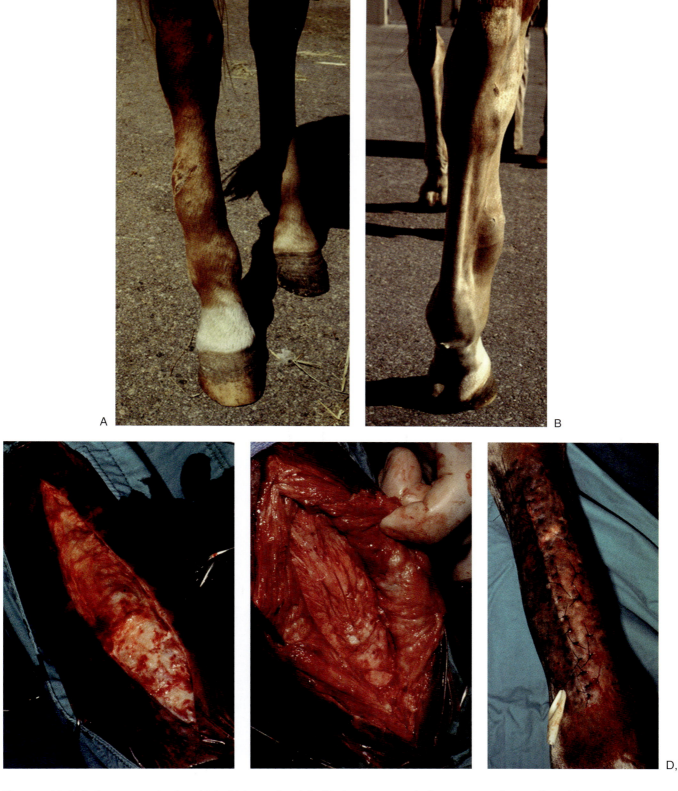

Figure 5.29. This horse sustained multiple kicks to the right hind metatarsus during transport in a trailer with another horse ~6 months earlier. The owner was interested in cosmetic reconstruction. (A) Dorsal view of the injury site. Note that the skin is intact but significant swelling is present deep to the skin. The horse was clinically normal at exercise. Radiographs revealed slight bone proliferation from the cortex of the third metatarsal bone. (B) Plantar view of the same. (C) At surgery a long fusiform skin excision was used to expose the underlying scar tissue. (D) Scar tissue was bisected down to the underlying tendon after which the skin was undermined and the scar was removed. (E) Closure complete. A lower limb cast was applied for 2 weeks.

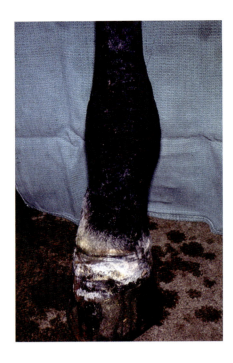

Figure 5.30. Appearance of reconstructed wound in Figure 5.27 2 months after surgery. The horse appeared normal at exercise, and flexion of the fetlock revealed it had a full range of motion.

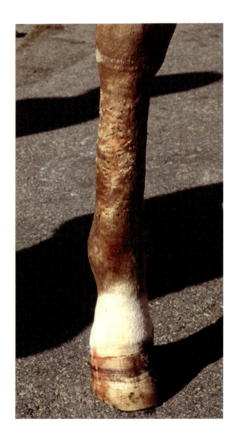

Figure 5.31. Appearance of the reconstructed site in Figure 5.28, at the time of dismissal 2.5 weeks after surgery.

While usually unnecessary in small animals (cats and dogs) that have relatively loose skin, the use of geometric measurements is most important in designing an H plasty in the horse. If two sliding flaps are used, the base of the triangles should equal at least half the width of the defect (Figure 5.32a), whereas with a single flap the base of the triangles should equal the width of the defect (Figure 5.33a). The skin flap(s) are undermined to separate their subcutaneous tissue attachments to the underlying fascia. For older wounds, removal (debulking) of scar tissue is usually required to allow skin mobility (Figures 5.34a,b). Tension sutures will be required in most cases. Vertical mattress sutures are placed in the mobilized skin flaps, the tension is taken up by applying towel clamps, and the sutures are tied (Figures 5.32b, 5.35a,b). Next, the base of the triangles is sutured (Figure 5.32c). A drain is often used under these flaps (Figures 5.35a,b). Primary suture apposition of the rest of the plasty then follows. A modification of the one-half H plasty can be used to cover unequal or irregularly shaped defects where limited skin is available for creating a sliding flap (Figures 5.36, 5.37a,b). An advantage to this technique is that, for a narrow defect, the base of a sliding flap can be made wider to ensure a good blood supply to the reconstructed site.

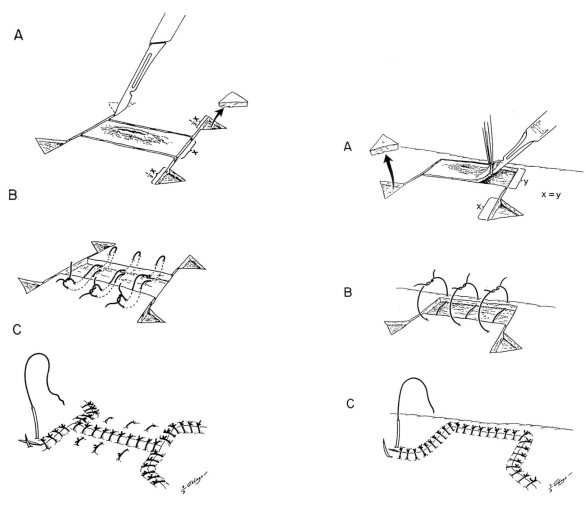

Figure 5.32. Sliding H flaps being used to reconstruct a rectangular defect. (A) Rectangular defect is excised (center- width = X) and the two arms of the H incision extend at least 1 to 1.5 base widths away from the excision site. Triangles whose base equals 1/2 X are created at the end of each arm to prevent puckering after the skin edges are sutured. (B) Following undermining, the skin flaps are drawn together with vertical mattress tension sutures. (C) Simple interrupted sutures complete the closure. A drain is often used under the skin flaps.

Figure 5.33. Example of a half H plasty being used when skin is available on only three sides of the defect. (A) Y = the width of the defect created by excision. Note the base of the triangle. X = the width of the excised defect, Y. (B) Following undermining, simple interrupted sutures are used to hold the top of the flap in place. The base of the triangles are then apposed. (C) Suturing is complete.

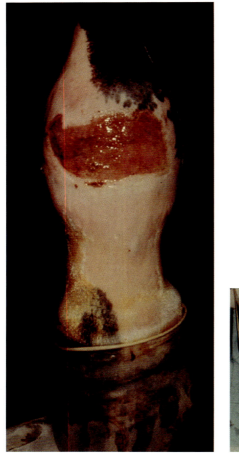
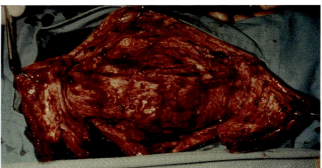

A   B

Figure 5.34. (A) Non-healing wound on the dorsal fetlock ~6 months' duration. (B) At surgery, the central lesion was excised, the skin flaps were undermined, and the scar tissue in the wound was removed in preparation for the closure of the H plasty.

Triangular Defects

Tissue adjacent to a triangular defect may be used to cover it (Figure 5.38). If there is excessive tension, one (Figure 5.39) or two inverted triangles (Figure 5.40) can be made two to three triangle base widths away from the lesion; and then skin flaps are undermined, pulled into position, and sutured. The decision to create one or two flaps is dictated by tension and the amount of available loose skin. In most cases two inverted triangles, each with a base of one-half of the width of the original defect, relieves more tension than one large inverted triangle.

V-shaped Defects

V-shaped wounds are fairly common and often the tip of the V-flap is lost or requires debridement prior to closure. Following debridement the chevron-shaped wound can be closed in a Y pattern similar to that of the V-Y plasty (Figure 5.13). An alternative for a long, narrow V-shaped wound with ample loose skin surrounding it would be to remove it using a fusiform excision (Figure 5.19), which would be closed as a linear defect (Figure 5.21).

Circular Defects

Pedicle flaps, rotation flaps, or transposition flaps (Table 5.1) can be used to close or cover circular wounds as depicted (Figure 5.41, see page 269). Although these techniques are best used in regions where the skin is

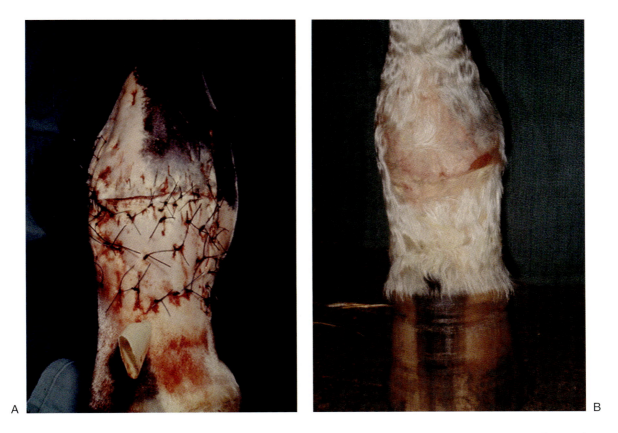

Figure 5.35. Same horse as in Figure 5.34a. (A) Following placement of a drain and skin closure. Three rows of vertical mattress sutures were required to sufficiently reduce the tension on the primary suture line. A lower (short) limb cast was used for 3 weeks. (B) Healed wound ~8 weeks post surgery. A small portion of the skin flap on the right side will have to heal by second intention. Note the dark skin pigmentation is markedly diminished just proximal to the surgical site on the right side, and the alopecia. It is conjectured that the loss of pigmentation and alopecia may be due to a reduction in blood supply either from the extensive undermining of the skin or as a result of the suture tension required for skin closure.

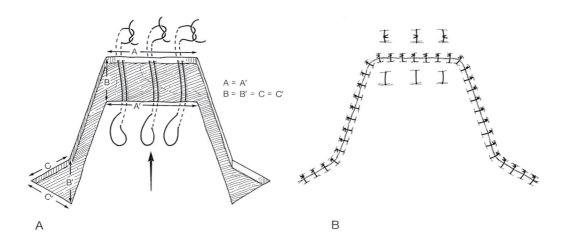

A = A′
B = B′ = C = C′

Figure 5.36. Modified half H plasty which can be used to cover an irregular (unequal) angular defect. (A) Following removal of an angular defect, incisions in normal skin are extended at the same angle from the defect. Triangles whose base B′ = that of B are incised. The skin flap has been undermined and vertical mattress sutures are preplaced. The arrow indicates the direction in which the skin flap will be pulled. (B) Vertical mattress sutures are tied and simple interrupted sutures are used for skin closure.

267

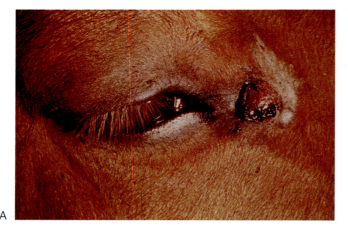
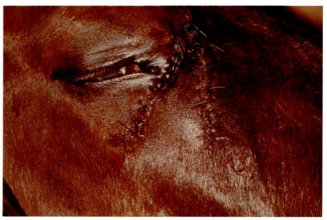

A

B

Figure 5.37. (A) A lesion adjacent to the medial canthus of the eye that would be amenable to removal and coverage with full thickness skin using a modified half H plasty. (B) Following excision of the lesion, the skin rostral to the medial canthus was mobilized to allow coverage of the defect.

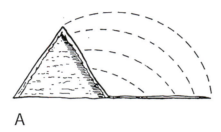
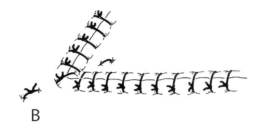

A

B

Figure 5.38. Triangular shaped defect with adjacent loose skin. (A) Adjacent skin is undermined (dotted lines). (B) A vertical mattress suture secures the apex of the flap and simple interrupted sutures are used for closure.

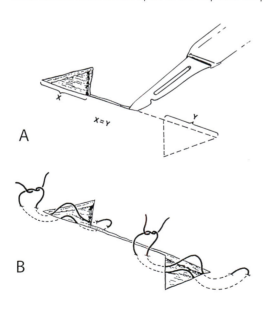

A

B

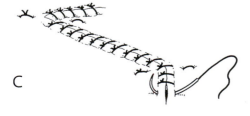

C

Figure 5.39. Triangular-shaped defect with loose skin available ventral to the defect. (A) One inverted triangle is created several base-widths away from the original triangular defect. (B) Following undermining of the skin, vertical mattress sutures are placed at the base of the triangles to pull them into apposition. (C) Simple interrupted sutures are used to appose the skin.

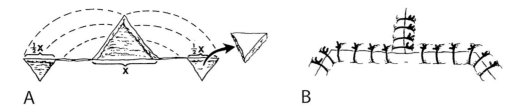

Figure 5.40. Triangular-shaped defect with loose skin available on either side. (A) Two inverted triangles, equaling 1/2 X, are created several base-widths away from the defect. The skin is undermined (dotted lines) in preparation for mobilization and closure. (B) Simple interrupted sutures are used for skin apposition.

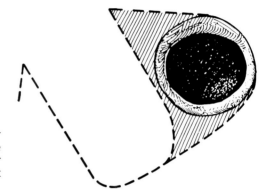

Figure 5.41. A transposition flap is created to cover a full-thickness circular defect (solid black). Dotted lines indicate incisions. The solid line indicates the circular defect. Oblique lines surrounding the circular defect represent further skin removal required to accommodate transposition of the skin flap from left to right.

more freely moveable, such as the neck and trunk, the transposition flap is occasionally used in tight-skinned regions, such as in the head, to cover a defect (e.g., nasocutaneous fistula) (Figure 6.44a). The length and width of a transposition flap should be slightly longer and wider than the defect itself. In the case of pedicle skin flaps, the work of Hinchcliff, et al. showed a positive correlation between flap width and viable length.[11] Since the transposition flap's length decreases as the arc of rotation increases and the horse's skin lacks the extensibility seen in small animals, the flap should be created as close to the lesion as possible (Figure 5.41). Often in tight-skinned regions, a small defect may remain and need to heal by second intention (Figure 6.44f). For more information regarding the use of a transposition flap for the repair of nasocutaneous fistula, see Chapter 6.

Vascularized Free Tissue Transfers

Large wounds, particularly those involving the distal limb, remain difficult to treat using reconstructive surgical techniques. Vascularized free tissue transfers, based on axial pattern flaps and using microvascular anastomosis, are commonly used in small animals.[17,53-55] Attempts have been made to adapt this approach for use in the horse.[56] In the horse, a large free axial pattern skin flap and microvascular anastomosis using the deep circumflex iliac artery and vein[57,58] and a smaller skin flap using the saphenous artery and medial saphenous vein have been described.[59] In these experimental studies none of the transferred skin flaps survived longer than 4 to 6 days. Failure was believed to result from ischemia reperfusion injury, vascular thrombosis, and poor perfusion as a result of vasospasm, known as a "no-reflow" phenomenon, within the skin flap. An experimental study showed no difference in the accumulation of neutrophils, a significant source of oxygen free radicals, between the control myocutaneous flap and those subjected to ischemia and reperfusion.[60] More work is needed to define the potential benefits of this approach.

Conclusion

The aim of reconstructive surgery is to shorten healing time, improve cosmesis of the site over that which would be achieved by second intention healing, and return the horse to performance as soon as possible.

Reconstructive techniques range from the use of simple tension-relieving measures to complex vascularized free tissue transplants. While most skin wounds should be closed using the simplest approach, considering the scarceness of loose skin in our equine patient, the various methods described in this chapter to mobilize surrounding skin to cover a defect are often overlooked in practice. By successfully applying these techniques, the potentially deleterious effects associated with second intention healing (e.g., slow contraction, excessive unsightly scarring, and reduced function) can be avoided. This chapter has attempted to provide the practical information required to safely apply the various techniques of reconstructive surgery in hopes that it will stimulate interest and encourage their use in practice.

References

1. Kirk MD: Selective scar revision and elective incision techniques applicable to the legs of horses; part 1. Vet Med Small Anim Clin 1976;71:661
2. Kirk MD: Selective scar revision and elective incision techniques applicable to the legs of horses. part 2. Vet Med Small Anim Clin 1976;71:801
3. Stashak TS: Reconstructive surgery in the horse. J Am Vet Med Assoc 1977;170:143
4. Stashak TS: Full thickness sliding skin flaps for reconstructive surgery in the horse. Proc Am Assoc Equine Pract 1978;24:395
5. McGuire MF: Studies of the excisional wound: I. Biomechanical effects of undermining and wound orientation on closing tension and work. Plast Reconst Surg 1980;66:419
6. Peyton LC: Reconstructive surgical techniques in the horse. J Am Vet Med Assoc 1981;179:460
7. Pavletic MM, Peyton LC: Plastic and reconstructive surgery in the dog and cat. In Joseph Bojrab, ed. *Current techniques in small animal surgery (2nd edition)*. Philadelphia: Lea and Febiger, 1983, p.424
8. Stashak TS: Mobilization of adjacent skin to cover full surface defects for the practice of large animal surgery. In Paul Jennings, ed. *Large animal surgery (1st edition)*. Philadelphia: WB Saunders, 1984, p.305
9. Bailey JV: Principles of reconstructive surgery. In Jorge Auer and John Stick, eds. *Equine surgery (3rd edition)*, St. Louis: Elsevier Saunders, 2006, p.254
10. Peyton LC, Campbell ML, Wolf GA, et al: The use of random skin flaps in equine reconstructive surgery. Equine Vet Sci 1983;3:80
11. Hinchcliff KW, MacDonald DR, Lindsay WA: Pedicle skin flaps in ponies: viable length is related to flap width. Equine Vet J 1992;24:26
12. Bristol DG: The effect of tension on perfusion of axial and random pattern flaps in foals. Vet Surg 1992;21:223
13. Smyth GB, Brown RG, Juzwiak JS, et al: Delayed repair of an extensive lip laceration in a colt using an Estlander flap. Vet Surg 1988;17:350
14. Taylor GI, Palmer JH: The vascular territories (angiosomes) of the body: Experimental study and clinical applications. Br J Plast Surg 1987;40:113
15. Taylor GI, Minabe T: The angiosomes of the mammals and other vertebrates. Plast Reconstr Surg 1992;89:81
16. Pavletic MM: Vascular supply to the skin of the dog. A review. Vet Surg 1980;9:77
17. Paveletic MM: Canine axial pattern flaps using the omocervical thoracodorsal and deep circumflex iliac direct cutaneous arteries. Am J Vet Res 1981;42:391
18. Lindsay WA: Wound treatment in horses: healing by third intention. Vet Med 1988;83:506
19. Hughes HV, Dransfield JW: The blood supply to the skin of the dog. Br Vet J 1959;l15:199
20. Borges AF: *Elective incisions and scar revision (1st edition)*. Boston: Little Brown, 1973, p.316
21. Swaim SF, Henderson RA: Management of skin tension. In Steven Swaim and Ralf Henderson, eds. *Small animal wound management (1st edition)*. Philadelphia: Lea and Febiger, 1990, p.87
22. Kraissl CJ: The selection of appropriate lines of elective surgical incisions. Plast Reconstr Surg 1951;l6:1
23. Irwin DHG: Tension lines in the skin of the dog. J Small Anim Pract 1966;7:593
24. Liang MD, Briggs P, Heckler FR, et al: Presuturing—a new technique for closing large skin defects: Clinical and experimental studies. Plast Reconstr Surg 1988;81:694
25. Gibson T, Kenedi RM: Biomechanical properties of skin. Surg Clin North Am 1967;47:279
26. Cartee RE, Cowles WR: Surgical implications of extensibility of the skin of the equine carpus. Am J Vet Res 1978;39:387
27. Gibson T, Kenedi RM, Carik JE: The mobile microarchitecture of dermal collagen: a bioengineering study. Br J Surg 1965;52:764
28. Madison JB: Tissue expansion. Vet Clin N Am Equine Pract 1989;5:633
29. Bigbie RB, Shealy P, Moll D. Presuturing as an aid in the closure of skin defects created by surgical excision. Proc Am Assoc Equine Pract 1990;36:613

30. Neves RI, Saggers GC, Mackay DR, et al: Assessing the role of presuturing on wound closure. Plast Reconstr Surg 1998;97:807

31. Harrison IW: Presuturing as a means of reducing skin tension in excisional biopsy wounds in four horses. Cornell Vet 1991;81:351

32. Scardino M, Swaim SF, Henderson RA: Enhancing wound closure on the limbs. Compend Contin Educ Pract Vet 1996;18:919

33. Swaim SF: Management of skin tension in dermal surgery. Compend Contin Edu Pract Vet 1980;2:758

34. Hirshowitz B, Lindenbaum E, Har-Shai Y: A skin-stretching device for the harnessing of the viscoelastic properties of skin. Plast Reconstr Surg 1993;92:260

35. Pavletic MM: Use of an external skin-stretching device of wound closure in dogs and cats. J Am Vet Assoc 2000;217:350

36. Barnea Y, Gur E, Amir A, et al: Our experience with wisebands: A new skin and soft-tissue stretch device. Plast Reconstr Surg 2004;113:862

37. Melis P, Noorlander ML, Bos KE, et al: Tension decrease during skin stretching in undermined versus not undermined skin: an experimental study in piglets. Plast Reconstr Surg 2001;107:1201

38. Wihelmi BJ, Blackwell SJ, Mancoll JS, et al: Creep vs. stretch: a review of the viscoelastic properties of skin. Ann Plast Surg 1998;41:215

39. Johnson TM, Brown MD, Sullivan MJ, et al: Immediate intraoperative tissue expansion. J Am Acad Dermatol 1990;22:283

40. Johnson TM, Lowe L, Brown MD, et al: Histology and physiology of tissue expansion. J Dermatol Surg 1993;19:1074

41. McKay DR, Saggers JC, Kotwal N, et al: Stretching skin: Undermining is more important than intraoperative expansion. Plast Reconstr Surg 1990;86:722

42. Hochman M, Branham G, Thomas RJ: Relative effects of intraoperative tissue expansion and undermining on wound closing tensions. Arch Otolaryngol Head Neck Surg 1992;118:1185

43. Austad ED, Rose GL: A self-inflating tissue expander. Plast Reconstr Surg 1982;70:588

44. Madison JB, Donawick WJ, Johnston DE, et al: The use of skin expansion to repair cosmetic defects in animals. Vet Surg 1989;18:15

45. Booth L: Tissue expanders for mobilizing skin. Proc Ann Surg Forum 1987;15:55

46. Morgan RF, Edgerton MT: Tissue expansion in reconstructive hand surgery: case report. J Hand Surg 1985;10:754

47. van Rappard JH, Molenaar J, van Doorn K et al: Surface-area increase in tissue expansion. Plast Reconstr Surg 1988;82:833

48. Austad ED, Pasyk KA, McClatchey KD, et al: Histomorphologic evaluation of guinea pig skin and soft tissue after controlled tissue expansion. Plast Reconstr Surg 1982;70:704

49. Bailey JV, Jacobs KA: The mesh expansion method of suturing wounds on the legs of horses. Vet Surg 1983;12:78

50. Vig MM: Management of integumentary wounds of extremities in dogs: An experimental study. J Am Anim Hosp Assoc 1985;21:87

51. Furnas DW, Fischer GW: The Z plasty: biomechanics and mathematics. Br J Plast Surg 1971;24:141

52. Bowman KF: Double apposing Z plasty for correction of stenotic nares in a horse. J Am Vet Med Assoc 1982;180:772

53. Fowler JD, Miller CW, Bowen V, et al: Transfer of the vascular cutaneous flaps by microvascular anastomosis: results in six dogs. Vet Surg 1987;16:446

54. Miller CW, Bowen V, Change P: Microvascular distant transfer of a cervical axial pattern flap in a dog. J Am Vet Med Assoc 1987;190:203

55. Remedios AM, Bauer MS, Bowen CV: Thoracodorsal and caudal superficial epigastric axial pattern skin flaps in cats. Vet Surg 1989;18:380

56. Bristol DG, Hudson LC, Spaulding KA: The use of a barium gelatin mixture to study equine vasculature with potential application to free flap transfer. Vet Radiol 1991;31:196

57. Lees MJ, Bowen CV, Fretz PB, et al: Transfer of deep circumflex iliac flaps to the tarsus by microvascular anastomosis in the horse. Vet Surg 1989;18:292

58. Lees MJ, Bowen CV, Fretz PB, et al: Identification of a free skin flap from the region vascularized by the deep circumflex iliac artery of horse. Am J Vet Res 1990;51:796

59. Miller CW, Hurtig M: Identification and transfer of free cutaneous flaps by microvascular anastomosis in the pony. Vet Comp Orthop Traumatol 1989;1:21

60. Scott MW, Fowler D, Matte G, et al: Effect of ischemia and reperfusion on neutrophil accumulation in the equine microvascular tissue flaps. Vet Surg 1999;28:180

6 | Management of Wounds of the Head

Spencer Barber, DVM, Diplomate ACVS, and Ted S. Stashak, DVM, MS, Diplomate ACVS

Introduction

Wounds of the head region are common in horses, particularly in those attempting to flee from a fearful situation. In the authors' experience head injuries are most likely to occur while the horse is being handled and restrained by a halter and lead rope, whereas injuries to the limbs and body more commonly occur while the horse is loose at pasture. This chapter will describe the various wounds and injuries occurring in the head region as well as the factors important to their successful management.

Lacerations

Lacerations are among the most common injuries seen in the head region. Although there are a number of important considerations regarding their management, most are treated by primary or delayed closure. There are several reasons for this:

(1) Because there is a limited amount of mobile skin on the face to provide for maximum wound contraction, wounds that heal by second intention are likely to develop a larger scar than if the wound edges had been apposed with sutures.
(2) Regions that heal primarily by epithelialization will lack hair and sebaceous and sweat glands, as well as pigmentation—an end result referred to as scar tissue epithelium.[1] Because scars and areas of hair loss on the head are highly visible, they are often considered esthetically unacceptable and can markedly decrease the horse's value.

(3) The head contains portions of several important body systems (e.g., respiratory, digestive, auditory, and ocular). Depending on the body system involved and the extent and seriousness of the injury, lacerations have the potential to interfere with the normal function that is important for performance and, in some cases, the life of the horse.[2] Consequently, lacerations involving the specific body systems are often repaired in an attempt to maintain/restore function.

Head wounds often present when they are fresh because they frequently occur during handling and are highly visible. There usually is minimal contamination because of their remote distance from the ground and fecal material. Clinical experience suggests that suturing is more successful in the management of head lacerations than those located on the limb or body. An abundant blood supply to the head has been suggested as contributing to this success.[3–5]

The subject of head wounds will be covered according to regions.

Lip

Although uncommon, lip lacerations are usually caused by sharp, protruding objects (e.g., nails) (Figure 6.1). Partial-thickness wounds can be treated either by primary or delayed primary closure or they can be allowed to heal by second intention.[5] If second intention healing is selected, the outcome, although functional, may not be cosmetically appealing. Full-thickness wounds can be difficult to treat and end-up with good cosmetic and functional results.[4–6] Left untreated, the buccal seal is often compromised, leading to feed and/or saliva drooling from the mouth.

Dehiscence, either partial or complete, is a common complication following repair but this can be overcome by using some basic reconstructive surgical principles (Figure 6.2). Excessive movement of the repair site appears to be the cause of the problem. This movement is due to the intimate attachment of the lip muscles to the dermis of the skin and the submucosa of the oral cavity. Sharply undermining the skin and mucous membrane from the muscle, in addition to employing a tension suture pattern to stabilize the repair, will largely overcome the problem of dehiscence.[4]

Lip lacerations rarely become infected following injury due to a copious blood supply. An exception to this is a split lip due to blunt trauma where the blood supply may be compromised. Although various types of

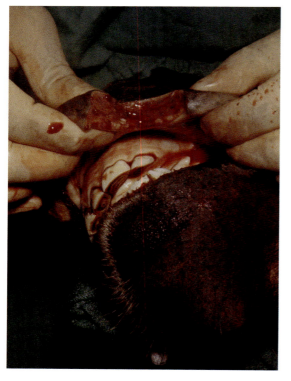

Figure 6.1. Acute sharp laceration of the rostral upper lip.

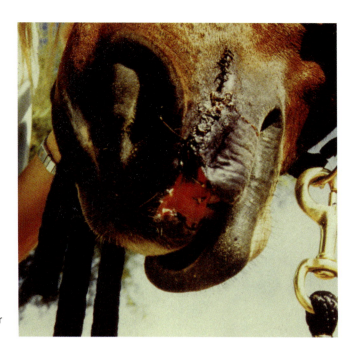

Figure 6.2. Sutured lip laceration that dehisced 6 days after reconstruction.

injury can affect the lips, we have selected an acute rostral laceration, a chronic laceration of the commissure and lower lip, and a droopy lip from facial paralysis to illustrate techniques of repair and reconstructive surgery of the region. Smyth GB, et al. (1988) described the use of a full-thickness axial pattern flap, called an Estlander flap, for the repair of an extensive laceration with loss of approximately 40% of the lower lip.[6] The reader is referred to this article for more information.

Treatment

Preoperative preparation in most cases includes the administration of penicillin G (22,000 units/Kg [10,000 IU/lb] IM) and a non-steroidal anti-inflammatory drug (NSAID). The tetanus status should be verified. The oral cavity is prepared by flushing out the feed and lavaging with a mild, sterile, antiseptic solution (e.g., 0.1%–0.2% [1–2 ml/100 ml] povidone iodine[PI]). Following removal of facial hair, the skin is prepared for surgery in a routine fashion.

Acute lacerations are draped similar to wounds in other regions except the draping material is often placed in the mouth to further isolate the wound from the oral cavity. Wound debridement and irrigation are also employed. Using a #10 Bard Parker scalpel blade, the skin and oral mucous membrane are undermined (1 to 1.5 cm) to separate them from their muscular attachments (Figures 6.3a and 6.3b). The muscles should be separated from all of the edges of the wound. Once complete, vertical mattress quill tension sutures of #0 or #1 monofilament non-absorbable sutures are preplaced so they penetrate the dissected muscles centrally and so the knots and supports will be on the outer surface of the lip when the sutures are tied later (Figures 6.3c,d).

The mucous membrane is apposed with simple interrupted or continuous sutures of 2-0–3-0 synthetic absorbable suture (Figure 6.3e). A vertical mattress pattern, using the same suture material, is used to secure the apposition of the mucocutaneous junction because this is the site where early separation often begins (Figure 6.3e). The preplaced vertical mattress quill tension sutures are then tied. The skin is apposed with interrupted vertical mattress sutures of 2-0 monofilament nylon or prolene. A vertical mattress pattern is preferred, because if simple interrupted sutures are used, inversion of the skin edges is often a problem. Soft rubber tubing (Penrose drain) is used to support the quill sutures (Figure 6.3f).

Chronic lacerations that have healed by second intention are managed in a manner similar to that used for acute lacerations. One notable difference is that scalpel dissection must begin at the scarred mucocutaneous junction and continue until the mucous membrane and skin are separated from the underlying scarred muscle (Figures 6.4a,b). Dissection should continue until approximately 1.5 cm–2 cm of the skin and mucous membrane

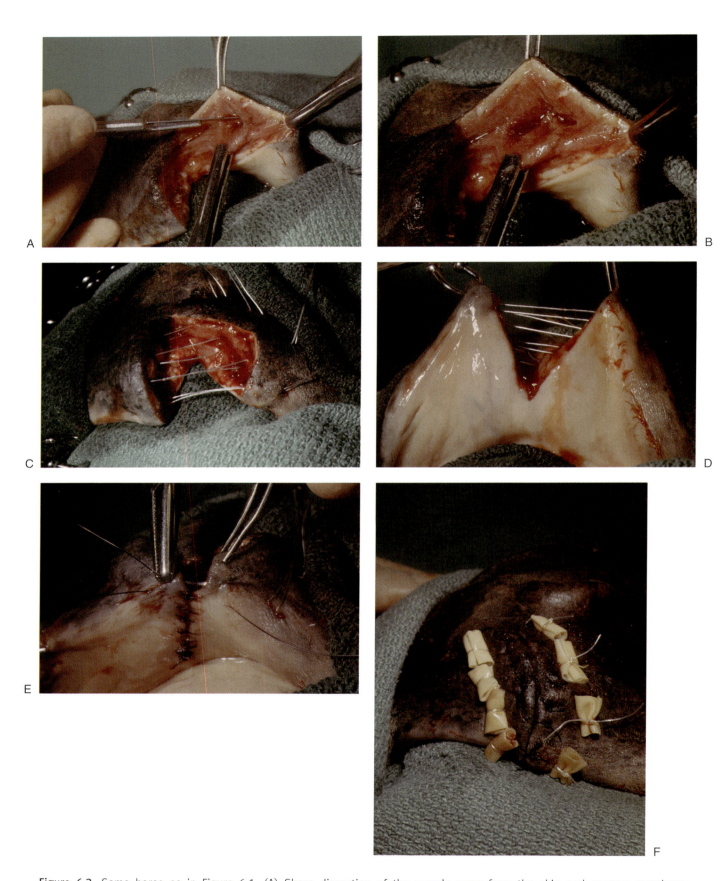

Figure 6.3. Same horse as in Figure 6.1. (A) Sharp dissection of the muscle away from the skin and mucous membrane. (B) Dissection is complete except for the muscle at the mucocutaneous junction. (C) External view of the placement of vertical mattress tension quill sutures. Both suture passages should go through the muscle. (D) Oral view of the placement of the vertical mattress tension quill sutures. (E) The mucous membrane of the oral cavity is apposed with simple interrupted sutures and the mucocutaneous junction is being sutured using a vertical mattress pattern. (F) Vertical mattress sutures appose the skin and vertical mattress quill sutures are tied over soft rubber tubing.

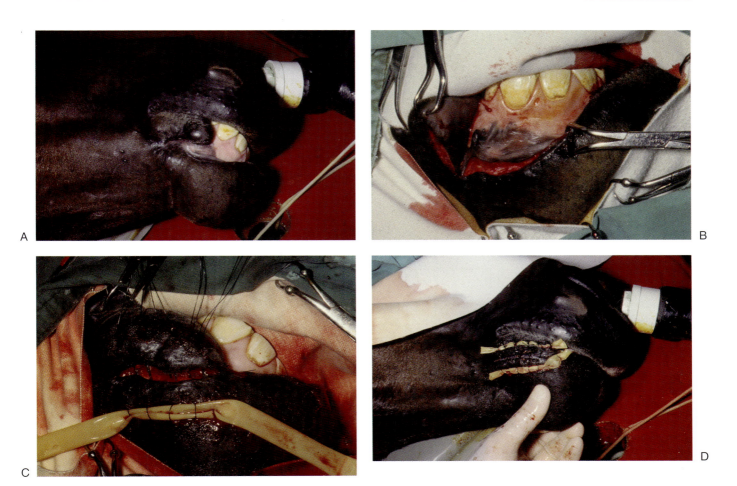

Figure 6.4. (A) Chronic lower lip laceration that was sutured on two separate occasions and dehisced following repair. (B) Incision at the mucocutaneous junction. The skin and mucous membrane must subsequently be dissected from the scarred muscle. (C) Placement of the quill vertical mattress tension sutures at least 2 cm from the repair site. The mucous membrane and scarred muscle have been apposed with sutures. (D) Repair completed.

have been undermined. Quill vertical mattress sutures are preplaced in a fashion similar to that described for the acute laceration except they penetrate the center of the scarred muscle and exit the skin at least 2 cm from the undermined skin edges (Figure 6.4c). The rest of the repair is similar to that used for acute lacerations (Figure 6.4d).

If the laceration involves the commissure of the lips an additional step should be taken to stabilize the repair site (Figures 6.5a,b). Because the lip commissure is under excessive tension when the mouth is opened, at least two additional quill vertical mattress sutures of #1 or #2 monofilament non-absorbable suture material should be placed in the intact (unaffected) lip rostral to the repair site to stabilize the region (Figures 6.5c,d).[4]

Postoperatively, antibiotics are usually continued for 24 hours and NSAIDs are recommended for 3 to 4 days or longer if needed. The patient may be cross-tied immediately or may be observed closely and cross-tied if there is any evidence of rubbing of the repair site. NSAIDs, and in some cases tranquilization, usually reduce the tendency to rub the surgical site. The first evidence of dehiscence is usually seen with separation of the lip at the mucocutaneous junction. Without signs of dehiscence, quill sutures can be removed in 7 to 10 days and skin sutures in 14 days. Feeding should proceed as normal.

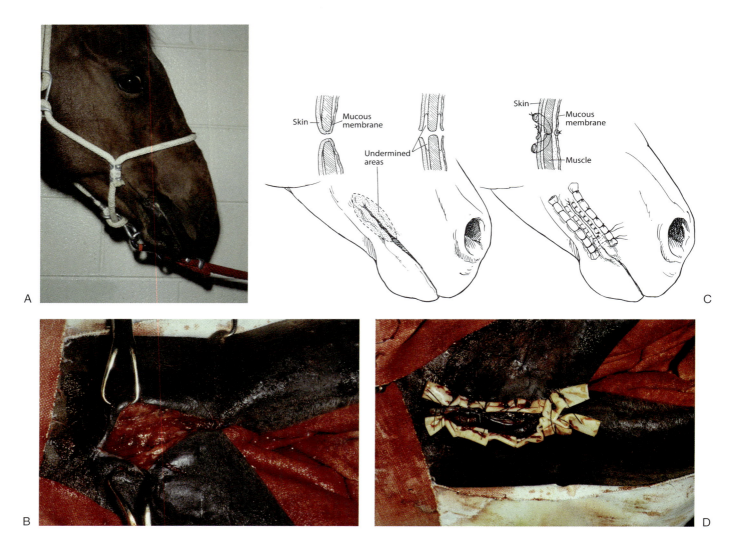

Figure 6.5. (A) Chronic laceration involving the left commissure of the lip and cheek region. (B) Dissection of skin off the cheek muscles. (C) Left bottom: dotted line and dotted area illustrate the extent of undermining of the lip and cheek; left top: two cross-sections illustrating the undermining procedures; right bottom: the laceration is sutured and two quill sutures are placed rostral to the repaired commissure to further stabilize the region; right top: cross-section illustrating suture apposition of the various layers. (D) Closure completed.

Facial Nerve

Lacerations involving the forehead region that transect the facial nerve cause a permanent sagging of the lower lip and a wry nostril and upper lip (Figures 6.6a,b). Affected horses usually maintain good body condition but paralysis of the lips results in unsightly slobbering of feed and water as well as drooling.

Treatment

Wedge resection of the lower lip is adequate to obtain an acceptable result.[4] This approach seems to seal the mouth sufficiently to prevent slobbering and drooling. Slight improvement in the wry lip and nostril also may result. The amount of lower lip to be removed is estimated at surgery by pushing the lower and upper lips back into their normal position. The lower lip should approximate the upper lip. Because the upper lip will droop slightly under the influence of general anesthesia, it also must be manipulated back into normal position. It is important to avoid pulling the lips into position by applying caudal tension at the commissure. Instead,

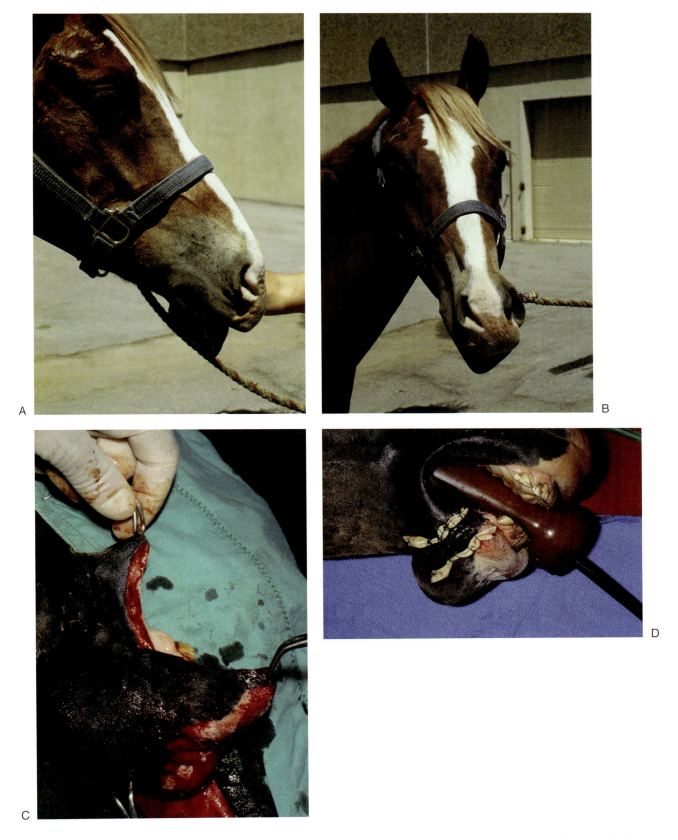

Figure 6.6. (A) Lateral view of a horse with transection of the facial nerve. The lips on the right side are droopy and the tongue protrudes slightly. Note the scar between the ear and the eye. (B) Frontal view of the same horse. Note the wry appearance to the right lips and nostril. (C) Wedge resection of the lower lip completed. (D) Sutured lip. (E) (next page) Lateral view 1 year follow-up. Note the good apposition of the lips. (F) (next page) Frontal view 1 year follow-up.

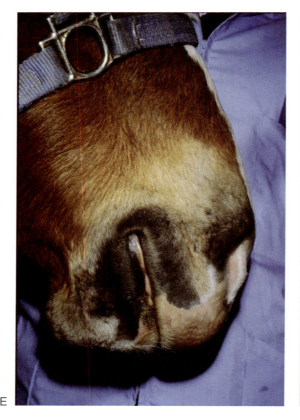
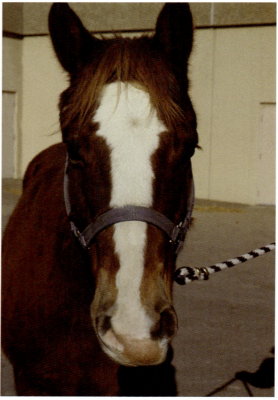

E   F

Figure 6.6. *Continued*

the lips are pushed back from their sagged position by applying pressure on the muzzle. By using this technique the lower lip will bulge laterally, allowing an estimate of the amount of tissue to be removed.

A full-thickness triangular wedge of lip is removed. The apex of this wedge is ventral, extending to the reflection of the mucous membrane onto the gum while the base is at the lip margin (Figure 6.6c). After the wedge of tissue is removed, the mucous membrane and skin are undermined to separate them from the underlying atrophied muscle. Vertical mattress quill tension sutures of #0 or #1 monofilament non-absorbable sutures are preplaced so they penetrate the dissected atrophied muscles centrally and so the knots and supports will be on the outer surface of the lip when the sutures are tied later. The mucous membrane is sutured from the oral cavity, so that the knots are oral, using 2-0 synthetic absorbable suture in a simple interrupted or continuous pattern. The skin is apposed with 2-0 non-absorbable monofilament sutures in a vertical mattress pattern, after which the preplaced tension quill sutures are tied (Figure 6.6d).

Postoperatively, antibiotics are continued for 24 hours and NSAIDs are continued for 2 to 3 days and in some cases longer if needed. The horse should be either cross-tied initially or observed closely for any signs of rubbing of the surgical site. In the latter instance, if rubbing is observed, cross-tying should be considered along with continued administration of NSAIDs and possibly tranquilization. The first evidence of dehiscence is usually seen with separation of the lip at the mucocutaneous junction. If healing progresses normally, tension sutures can be removed in 7 to 10 days and skin sutures can be removed 14 days postoperatively. According to the horse's disposition, sutures within the oral cavity can also be removed. Generally, a cosmetic and functional end result is achieved (Figures 6.6e,f).

Tongue

Lacerations of the tongue may occur during recovery from general anesthesia, when a horse rears or pulls away when tied fast by the reins with the bit in its mouth, or when sharp objects are placed in the mouth.[4,5] The lacerations normally run transversely across the dorsal surface and extend a variable distance into the tongue's

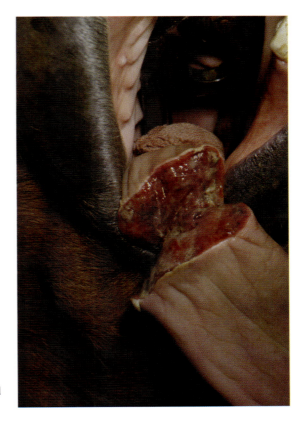

Figure 6.7. Deep laceration of the tongue, which would likely become flail if not sutured.

musculature. If left to heal by second intention, the constant motion of the tongue, saliva, and irritation to the wound repair site from feed will produce a variably sized (i.e., width and depth) defect or groove at the tongue's surface.

This defect can cause two problems: (1) The bit may periodically lodge in the defect, causing problems with head control and performance or causing periodic re-injury and bleeding. (2) If the defect is deep the tongue may not remain straight between the dental arcades (e.g., flail tongue) and can subsequently be injured by the teeth. So while most lacerations heal without suturing, long-term problems may develop with some that are unsutured. The depth and extent of the laceration, its location, and the intended use of the horse will determine if the wound is to be sutured. While lacerations involving <30% of the tongue's depth can be left to heal by second intention, deeper lacerations definitely should be sutured (Figure 6.7).

Because the tongue's vascular and nerve supply is located in the ventral half of the tongue, even very deep lacerations can be successfully sutured. However, in some cases amputation will be required due to complete loss of the blood supply. In most cases the color, temperature, and the cutting of the tongue with a blade to see if it bleeds can provide a reasonable assessment of the vascular supply. If a question still exists, fluorescein dye (1.2 mg/kg) can be administered intravenously. In a limited number of cases where amputation was required, even back to the junction of the frenulum, no functional abnormalities were observed in the postoperative period. Because of the copious blood supply, most tongue lacerations can be repaired regardless of the duration since injury.

Treatment

Preoperative preparation includes the administration of penicillin G, (22,000 units/Kg [10,000 IU/lb] IM) and NSAIDs. The oral cavity is prepared by flushing out the feed, scrubbing the tongue, and lavaging caudal to the laceration with a mild, sterile, antiseptic solution (e.g., 0.1%–0.2% [1–2 ml/100 ml] povidone iodine). The portim of the tongue can be exteriorized and stabilized using towel clamps.

Small lacerations at the tip of the tongue can sometimes be repaired in a standing sedated horse; however, general anesthesia is preferred for more extensive injuries or those that are located more caudally on the tongue.

Under general anesthesia the tongue is exteriorized by traction with a towel clamp placed in the dorsum of the tongue or by a gauze loop placed around the tongue caudal to the laceration. The exposed portions of the tongue can be isolated by draping (Figure 6.8a).

Debridement of a thin margin of the wound edges with a scalpel is usually all that is required to produce viable wound edges; however, this must be done without excessive removal of tissue to prevent a dorsal or lateral deviation. Because of the constant movement of the tongue and the presence of saliva, bacteria, and feed at the sutured site postoperatively, it is important to close as much dead space as possible and accurately approximate the tongue's surface to reduce the risk of dehiscence.

The dorsal surface of the tongue has the greatest strength and will hold tension sutures well, but the tissue edges on all sides must be accurately sutured. The lacerations normally run transversally across the tongue and extend from the dorsal surface down into the depths of the tissue. Absorbable suture material is preferred because it prevents the necessity for suture removal. Vertical mattress tension sutures of #0 monofilament synthetic absorbable sutures that penetrate the laceration in the muscle to at least half the depth of the wound are placed, with the knots tied on the external surface (Figure 6.8b). This layer gives greater strength to the repair. Above this, synthetic absorbable monofilament sutures (0 or 2-0) that are buried are used to appose the lacerated muscles and eliminate dead space. The mucous membrane is apposed with a similar suture placed in a vertical mattress pattern (Figures 6.8c,d) or a combination of vertical mattress and simple interrupted sutures.

If the laceration is severe and the blood supply is lost, amputation followed by oversewing the remaining stump with mattress sutures is indicated. Incision of a transverse wedge-shaped piece of tissue from the viable tip facilitates suturing of the dorsal and ventral aspects of the tongue.[5]

Postoperatively, antibiotics are continued for 24 hours and NSAIDs for 2 to 3 days; however, if the tongue's blood supply is marginal, these medications can be continued longer. Eating does not appear to be affected after repair or amputation; however, food that is soft is recommended. A good functional end result is expected in most cases (Figure 6.8e)

Nostril

Lacerations of the nostril are usually caused by a protruding object. The object may be blunt or sharp and lacerate the nostril from within or from the outside. A common offender is an angled bolt protruding from a gate or a horse trailer.[4] Horses predisposed to these lacerations are often "head shy."

If the laceration is extensive and full-thickness, the soft tissues will collapse during inspiration and flutter during expiration. The collapse is due to an inability to properly dilate the nostril and the negative inspiratory pressure. As with other regions of the head, the nostrils benefit from a good blood supply which ensures that repair will be successful even when carried out days after injury.

Laceration at the lateral margin (base) of the nostril can be problematic following repair, however, because of tension/shearing forces applied to the surgical site and a tendency to rub the area. Tension/shearing forces result from muscle contractions associated with movement of the lips and those associated with movement of the alar cartilages when the nostrils dilate. Rubbing the site can be discouraged by administering NSAIDs, cross-tying, and/or the application of a half-muzzle. Repair of a full-thickness laceration to the arch of the nostril is fairly straightforward and rarely problematic. In both cases, however, the horse may attempt to rub the repair site postoperatively; therefore, it must be closely observed during this period or cross-tied. Administration of penicillin G, (22,000 units/Kg [10,000 IU/lb] IM) and NSAIDs is recommended.

Occasionally, a horse will present with a history of trauma to a nostril that has been allowed to heal by second intention (Figure 6.9a) or it was sutured and the end result is a stenotic nostril. If the stenosis occurs following second intention healing, and only the most rostral aspect (external orifice) of the nostril is involved, two Z plasties may be used to increase the diameter of the opening (Figure 6.9b).[7] However, if the stenosis occurs following closure of a full-thickness laceration that extended caudal for at least two-thirds the length of the false nostril, the sutured site will have to be incised and re-apposed in such a fashion so that the normal arch of the nostril is restored.

Treatment

Acute lacerations of the dorsal arch of the nostril (Figure 6.10a) are best managed by suturing the defect with #2-0 monofilament nylon in an interrupted pattern placed in a modified figure-8 fashion (Figure 6.10b).[4]

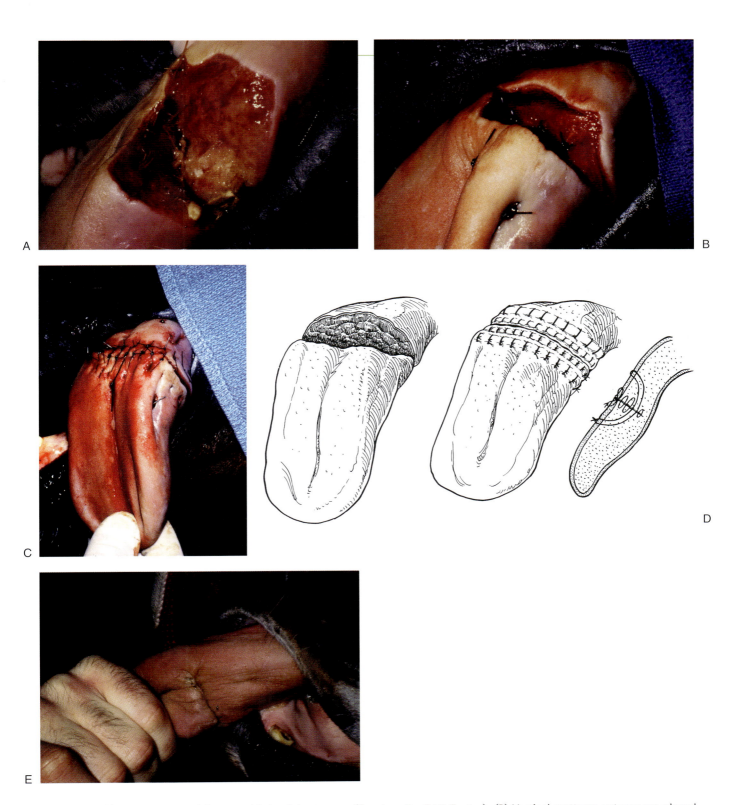

Figure 6.8. (A) Laceration involving two-thirds of the tongue (Courtesy Dr. G.W. Trotter). (B) Vertical mattress sutures are placed and the muscles are apposed with a simple interrupted suture pattern. (C) Repair completed. (D) Combination of vertical mattress and simple interrupted suture patterns. (E) Top view of healed tongue laceration.

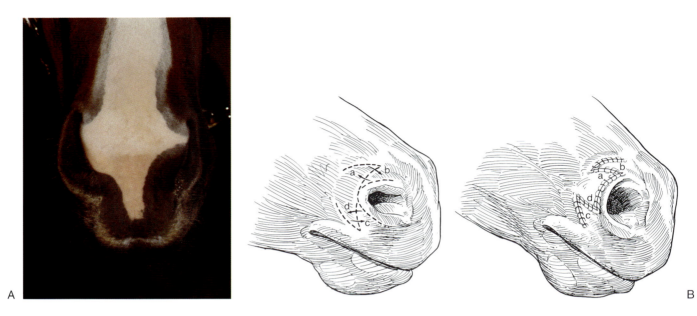

A   B

Figure 6.9. (A) Limited left nostril opening following suture repair 3 months earlier. This racehorse was presented for inadequate and noisy air flow through the left nostril. (B) Left: constricted nostril due to scarring (dotted lines illustrate incisions for Z plasties); right: Z plasties completed and sutured. The diameter of the nostril is enlarged.

The suture begins on one side of the skin and is passed halfway through the thickness of tissue, crosses the laceration to enter the opposite side at a similar location, and then penetrates the skin of the false nostril (Figure 6.10c). The suture is then passed through the opposite skin surface and penetrates the tissue in a similar fashion, yet reversed from what is previously described (Figure 6.10b). Once the skin on the outer surface of the nostril has been penetrated, the suture is tied (Figure 6.10d). The advantages of this approach are speed of application, good apposition of all tissue layers, and the ability to remove the sutures by cutting a single loop. Alternatively, simple interrupted sutures may be used; however, a tendency for gaping of the wound between those sutures is common.

Acute lacerations of the base of the nostril are best handled by primary closure in most cases (Figure 6.11a).[4] After cleansing and lavage, the nostril is packed with sterile gauze after which the surgical field is draped (Figure 6.11b). The wound should be debrided but care must be taken not to further compromise the blood supply to the flap of tissue (Figure 6.11c). Because the tissue at the base of the nostril is influenced by movement of the muscles of the upper lips and movement of the alar cartilage—thus it is more mobile than that at the arch—a three-layer closure is strongly recommended (Figure 6.11d). A three-layer closure provides greater security and better approximation of tissue than a single- or double-layer closure. The mucous membrane is sutured from within the nostril using a continuous horizontal mattress suture of 2-0 synthetic absorbable suture material (Figure 6.11d, right). The deep tissue should be apposed with a similar suture material placed in a simple interrupted fashion and the skin apposed with 2-0 monofilament nylon in an interrupted vertical mattress suture pattern (Figures 6.11d,e).

Chronic lacerations of the base of the nostril that have healed by second intention, without treatment or following dehiscence, present special problems (Figures 6.12a,b).[4] Because the wound edges have epithelialized and contracted, the flap of tissue may be smaller than its original size and without fresh edges for closure. Therefore, incision and undermining are required to reform the inner and outer epithelial layers of both the nostril base and the flap. However, care should be taken during preparation of the free edges to remove a minimal amount of tissue (Figure 6.12c).

The first step is to make an incision in the nostril base that extends along the line of injury from the base of the flap rostrally to the site where the most rostral tip of the flap will lay without reducing luminal diameter. The tissue is then undermined laterally and medially to produce two fresh edges of epithelialized tissue, one

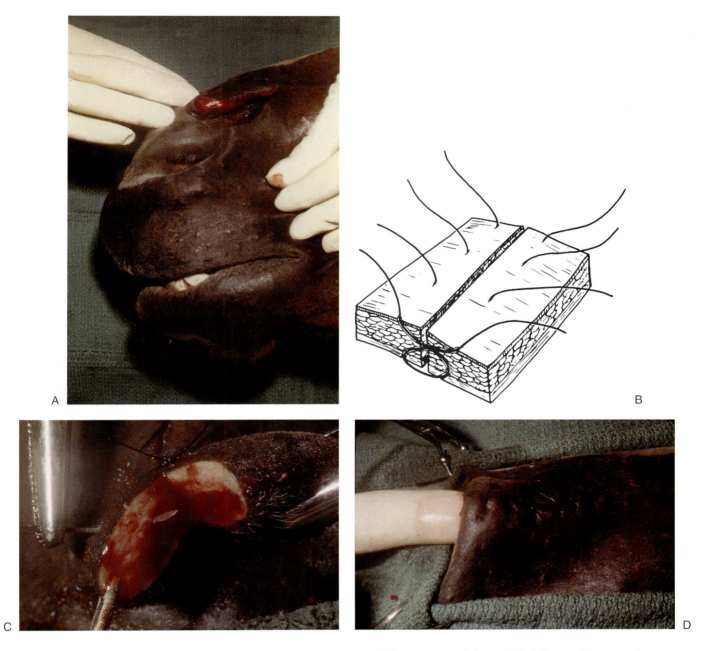

Figure 6.10. (A) Sharp laceration of the dorsal arch of the left nostril. (B) Placement of the modified figure-8 interrupted suture pattern that apposes both epithelial surfaces. (C) Passage of the suture through half the thickness of tissue. It then will enter the tissue on the opposite side and exit through the skin within the false nostril. (D) Suturing is complete.

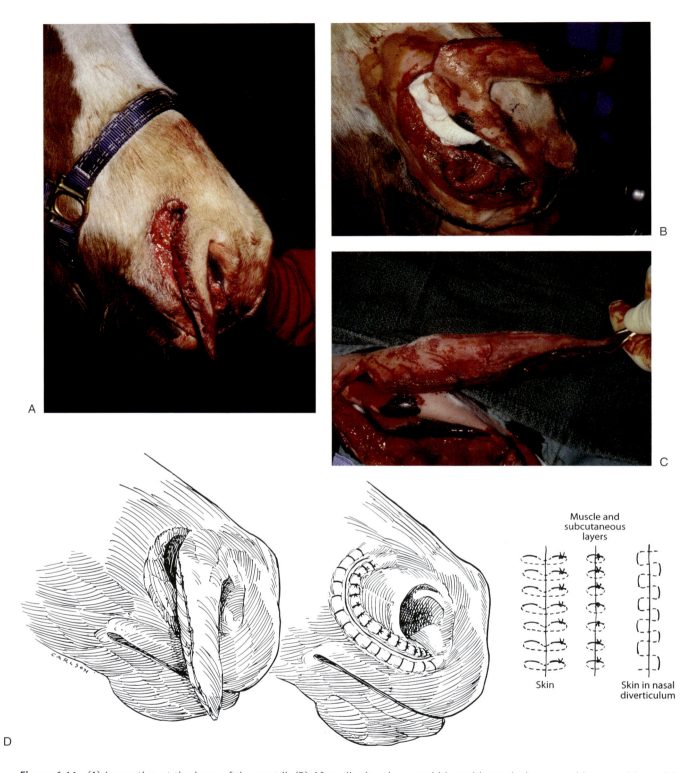

Figure 6.11. (A) Laceration at the base of the nostril. (B) After clipping then scrubbing with surgical soap and lavage with a mild antiseptic solution, the nostril is packed with sterile gauze. (C) Debridement is complete. Note the limited attachment of the caudal extent of the skin flap. (D) Left: laceration; middle: suture of the nostril; right: suture patterns used for the three-layer closure. (E) (next page) Suturing completed.

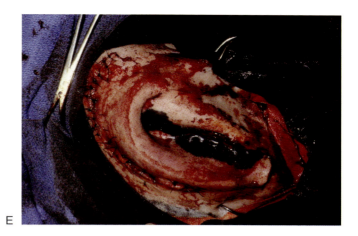

Figure 6.11. *Continued*   E

external the other inside the false nostril (Figure 6.12c, top). Then in a similar manner an incision is made in the tissue flap to create inner and outer edges (Figure 6.12c, top). The fresh edges produced by these incisions are sutured as described for acute lacerations. Closure is usually performed by suturing from the base of the flap toward its tip (Figures 6.12d,e).

Alternatively, the closure may start by suturing the tip of the flap to the appropriate spot on the nostril base. Remember that pulling the flap too rostral can result in stenosis of the nostril and will place increased tension on closure of the remainder of the wound. In addition, a muzzle that covers the nostril but also allows the horse to eat and drink can be applied to prevent the horse from rubbing the surgical site (Figure 6.12f).

Postoperatively, antibiotic therapy is continued for 24 hours and NSAIDs are recommended for 3 to 7 days. If the horse begins to rub the surgical site, it should be cross-tied or muzzled. The administration of NSAIDs for a longer period should be considered; occasionally, tranquilization may also be beneficial. Sutures are removed in 10 days for a repaired arch laceration and 14 days for a repaired laceration at the base of the nostril. Without rubbing, healing is usually problem-free and a good cosmetic end result can be expected.

Eyelid

Eyelid lacerations are relatively common and are often caused by sharp or blunt protruding objects.[4,8–11] The horse either runs into the object, lacerating the eyelid, or hooks the object underneath the lid and pulls away rapidly, tearing it. If a lid laceration is caused by a kick from another horse or is the result of running into or being hit by a blunt object, it is critical to examine the bony orbit for fractures (see management of fractures of the Medial Orbital Rim and Zygomatic [Supraorbital] Process in this chapter). In all cases, the eye must be assessed for trauma and a general physical examination should follow. Both the upper and lower eyelids can be affected. Because of a generous blood supply, most severe lacerations, including skin flaps of the eyelid, can be salvaged for repair. Even in the case of a very small base, it often survives such that every attempt at repair is made (Figures 6.13a–d).[8,9] This is critical because no available tissue can duplicate the function of the muco-cutaneous junction of the eyelid.[8,9]

Generally speaking, eyelid lacerations <3 hours in duration can be prepared for surgery immediately. Lacerations between 3 and 12 hours old may be treated surgically immediately unless there is excessive edema and severe contamination. Because swelling is often severe and infection may be a problem, lacerations >12 hours in duration are usually treated the following day by delayed primary closure. Following sedation, the eye and cornea are examined more closely. Fluorescein stain should be used to assess the corneal surface for defects or ulcerations. A tractable horse with a simple wound may be treated standing while under sedation and local anesthesia. In general, repair of lacerations extending through all layers of the eyelid and of skin flaps involving eyelid margins will require general anesthesia.

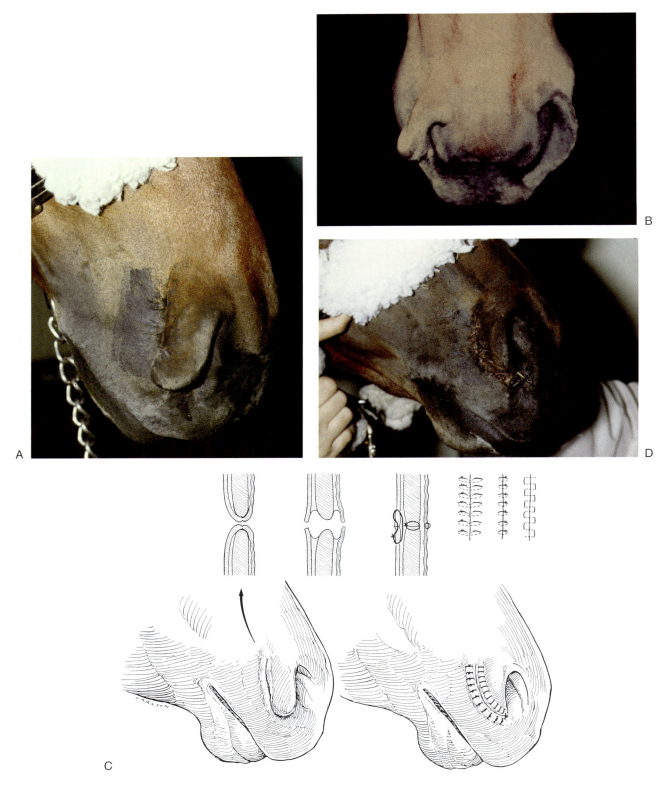

Figure 6.12. (A) Side view of a chronic laceration at the base of the right nostril. (B) Cranial view of this chronic laceration. Note the reduction in diameter of the external nares. (C) Top: dissection planes and layers of closure; bottom left: laceration at the base of the nostril; bottom right: nostril reconstruction is complete. (D) Lateral view of the reconstructed nostril. (E) (next page) Cranial view of the reconstructed nostril. Note the nostril diameter which is almost equivalent to that of the opposite normal side. (F) (next page) A half-muzzle covering the nares to protect the repair site from trauma. It was attached to the halter and because it only covered the nostrils, the horse could still eat and drink.

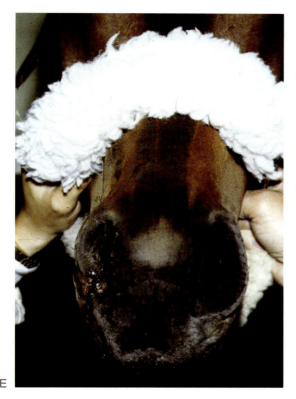
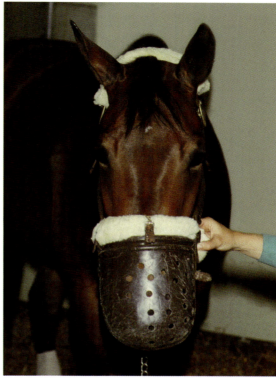

E

F

Figure 6.12. *Continued*

Treatment

Preoperative medication for acute wounds includes penicillin G, (22,000 units/Kg [10,000 IU/lb] IM) and flunixin meglumine (10 mg/kg IV). Preparation of the eyelid for surgery differs from that of other regions. The hair is clipped minimally (be gentle) but not shaved because this would create enough irritation to result in swelling. Scissors are used to trim the eyelashes. The skin and wound are gently cleaned with a 0.1%–0.2% dilute povidone iodine sterile saline solution. The solution for the final preparation is left on the skin to dry.

After appropriate isolation of the surgical field, the edges of the wound are debrided minimally, only removing tags of obviously dead tissue. Although ophthalmologic instruments are ideal, much can be done with straight and curved mosquito hemostats; Brown Addison thumb tissue forceps; and a #10, #11, or #15 Bard Parker scalpel blade.

Basic principles for surgery of the eyelid include:[4,5,8–11]

- Removal/debridement of as little tissue as possible (Figures 6.13c,d)
- Accurate alignment and careful apposition of the tissues
- In the case of a lacerated conjunctiva, the laceration should first be sutured (#4-0–6-0 synthetic absorbable suture material is recommended) so that the knots are buried in the tissue and do not rub on the cornea (Figure 6.14, a and b).

In some cases, a support skin suture must be placed first to align the tissues and reduce tension. The first skin suture is placed along the sharp edge of the lid through the meibomian gland and tied so that the knot does not contact the cornea (#4-0–6-0 non-absorbable suture material is recommended) (Figures 6.14, c and d, and 6.15a). This suture assures correct apposition and restoration of eyelid function. The next suture should be

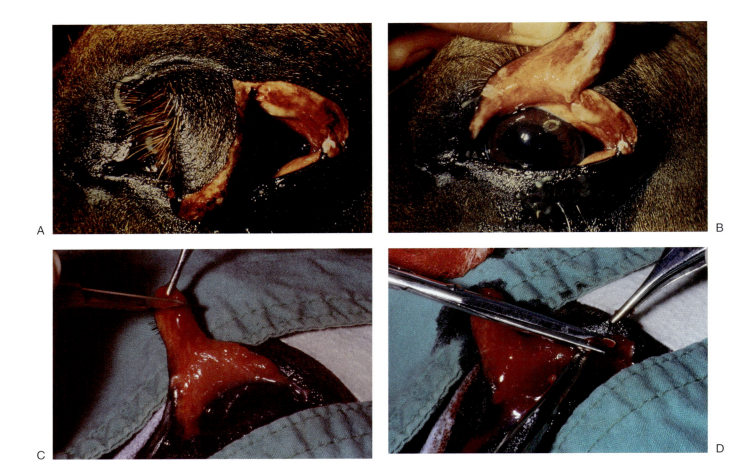

Figure 6.13. (A) Acute, full-thickness, oblique upper lid laceration. (B) Lacerated margin is elevated to expose the laceration of the conjunctiva. (C) A #11 Bard Parker blade is used to debride the laceration. (D) Scissors are used to complete the debridement. Courtesy of Dr. G. Severin.

placed deeply, 2 mm from the eyelid edge, to penetrate the tarsal plate (Figure 6.14 d,g,h). This suture takes up most of the tension. Alternatively, a figure-8 pattern can be used (Figure 6.14 i and j). The rest of the closure is routine, using either an interrupted or continuous suture pattern (Figure 6.15b).

If delayed primary closure is elected, the laceration and skin are cleaned with dilute PI solution after which the wound is treated liberally with Furacin ointment then bandaged (Figures 6.16a–d). Penicillin G IM and flunixin meglumine IV are administered. This approach is very effective in reducing the edema and in most cases the wound can be sutured after 24 hours of treatment. Wound preparation and suturing follows the steps just described for primary closure (Figures 6.16e,f).

Postoperatively, systemic antibiotic therapy is recommended for 24 hours in treating a "fresh" wound without signs of infection and should be prescribed for 5 to 7 days if the wound was infected. NSAIDs can be administered for 3 to 5 days to reduce local inflammation and patient discomfort. Longer treatment with NSAIDs should be recommended if the eye had signs of uveitis. Avoid excess manipulation of the eyelid to reduce the risk for misalignment of the mucocutaneous eyelid junction. Disruption of the eyelid margin will cause a notch defect, which could contribute to future corneal disease.

Local antibiotics are not recommended unless the cornea was injured and/or the eyelid wound was infected. If deemed necessary and the upper eyelid was sutured, then the antibiotic can be instilled under the lower

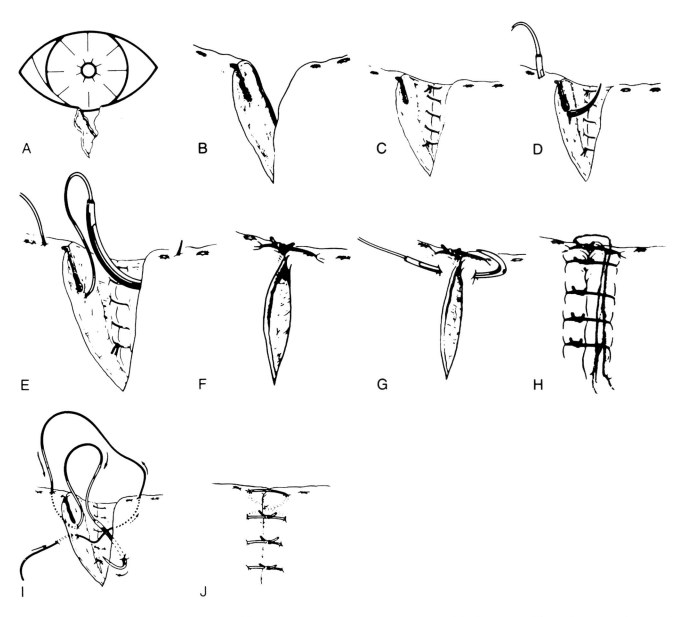

Figure 6.14. Repair of an eyelid laceration. (A) Full-thickness lower eyelid laceration. (B) Close-up of (a). Dark lines at the eyelid margin illustrate the tarsal plate. (C) Continuous sutures are used to appose the conjunctiva. Note that the knots are placed so they are buried in tissue and will not rub on the cornea. (D, E, and F) Suture is placed along the lid margin through the meibomian gland and tied so the knot does not contact the cornea. (G) The second skin suture is placed through the tarsal plate and tied to take up the tension. (H) Simple interrupted sutures appose the skin. (I) Illustrates a figure-8 suture to appose the lid margin and suture the tarsal plate. (J) Simple interrupted suture closure. Courtesy of Dr. G. Severin.

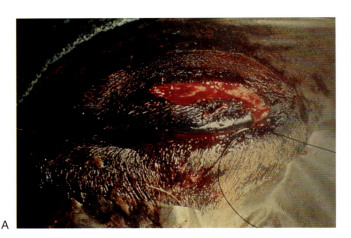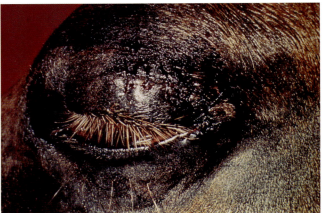

A   B

Figure 6.15. Same horse as in Figure 6.13. (A) The apex of the laceration was sutured into its normal position to assure good alignment. (B) The eyelid 14 days post-operatively. Courtesy of Dr. G. Severin.

eyelid by displacing only the lower lid rostrad. If the lower eyelid was sutured, topical medication can be administered via a subpalpebral lavage system placed under the upper eyelid. Application of warm compresses and cleansing debris from the medial canthus reduce discomfort and additional contamination risks. Bandaging, a fly mask, and/or protective goggles or cup ("Eye Saver") might be necessary to protect the wound and reduce self trauma.[5,8] Cross-tying should be considered if rubbing and self trauma is a problem. Skin sutures can be removed 14 days following closure.

Ears

Injury to the ears, although uncommon, can be the result of freezing due to very cold weather, bites, and lacerations.[4,5,12] Usually only the tips of the ears are involved in the cases of freezing and bite injuries (Figures 6.17 and 6.18).

Occasionally, greater portions of the ear are affected (Figure 6.19a). Because the ears are flexible and mobile, they are not frequently lacerated but when they are, it is usually by sharp, protruding objects. If left untreated, lacerated ears tend to curl or flop over and become unsightly and non-functional in some situations (Figures 6.19a and 6.20).[4,13,14] As with other regions of the head, the ears are well vascularized and therefore, if properly treated, a good functional result is usually achieved.

Treatment

General principles in handling ear lacerations include:

- Minimal debridement of the soft tissues (Figures 6.21a,b)
- Removal of a narrow edge of the cartilage on both sides
- Suturing of only the soft tissues without penetrating the cartilage (Figures 6.19b, 6.21c,d) except if a stent is applied, in which case sutures must penetrate the ear some distance from the wound (Figure 6.21e). If the ear bends, curls, or flaps over due to the injury (Figure 6.19a), a support stent made of X-ray film, rolled gauze, or thermoplastic material can be applied to the inside of the ear (Figure 6.19b) following suture repair (Figure 6.19c).[4,12–14] An ear stent may need to be left in place for 4 weeks. This period is necessary to provide support until the ear cartilage has healed enough to hold the ear in an upright position.[14]

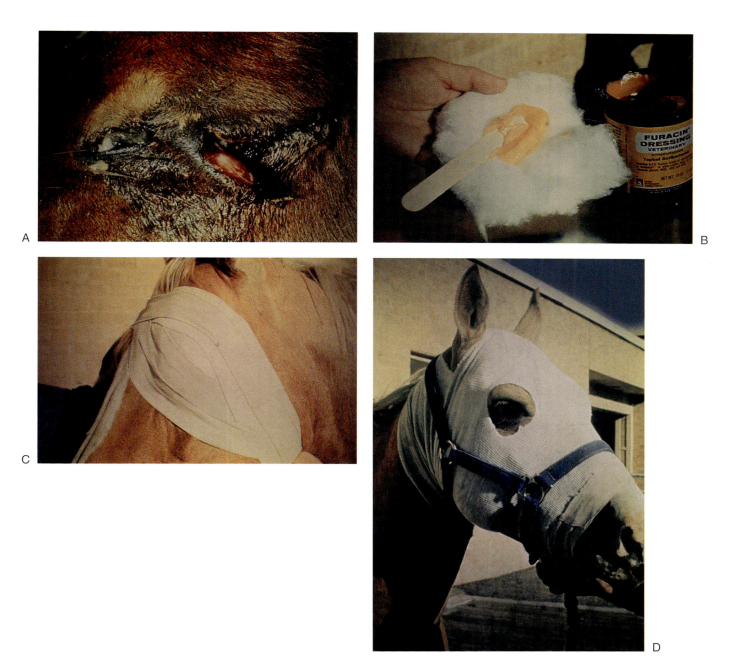

Figure 6.16. (A) Full-thickness laceration of the upper eyelid. Delayed primary closure was the selected approach due to a period since wounding of >12 hours and due to the amount of swelling and contamination (Courtesy of Dr. Glenn Severin). (B) Furacin ointment is being applied liberally to cotton dressing. (C) Elastic adhesive bandage material holds the cotton/Furacin ointment dressing in place. (D) Six-inch orthopedic stockinet head bandage is applied to further protect the region. (E) (next page) Sutured laceration. (F) (next page) Fourteen days postoperatively, sutures are removed. A cosmetic and functional end result was achieved.

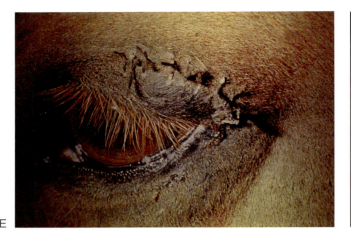
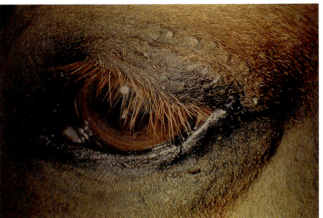

E   F

Figure 6.16. *Continued*

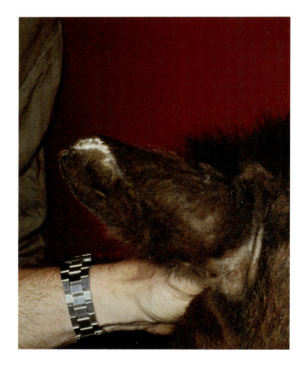

Figure 6.17. The tip of an ear was lost due to frostbite.

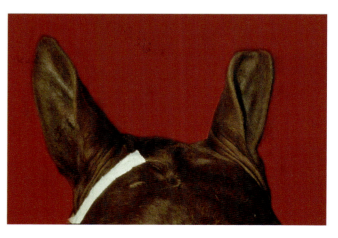

Figure 6.18. The tip of the left ear was bitten off by the dam.

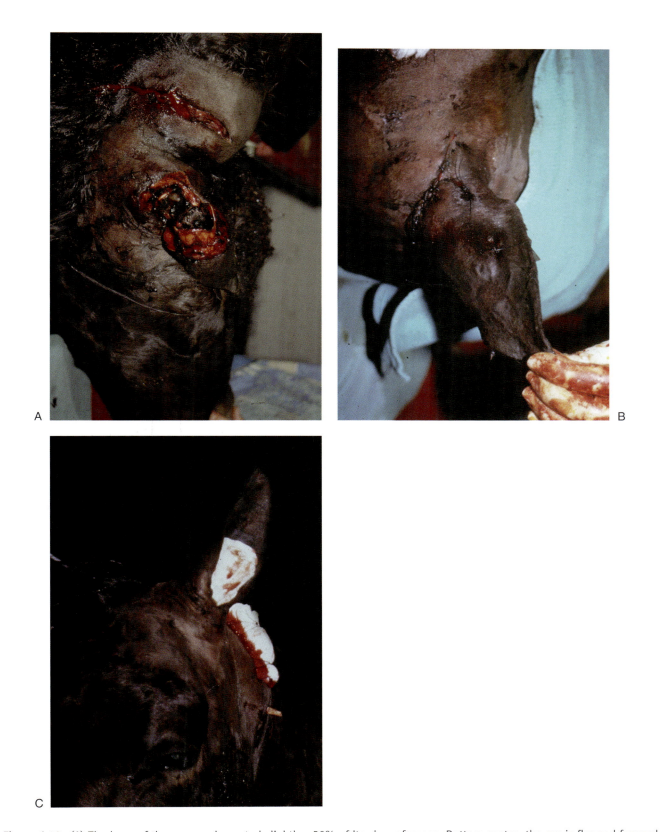

Figure 6.19. (A) The base of the ear was lacerated slightly >50% of its circumference. Bottom center: the ear is flopped forward and the tip resides above the lateral canthus of the eye. Muscles transected included parietoauricularis, scutuloauricularis superficialis, and scutuloauricularis supeficialis accessories. Another laceration is seen caudal (upper center) to the lacerated ear. (B) Following suturing of the muscles, the skin at the base of the ear was sutured. (C) Rolled gauze was packed in the ear canal and sutured to support the ear in an upright position until healing was complete. A head bandage was applied to encircle the affected ear. The drain was removed within 2 days. The gauze stent was removed 4 weeks postoperatively.

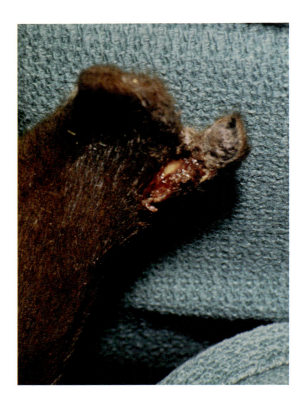

Figure 6.20. A chronic ear laceration, if left untreated, would become thickened and curled and have a forked tip. Courtesy Dr. G.W. Trotter.

Owners occasionally are interested in cosmetic reconstruction if the tip of the ear is lost due to bite injury or both tips are lost due to freezing. The ears should be completely healed before attempting reconstruction so that inflammation and infection, which could be detrimental to repair, are no longer present (Figures 6.17 and 6.18).[4]

If only one ear is involved, the opposite ear will serve as a template. Sterile paper or sterile X-ray film works well for this purpose. After the normal ear is laid flat, the template is cut to duplicate the normal ear contour. The template is then reversed and applied to the affected ear.

Because the affected ear is shorter than normal, the height of the template must be adjusted appropriately. To do this, the length of the affected ear is measured from its base to its tip. The template is then cut to that length, by trimming the base portion of the template, repositioned in a reverse fashion (mirror image) on the affected ear, and the contour drawn on the ear with a sterile marker or sterile methylene blue (Figure 6.22a). Because cosmesis is important, the measurements should be rechecked to prevent error. Once the symmetry appears satisfactory, the ears are trimmed following the previously drawn image (Figure 6.22b).

The thumb and forefinger are used to tighten the skin by pulling it toward the side opposite that to be cut. This not only facilitates cutting because the ear is held rigid, but also ensures that enough skin will be available to cover the exposed cartilage. Sharp, straight, or curved Mayo scissors are used to trim the excessive skin and cartilage. Trimming all layers of the ear at once with the scissors helps reduce the amount of bleeding and prevents retraction of the skin edge relative to the cartilage surface that would occur if they were cut independently. After the edge has been trimmed, the edge of the opposite side is trimmed in a similar fashion except the skin is pulled in the other way. The two skin surfaces are then apposed, in close approximation, with a continuous suture pattern of #3-0 synthetic monofilament non-absorbable suture (Figures 6.22c,d).

Postoperatively, antibiotic therapy is continued for 24 hours while NSAIDs and possibly tranquilizers may be required to stop the horse from rubbing its ears. In some cases, cross-tying will be necessary.

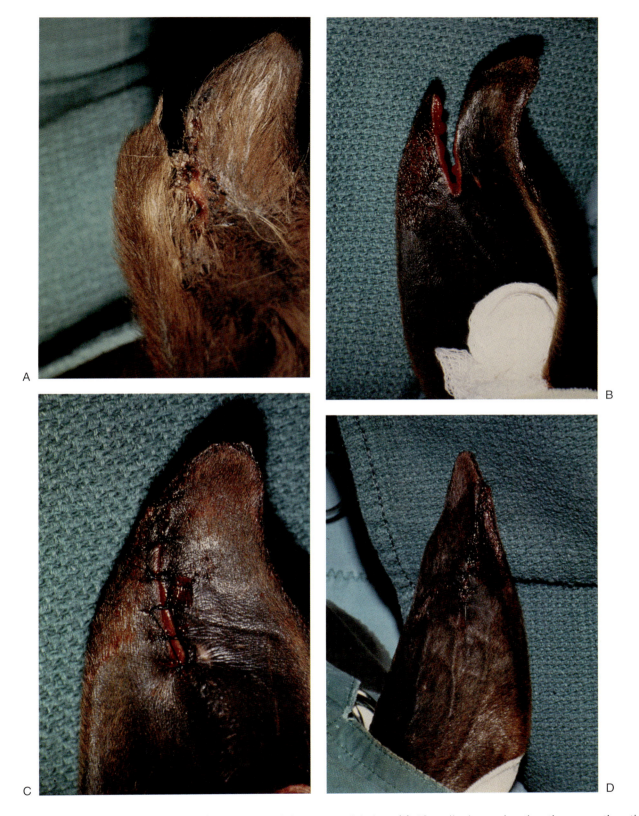

Figure 6.21. Same case as Figure 6.20. (A) Laceration of the ear, cranial view. (B) After clipping and antiseptic preparation, the laceration (skin and cartilage) was debrided. The ear canal was packed with sterile gauze. (C) The skin, only on the inner surface of the ear, is apposed with simple interrupted sutures of #3-0 nylon. (D) The skin, only on the outer surface of the ear, is apposed with simple interrupted sutures of #3-0 nylon. (E) (next page) Widely placed through-and-through #2-0 nylon sutures are used to hold a piece of X-ray film on the inner surface of the ear to hold it in an upright position. Courtesy Dr. G.W. Trotter.

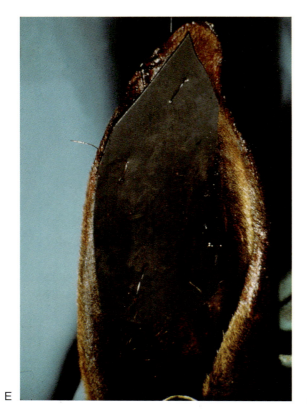

E

Figure 6.21. *Continued*

Scalping and Degloving Injuries of the Head

Forehead

V-shaped "scalping" injuries are one of the most common types of laceration seen on the head. They are often located on the forehead overlying the neurocranium (Figures 6.23a and 6.24a). These lacerations usually occur during handling when the horse throws its head and contacts the roof of a trailer or the archway of a doorway or overhead gate.[2]

The flap of tissue is typically restricted to the skin and subcutaneous tissue, and the V of the flap can be pointed either caudal or rostral while it usually has a broad base ensuring a good blood supply. The periosteum of the frontal or nasal bones may also be exposed or elevated (Figures 6.23a–d and 6.24a,b). Movement of the head causes repeated displacement of the flap, the tip of which may curl under, exposing a portion of the wound surface and possibly the bone. Generally there is minimal skin retraction immediately following the injury, allowing easy apposition of the skin edges. Suturing is indicated to prevent a major blemish.

Treatment

Acute wounds, which are usually very fresh and minimally contaminated, can be sutured in the standing sedated horse with—in some cases without—infiltration of a local anesthetic solution. The wound is prepared for surgery in a routine fashion following the principles outlined in Chapter 2.

If the periosteum is elevated, there are some additional issues to consider. The periosteum plays several roles, in particular supplying blood to the external bone cortex and acting as a protective barrier for the underlying bone should the skin be lacerated. If the periosteum has been elevated from the frontal or nasal bones, the external cortex may be ischemic.[4] Both the irregular surface of the cortex and the Volkmann canals that open at the cortical surface provide locations for bacteria to hide or gain access to the interior of the cortex. Ischemia and contaminated bone may become infected and cause sequestrum formation.[15–18]

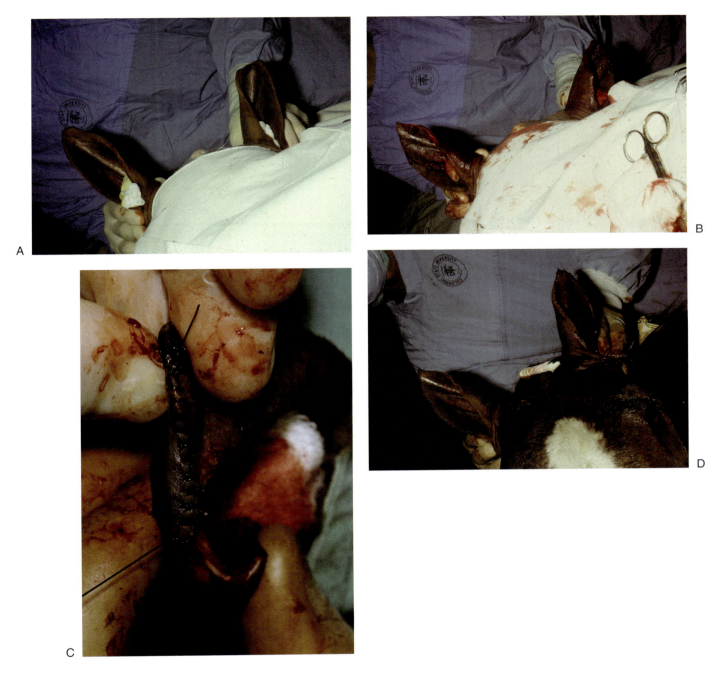

Figure 6.22. Same horse as in Figure 6.18. (A) Sterile methylene blue was used to draw the contour on the inner surface of the ear to adjust the height of the affected ear. (B) Both ears trimmed and rechecked for symmetry. (C) Ear is being sutured so that the skin completely covers the cartilage. The suture bites should be placed close enough together so that the subcutaneous tissue is completely covered. (D) Suturing completed.

The authors believe that curettage alone is ineffective at removing bacteria from the bone surface due to its irregularity, and prefer low-pressure lavage (15 PSI) or "partial decortication"—the removal of the outer ischemic and contaminated bone cortex with a pneumatic-driven burr or a hip arthroplasty rasp (Fig. 2.23). In acute wounds low-pressure lavage is likely adequate but partial decortication is preferred if there is gross contamination or if the bone is discolored or looks chalky (Figure 6.25a). Only a thin layer can be removed because these

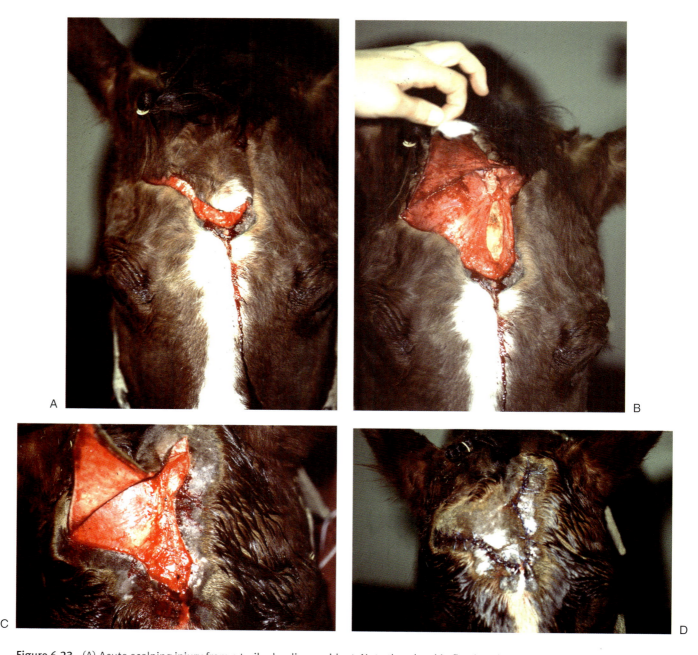

Figure 6.23. (A) Acute scalping injury from a trailer loading accident. Note that the skin flap is only slightly retracted from its normal position. (B) The wound is fresh (<3 hours) and minimally contaminated but the periosteum has been lacerated and a portion of the frontal bone is exposed. (C) Following low-pressure lavage of the bone surface, the periosteum was closed over the bone. (D) The wound is closed by suturing the flap with an interrupted suture pattern placed without excessive tension. A drain was not needed.

flat bones are thin. Once the cortical surface has been debrided, it is irrigated with a dilute PI solution applied at 10–15 PSI (Figure 6.25b), after which it is covered with viable tissue (muscle, subcutaneous tissue, or skin) to avert sequestrum formation (Figure 6.25c). For more information regarding the effects of lavage pressure and debridement on the incidence of wound infection, see Chapter 2.

In some cases there is insufficient subcutaneous tissue to be closed as a separate layer. With acute flaps the skin edges can usually be easily apposed with a synthetic non-absorbable (e.g., #2-0 nylon or Prolene or Novafil)

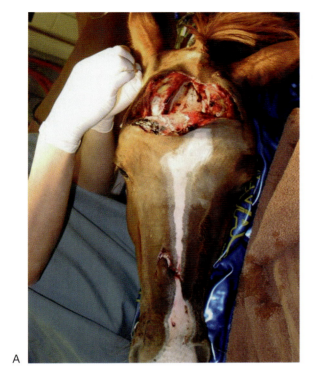
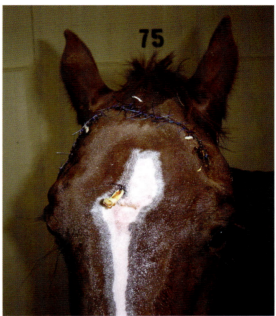

A   B

Figure 6.24. (A) Large scalping injury in a foal. The periosteum was elevated with the skin flap, but the temporal muscles were intact. Following lavage and partial decortication of the bone surface, a Penrose drain was placed deep in the wound to drain the dead space underlying the base of the flap. (B) Because there was some tension upon closure a few sutures placed in a near-far-far-near pattern were used along with a simple interrupted suture pattern.

suture material placed in a simple interrupted pattern. A near-far-far-near pattern can be used along with sub-cutaneous undermining of the wound edges if there is excessive tension during closure. Because the arms of the V are often of different lengths and the flap is retracted, complete closure of the defect is obtained if the repair is started by pulling the tip of the flap into position at the point of the V. Dead space is minimal and a drain is rarely necessary.

Chronic wounds differ in that they are desiccated and contaminated, and the skin flap can become fibrotic and fold over. In these cases general anesthesia is recommended to ensure optimal repair. Extensive layered/excisional debridement, partial decortication of any exposed cortical bone, and pressure lavage are often required. Skin closure can be challenging after a few days because both the flap and surrounding skin become less extensible. A 2 mm–3 mm strip of skin should be removed from the wound edges to create viable tissue for closure. Extensive subcutaneous dissection can safely be performed to relieve tension as long as the subcutaneous tissue is elevated with the skin and major vital structures are avoided. If tension is still a problem, mesh expansion of the surrounding skin edges (preferred) or the development of the skin flap can be useful.[19]

If there is loss of a portion of the skin flap, the defect may only be closed by using either a transposition flap or a single or bi-pedicle advancement flap.[4,19] The latter technique will leave a skin defect adjacent to the wound; however, this is preferable to leaving cortical bone uncovered.[4]

Nasal Region

Degloving injuries, which expose bone, are very similar to "scalping" injuries except they occur in the rostral portion of the head. They can involve the dorsal rostral face or the lower lip regions (Figures 6.26a–c, 6.27a,b). When the dorsal face is involved, the V of the skin flap is usually pointed caudal with reflexion of the skin and subcutaneous tissue rostrad, exposing the nasal bones which may be stripped of their periosteum or even fractured.

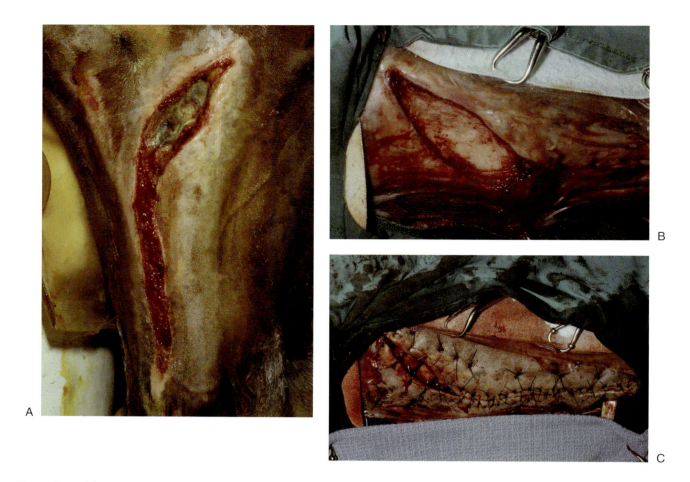

Figure 6.25. (A) Four-day-old scalping injury to the face with exposed discolored bone. (B) Forehead to the left. The wound, after debridement of the soft tissues and partial decortication of the discolored bone using a hip arthroplasty rasp. Following debridement, the wound edges were undermined and mobilized to reduce skin tension for wound closure. (C) The skin was apposed using a combination of widely placed vertical mattress and simple interrupted sutures. Alternatively, a near-far-far-near suture pattern could have been used. Only a narrow strip of the facial bone remains exposed. The region of exposed bone healed uneventfully by second intention.

Treatment

The comments regarding debridement and closure of scalping injuries generally apply to these lacerations, as well. However, if the nasal bones are fractured and displaced, fracture reduction is necessary for a cosmetic repair and to prevent impairment of air flow through the nasal passage. The fragments should be levered or elevated back into position using a bone hook and the nasal septum examined and repositioned if necessary. More commonly, nasal bones fracture and separate from their dorsal attachments to the nasal septum without damaging the latter. In the case of instability, the fragments can be secured with either stainless steel wire or suture material placed through holes drilled in the bone. If a small fragment of the nasal bone is lost, the soft tissue can usually be closed over the osseous defect without any loss of function. Penrose drains are often placed deep in the wound to allow drainage of the dead space located under the rostral aspect of the skin flap.

Lower Lip

Degloving injury of the lower lip, with displacement of the tissue from the rostral mandible, is seen occasionally and the cause is believed to be from falling and contact of the lower lip and chin with the ground.[4] The

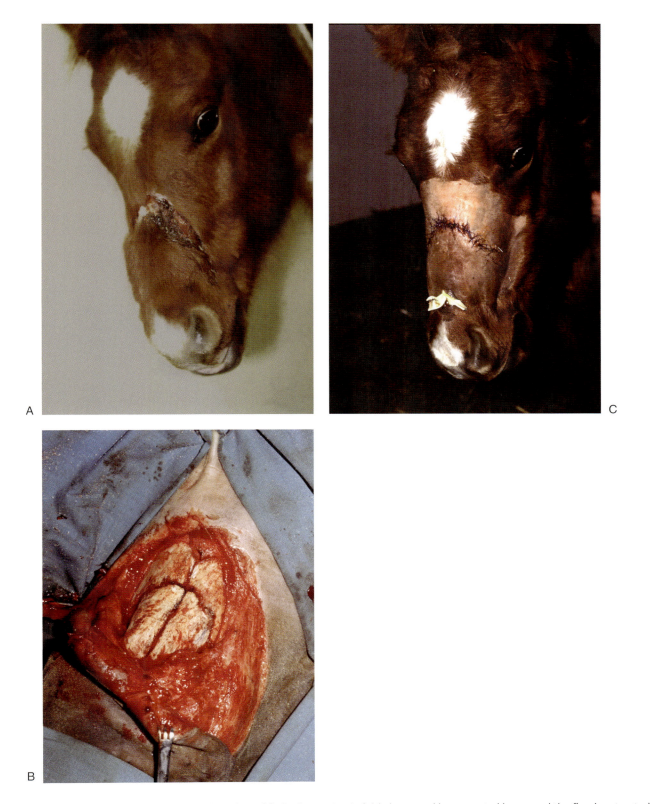

Figure 6.26. Typical degloving laceration of the face. (A) The laceration is fairly large and has a rostral base, and the flap is retracted to expose the nasal bones. The wound is <12 hours old. (B) Wound following debridement. Periosteum is lost from the nasal bones, which nonetheless look healthy after partial decortication. There was a non-displaced fracture of both nasal bones, which was stabilized with suture material placed through holes drilled in the nasal and adjacent frontal bones. (C) Soft tissue was closed over the exposed fracture site in two layers. Penrose drains were inserted to provide ventral drainage.

injury results in exposure of the rostral (Figures 6.27a and 6.27b, top). If the wound is left untreated, the horse cannot eat properly and an unsightly deficit remains.

Treatment

Reconstruction usually involves drilling holes in the rostral mandible between the incisor teeth roots and placing a single row of through-and-through modified quill tension sutures of #2 monofilament nylon (Figure 6.27b, top and bottom left). The sutures are placed in a rostral-caudal direction in a mattress pattern through the lower lip, through bone, into the oral cavity, and in a reverse fashion from the oral cavity out through a bone hole and the skin (Figure 6.27b, top and bottom left). Once all of the sutures are placed they are tied over a Penrose drain to act as modified quill sutures which ensure stability of the lip flap so the mucosa can be reconstructed. Generally, a single row of the modified quill sutures is all that is needed; however, if the lip appears unstable after their placement, more rows of these sutures can be added.

In some cases the mucosa must be undermined on the flap to free it sufficiently for suturing. The mucous membrane is apposed with a simple interrupted pattern of #2-0 synthetic absorbable suture material (Figure 6.27b, bottom right). Although the sutured membrane may partially dehisce, healing occurs in most cases without major problems. A Penrose drain, exiting ventrally, should be employed because there may be a large dead space remaining underneath the avulsed flap (Figure 6.27b, bottom left).

Postoperatively, a moist gruel is fed and in between feedings, the mouth should be lavaged with a dilute antiseptic solution followed by the application of a muzzle. The Penrose drain, used to drain the dead space, is usually removed within 48 hours but can be left in longer if drainage persists. Antibiotic therapy is continued for 5 to 7 days and NSAIDs are administered as needed. The modified quill sutures can usually be removed in 7 to 10 days. Complete healing can be expected to occur in 15 to 21 days.

Ear

Degloving injury to the ear, although uncommon, usually involves the outer surface with loss of skin and exposure of the underlying cartilage (Figure 6.28a). The injury is most commonly seen in foals and weanlings and is most often caused by either the dam or pasture mate biting the ear. If the wound is untreated and heals by second intention, the ear develops a curling defect from the scar that forms.

Treatment

Preoperative preparation includes antibiotic and NSAID therapy as well as bandaging the head and ear until a healthy bed of granulation tissue covers the exposed cartilage (Figure 6.28a).

In the authors' opinion, skin grafting is the best option. Either a full-thickness or a meshed full-thickness graft is preferred (for more information regarding the techniques of skin grafting, see Chapter 11). Full-thickness grafts are preferred because they are better at preventing secondary graft contraction and are less susceptible to tissue mismatch than are split-thickness grafts.[20] At surgery, a template of the auricular skin defect can be obtained using sterile X-ray film or paper that covered the surgical gloves (Figure 6.28b). The skin graft is held in place with the least number of sutures possible (Figure 6.28c).

Post-operative bandaging of the ear and head are important. The graft must be covered with a non-adherent primary dressing and the ear should be splinted to prevent it from curling. A non-adherent semi-occlusive dressing, or one that has its contact layer lightly coated with triple antibiotic ointment, usually suffices as the primary dressing. The ear can best be splinted by placing rolled gauze in the ear canal, followed by bandaging with conforming gauze, which is secured in place with elastic adhesive tape that is applied with minimal circumferential pressure to prevent ischemia of the graft. In addition, the elastic adhesive tape will have to encircle the throat latch region to secure the bandage in place. This first bandage is usually left in place for 5 to 7 days.

Antibiotic therapy is continued for 24 hours and NSAIDs are administered for 5 to 7 days. Tranquilization may be required to prevent the horse from rubbing its ears. In some cases, cross-tying will be necessary. Sutures holding the graft in place are removed 10–12 days after surgery. Bandaging is usually continued for at least 3 weeks, after which the graft site should be protected from direct sunlight, which may cause a burn of the new tissue at the graft site, for at least 2 months.

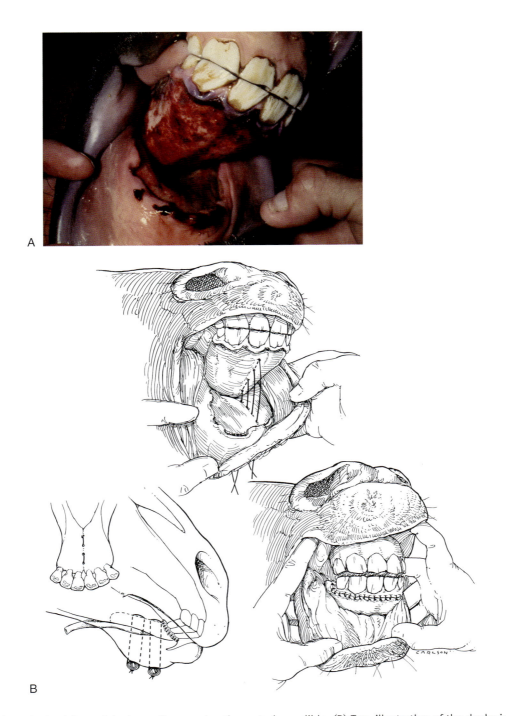

A

B

Figure 6.27. (A) Degloving injury of the lower lip exposing the rostral mandible. (B) Top: illustration of the degloving injury; holes have been drilled through the rostral mandible and nylon sutures have been inserted through the holes; bottom left: illustrates placement of the mattress sutures as quills and the location of the Penrose drain; the mucous membrane has been sutured; bottom right: frontal view illustrating sutures in the mucous membrane.

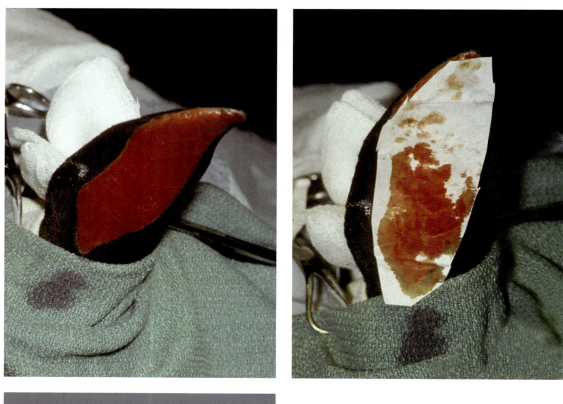

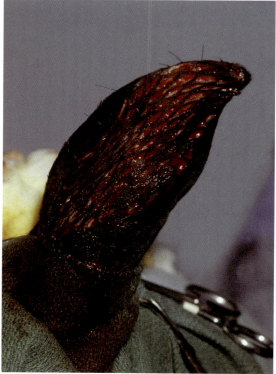

Figure 6.28. Avulsion injury to the ear of a foal caused by a bite from the dam 4 days earlier. The ear had been bandaged following the injury. (A) At surgery, note the healthy bed of granulation tissue which will facilitate graft take. (B) A template using surgical glove paper is made to document the dimensions of the degloving defect so a piece of skin of appropriate size can be harvested from the pectoral region for the grafting procedure. (C) The full-thickness meshed skin graft is held in place with a few sutures. Although there were no follow-up pictures taken, the referring veterinarian reported that the graft took and the ear healed without a tendency to curl.

Fractures of the Facial Bones

Fractures of the flat facial bones occur fairly commonly in horses. They result from external trauma—either impact with a solid stationary object or an external blow such as a kick. Because of the complex anatomy of the head, clinical signs may vary and treatment can be challenging.[2,15,18]

Anatomical Considerations

The bones most commonly fractured are the nasal, maxillary, lacrimal, frontal, and malar (zygomatic) (Figures 6.29a,b).[2] These bones are relatively thin, form the external limits of the nasal passage and paranasal sinuses, and are sparsely covered with muscle, hence exposed to external trauma.

The nasal passage is covered by the nasal bones, while the frontal bones overlay the frontal sinus. The bones that form the external wall of the maxillary sinus are the maxillary, lacrimal, and malar (zygomatic) bones. The limits of the maxillary sinus are important clinically (Figures 6.29a,b); they are the orbital rim caudally, the facial crest laterally, a line from the infraorbital canal to the facial crest cranially, and a line from the infraorbital canal to the medial canthus of the eye dorsally. The maxillary sinus is divided into rostral and caudal compartments and the dividing septum is both variable in location and often incomplete. Each compartment of the maxillary sinus drains into the middle meatus of the nasal passage through a separate slit-like opening. The frontal sinus does not drain directly into the nasal passage; secretions must first pass via the fronto-maxillary opening into the caudal maxillary sinus.[18]

The lacrimal and malar (zygomatic) bones form a large portion of the medial orbital rim. The lacrimal bone contains the fossa for the lacrimal sac and the nasolacrimal duct traverses the maxillary and lacrimal bones in a direction parallel to the facial crest and slightly above the infraorbital foramen.[18]

Flat Bones

A perpendicular external blow to the flat facial bones commonly causes a fracture. The impact may produce a complete fracture in which there is separation of the fracture fragment from the parent bone on all sides, or the fracture may be incomplete with attachment of the fragment along one of its sides. Incomplete fractures are usually depressed into the nasal passage or paranasal sinuses and are stable, while the fragments from complete fractures may be depressed but more commonly are unstable. Often a combination of complete and incomplete fracture fragments is present.[2]

The flat bones of the skull are formed by intramembranous ossification. They have a diffuse blood supply and the blood flow to them has been shown to be greater than that to other bones of the skeleton.[18] This may explain the clinical impression that fractured facial bones heal more rapidly than other bones.

The clinical signs depend on the anatomical location of the injury and the severity and nature of the damage. If the injury is caused by a sharp object the skin usually is lacerated and the bone exposed (Figures 6.30a–d). Digital and visual examination will often reveal if there are fractures and if the sinus or nasal passage is involved, but the full extent of damage seldom can be determined in this manner.

More commonly, the injury is caused by a blunt object and the skin is intact (Figure 6.31).[6,7] Asymmetry of the face indicates displacement of the fragments, but in some acute cases the swelling obscures this sign.[2,3,15] Crepitus is present if the fracture is comminuted and unstable but will not be felt with depressed stable fractures. Tenderness also prevents a very thorough digital examination unless sedation is used.[2,3] In chronic cases asymmetry is obvious with the fragments having healed in malposition.

Epistaxis is a common clinical sign indicating damage to the mucosal lining of either the nasal passage or paranasal sinuses.[2,3] Bilateral epistaxis indicates bleeding has occurred into either both nasal passages or both paranasal sinuses, or there is damage to the nasal septum. Dyspnea is uncommon but can occur if there is sufficient narrowing of the nasal passage or damage to the nasal septum to interfere with airflow, or if there is a large blood clot in the nasal passage. Subcutaneous emphysema has been seen occasionally when a fragment has penetrated the airway.

Fractures of the orbital rim can cause several signs attributed to abnormal configuration and function of the orbital structures, and are common with fractures to the maxillary, malar (zygomatic), and lacrimal bones located cranial to the orbit.[2] Depressed fragments of the orbital rim or orbit can impinge upon the globe or its muscles and prevent normal movement of the eye within the orbit when the head is moved.[2,4,21] The eye may

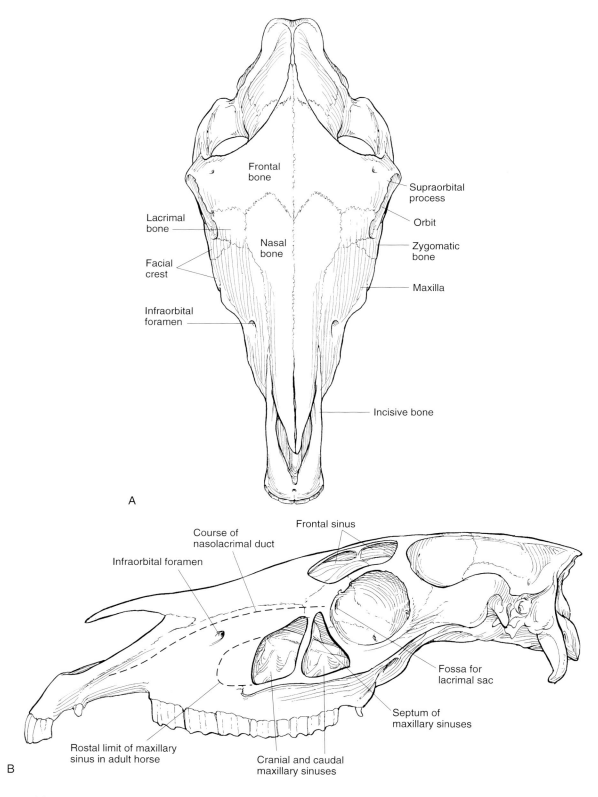

A

B

Figure 6.29. (A) Dorsal view: horse skull showing the bones of the face that commonly are fractured by facial trauma. (B) Lateral view of the skull with portions of the facial bones removed to demonstrate the location of the sinuses. Note the location of the rostral limit of the maxillary sinus and the location of the nasolacrimal duct.

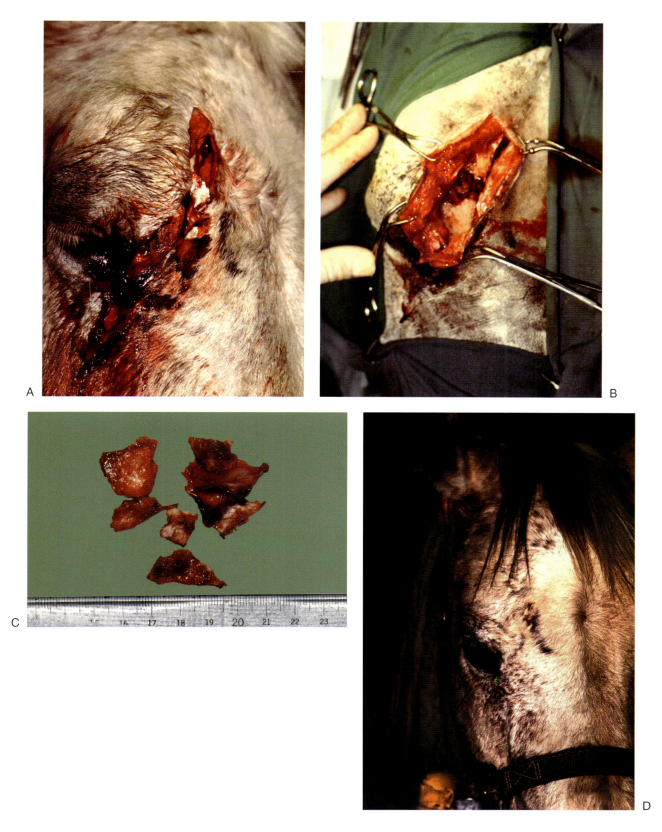

Figure 6.30. (A) This horse impaled its head on a metal bolt, lacerating the skin and fracturing the frontal and lacrimal bones over the frontal sinus. (B) The laceration, when slightly enlarged, gave excellent exposure for surgical manipulations. The supraorbital process had to be stabilized with wire sutures. (C) Several small fragments of loose bone were removed and the defect was covered with soft tissue. (D) Excellent appearance 13 weeks post-operatively.

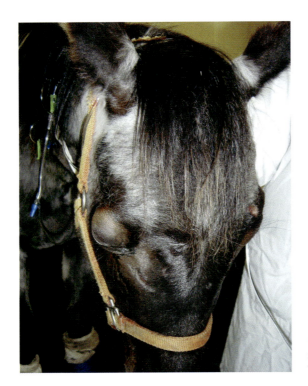

Figure 6.31. Yearling kicked in the face by an older horse. Note the intact skin and depression in the facial bones rostral to the right eye. The eye was entrapped and partially proptosed.

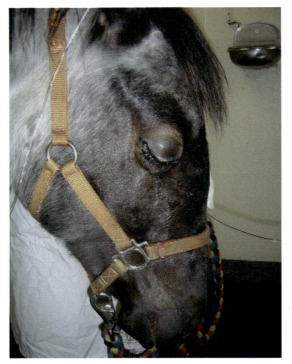

Figure 6.32. Same horse as in Figure 6.31. Note the swelling in the orbital area. The swollen eyelids could no longer completely cover the cornea, which developed an exposure keratitis. Following reconstruction of the facial bones the eye was no longer entrapped or proptosed, and the corneal defect healed after topical medication was administered via a subpalpebral lavage system.

also protrude from the orbit and swelling of the eyelids may prevent their closure (Figure 6.32). Transection of the nasolacrimal duct within the lacrimal bone or maxilla may not be readily apparent on initial examination as lacrimal secretions will be discharged into the open wound. Epiphora is seen in chronic cases after the transected nasolacrimal duct is occluded by the healing process.[2,22]

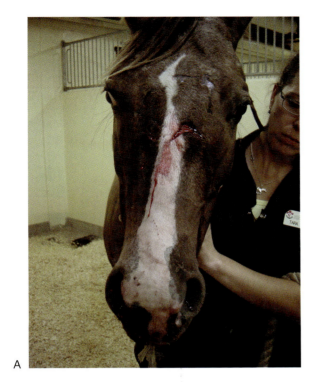
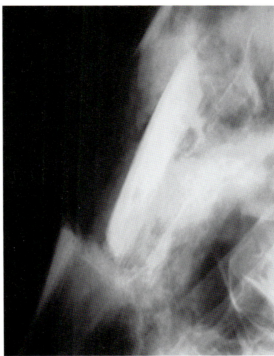

Figure 6.33. (A) This horse ran into a heavy metal gate head first. The only abnormality seen clinically was a small cut and some exposed nasal bone. (B) Radiographs show a very large fragment of bone that was greatly displaced into the frontal sinus. No cavitation of the face was seen clinically, likely due to swelling.

Passing a nasogastric tube is a simple and effective method of checking the patency of the nasal passage. Endoscopic examination of the nasal passage provides valuable information about the integrity of the nasal septum as well as the bones that form the nasal passage, and whether there is drainage or hemorrhage from the maxillary sinus into the middle meatus.

A detailed digital exam, under sedation, is indicated to check the orbit and orbital rim. A bilateral ocular exam is also advised because severe injury to the globe, including retinal detachment of the contralateral globe, has been recorded.[22] The patency of the nasolacrimal duct can be checked by passing a catheter in a retrograde fashion, by lavage, or with the use of fluorescein dye.[2,22]

Radiography is indicated in all cases of suspected facial trauma (Figures 6.33a,b). The paranasal sinuses normally are filled with air such that the presence of a fluid line within them indicates hemorrhage into the sinus.[2,3,19] The integrity of the nasal septum can be checked with a dorsoventral radiographic projection of the head. Displaced fractures are identified as sharp alterations in the facial contour. Several radiographic views of varying obliquities are often needed to identify a fracture.

The full extent of the fractures often cannot be determined radiographically because the head is a very complex bony structure, the bones are thin and may be minimally displaced, and it can be difficult to profile the area of trauma.[2] Fractures of the nasal bone and lateral orbital rim are the easiest to profile but are not seen as often as the more common fractures of the maxillary, lacrimal, and malar bones cranial to the orbit, which are harder to profile. Radiographs are used primarily to determine whether there is fluid in the maxillary sinus and to confirm the existence of a fracture rather than to determine the number of bony fragments and their relationship to one another. Additional fractures are usually identified at surgery.[2] Computerized tomography (CT scan) is excellent for providing greater detail but its use is not required for successful treatment. If available, it should be considered in complicated cases, especially those involving the orbital rim.

Indications for Surgery

Those cases that have an open sinus or nasal passage, an entrapped or damaged eye, abnormalities to the nasal cavity or nasal septum, or where cosmesis is a concern should be treated surgically.[2] While most cases will heal without surgery, except those involving imbedded foreign bodies, surgical treatment will minimize the chance of the following complications: (1) accentuation of the facial deformity, upon resolution of edema, to an extent that is unexpected and unacceptable to the owner; 2) bone sequestration of small comminuted fragments in some fractures that are compound and contaminated. These are accompanied by laceration of the skin or the nasal or sinus mucosa; (3) formation of blood clots in the sinus which may occlude the normal slit-like openings required for drainage and lead to maxillary sinus infection. For these reasons, the authors recommend surgical treatment of most cases of facial fractures mentioned above.

Treatment

All patients should be given antibiotics systemically and NSAIDs for several days. If an open fracture extends into the maxillary sinus or the sinus contains blood, a lavage system should be placed into the cavity to allow it to be flushed twice daily with physiological saline or a dilute antiseptic solution.[2] The horse should be fed off the ground to enhance natural drainage. A lavage system can be easily installed in a standing sedated or recumbent anesthetized horse.

A small stab incision is made in the skin where the catheter will be placed. An intramedullary pin just slightly larger than the catheter to be inserted is placed through the bone, adjacent to the fracture, using a hand chuck.[2] A hole pierced through the maxillary bone will place the catheter directly into the maxillary sinus. If the hole is created more dorsal, through the nasal or frontal bones, the catheter will pass through the frontal sinus and fronto-maxillary opening into the maxillary sinus. A silastic catheter is fed several inches into the sinus and secured by suturing butterfly tape to the skin. Extension sets can be attached to the withers or neck region to facilitate lavage of the sinus from a remote site. Following lavage, usually for approximately 5 days, the tubing can be removed and the skin opening closed with a suture or skin staple.

Surgical Approaches

The selected surgical approach depends on the location, type, and extent of injury as well as surgeon preference.[2,3,19] In the case of large open wounds, retraction of the wound edges may be all that is required for adequate exposure, while enlargement of the wound opening is sometimes necessary for smaller wounds (Figure 6.30). These approaches provide excellent exposure to the fracture site but force wound closure to take place directly over the fracture repair, making it more likely that the sutured wound will subsequently dehisce. With a closed fracture or an open fracture with a small skin opening, the authors' preference is to make a curved skin incision adjacent to, but removed from, the area of trauma (Figures 6.34a–f and 6.35a–d).[2,3]

The skin and subcutaneous tissue are undermined and reflected to expose the fracture site. If a small hole from the original injury is present in the skin flap it is debrided and closed (Figures 6.34a–f). While a more invasive approach is necessary for management of complex, unstable, comminuted fractures, simple incomplete depressed fractures may be reduced through one or more small stab incisions (Figures 6.36a,b).[4,19]

If the periosteum has been torn and elevated from the depressed bone fragments, it may be necessary to reflect a large piece of it to gain access to the underlying comminuted fracture sites for repair (Figures 6.34a–f). Subperiosteal dissection should be kept to a minimum so as not to interfere with the blood supply.

Reduction. Blood clots present at the fracture site should be removed prior to attempting reduction of the fracture while blood in the sinus should likewise be removed by lavage and suction (Figure 6.34a–f). In the case of fractures that are several days old, the fibrin must be removed to obtain an accurate anatomical reduction. Repairing older fractures that have started to heal may necessitate cutting or breaking the bones to accurately reposition them.

Complete fractures with highly mobile fragments are usually easy to reduce, but the fragments may be depressed into the sinus or nasal passage. They will need to be retrieved and the edges cleaned prior to stabilization. Incomplete depressed fractures are usually stable and once the fragments have been elevated into position may not require further stabilization.[2,3,19] Many of these fractures are made up of a combination of complete unstable and incomplete depressed stable fragments.

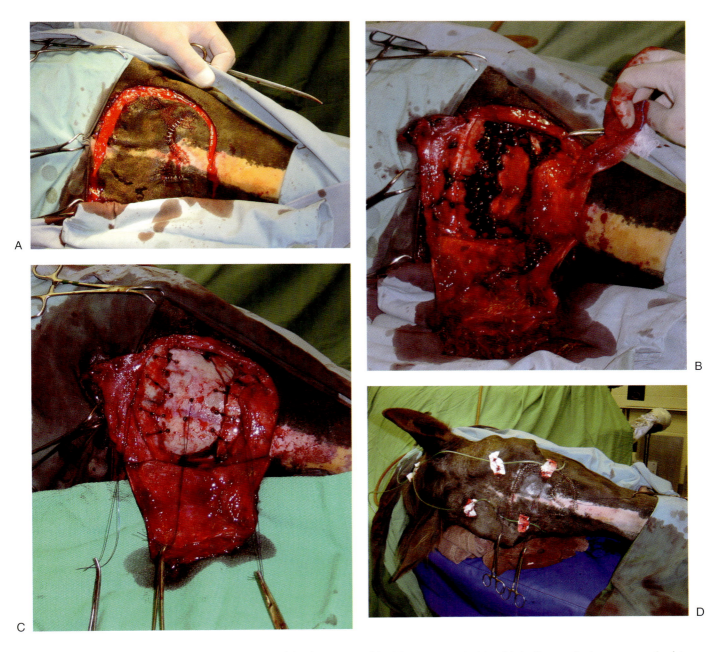

Figure 6.34. Same horse as seen in Figure 6.33. (A) A large curved incision was needed to obtain the surgical access required to reduce the large fracture seen on the X-ray in Figure 6.33b. Note: the small wounds over the nose were debrided and closed with staples. (B) While the periosteum was torn during injury it was still necessary to make a large periosteal flap to expose the fracture. Notice the large piece of nasal bone imbedded in the frontal sinus and the large blood clots. (C) The large fragment has been reduced and stabilized with suture material placed through pre-drilled holes. Note the bony defects left from discarding small bony fragments. Three horizontal mattress sutures, in the fragment and surrounding stable bone, have been preplaced through the bone to secure an external splint following closure of the skin. (D) The skin flap has been closed and lavage systems were placed in both sinuses with extensions along the neck. (E) (next page) The horse on the first postoperative day. Note the external plastic splint which is secured with the horizontal mattress sutures that were preplaced through the bone at surgery and extend through the skin. (F) (next page) Radiographic appearance of the head postoperatively. The fragment had been stabilized with absorbable suture material. Note the metal skin staples.

313

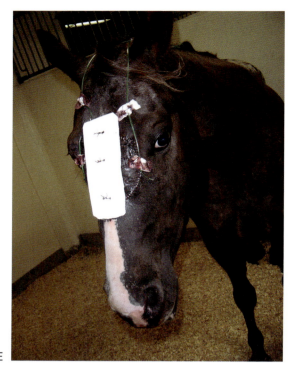
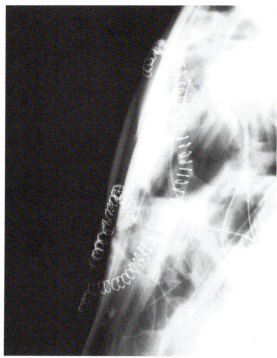

E   F

Figure 6.34. *Continued*

There are numerous ways to reduce incomplete fractures. Various instruments can be used to lever and pry the displaced fragment back into position. These can include periosteal elevators, retractors, bone hooks, or even scissor blades (Figure 6.36c).[2-4,19] The instrument can be inserted into the fracture line or through a space created by a displaced or discarded small fragment.[2] Care should be taken to avoid prying on the edge of the fragment because this can cause fragmentation. If a space is not present one can be made at the edge of the fracture line with a rongeur, or a hole can be drilled into the fragment to allow insertion of an instrument to be used for lifting. A bone hook or an intramedullary pin that is bent to form a retractor will work well.[3,19] Another approach is to insert a screw into the fragment and then lift on the head of the screw.[2,5]

Once reduced, incomplete depressed fracture fragments usually have a sufficient number of interdigitations along their edges to become stable (Figures 6.36a–e).[2,3,19] Some fractures occur obliquely through the bone and small pieces of the bone's edge may need to be removed with a rongeur to obtain reduction.[2] In cases where the fracture remains somewhat unstable after repair, particularly those involving bony prominences, it is advisable to create a cast helmet to protect the reduced fracture region for recovery if general anesthesia was used (Figure 6.36d).

Stabilization. Unstable fracture fragments should be secured with either monofilament synthetic suture material (#0–#1) or orthopedic wire (20 gauge) placed through drill holes made along the edge of the fragment and the stable parent bone (Figures 6.34c and 6.35b). Suture material is preferred because it is easy to work with, absorbable, the ends are less irritating to the overlying soft tissue, does not cut through the bone like wire can if pulled too tight, and is easier to preplace. Once the fragments are reduced it doesn't take many sutures to hold them in position. The holes for placement of the wire or suture are best made before complete fracture reduction. If the fracture remains unstable a bone plate(s) can be used; however, complications with drainage, screw loosening, and the need for implant removal have been reported.[23,24]

Following the repair of some comminuted fractures with wire or suture, the fragments tend to collapse into the sinus. These fractures can be stabilized in a reduced position with an external splint (Figures 6.34e and

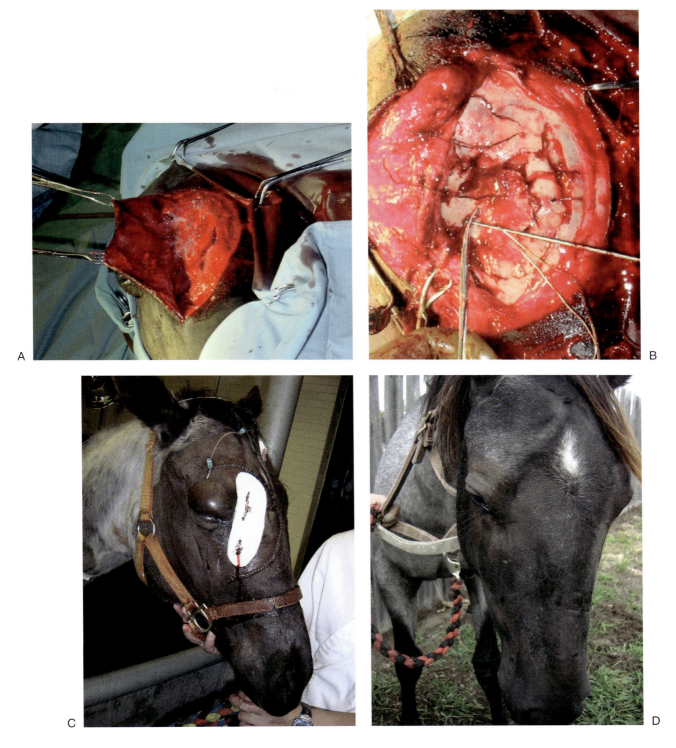

Figure 6.35. Same horse as seen in Figures 6.31 and 6.32. (A) A large skin flap was required to gain sufficient access for visualization and fracture reduction. (B) There were several comminuted and depressed fragments. Reduction was difficult and the fracture fragments remained somewhat unstable, even following wiring. (C) Appearance of the horse on postoperative day 1. Note the external plastic splint that was used to prevent collapse of the fracture fragments, the lavage system into the frontal sinus (located axial to the plastic splint), and the catheter in the medial canthus of the eye that passes through the lacrimal duct into the maxillary sinus. (D) Appearance 4 months after surgery. The face looks symmetrical, there is minimal blemish from the surgical repair, and epiphora is absent.

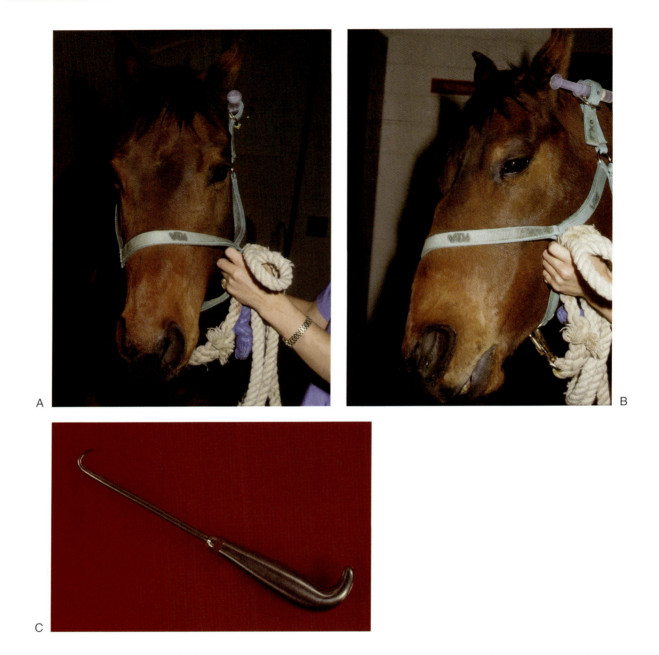

Figure 6.36. (A) Example of a simple depressed incomplete fracture of the facial bones that may be reduced without using wire or bone plates for stabilization. (B) Side view of the same fracture. (C) Example of a bone hook that was used to elevate the depressed incomplete fracture. Several small stab incisions were used to gain access to the fragment and a bone rongeur was used to create an opening in the parent bone to allow introduction of the bone hook. (D) (next page) Illustrates the cast helmet used to recover this horse from general anesthesia. (E) (next page) Lateral view taken the day following surgery. Note the cosmetic effect.

6.35c).[2] Holes are drilled in the fragments and adjacent stable bone for the preplacement of heavy suture material (#1–#2) or orthopedic wire in a mattress pattern. The ends of the wire are extended through the periosteum, subcutaneous tissue, skin, and holes made in the splint. Although many materials can be used to create the splint, moldable plastic works well and can be shaped and trimmed to fit the face.[2] Little force is usually needed to maintain reduction and it is important not to apply the splint too tightly against the skin surface. The splint is easily removed in 1 to 2 weeks when healing has produced sufficient stability.

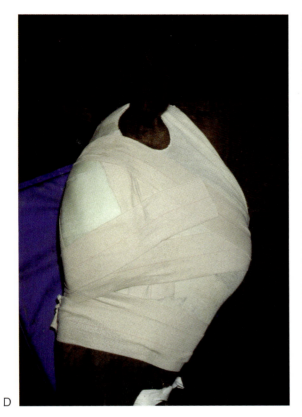
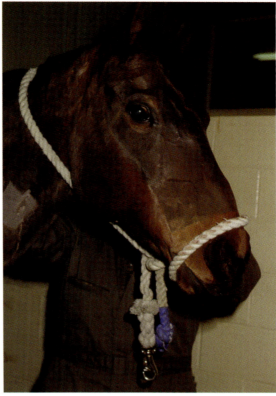

D

E

Figure 6.36. *Continued*

Small fragments that are completely free and would be difficult to stabilize are commonly discarded (Figures 6.30c and 6.34b,c).[2,3] Healing occurs as long as there is viable soft tissue to close over the defect. If the defect created by the removal of the loose fragment is located in a dependent aspect of the sinus, post-operative lavage may be impossible or limited in volume to prevent drainage of liquid into the subcutaneous tissue. This might predispose to infection and/or wound dehiscence. Large pieces of bone completely devoid of periosteum are reduced, stabilized, and covered with soft tissue. Although lacking a blood supply they are needed for structural support of the soft tissues to prevent deformity. With systemic antibiotic therapy, vigorous lavage of the surgical site and sinus, fragment stabilization, and covering of the bone with viable soft tissue, sequestration is very uncommon.

Closure. All available portions of the periosteum, including that which was elevated, should be closed over the fracture site. The periosteum protects and supports the repair, may enhance blood supply, and has osteoprogenitor cells in its cambial layer which may facilitate fracture healing. If a large bony defect is present, a flap of periosteum from adjacent intact bone can be reflected over the opening.[25] Another technique is to bridge the opening with synthetic mesh which is then covered with skin.[26] Absorbable mesh (e.g., Vicryl [polyglactin 910] Mesh, Ethicon, Inc. or Dexon [polyglycolic acid] Mesh, Davis and Geck) is preferable because of the risk of infection.

It is important to cover the repaired fracture site with viable soft tissue for healing and protection. This tissue provides nourishment to the devitalized fragments after periosteal elevation. There is often minimal skin for closure but subcutaneous undermining usually allows the incision to be closed without excessive tension. In cases where there is loss of skin, relieving incisions, transposition skin flaps, or single pedicle or bi-pedicle advancement flaps can be used.[4] Any subcutaneous defect created by these techniques can be closed with other plastic reconstructive surgical techniques or left to heal by second intention. It is better to have a cutaneous defect a few centimeters adjacent to the fracture site than directly over it. For more information regarding reconstructive surgical techniques, see Chapter 5.

Medial Orbital Rim

Comminuted and depressed fractures of the facial bones rostral to the medial canthus are common. If the malar (zygomatic) bone, or more commonly the lacrimal bone, is depressed, a portion of the bone that either forms the orbital rim or lies within the orbit can be displaced and interfere with or damage the globe. This can result in proptosis or entrapment of the eye in a fixed position when the head is moved (Figure 6.31).[2,27]

Pieces of bone that form the orbit should be elevated into position and stabilized as previously described. The impinging fragment is often a portion of bone from along the walls of the orbital canal. If reduction is impossible, the fragment should be attended to either by dissecting subconjunctivally and removing it with a rongeur or by breaking off and eliminating the impinging portion. A thorough examination of each globe is indicated because injuries to both the ipsilateral and contralateral eye have been reported.[21]

The lacrimal system can also be injured by fractures of the facial bones. The lacrimal sac is contained within the lacrimal fossa of the lacrimal bone, while the nasolacrimal duct is protected by its passage through the maxilla and lacrimal bone[18] such that fracture of either of the latter can result in damage to the duct. No associated clinical signs will be seen in an acute injury because the lacrimal fluid drains into the wound or a sinus. Epiphora develops once the transected duct becomes occluded by fibrosis or bony callus.[2,3]

In the authors' experience, comminution of these bones with minimal displacement does not usually result in loss of integrity of the nasolacrimal duct. However, the patency of the duct should always be checked by catheterization or by flushing with fluorescein dye. If the duct is transected, silicone tubing can be placed through it to act as an internal splint during healing,[21,26] providing both ends of the duct can be identified within the fracture site.

Another technique is to create a permanent communication into the maxillary sinus. To do so, a segment of silastic tubing is placed through the orbital puncta and into the maxillary sinus, either through a bony defect created by the fracture or through a hole made by the surgeon (Figure 6.35c).[2,21] The latter is less likely to become occluded by fibrosis or bony callus. With either approach the catheters are left in place for 2 to 3 weeks. Because horses have a tendency to rub the catheters out, cross-tying during this period is indicated to prevent premature removal.

Zygomatic (Supraorbital) Process

The zygomatic (supraorbital) process is that portion of the frontal bone which forms the dorsal and caudal segments of the orbital rim.[18] Its prominence predisposes it to external trauma. While it may be fractured along with other facial bones, it is often injured separately. The skin is usually intact and characteristically a single fragment is displaced medially and ventrally.[3,19]

Asymmetry of the orbital region along with swelling and tenderness over the zygomatic process are common.[3] The depressed fragment may cause damage to or entrapment of the eye. In these cases the eye will be fixed in position when the head is moved, and there may be ocular swelling or proptosis. Skyline oblique radiographs will usually identify fracture of the zygomatic (supraorbital) process (Figure 6.37).[3,4]

Fractures that do not interfere with the globe can be left untreated and will heal, albeit not always cosmetically. However, the authors recommend surgical treatment to reduce the likelihood of eye damage caused by further displacement of the fragment before it heals.

Repair can be achieved via non-invasive or invasive techniques. Simple fractures can be managed non-invasively by reduction with a bone hook (Figure 6.36c).[28] A detailed digital exam of the interior of the orbit can be performed by palpating through the conjunctiva with the horse under general anesthesia. Using a finger as a guide, the surgeon then places the end of the bone hook on the ventral aspect of the fragment. Reduction is achieved by lifting on the bone hook, which can be repositioned under the fragment to provide elevation from more than one site (Figures 6.38a–c).

The accuracy of the reduction is determined by visual inspection of the external orbital rim and by palpation of the internal and external orbits. If the reduced fragment is stable no further treatment is necessary. Fragments that are unstable following use of the bone hook or are more comminuted can be approached by incising over the area of fracture.[3,4] The fragments are elevated and stabilized by passing wire or absorbable suture through holes drilled in them and in the adjacent parent bone (Figures 6.39a–d). Very unstable fractures can be repaired with reconstruction plates.[29] Adequate protection of the head with a padded hood or cast helmet during recovery from anesthesia in indicated (Figure 6.36d). Alternatively, the horse can be hand recovered.

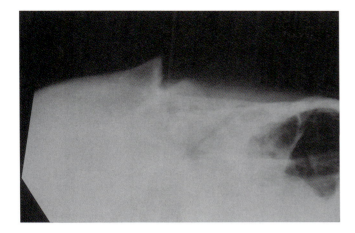

Figure 6.37. Oblique radiograph showing a displaced fracture of the supraorbital process.

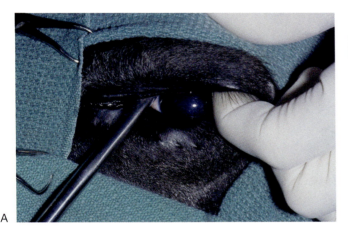

A

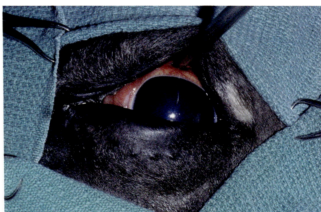

B

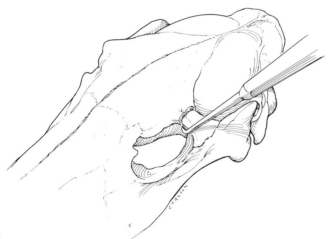

C

Figure 6.38. A gloved finger is used to palpate the fornix of the conjunctiva prior to placement of the bone hook. (A and B) The bone hook is positioned beneath the fracture fragment for elevation. (C) Drawing showing the positioning of the bone hook for elevation of the fracture fragment.

Antibiotic and NSAID therapy as well as sinus lavage are continued for several days, and the horse should be fed on the ground to encourage ventral drainage. Cross-tying may be necessary to prevent the horse from rubbing lavage catheters or those placed in the nasolacrimal duct. The lavage catheters are removed in 4 to 5 days if the sinus can be flushed easily and the solution drains cleanly. A single stitch or skin staple can be

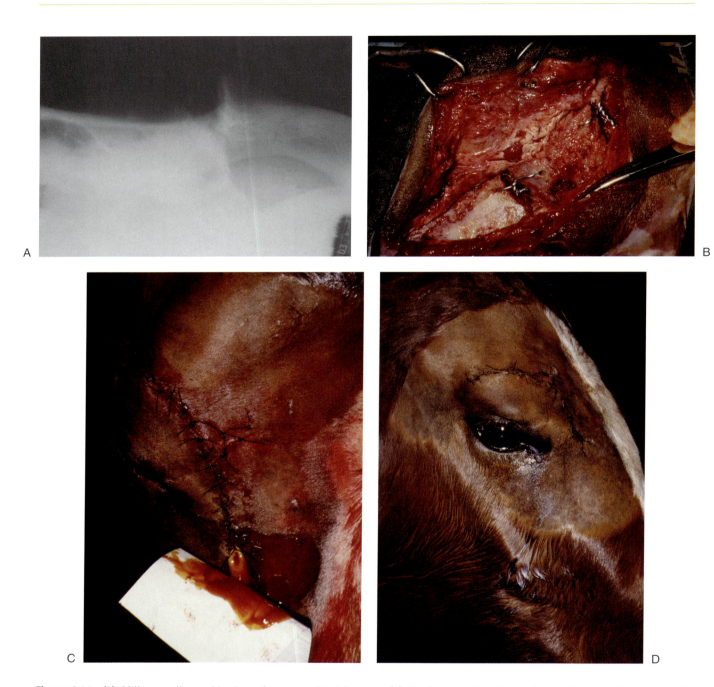

Figure 6.39. (A) Oblique radiographic view of a supraorbital fracture. (B) The fragment has been elevated into position and stabilized with orthopedic wires placed at each end. (C) Immediately following surgery. Note the size and location of the incision required for surgical exposure and the placement of the Penrose drain. (D) Two days postoperatively. A stent bandage, originally placed over the incision, and the Penrose drain have been removed. Cosmetic and functional outcomes were achieved.

used to close the skin hole after catheter removal. The complication rate following aggressive therapy is very low and the cosmetic results are often excellent (Figure 6.35e).

Imbedded Foreign Bodies

Occasionally, a horse will suffer from a foreign body that has become imbedded in the skull (Figure 6.40a). The challenge is to establish which structures have been penetrated by the object. Lateral and dorsal radiographs

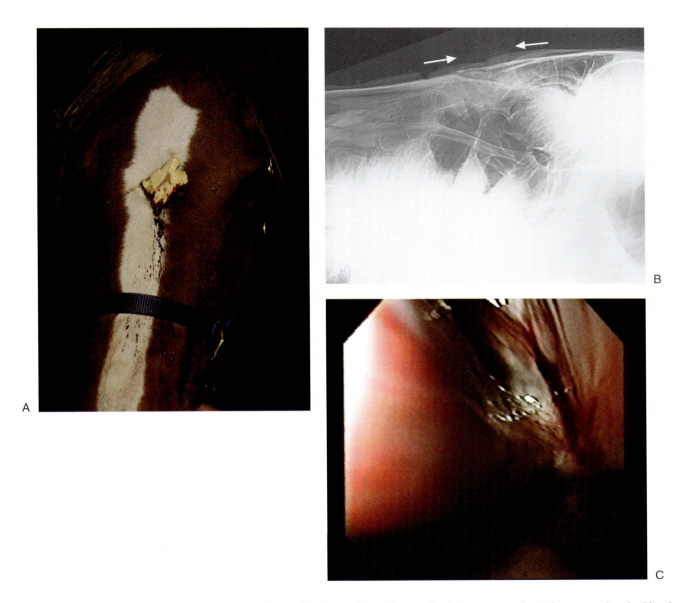

Figure 6.40. (A) Example of an imbedded piece of wood in the skull of a horse. The injury occurred <12 hours previously. Blood was dripping from the horse's left nostril. (B) Radiographic examination identified fluid in the left dorsal conchal and rostral maxillary sinuses. The outline of the piece of wood is seen (arrows) with what appeared to be an incomplete depressed fracture of the nasal bone. (C) Endoscopy of the left nasal passage revealed blood draining from the nasomaxillary opening. (D) (next page) Removal of the piece of wood using channel-lock pliers. (E) (next page) Wound following removal of the imbedded wood fragment. The tract was debrided, lavaged, and packed with Kerlix AMD gauze. The packing was changed daily for 2 days, after which the incomplete fracture was elevated into position using a bone hook. (F) (next page) Appearance of the bone following reduction. While it would have been ideal to suture the soft tissues, the owner did not wish to incur the additional expense. (G) (next page) Follow-up, 1 year. Note the dimple-like scar. This may have been prevented by suturing the wound after reduction of the bone flap.

are used to determine the depth and location of the foreign body and if there is evidence of hemorrhage or exudate in the paranasal sinuses (Figure 6.40b). Endoscopy will identify the presence of the foreign body in the nasal cavity, hemorrhage, or exudate coming from the nasomaxillary ostia and or the guttural pouches (Figure 6.40c). Direct sinus endoscopy can be helpful in identifying the foreign body and fracture fragments in some cases.

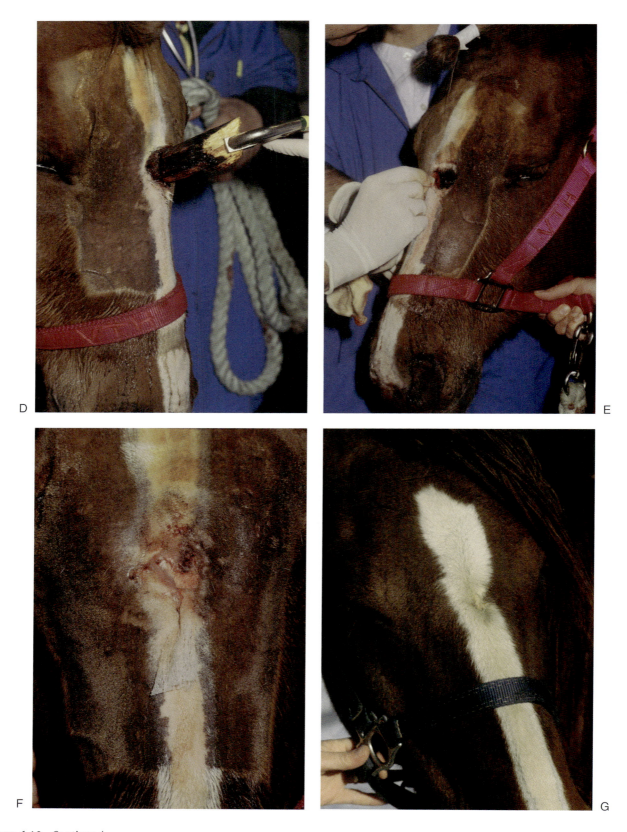

Figure 6.40. *Continued*

Preoperative preparation includes the administration of antibiotics and NSAIDs. Many of these foreign bodies can be extracted in the standing sedated horse. As with other injuries to the head region, a neurologic exam should be done prior to sedating the patient.

Imbedded foreign bodies can usually be extracted with a pair of large bone-holding forceps or channel-lock pliers (Figure 6.40d). Appropriate material should be available to pack the site if substantial hemorrhage occurs following extraction of the object. The packing should be left in place until the hemorrhage is under control (usually 2 to 4 hours). In most instances hemorrhage is not a problem, in the authors' experience. After removing the object, the wound should be examined to identify the nature of the soft tissue injury and the fracture. Subsequently, the wound is lavaged and debrided and a decision regarding the management is made.

In many cases dirt, hair, and debris have been driven into the depths of the wound, making it inadvisable to reduce the fracture and suture the wound; in such instances delayed reduction and closure are usually selected. An antimicrobial dressing (e.g., Kerlix AMD®, Covidien Animal Health/Kendall, Dublin, OH) can be used to pack the cavity. The packing is changed daily and is usually effective in removing hair, necrotic tissue, and debris within 48 hours. Remaining fragments of devitalized tissue, hair, and debris can be removed with lavage, forceps, and a gauze sponge in some instances.

The wound is ready for repair once a healthy bed of granulation tissue is present. These types of injuries often cause incomplete fracture of a facial bone (Figure 6.40b). If this is the case the bone can be elevated in the standing and sedated horse. A notch may have to be created in the adjacent parent bone to allow insertion of a bone hook or other instrument to elevate the bone flap. The notch can easily be created with a bone rongeur. Once the fracture has been reduced (Figure 6. 40f), the wound, including any available periosteum, can be sutured. Alternatively, the wound can be left to heal by second intention, though this is not ideal (Figure 6.40g).

Nasocutaneous and Sinocutaneous Fistulas

A fistula, by definition, is an abnormal passage from one epithelialized surface to another. Trauma to the facial bones can result in a full-thickness wound that enters the nasal passage or a paranasal sinus. Contamination and infection of the wound, along with sinus or sequestrum formation or a large facial bone defect, may lead to the formation of a permanent fistula (Figures 6.30 and 6.41).[2–4,22]

Surgical closure (primary or delayed primary) of the defect is recommended in most cases; however, many small defects (<3 cm) will heal without surgery. With conservative treatment the wound opening decreases in size as the granulation tissue forms and proceeds toward the center of the wound. Many defects will close spontaneously through the processes of epithelialization and wound contraction. There is, however, a tendency for some to form a permanent fistula if the mucosa and the epithelium heal over the advancing edge of granulation tissue.[3,4] This can be prevented, to a large extent, by frequent curettage of the wound edges and possibly the application of an extracellular matrix scaffold which is strongly angiogenic (see Extracellular Matrix as a Scaffold for Tissue Engineering in Veterinary Medicine in Chapter 3).[30] While conservative management may be successful, it is time consuming and labor intensive, and may result in a significant scar. In the absence of financial constraints, surgical repair is encouraged by the authors.

A number of techniques can be used to cover an opening into the nasal passage or paranasal sinus in either an acute wound or a fistula.[4,25,26,31–34] An important principle that applies to the acute wound or fistula involving a contaminated cavity (e.g., nasal or sinus) is that whenever possible a tissue barrier should be created between the contaminated cavity and the skin that covers the defect. The barrier will decrease the chance of the overlying sutured skin becoming infected, which would result in wound dehiscence. The barrier in the acute injury can be composed of a layer of subcutaneous tissue, fascia, or muscle (Figures 6.42a,b).

In the case of a permanent fistula, a barrier can be created using either the mucosa (Figure 6.43c), inverted or reversed skin flaps (Figures 6.44b,c) or periosteum (Figures 6.45c,d) and/or muscle flaps (Figure 6.46). In either case (acute injury or permanent fistula), once the barrier has been created an attempt is made to mobilize the skin to cover the defect.

Management of the Acute Injury

In the acute injury, once the wound has been lavaged and debrided it must be decided whether the wound will be closed primarily or in a delayed fashion. In either situation, antibiotic and NSAID therapy are begun.

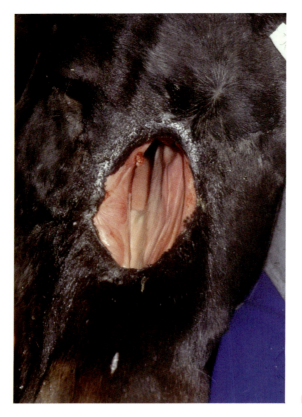

Figure 6.41. Example of a large nasocutaneous fistula in a horse.

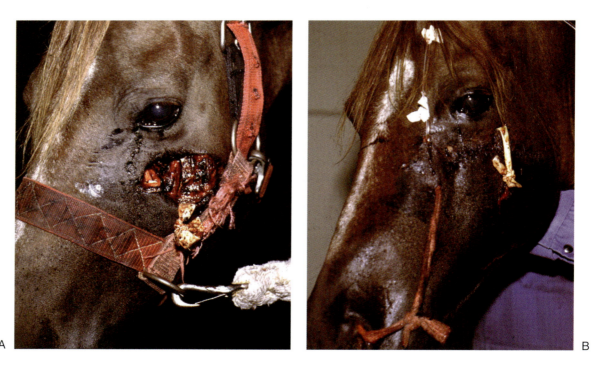

A

B

Figure 6.42. (A) Example of a facial injury with loss of several bone fragments and a large opening into the maxillary sinus. Note the Penrose drain placed for drainage. (B) Postoperative appearance following wound debridement, sinus lavage, and wound closure. The soft tissues could be apposed over the bony defect after the subcutaneous tissue was undermined. Note the lavage system placed in the sinus, the gauze placed through the sinus and nasal passage to assure drainage into the latter, and the Penrose drain in the subcutaneous tissue.

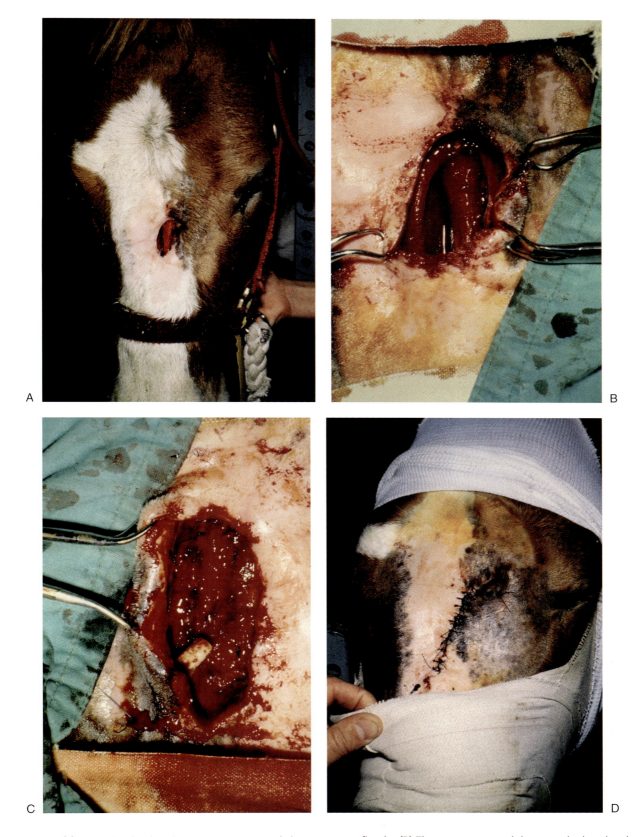

Figure 6.43. (A) Example of a chronic nasocutaneous and sinocutaneous fistula. (B) The mucosa around the wound edges has been separated from the epithelium. The mucosa will be undermined from the nasal septum (left side) and the maxillary sinus (right side). The mucosa overlying the dorsal concha (central) will be incised and undermined to create two mucosal flaps—one lateral, the other medial. (C) The mucosal flap from the nasal septum has been sutured to the medial mucosal flap from the dorsal nasal concha, and the mucosal flap from the maxillary sinus has been sutured to the lateral mucosal flap of the dorsal nasal concha. Note the Penrose drain. (D) The skin was undermined to allow closure of the defect.

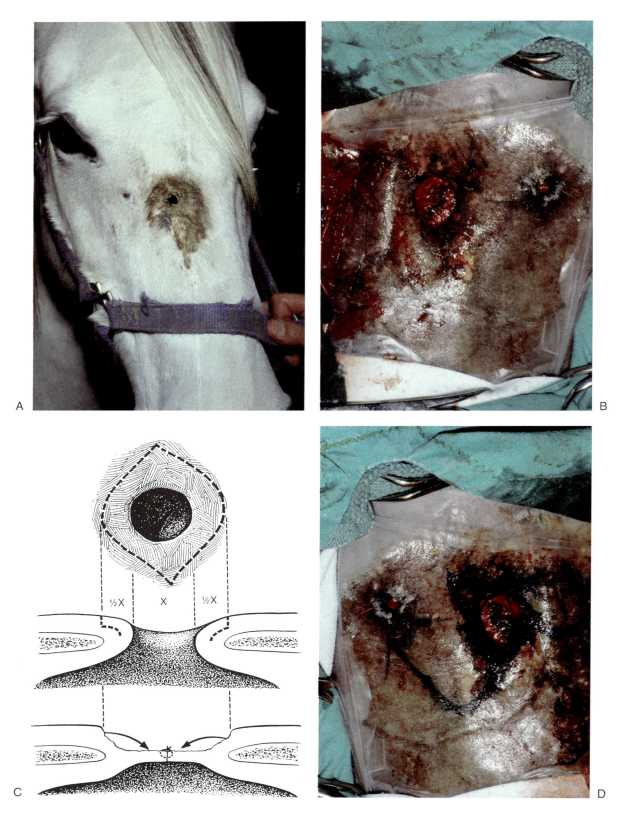

Figure 6.44. (A) Chronic nasocutaneous fistula. (B) The nasocutaneous fistula has been closed with two inverted skin flaps. (C) Illustration of inverted skin flaps: Top: the dotted lines indicate the fusiform skin incision adjacent to the fistula necessary to create two skin flaps. Middle: cross-sectional view of the fistula; X = the width of the fistula; ½X = the distance the skin incisions must be located adjacent to the fistula to create flaps large enough to close the defect; the heavy dotted line indicates the depth and direction of the dissection to create the skin flaps; bottom: the flaps have been everted to close the defect, resulting in the cutaneous tissue now lining the nasal passage. (D) Transposition flap developed from adjacent tissue. The outline of the flap has been drawn to the left of the fistula.

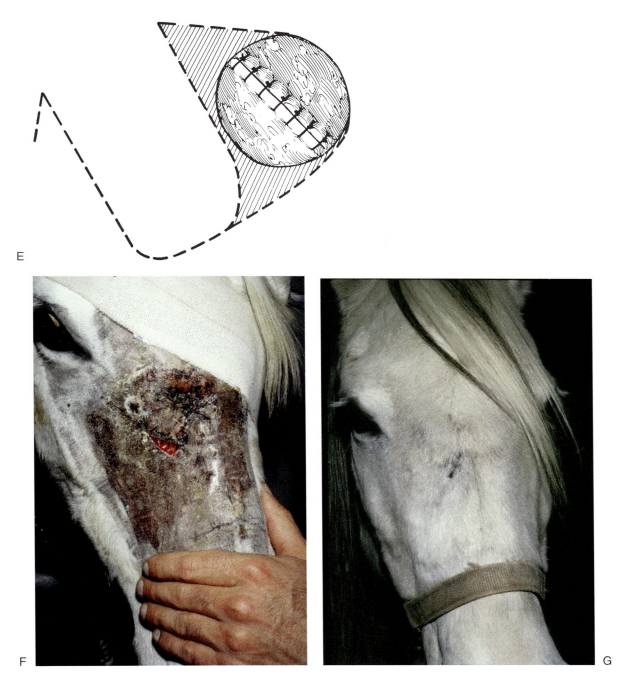

Figure 6.44. (*Continued*) (E) Illustration of the formation and mobilization of a transposition skin flap. The transposition flap is developed as close to the repair site as possible to minimize required rotation. Oblique lines surrounding the closed fistula represent further skin removal to accommodate the skin flap. (F) The transposition flap has been sutured in place. Vertical mattress sutures were used to reduce the size of the remaining defect lateral to the transposition flap. Four days after surgery. (G) Follow-up at 3 years. A reasonably good cosmetic and functional end result was achieved.

If primary closure is selected a barrier should be created at the site of the bony defect, using any and all of the tissues previously mentioned. Because there may be limited tissue to create this barrier it is important to restrict debridement to only that tissue which needs to be removed. Once the tissue barrier has been created, the surgeon must decide how to mobilize skin to cover the defect (see Selected Techniques for Mobilizing Skin (page 330) and

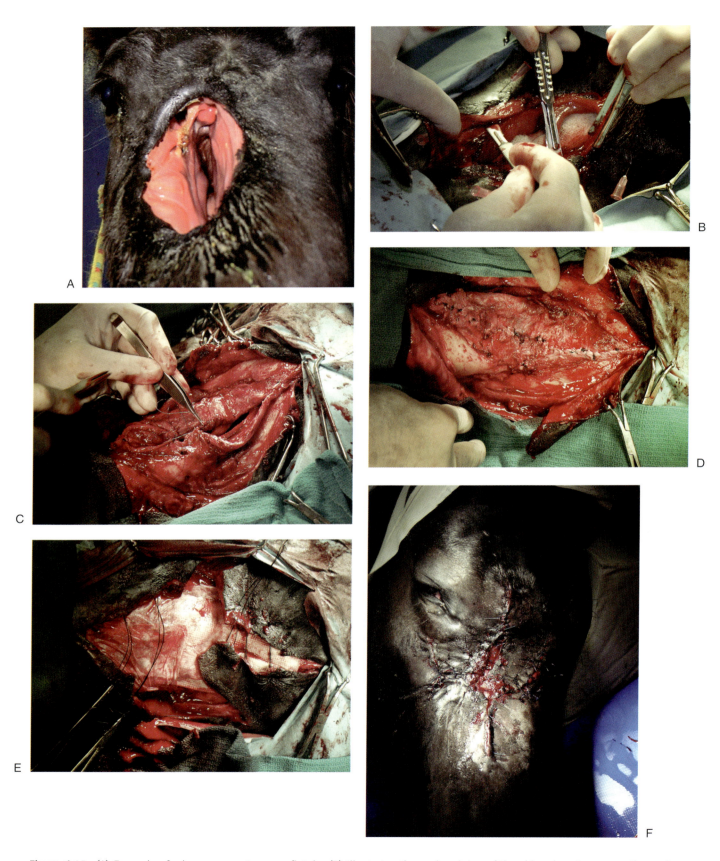

Figure 6.45. (A) Example of a large nasocutaneous fistula. (B) Illustrates the undermining of the skin edges to expose the periosteum. (C) Illustrates the formation of large reversed periosteal flaps. (D) The periosteal flaps are sutured. (E) Application of an ECM scaffold (ACell Vet® Scaffold, ACell, Inc, Jessup, MD) over the reversed sutured periosteal flaps. (F) Skin flaps were created to increase skin coverage of the wound. Skin and skin flaps were sutured with vertical mattress tension sutures. (G) (next page) Appearance of the forehead 1 year following several surgeries.

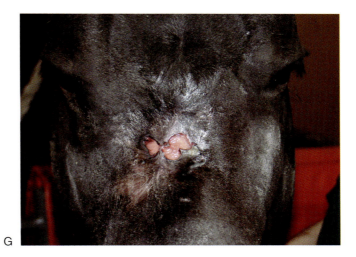

Figure 6.45. *Continued* G

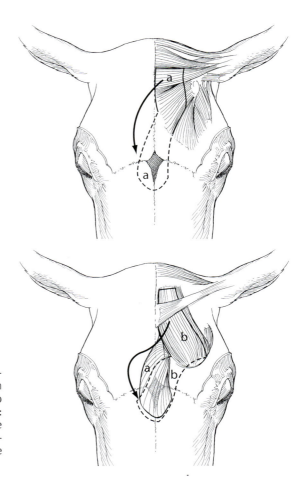

Figure 6.46. Illustrates a frontocutaneous fistula (center black rectangle). Top: The interscutularis muscle and fascia (a) are separated from their origin and incised laterally to form a muscle flap. The muscle flap is rotated to cover the fistula and sutured to the periosteum. Bottom: The interscutularis muscle (a) is sutured in place. The temporalis muscle (b) is incised in a saggital plane, then rotated to overlie the interscutularis muscle and the fistula. Campbell ML, Peyton LC: Muscle Flap Closure of a Frontocutaneous Fistula in a Horse. Vet Surg 1984;13:185

Chapter 5 for a more complete discussion). When a sinus cavity is involved a lavage system is usually placed to allow flushing of the cavity during the postoperative period (Figure 6.42b).

Delayed closure requires the administration of antibiotics and NSAIDs, along with wound irrigation and debridement as needed, for several days. In some cases it is helpful to pack the wound (including the sinus) with an antiseptic dressing (e.g., Kerlix AMD®, Covidien Animal Health/Kendall, Dublin, OH) for a few days.

Once granulation tissue begins to fill the wound, (usually within 4 days) the same steps as described for primary closure are used to close the bone defect and wound.

Management of Chronic Fistulas

Inverted or reversed periosteal flaps and skin flaps have been used to close fistulas resulting from bony defects (Figures 6.44a–g, 6.45a–g, 6.46).[4,25,32,33] Both provide a viable soft tissue barrier originating from the wound margins to cover the nasal or sinus opening and a healthy environment upon which to place a transposition flap or skin graft. Moreover, the osteoprogenitor cells of the cambial (inner cellular) layer of periosteal flaps have the potential to produce bone. A bone graft can also be placed between these barrier flaps and a transposition skin flap to encourage bone formation. Successful repair of a sinocutaneous fistula was achieved using a mucosal lined myocutaneous transposition flap.[34] The flap was composed of skin and muscle lined with a free, autologous mucosal graft, the latter of which formed the barrier to the sinus.

To create inverted skin flaps an elliptical skin incision is made along the periphery of the wound (Figures 6.44a–g).[4] To ensure sufficient skin for closure, the incision must be made at least one-half the diameter of the opening into the sinus or nasal passage, away from the defect. The skin edges along the wound are then undermined and reflected toward the center of the defect, where they are sutured together and covered with a transposition flap.[4]

Periosteal flaps are made in a similar manner. Either a single large periosteal flap that covers the entire defect is created from one side or periosteum is elevated on two sides of the wound and reflected to the center, where it is sutured (Figures 6.45c,d).[3,25] The advantage of a single large flap is the absence of holes over the covered defect. Both techniques require elevation of the skin and subcutaneous tissue for access to the periosteum. To harvest a single large periosteal flap, a larger incision of the surrounding skin is necessary. A cancellous bone graft can be placed over the periosteum before it is covered with a skin flap.[25] Alternatively, an extracellular matrix scaffold (ACell Vet® scaffold, ACell, Inc, Jessup, MD) may be placed over the periosteum to facilitate constructive, tissue-specific replacement of the tissue within the wound.[30]

The use of flaps created from the interscutularis and temporalis muscles has been reported for closure of a frontocutaneous fistula.[31] The caudomedial attachment of the superficial interscutularis muscle and fascia was elevated to create a flap. The flap was rotated to cover the fistula and was sutured to the periosteum. The ventral border of the temporalis muscle and fascia was incised (split) in a saggital plane to create a split-thickness muscle flap which was rotated over the interscutularis muscle to support coverage of the fistula (Figure 6.46). Because the flap(s) retain their blood supply, they can be covered with a skin graft or a skin flap, or they can be allowed to heal by second intention. Muscle flaps are not commonly used in equine practice because there are few head muscles available for creating a flap located close to the defect.

Selected Techniques for Mobilizing Skin

Undermining the skin adjacent to the defect works well, particularly for small defects (Figures 6.42a,b, 6.43a–d).[4,19] The skin can be undermined several centimeters without the risk of producing necrosis as long as the subcutaneous tissue is elevated with the skin. Undermining releases the skin from some of its normal attachments, thus allowing it to be mobilized. The subcutaneous tissue, and skin if possible, are closed as separate layers. A Penrose drain should be placed if dead space remains (Figures 6.42b and 6.43c).

"Meshing" the skin adjacent to a wound is an excellent technique to mobilize skin for wound closure, especially when used with undermining (Figure 5.12). Unfortunately, it is of limited use for many of these wounds because the mesh incisions should not be placed over the defect.[19] If meshing is used, the stab incisions should be placed in the undermined skin in such a manner that mesh openings will not directly overlie the defect when the wound is closed. Pre-suturing is based on the principle of stress relaxation, whereby the skin stretches (lengthens) to release tension placed upon it.[33] Sutures can be placed in the skin adjacent to the defect 2 to 8 hours prior to repair. The additional length gained in this manner will decrease the tension upon closure. This technique is probably most applicable for body, upper limb, and neck wounds (see Figure 5.5).

The use of skin expanders has been reported in horses (Mentor Tissue Expanders, Mentor Corporation, Santa Barbara, CA).[19,32] The expanders are inserted subcutaneously, adjacent to the defect, and gradually expanded. Because of stress relaxation the skin slowly stretches, producing more skin that can be used for a reconstructive procedure. While this may be useful in selected cases it requires more than one surgical procedure, is expensive, and has had numerous complications associated with it.[32] For more information on this topic, see Chapter 5.

Skin Flaps

Skin flaps are indicated primarily for situations in which a skin deficit exists. A bi-pedicle advancement flap is created by making a linear incision in the skin a few centimeters adjacent to the defect.[19] The skin and subcutaneous tissue between the defect and the incision are undermined and the flap is slid over the defect. This will result in a skin defect at the site of the mobilized skin, which may be closed with other plastic techniques or allowed to heal by second intention.

Rotational skin flaps are of limited use in horses because of the tautness of the skin, but they may work for small defects.[4,19] Following semicircular incision of the skin and subcutaneous tissue at the wound edge, the undermined skin is rotated over the defect. An advantage of this technique is that it does not result in a skin defect; however, it does require sufficient skin for rotation, which limits its use on the horse's head.

Transposition skin flaps are rectangular pieces of skin and subcutaneous tissue that are created adjacent to the defect and rotated over the wound.[4,19] A skin defect beside the wound is created by movement of the skin. This defect is usually allowed to heal by second intention (Figure 6.44). For a more complete discussion of skin flaps, see Chapter 5.

Conclusion

The horse is a flight animal and commonly sustains injuries to its head that usually result from its artificial environment or are associated with its handling or use for work or sports activities. The head is a very complex area that has several body systems that can be injured. These injuries can result in serious health problems, greatly impair performance, or cause serious cosmetic deformities. However, many of these injuries can be treated successfully. Early identification and appropriate treatment of the injuries enhance the chances of a successful outcome. This chapter has attempted to provide useful information on the common injuries of the head to aid the reader in making an accurate diagnosis and selecting the appropriate treatment for the best possible recovery.

References

1. Stashak TS: Principles of wound healing. In Ted Stashak, ed. *Equine wound management (1st edition)*. Philadelphia: Lea and Febiger, 1991, p.1
2. Barber SM: Management of neck and head injuries. Vet Clin N Am Equine Pract 2005;21:191
3. Bailey JV: Principles of Reconstructive and plastic surgery. In: Jorge Auer and John Stick, eds. *Equine Surgery (3rd edition)*. Philadelphia: WB Saunders, 2006, p.254
4. Stashak TS: Wound management and reconstructive surgery of the head region. In Ted Stashak, ed: *Equine wound management (1st edition)*. Philadelphia: Lea and Febiger, 1991, p.89
5. Wilson DA: Management of head and neck injuries. Proc N Am Vet Conf 2006;20:252
6. Smyth GB, Brown RG, Juzwiak JS, et al: Delayed repair of an extensive lip laceration in a colt using an Estlander flap. Vet Surg 1988;17:350
7. Bowman KF: Double opposing Z-plasty for correction of stenotic nares in a horse. J Am Vet Med Assoc 1982;180:772
8. Lavach JD: *The Handbook of equine ophthalmology*. Fort Collins, Colorado: Giddings Studio Publishing, 1987, p.62
9. Barnett KC, Crispin SM, Lavach JD, et al: Ocular and adnexal emergencies and trauma, In *Equine ophthalmology (2nd edition)*. Philadelphia: Saunders, 2004, p.36
10. Milne FJ: Plastic surgery of the eyelid. Proc Am Assoc Equine Pract 1964,10:326
11. Blanchard GL, Keller WF: The rhomboid graft flap for the repair of extensive ocular adnexal defects. J Am Anim Hosp Assoc 1976;12:576
12. Titus RS: Ear. In FW Oehme and JE Prier, eds. *Textbook of large animal surgery (1st edition)*. Baltimore: Williams and Wilkins Co, 1974, p. 574
13. Howard RD, Stashak TS: Reconstructive surgery of selected injuries of the head. Vet Clin Equine Pract 1993;9:185
14. Massoni S, Vlaminck LE, Cokelaere SM, et al: Surgical correction of ear curling caused by scar tissue formation in a horse. J Am Vet Med Assoc 2005;227:1130
15. Tremane H: Management of skull fractures in the horse. In practice 2004;26:214

16. Wilson JW: Blood supply to developing, mature and healing bone. In G Sumner-Smith, ed. *Bone in clinical orthopedics (2nd edition)*. New York: Thieme Stuttgart, 2002, p.23

17. Clem MF, Debowes RM, Yovich, et al: Osseous sequestration in horses. Comp Cont Educ 1987;9:1291

18. Hillmann DJ: Equine osteology. In Robert Getty, ed. *Sisson and Grossman's, the anatomy of the domestic animals (5th edition)*. Philadelphia: WB Saunders, 1975, p.255

19. Auer JA: Craniomaxillofacial disorders. In: Jorge Auer and John Stick, eds. *Equine surgery (3rd edition)*. Philadelphia: WB Saunders, 2006, p.1341

20. Pham TV, Early SV, Park SS: Surgery of the auricle. Facial Plast Surg 2003;19:53

21. Caron JP, Barber SM, Bailey JV, et al: Periorbital skull fractures in five horses. J Am Vet Med Assoc 1986;188:280

22. Cruz AM, Barber SM, Grahn BH: Nasolacrimal duct injury following periorbital trauma with concurrent retinal choroidal detachment in a horse. Equine Pract 1997;19:20

23. Dowling BA, Dart AJ, Trope G: Surgical repair of skull fractures in four horses using cuttable bone plates. Aust Vet J 2001;79:324

24. Burba DJ, Collier MA: T-plate repair of fractures of the nasal bones in horses. J Am Vet Med Assoc 1991;199:909

25. Schumacher J, Auer JA, Shamis L: Repair of facial defects with periosteal flaps in two horses. Vet Surg 1985;14:235

26. Martin GS, McIlwraith CW: Repair of a frontal sinus eversion in a horse. Vet Surg 1981;10:149

27. McIlnay TR, Miller SM, Dugan ST: Use of canaliculorhinostomy for repair of nasolacrimal duct obstruction in a horse. J Am Vet Med Assoc 2001;218:1323

28. Blackford JT, Hanselka DV, Heitmann JM, et al: Noninvasive technique for reduction of zygomatic process fractures in the horse. Vet Surg 1985;14:21

29. Brooks DE: Orbit. In Jorge Auer and John Stick, eds. *Equine surgery (3rd edition)*. Philadelphia: WB Saunders, 2006, p.755

30. Badylak SF, Park K, Peppas N, et al: Marrow-derived cells populate scaffolds composed of xenogeneic extracellular matrix. Experimental Hematology 2001;29:1310

31. Campbell ML, Peyton LC: Muscle flap closure of a frontocutaneous fistula in a horse. Vet Surg 1984;13:185

32. Madison JB, Donawick WJ, Johnston DE, et al: The use of skin expansion to repair cosmetic defects in animals. Vet Surg 1989;18:15

33. Bristol DG: Skin grafts and skin flaps in the horse. Vet Clin N Am Equine Pract 2005;21:125

34. Waldridge BM, Bradley DM, Scardino MS, et al: Repair of a sinocutaneous fistula in a horse using a mucosal-lined myocutaneous transposition flap. Equine Pract 1997;19:7

7 | Management of Wounds of the Neck and Body

Spencer Barber, DVM, Diplomate ACVS

Introduction

A wide variety of wounds involving the neck and body are encountered in horses, and many of the factors determining the incidence of these injuries are related to the domestication and use of the horse. As a "flight" animal, the horse often reacts to frightening circumstances by running into objects (e.g., wooden post or fence or barbed wire). Horses used at high speed carry some inherent risk of impact with objects. Additionally, horses housed on premises that are not properly maintained (e.g., protruding nails, broken boards, broken tin sheds) are at a greater risk of injury. Because the horse's skin is relatively thin, impact with objects commonly leads to large skin wounds. Although most wounds of the neck and body are superficial, primarily involving the skin, many involve deeper structures.

Understanding the biology of wound repair—especially that involved in second intention healing—as well as possessing a solid knowledge of the principles of wound management and the factors that affect healing will ensure successful management of these wounds. This chapter will describe wounds occurring at specific locations on the neck and body as well as the factors that are important for their successful management.

Wounds of the Neck

Lacerations

Lacerations to the neck resulting from impact with a variety of sharp objects are especially common when horses are placed in pastures fenced with barbed wire. The injuries occur when the horse runs into the fence, causing a laceration that is usually located at the base of the neck in a horizontal plane.[1] As a result of the elastic fibers in skin, the direction of Langer's lines of tension in this area, and the natural movement of the neck, the skin edges retract.[2]

Wound Evaluation

Lacerations caused by wire often involve only the skin and subcutaneous tissue and are characterized by minimally retracted, relatively sharp skin edges (Figure 7.1). Although the brachiocephalicus, sternocephalicus, and sternothyrohyoideus muscles may be involved, they are rarely completely transected. If the laceration crosses the entire width of the neck and transects these "strap" muscles there can be considerable retraction of skin and muscle edges and subsequent loss of function.[1] If the injury is caused by contact with a wooden object (e.g., tree branch or corral fence) the wound edges are often ragged, irregular in depth, and more highly contaminated.

Treatment

Treatment options include primary closure, delayed closure, and second intention healing. Many factors must be considered prior to selecting the most appropriate treatment.[3,4] Although these wounds are classified as contaminated they often are presented in a timely fashion, are minimally contaminated, and have sharp and viable skin edges. While the tension produced upon closure of the wound edges and that produced by movement of the head and neck is an important factor, primary closure is the ideal treatment in many cases. If the wound is narrow (2 cm–3 cm wound gap) it usually can be successfully closed without excessive tension.[3] If the wound is fresh it can be debrided and closed in a standing, sedated horse.

These wounds do not usually involve underlying muscle, but if they do the muscle layer does not require closure. The subcutaneous tissue and skin are closed in one or two layers with interrupted sutures. In some cases the number of small wounds is so great that primary closure would be impractical and cost-prohibitive; in these cases the wounds will usually heal uneventfully by second intention (Figure 7.1). With intermediate-sized lacerations (10 cm–15 cm wound gap), tension suture patterns (e.g., widely placed vertical mattress or near-far-far-near) and possibly quill sutures (supports under the sutures) are needed to counteract the skin tension. Quill sutures can cause skin necrosis if they are applied too tightly or too close to the wound edges.[5] Wounds that are several days old require more extensive debridement and often are more difficult to close because of loss of pliability of the skin edges (Figure 7.2). Because these intermediate-sized wounds will heal by second intention with a cosmetically acceptable outcome, many clients choose this option over primary closure.

Fortunately, large wounds (wound gap > 15 cm), or those with complete transection of the "strap" muscles are uncommon (Figure 7.3a). They usually are treated by primary or delayed closure, if possible, because second intention healing is often very protracted and labor-intensive and because these wounds could result in significant scarring or loss of function. If, in the standing horse, wound edges can be approximated without generating excessive tension, prognosis for primary repair is reasonable as long as the patient is cooperative. Patients that accept the use of a Martingale to limit head elevation are better candidates. In others, surgical repair is best done under general anesthesia to ensure optimal debridement and closure. Thorough layered (excisional) debridement of the entire wound is important; techniques are discussed in Chapter 2.

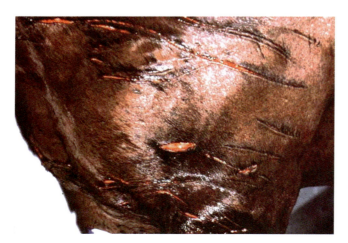

Figure 7.1. Multiple lacerations of the neck and chest caused by barbed wire fencing. These wounds, which are fresh and display sharp edges, are minimally retracted. Although they could be successfully sutured, they will also heal rapidly by second intention.

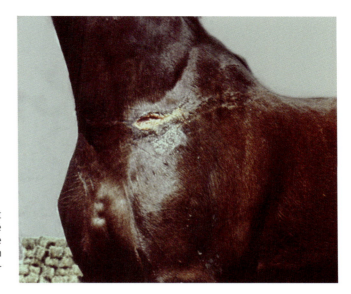

Figure 7.2. Based on the presence of granulation tissue it is estimated that this laceration is several days old. While primary closure is still possible, healing/thickening of the retracted skin edges would produce tension on the closure. With appropriate care this wound will produce minimal blemish following second intention healing.

If a strap muscle is completely transected (Figures 7.3b,c), its ends should be apposed or approximated with tension sutures, incorporating as much fascia as possible. The use of a drain is necessary because dead space will remain. Penrose drains are inexpensive and easy to place and provide good passive drainage (Figure 7.3d). Most commonly, they are used as a single-exit drain, whereby the proximal end is sutured in the depth of the wound and the distal end exits through a separate skin opening ventral to the wound. With a double-exit technique, one end exits above the wound and the other below the wound. The advantage to the double-exit technique in the ventral neck region is that drainage occurs no matter the position of the neck—flexion, neutral, or extension.

To protect the wound and Penrose drain exit site(s) from contamination and the sutures from excessive tension, a stent bandage is recommended. Umbilical tape fed through suture loops fixed in the skin adjacent to the closed incision can be used to secure a dressing over the closed laceration (Figure 7.3d). The stent bandage should be pulled tightly enough to produce some discomfort for the conscious horse because this will help restrict head movement. The use of a Martingale is also advised (Figures 7.3e,f). The stent bandage can be loosened and the dressing changed under sedation. The Penrose drains are generally removed in 2 to 3 days if there is minimal drainage, but can be retained for 5 to 7 days if drainage persists. Importantly, the longer the drains are left in place the greater the risk of ascending infection; thus, exit sites need to be maintained in a sterile environment and handled aseptically.[6–8] Anti-inflammatory drugs can be used in the first postoperative week, though some tenderness at the wound site might help limit head extension.

Neck wounds that are not sutured heal by second intention, which consists of granulation tissue formation, wound contraction, and epithelialization[9] (Figures 7.4 and 7.5). Regardless of the choice of treatment, all wounds should be thoroughly debrided and lavaged. Treatments should aim to stimulate granulation tissue formation and provide an environment in which epithelialization and wound contraction are enhanced.

Hydrotherapy of the acute wound is effective for cleansing and debridement[4] and is thought to enhance second intention healing by preventing wound dessication and stimulating granulation tissue formation, although this has not been confirmed by research. In fact, horse wounds treated with saline and water administered by gentle pressure from a syringe or rubber hose showed decreased fibroblastic activity, increased collagen production, a blunted edge to the epithelium, and no enhancement of healing rates.[10] On the other hand, it is speculated by the author that stronger pressure might enhance granulation tissue formation through increased circulation or via micro-damage to wound cells, causing them to release beneficial growth factors. The author thus advocates high-pressure hydrotherapy for the latter reason and suggests it be administered via a rubber hose with the pressure turned up high, and if necessary increased by either partially occluding the tip of the hose or by using a nozzle. Pressure sufficient to cause slight bleeding of fresh granulation tissue is recommended.

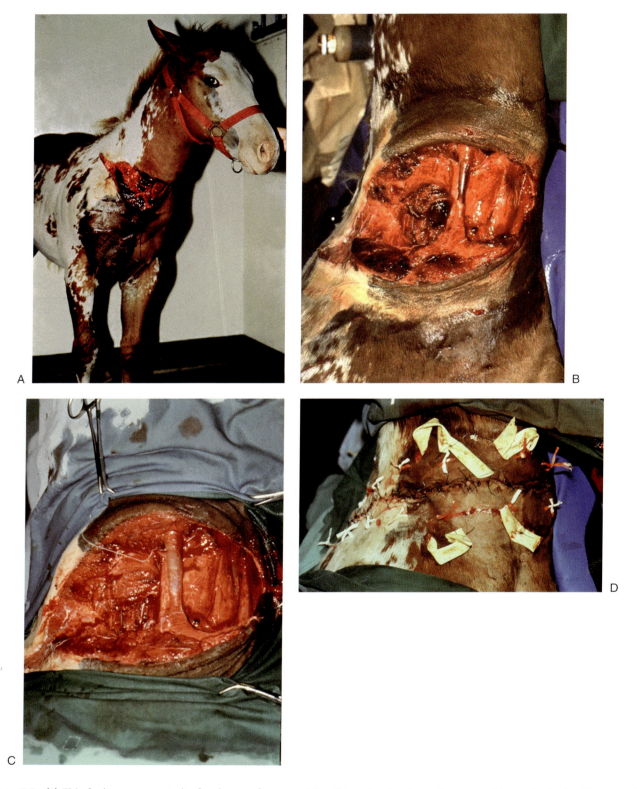

Figure 7.3. (A) This foal was presented a few hours after sustaining this extensive laceration caused by barbed wire. The wound appeared clean and fresh, and the skin edges, which were sharply cut, could be easily apposed. (B) The foal positioned in dorsal recumbency for wound reconstruction. The exposed jugular vein is viable but is missing much of its perivascular tissue. Notice the dark surface of the transected "strap" muscles (bottom left). The proximal ends of the transected muscles are retracted under the skin edge. (C) Appearance of the wound following debridement in preparation for primary closure. (D) Two Penrose drains were placed in the depth of the wound and their ends exited through slits in the skin proximal and distal to the wound. Care was taken to not place the drains in close proximity to the neurovascular structures. The strap muscles were apposed with interrupted near-far-far-near sutures without excessive tension. The jugular vein was covered with viable tissue while subcutaneous tissue and skin were closed with interrupted sutures. Umbilical tape loops were placed parallel to the skin closure in view of securing a stent bandage.

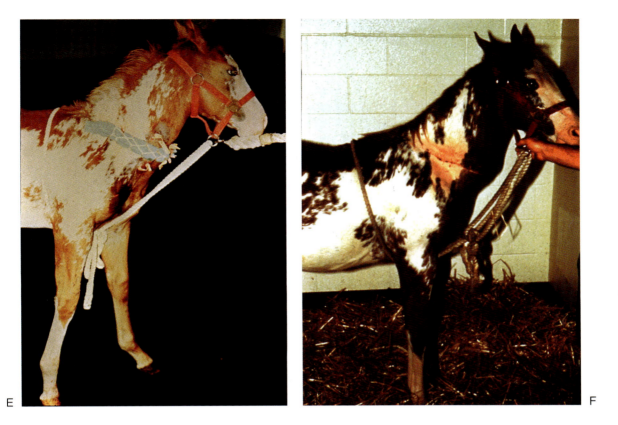

Figure 7.3. (*Continued*) (E) The wound is protected by a stent bandage made from a sterile towel, and by a "homemade" Martingale whose role is to prevent excessive upward movement of the head. The drain exit sites were cleaned QID with an antiseptic to minimize the chance of dust/dirt, other contaminants, and bacteria from entering them. (F) Healing of the wound 3 weeks after primary closure. The stent bandage was removed but the Martingale was used for another 3 weeks.

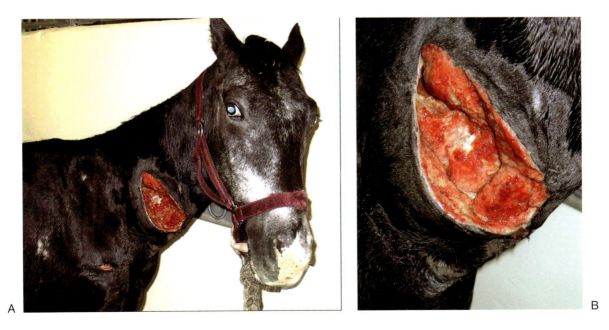

Figure 7.4. (A) A wound of the neck, presented a week after injury, healing by second intention. (B) The wound cavity should be encouraged to fill with granulation tissue for epithelialization and contraction to proceed rapidly and to a maximum extent to produce a cosmetic repair.

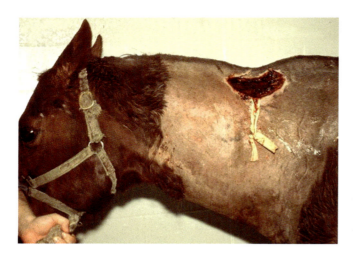

Figure 7.5. This gelding was attacked by a stallion and sustained bilateral bite wounds to the dorsolateral neck region that could not be closed. A drain was placed to ensure ventral drainage from the dorsally located wound. The blemish following healing should be minimal.

The author also advises scraping the surface of the granulation tissue lightly with the fingertips of a gloved hand or with a sterile 4×4 gauze sponge to produce light surface bleeding. As long as a defect remains in the wound it is important to stimulate granulation tissue formation to produce a level surface for optimal wound contraction and epithelialization, leading to a better cosmetic outcome. Topical application of live yeast cell derivative (Preparation H, Whitehall Laboratories, New York, NY) was shown to enhance granulation tissue formation[11] in equine limb wounds and is favored by the author after hydrotherapy.

Bandaging wounds in horses enhances granulation tissue formation and healing by maintaining a moist environment, lowering the wound pH, and providing an increased oxygen debt at the wound surface.[12,13] Conversely, exposed wounds are subject to desiccation, contamination, and slower healing rates. Because it can be difficult or impossible to bandage wounds on the neck of horses, the author covers the wound surface with a cream or sprays it with an oil-based preparation (Red Kote, H.W. Naylor Co., Morris, NY) after hydrotherapy in an effort to provide a moist environment with an increased oxygen debt. Despite the number of commercially available topical wound products, there is little scientific evidence based on controlled studies in horses upon which to base treatment selection. Hence, the choice of therapies relies on extrapolation of results from research in other species, anecdotal evidence, and evidence obtained from healing studies done in other regions of the body in horses.

Injuries of Vessels and Nerves

Laceration to the cranial aspect of the neck has the potential to damage important neurovascular structures including the jugular vein, common carotid artery, recurrent laryngeal nerve, and vagosympathetic trunk (Figure 7.6). Of these structures, the jugular vein is the most superficial. Fortunately, it is protected within the jugular groove formed by the sternocephalicus and brachiocephalicus muscles. Wounds that transect these muscles can expose the vessels and lacerate them, resulting in severe hemorrhage. More commonly, the vessel remains intact while the perivascular tissue is stripped away, subjecting its wall to ischemia and delayed rupture (Figure 7.3b).

Deep wounds may affect the carotid artery, whose complete laceration would result in rapid exsanguination. If at all possible, viable soft tissue should be apposed over these vessels during wound management to protect its wall from desiccation and trauma and to provide a source of nourishment. Neither the jugular vein nor the carotid artery are necessary for survival and if there is any concern over the integrity of the vessel it should be ligated prophylactically.[14]

The recurrent laryngeal nerve and vagosympathetic trunk are most likely to be injured in wounds of the lower cervical region, where they are closer to the skin surface and no longer covered by the omohyoideus muscle. Endoscopic examination of the larynx allows evaluation of arytenoid abduction, which is dependent upon innervation by the recurrent laryngeal nerve. Numerous clinical signs accompany damage to the vagosympathetic trunk, including abnormal intestinal motility, colic, alteration in heart rate, abnormal esophageal

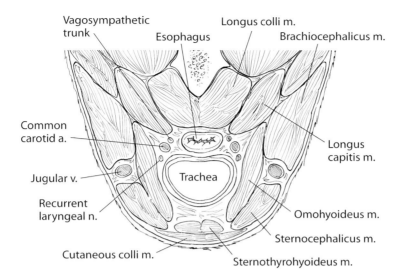

Figure 7.6. Cross-sectional drawing of the proximal cervical region showing the location of the esophagus, trachea, overlying musculature, and neurovascular structures. Lacerations to the cranial neck could result in injury to these structures.

function, sweating, and changes in skin temperature. If the carotid artery or jugular vein is prophylactically ligated, as mentioned previously, care must be taken to prevent injury to these nerves.

Injuries of the Trachea

The location of the trachea on the ventral aspect of the neck predisposes it to various forms of injury. It is located on the midline throughout the cervical region with the common carotid artery, recurrent laryngeal nerve, and vagosympathetic trunk on its dorsolateral surfaces (Figure 7.6). The esophagus is dorsal to the trachea in the proximal cervical region, on its left at the mid-cervical region, and ventral to it at the base of the neck. Throughout the entire cervical region the trachea is covered with musculature which is especially thick in the caudal aspect. The cranial cervical region is more susceptible to injury because the left and right sternocephalicus muscles have diverged and the trachea is easily palpated subcutaneously.[15]

The trachea is a flexible tube composed of hyaline cartilaginous rings that are incomplete dorsally where they are bridged by the tracheal membrane. The tracheal rings are joined to one another by the annular tracheal ligament. The trachea does not collapse in response to the negative internal pressure induced by inspiration because of these cartilaginous rings. The incomplete structure of each ring allows for lumen expansion which enhances air flow during exercise. The shape and size of the cartilaginous rings vary; proximally the rings are circular with a diameter of 5.5 cm, whereas distally they are flattened with a transverse diameter of 7 cm and a dorsoventral diameter of 5 cm.

While the trachea could be injured by a laceration, its rigid structure makes it more susceptible to damage by external forces arising from a kick, pressure from a rope, or impact with a sharp or solid object.[16–19] Other causes of tracheal injury are punctures from internal or external foreign bodies as well as excessive pressure exerted by an endotracheal tube.[20]

Trauma can result in injury to the tracheal mucosa, cartilaginous rings, tracheal membrane, and/or annular tracheal ligament. There is a wide variance of clinical signs, depending on the structures involved and the nature of the injury. The most commonly reported clinical signs are subcutaneous emphysema and changes to the respiratory rate and sounds. The clinician should check closely for tracheal damage in any deep wound that exposes the trachea in the cervical region. External examination of the trachea may be difficult in small open wounds and those with intact skin, or if there is swelling and tenderness.

Any hole of the tracheal wall will result in air escaping subcutaneously. If the skin is open, subcutaneous emphysema can be absent or minimal, but if the skin is intact the amount of subcutaneous emphysema can be extensive.[18,19] If cartilaginous rings or the tracheal membrane are ruptured and invaginate into the tracheal lumen, increased inspiratory and expiratory noises will be present over the site of injury. With marked obstruction there can be an elevated heart rate and occasionally respiratory distress.[16]

Radiographic and endoscopic examinations are indicated in any horse with a suspected tracheal injury. Radiographs of the tracheal region can readily identify a narrowed lumen, intraluminal masses, or the presence of peritracheal gas in cases with intact skin. Radiographs should also be taken of the thorax to check for pneumomediastinum, which can lead to pneumothorax. Endoscopic examination of the trachea is useful to confirm disruption of the tracheal wall, determine the size of the defect, and identify any tissues protruding into the lumen.

Treatment selection depends on the structures involved and the severity of the injury. Small, full-thickness tears accompanied by minimal subcutaneous emphysema often heal spontaneously.[17,18] Repair can be assisted by stall confinement and a pressure bandage applied over the involved site. Larger wounds with minimal subcutaneous emphysema and open wounds similarly heal well by second intention.

If the skin is intact but subcutaneous emphysema extensive, the defect may be treated in one of three ways: (1) the skin and soft tissue over the tracheal hole can be incised to enlarge the opening, (2) a tracheotomy can be performed adjacent to the rupture site, or (3) the tracheal defect can be sutured if adequate tissue is available for closure. The former two approaches are allowed to heal by second intention. Prolapse of tracheal membrane or extraluminal connective tissue into the lumen is an indication for surgical debridement and closure of the defect if possible.[18]

A large defect or complete transection of the trachea occurs rarely, can cause severe respiratory distress, is an emergency, and has been successfully repaired by primary closure.[16,19] Absorbable suture material (e.g., #2 polydioxanone) is recommended over stainless steel (25–30 gauge), which has a tendency to cut the cartilaginous rings and damage the soft tissues. Furthermore, it is important to avoid penetrating the tracheal mucosa when suturing.

Broken tracheal rings can be problematic. They may project into the tracheal lumen and obstruct airflow, act as a stimulus for granuloma formation, or cause the trachea to be unstable and collapse. If the trachea is stable, the portions of the ruptured ring protruding into the lumen can be excised and the wound allowed to heal by second intention. If several tracheal rings are ruptured on the ventral aspect but the trachea is stable, a permanent tracheostomy may be performed. This surgery is usually executed to provide a patent airway in horses with a permanent laryngeal obstruction and has been shown to yield good success.[21,22] If the ruptured tracheal rings cause collapse or instability of the trachea, an external splint of polypropylene can be applied.[23,24]

In cases with advanced tracheal damage, complete resection and anastomosis have been reported.[25] Up to four or five tracheal rings can be removed, while amputation of more usually leads to excessive tension upon anastomosis, resulting in disruption of the repair and requiring euthanasia of the patient. Conditioning the horse to a Martingale prior to surgery helps manage post-operative tension.[25]

Tracheal Stenosis

Tracheal stenosis can be divided into two categories. Primary stenosis occurs with injury to any of the tracheal structures, leading to a decreased luminal diameter, while secondary stenosis is the result of external structures impinging upon and decreasing the luminal diameter of a normal trachea[26] (Figures 7.7a,b). Because primary tracheal stenosis is a result of injury, usually subsequent to external trauma, it is most often seen in the cervical area. Regrettably, most causes of primary tracheal stenosis are iatrogenic. Mucosal injury caused by endotracheal intubation is well documented.[20,26] Intraluminal tracheal masses have been seen secondary to penetration of the tracheal wall for intratracheal administration of medication or following transtracheal aspiration.[27]

The most commonly reported cause of primary tracheal stenosis is an improperly performed tracheotomy.[20] The tracheal lumen is normally entered by incising horizontally through the annular tracheal ligament on the cranial or ventral aspect of the trachea. This must be done while avoiding incision of the cartilaginous rings[28] because these are incomplete and if transected will no longer maintain structural support, resulting in side-to-side collapse of the lumen.[20,23] The narrowed tracheal lumen restricts air flow; furthermore, the mucosa will heal in this abnormal position, possibly leading to web formation across the lumen.[20]

Another major surgical mistake committed upon tracheotomy is to incise greater than 180° of the circumference of the trachea, which allows the adjacent tracheal rings to retract excessively, producing a large defect.

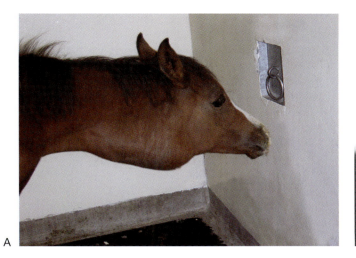
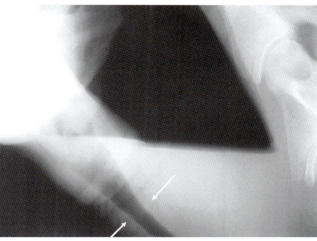

A B

Figure 7.7. (A) This foal had chronic severe bilateral guttural pouch tympany resulting in dysphagia and marked respiratory difficulty upon light exercise. (B) The markedly enlarged air-filled guttural pouches are seen as large black areas in the center and top of the radiograph. A horizontal fluid line is visible in the ventral part of guttural pouch. The tracheal lumen is stenotic secondary to the external pressure exerted by the enlarged guttural pouch.

Once again, the mucosa may heal over this defect, producing a web or invaginating into the lumen and causing obstruction upon inspiration.[20] Secondary tracheal stenosis has been reported following external pressure exerted by a peritracheal abscess,[29,30] abscessed lymph nodes,[31] lymphoma,[24] and guttural pouch tympany (Figures 7.7a,b).

The clinical signs of tracheal stenosis depend on the degree of narrowing and the demands placed upon the respiratory tract. Clinical signs may be absent in horses that have a sedentary lifestyle if there is only mild stenosis; however, the horse may show an intolerance to exercise.[20,26] Poor exercise performance, increased respiratory rate, and increased inspiratory and expiratory noises have been noted. With marked tracheal narrowing, clinical signs of dyspnea including flared nostrils, loud respiratory sounds that are primarily inspiratory, and an occasional cough can occur. As with tracheal collapse, auscultation helps localize the area of turbulent air flow. Intraluminal masses or broken and protruding tracheal rings can be identified by endoscopic examination, as will be flattening of the tracheal lumen associated with external masses.[20] Radiographs are helpful in localizing the area and the length of tracheal narrowing and in identifying intraluminal or external masses (Figure 7.7b) as well as broken tracheal rings. In some cases, abscesses or tumors may be identified externally or upon deep palpation.[24,31]

The management of tracheal stenosis will depend on the type of obstruction present. The goals of treatment are to remove any intraluminal mass, eliminate any external mass causing compression, and maintain integrity of the tracheal wall if structural support is lost. Transendoscopic laser treatment has been used successfully to remove small intraluminal masses.[27] The treatment of abscesses with drainage and antibiotics has successfully resolved secondary tracheal stenosis;[30,31] however, permanent damage to the trachea from external compression has also been reported.[24,29] In one case, an extraluminal polypropylene prosthesis was used to successfully prevent occlusion when three tracheal rings were damaged.[24] Complete transection of the tracheal rings during a tracheotomy procedure caused a deformity of the trachea, seen endoscopically as ventral narrowing with a "key-hole"-shaped lumen.[23] This was treated successfully by applying an extraluminal prosthesis.[23] Partial chondrotomies may be necessary to remodel the deformed tracheal rings in chronic cases.[23] A complete circumferential extraluminal prosthesis should not be placed in young animals, because secondary stenosis has been induced when the growing tracheal tissue is forced to fold inward, causing secondary luminal stenosis.[32]

Tracheal resection and anastomosis, as well as permanent tracheostomy, may occasionally be useful in treating tracheal stenosis.[21,22,25] If luminal patency and tracheal wall stability cannot be obtained with an extraluminal prosthesis, tracheal resection and anastomosis may be indicated for cervical lesions. Lesions restricted to five tracheal rings in ponies and three tracheal rings in horses have been treated successfully.[25] Following surgery it is important to restrict head movement, maintaining the head at a 90° angle to the neck to prevent disruption of the anastomosis.[25] A permanent tracheostomy is usually performed when a lasting severe respiratory tract obstruction exists rostral to the trachea.[21,22] However, this technique may also be used to treat tracheal stenosis if removal of the ventral one-third of the tracheal rings relieves the obstruction; for example, in the case of granulomas or cartilaginous tumors. Removal of the ventral aspect of four tracheal rings has also been reported.[21] A permanent tracheostomy is, however, not indicated for tracheal stenosis resulting from transected tracheal rings that have caused deformity of the lumen. In fact, tracheal stenosis secondary to "collapse" is occasionally seen following a permanent tracheostomy; however, most animals have productive lives—some can be used as brood mares while others may even be returned to riding activities.[21,22]

Esophageal Trauma

Both intraluminal trauma caused by an impaction or a foreign body and extraluminal trauma caused by impact with sharp or blunt objects may injure the esophagus (Figure 7.8a). Knowledge of the clinical signs,

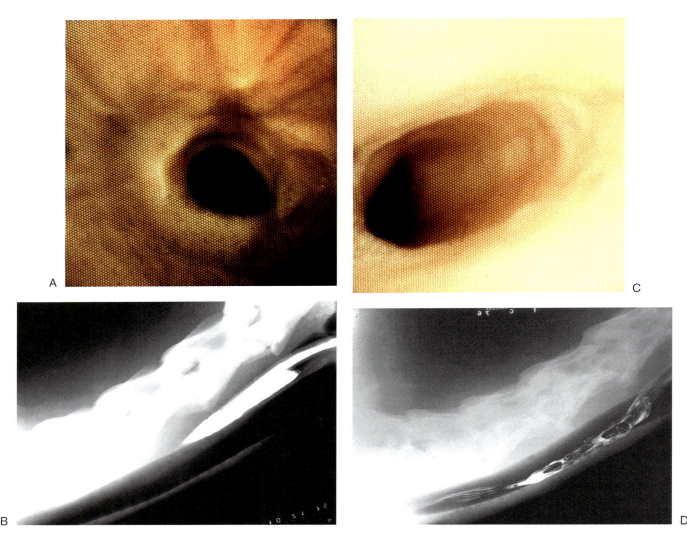

Figure 7.8. (A) Endoscopic view of the mid-cervical segment of the esophagus showing a chronic stricture secondary to a food impaction. (B) Positive contrast esophagram. Barium administered via a stomach tube cannot pass caudally because of the stricture and is refluxing proximally along the tube. (C) Endoscopic view showing enlarged esophageal luminal diameter following esophageal patch grafting with the sternocephalicus muscle. (D) Positive barium study. Note the patency of the esophageal lumen following an esophageal patch graft procedure.

diagnostic procedures, and available treatment options is important for optimal management. This section will focus on extraluminal trauma.

Anatomical Considerations

The cervical portion of the esophagus is the segment most often traumatized. It is covered by musculature over its entire length and is well protected from external trauma proximally by way of its location dorsal to the trachea. However, its location lateral to the trachea in the mid-cervical region and ventral to the trachea in the caudal neck subject it to external blows or lacerations. Adjacent to the esophagus are the recurrent laryngeal nerves, vagosympathetic trunks, and common carotid arteries, which could be injured simultaneously (Figure 7.6). The esophagus, a musculomembranous tube capable of dilation, is lined by abundant mucosa arranged in longitudinal folds. The mucosa and submucosa possess the greatest amount of collagen and are considered the strongest layers for surgical closure. The cervical esophagus is composed of two layers of striated muscle covered by a tunica adventitia.[33]

Clinical Signs

Clinical signs of esophageal trauma depend on the nature of the injury. Rupture of the esophageal musculature from blunt trauma, producing a pulsion diverticulum, causes a swelling that is more discrete and fluctuates in size in association with the intake of food and water. A full-thickness rupture or laceration of the esophageal wall causes discharge of saliva, food, air, and bacteria into the peri-esophageal fascial planes. If the skin is intact a cervical swelling that is diffuse, hot, painful to digital pressure, and presenting crepitus may develop. If the skin has been lacerated the signs of infection may be less evident but saliva and food material will be seen exiting the wound. In either case cellulitis is present and infection may gravitate toward the thoracic inlet. Increased respiratory rate and abnormal respiratory sounds, if present, suggest aspiration pneumonia or extension of the cervical infection into the mediastinum or pleura.[33,34]

Injury to an adjacent carotid artery can cause profuse and fatal hemorrhage,[35] while damage to a recurrent laryngeal nerve causes laryngeal hemiplegia[36] and injury to the vagosympathetic trunk causes Horner's syndrome. Lacerations of the esophagus cause loss of large volumes of saliva, and, without continued intake of food and water, hyponatremia, hypochloremia, metabolic alkalosis, and dehydration will ensue.[33]

Diagnostic Considerations

If a laceration is present the esophagus may be evaluated visually and digitally, using care to avoid injuring adjacent neurovascular structures. Passing a nasogastric tube is useful to check the patency and integrity of the esophagus. With a pulsion diverticulum or esophageal rupture the nasogastric tube may occasionally be passed normally, while at other times the tip of the tube may lodge itself in the diverticulum or exit the lumen into the peri-esophageal tissue or the open wound.

Endoscopic examination is important both diagnostically and for evaluating the severity of the injury. A flexible endoscope of approximately 2 m–3 m in length, with both irrigation and insufflation capabilities, is used in the standing horse. The normal esophageal mucosa is white to light pink in color, and except at the most proximal aspect it presents longitudinal folds that flatten when the lumen is dilated with air. If saliva or food material is present in the lumen it should be removed by lavage to allow a more detailed inspection of the esophagus. A defect of the wall may be seen with a pulsion diverticulum or ruptured esophageal wall, the latter allowing passage of the endoscope tip into the peri-esophageal tissues.[33]

Plain radiographs are important for identifying the nature of the injury even though a normal esophagus is not radiographically visible. With a pulsion diverticulum gas, food, and saliva can mix together proximal to the obstruction, producing either an irregular mottled gas shadow or a gas dilation of the proximal esophagus. Metallic foreign bodies or masses external to the esophagus (e.g., abscess) are rare but may also be identified radiographically. With intact skin, the presence of air outside the esophageal lumen suggests rupture of the esophageal wall.

However, when the skin has been penetrated, air in the depth of the wound is normal and contrast radiographs are required to demonstrate a luminal defect. A negative contrast radiograph, obtained by passing a cuffed nasogastric tube into the proximal esophagus and injecting air to dilate the esophagus, helps to identify foreign bodies, a diverticulum, or full-thickness wall perforations. In a positive contrast radiograph, barium sulfate paste given orally coats the normal longitudinal folds of the esophagus (Figure 7.8b). A pulsion diverticulum will allow collection of contrast material within the lumen, while a rupture permits dissemination into the fascial planes.

A double contrast study can be performed by injecting barium sulfate followed by air through a cuffed nasogastric tube. This dilates the esophagus and then coats the longitudinal folds with contrast material and is considered the method of choice to evaluate mucosal lesions. Swallowing during distention can produce peristaltic waves that can be misinterpreted as a stricture; this can be prevented by pre-medicating with xylazine (Rompun, Bayer Inc., Toronto, Ontario).[33]

Esophageal Healing

Constant tension, motion, and dilation, as well as the presence of saliva, food, and bacteria, challenge healing. Tissue strength is also limited by the absence of a serosal layer and a less than abundant blood supply. Furthermore, the healed esophagus must be dilatable to ensure proper function. The most common complications are dehiscence and stricture formation, and the long-term survival rate after esophageal injury is low.[37]

Injuries that cause destruction of only the epithelial component of the mucosal layer (similar to epithelial defects of the skin) heal without scar formation because of the epithelium's excellent regenerative capabilities.[38] However, all injuries, whether surgical or not, that involve any of the submucosal, muscular, or adventitial layers lead to the formation of granulation tissue with subsequent wound contraction and scar formation.[38]

Experimental studies in horses have shown that linear esophagostomy sites can heal without clinically significant strictures.[39] This suggests that the amount of trauma produced by experimental incisions is likely minor compared to naturally-occurring injuries and emphasizes the fact that most traumatic injuries are not linear. Because scar contracture is a concern during esophageal healing, circumferential injuries would potentially be more serious than linear ones. Indeed, when a 3 cm long mucosal resection and anastomosis was performed experimentally, mucosal repairs dehisced and all animals subsequently developed strictures.[40] Fortunately, the severity of the stricture often decreases over time. For example, maximal reduction in luminal diameter was shown in clinical cases to occur at approximately 30 days, followed by a spontaneous increase to reach a normal diameter in five of seven horses by day 60.[41] This no doubt results from normal scar remodeling and dilation from eating. If surgical correction of a stricture is contemplated, it likely should be delayed until at least 60 days post-injury.

In experimental horses, sutured linear esophagostomies healed faster than non-sutured lesions and had a lower incidence of traction diverticulum, but had a higher complication rate, including death, because of dehiscence, fistula formation, and abscessation of the sutured esophagostomies.[39] Sutured esophagostomy incisions are more likely to dehisce if a nasogastric tube is retained within the esophageal lumen following repair.[40] Diet can directly affect esophageal healing, with a high dehiscence rate in horses fed hay compared to a soft diet.[42] Placement of an esophagostomy tube caudal (aboral) to a sutured esophagostomy site allows better healing of the repair site, but complications and even fatality have been reported following placement of an esophagostomy tube as a result of cervical infection, thrombophlebitis, and thoracic infection.[40,43]

Management of Esophageal Lacerations and Ruptures

Laceration or puncture of the esophagus is uncommon but most likely to occur following injury to the lower half of the cervical region.[44] Ruptures of the esophagus have been caused by kicks, penetration with a foreign body, following forceful passage of a nasogastric tube, chronic obstruction, or by extension of an infectious process.[36,45,46] Ruptures are seen more commonly in the cranial esophagus and have been reported to be 2 cm–5 cm long.[36,44–46] Both lacerations and ruptures result in the escape of food, saliva, and bacteria into the peri-esophageal tissue (Figure 7.9).

The defect must be treated either by primary closure or second intention healing. Important elements to be considered when selecting the approach include the size, type, and degree of damage to the esophageal wall; the age of the injury; the degree of contamination; and the presence of infection or necrosis of the peri-esophageal tissue. Linear lacerations or acute ruptures with minimal esophageal trauma and contamination and with no established infection or necrosis have been treated successfully by primary closure.[44,45]

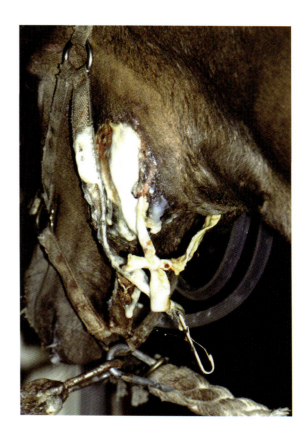

Figure 7.9. Discharge of saliva from a ruptured proximal esophagus.

If the esophagus is not exposed following laceration, it is approached by an incision created either over the jugular groove or on the ventral midline. General anesthesia and dorsal recumbency are recommended, while placement of a nasogastric tube helps to identify the esophagus. Debridement of esophageal tissue should be conservative to limit tension generated by closure. The mucosa and submucosa are closed in a simple continuous pattern using 3-0 polypropylene with the knots tied in the lumen, and the muscular layers are closed with interrupted sutures of 2-0 polydioxanone.[33] If there are concerns regarding the degree of contamination of the peri-esophageal tissue, the layers superficial to the esophagus can be left to heal by second intention. To protect the repair, feed should be withheld for a couple of days after which the horse may be fed water-soaked pelleted feed. Alternatively, an esophagostomy tube may be placed distal to the repair site; this port is then left to heal by second intention.[33]

If there is extensive damage to the esophageal wall, closure likely will fail and should not be attempted. With intact skin, feed, saliva, and bacteria will become trapped within the fascial planes, resulting in a marked cellulitis that in chronic cases can cause rupture of the overlying skin or dissect distally into the mediastinum or pleura. In this case, establishing ventral drainage followed by lavage of the fascial planes is paramount to success. An esophagostomy tube placed either through the rupture site or distal to the defect can be used to provide nutritional support and prevent further contamination that occurs from continued leakage of feed from the rupture site.[33,36] Loss of food, water, and saliva from the esophagotomy site, while it is healing by second intention, can be prevented by placing a temporary patch made of dental acrylic over the hole.[36] Esophagostomies have been associated with complications including mucosal web obstruction from a traction diverticulum, peri-esophageal diverticulum, and death.[36,43]

Broad-spectrum antibiotics, including those ensuring anaerobic coverage, must be administered for an extended time while fluid and electrolyte imbalances must be corrected. Indeed, the loss of large volumes of saliva leads to hyponatremia, hypochloremia, and metabolic acidosis.[33] Attention must also be paid to providing appropriate nutritional support.[36] Despite the best efforts and care, the prognosis following esophageal rupture remains poor.[37]

Management of Esophageal Diverticula

There are two types of esophageal diverticula: traction (true) and pulsion (false). A traction diverticulum forms following contraction of peri-esophageal fibrous tissue, usually secondary to surgical or non-surgical penetration of the esophagus, especially in sites healing by second intention. Traction of this fibrous tissue on the esophageal wall causes an outward deviation of the latter. While traction diverticula usually impart minimal clinical consequences,[33] esophageal obstruction was seen following formation of a mucosal web constriction in a traction diverticulum occurring at an esophagostomy site.[36] In this particular case, the obstruction was relieved initially by dilation over 14 days with an indwelling nasogastric tube, which favored scar tissue remodeling. The obstruction, which recurred a week later, was successfully treated with repeat linear incisions of the mucosa through the esophagostomy fistula, accompanied by dietary changes to increase roughage content. No luminal strictures or diverticula were identified on endoscopic examination 40 days later.[36]

Pulsion diverticula are much more likely to cause clinical problems. They result from loss of integrity of the esophageal muscular layer, possibly by overstretching and rupture of the latter secondary to esophageal impactions, but are more commonly seen as a result of blunt trauma such as a kick.[33,37] The mucosa bulges through the muscular defect into the peri-esophageal tissue, creating a cavity usually characterized by a narrow base. The prominent clinical sign is a cervical swelling that enlarges when the horse eats and diminishes after eating or upon massage of the swelling.[33,47] Repeated dilation may cause enlargement of the diverticulum and clinical swelling, which sometimes persists for several years.[33] The defect in the esophageal wall can occasionally be seen endoscopically. A contrast study will demonstrate the presence of a spherical diverticular sac and help define the size of both the sac and the diverticular opening.

Complete impaction of the diverticulum and obstruction of the esophagus with the classical signs of choke and secondary aspiration pneumonia have been reported.[48] Surgical correction is recommended to prevent complete esophageal obstruction or impaction of the diverticulum and its subsequent rupture. This can be accomplished by mucosal inversion or a diverticulectomy.

The preferred treatment is inversion of the mucosa and closure of the muscular layer because this preserves mucosal integrity.[33] In chronic lesions or any diverticula with a large sac and narrow base, inversion of the mucosa may, however, lead to esophageal obstruction in response to excessive tissue in the esophageal lumen. In these cases, a diverticulectomy is recommended.[47] Care must be taken to prevent contamination during surgery, and all layers of the wall must be closed meticulously to reduce the likelihood of esophageal leakage and subsequent infection or stricture. Modifying the diet, such as offering pelleted feed soaked in water for several days, is recommended post-operatively to reduce the risk of esophageal dehiscence.

Management of Esophageal Strictures

While experimentally created longitudinal incisions can heal without stricture formation,[39] esophageal strictures are a frequent complication of naturally occurring esophageal trauma or surgery because the injury is usually circumferential and all layers of the esophagus, except the mucosal epithelium, heal by fibroplasia and contraction. Different types of esophageal strictures have been described:[33] those involving only the mucosa and submucosa are known as esophageal rings or webs and those of only the muscular wall are called mural lesions, while those involving all layers of the wall are referred to as annular stenosis.

Conservative management using bougienage or pneumatic or hydrostatic dilators has been used with limited success in the horse. A mucosal stricture in a foal was nonetheless successfully treated with a balloon dilation procedure,[49] a technique previously used effectively in small animals and humans. Balloon dilation may be a superior technique because it uses radial forces rather than the longitudinal shearing forces generated by bougienage, which could cause esophageal perforation and diverticulum formation.

Because scar tissue is dynamic and can undergo considerable remodeling, surgical treatment of strictures should be delayed more than 60 days following injury, in case natural remodeling is sufficient to alleviate clinical signs.[41,50] A number of surgical procedures have been employed, with varying degrees of success, to treat esophageal stricture. These include esophagomyotomy, partial resection and anastomosis (of the mucosa), complete resection and anastomosis of the esophageal wall, as well as muscular patch grafting[33,51–58] (Figures 7.8c,d).

An esophagomyotomy was used successfully to treat mural strictures.[33,52,56] In this case, a linear incision that extends 1 cm oral and 1 cm aboral to the stricture is made through all layers of the esophageal wall except the mucosa. The muscularis is separated from the mucosa around the entire circumference of the esophagus and the muscular defect is left open. While mural strictures are thought to respond favorably to this treatment, some horses have developed recurrent obstructions when on a roughage diet.[56]

Esophageal rings or webs and annular stenosis present more formidable challenges for treatment. At this time, it is recommended that esophageal web constrictions be treated by resection of the mucosal scar, through a longitudinal esophagotomy, followed by anastomosis of the mucosa if it can be approximated without excessive tension. Otherwise, the mucosal defect is allowed to epithelialize naturally.[33] Unfortunately, mucosal resection and anastomosis, both experimentally[40] and clinically,[55] led to mucosal dehiscence and esophageal stricture formation in all treated horses.

Surgical closure of the mucosa without closure of the muscularis, which may be done for treatment of annular stenosis, usually results in mucosal dehiscence but the defect may still heal with an enlarged esophageal lumen.[53] In contrast, complete resection and anastomosis is indicated only when there is complete transection of the esophageal wall or when the wall of the esophagus is non-viable. Training a horse, prior to surgery, to accept a Martingale may help limit tension on the esophageal repair. Successful outcomes have been reported following removal of 3.5 cm and 5 cm segments of the esophagus in two foals.[57] Conversely, two other cases required long-term use of a modified diet to prevent recurrent obstructions, while complete failure and euthanasia has also been reported.[51,54] Enlargement of the esophageal lumen via the use of a sternocephalicus muscle patch has also been described and may be indicated when the stricture is extensive in length (Figures 7.8c,d),[58] yet success with this technique has also been mixed.[37,58]

In conclusion, while there are isolated reports of "success," complications abound and lead to a low long-term survival rate.[37] There is currently no consistently reliable surgical treatment for esophageal web and annular stenotic lesions.

Wounds of the Body

Wounds of the body are seen frequently in equine practice. In some geographical locations they are primarily caused by the horse coming in contact with barbed wire; however, any sharp or protruding object can inflict injury. Objects that are narrow (e.g., wire) or sharp (e.g., nail or tin) usually cause linear lacerations of the skin with either retraction of the wound edges or production of a skin flap. If the horse collides with a blunt object (e.g., post or rail), the tissues may suffer more trauma and have less regular wound edges, with the skin being the primary tissue injured. Lacerations that extend into the underlying musculature frequently produce multiple dissection planes and retraction of the cut portion of the muscle belly. Nevertheless, it is uncommon for this type of injury to cause complete transection of a muscle or damage to a sufficient amount of muscle belly to lead to a permanent loss of function. Because injuries are primarily caused by the horse running into or through a fence, the most common locations for wounds are the forearm (antebrachium), pectoral region, axilla, medial thigh, ventral abdomen, and lateral thorax.

Treatment selection depends on many factors. Generally, these wounds are less contaminated than those afflicting the distal limb; however, a repair cannot usually be protected with or covered by a bandage. Furthermore, loss or retraction of tissue, as well as excessive blunt trauma or multiple adjacent lacerations, may preclude primary closure. Additionally, the wounds may be located in areas of high motion where protection of the repair from tension is difficult. Thus, while primary or delayed closure of any wound is preferable, it often is impossible to close many body wounds (Figures 7.10a,b).

Another important consideration is the difference in healing between body wounds and distal limb wounds in horses. Wounds of the body, in most cases, do not develop exuberant granulation tissue and the associated complications seen in distal limb wounds. Moreover, body wounds benefit from more rapid and pronounced contraction than do wounds located on the distal limb.[59] Hence, second intention healing of body wounds occurs more rapidly and with fewer complications than that of distal limb wounds of similar size and nature (Figures 7.11a,b,c). Financial considerations also represent an important factor. If a horse suffers an injury that is capable of healing by second intention the client will often chose the latter over a more costly repair. Many of these body wounds heal with good cosmetic and functional results by second intention healing.

All wounds should be evaluated closely and debrided as thoroughly as possible, regardless of the chosen treatment (see Chapter 2 for a more complete discussion). The objectives of treating a wound healing by second intention are to stimulate granulation tissue formation and enhance wound contraction and epithelialization. When there is a muscular defect, it is desirable to have it fill with granulation tissue for two reasons:

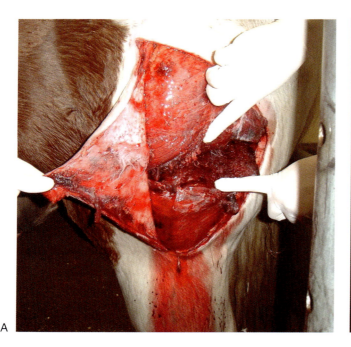
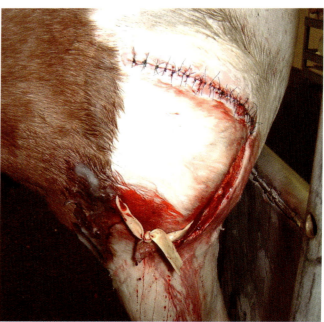

A   B

Figure 7.10. (A) This horse impaled itself upon a large metal gate hinge. There is a sizable L-shaped skin laceration and a large horizontal 6 cm deep rupture of the biceps femoris muscle. (B) A partial primary closure was performed. The wound was clean, there was minimal fraying of muscle tissue, and all except the caudal edge of the skin flap appeared viable. Following debridement a Penrose drain was placed to facilitate drainage. The muscle was not sutured but the subcutaneous tissue and skin were closed along the proximal aspect of the wound. The caudal edge of the skin flap died and was removed a few days later. The wound healed with minimal blemish.

granulation tissue contains myofibroblasts that contribute to wound contraction and the final appearance of the scar will be superior.

Hydrotherapy delivered at 15 PSI is helpful during initial wound management as a means to debride the wound. High-pressure lavage (≥15 PSI) is often avoided at the outset to prevent driving bacteria and contaminants into exposed tissue planes. When the wound surface is covered with granulation tissue, lavage with high pressure may enhance the formation of further granulation tissue. The author continues hydrotherapy until the wound is completely healed.

Wound contraction and epithelialization rates are faster in wounds that are dressed/bandaged because of reduced contamination, less desiccation, and a warmer environment, which favor the migration of keratinocytes. Because body wounds often cannot be bandaged, an attempt is made to prevent or reduce desiccation by applying an ointment to the wound surface following hydrotherapy. While many products are commercially available, most lack scientific proof of efficacy. Preparation H (containing BioDyne) has been shown experimentally to enhance granulation tissue formation in the distal limb wounds of horses and, in the author's experience, enhances wound contraction.[11]

Lacerations of the Forearm

The forearm is one of the most common locations for body lacerations. The wound is typically positioned on the cranial surface of the proximal forearm in a horizontal (transverse) plane (Figures 7.12a,b). The skin edges usually retract proximad and distad over a considerable distance because of the normal skin tension lines. Most often only the skin and subcutaneous tissues are involved but superficial lacerations of the extensor carpi radialis muscle and sometimes the common digital extensor muscle may occur. In these cases, the distal muscular segment can protrude cranially over the distal skin edge.

With more severe lacerations there can be loss of a sizeable portion of skin and muscle (Figures 7.13a–d) or creation of a large, ventrally-based flap of skin and muscle (Figures 7.14a,b). Because of the high degree of

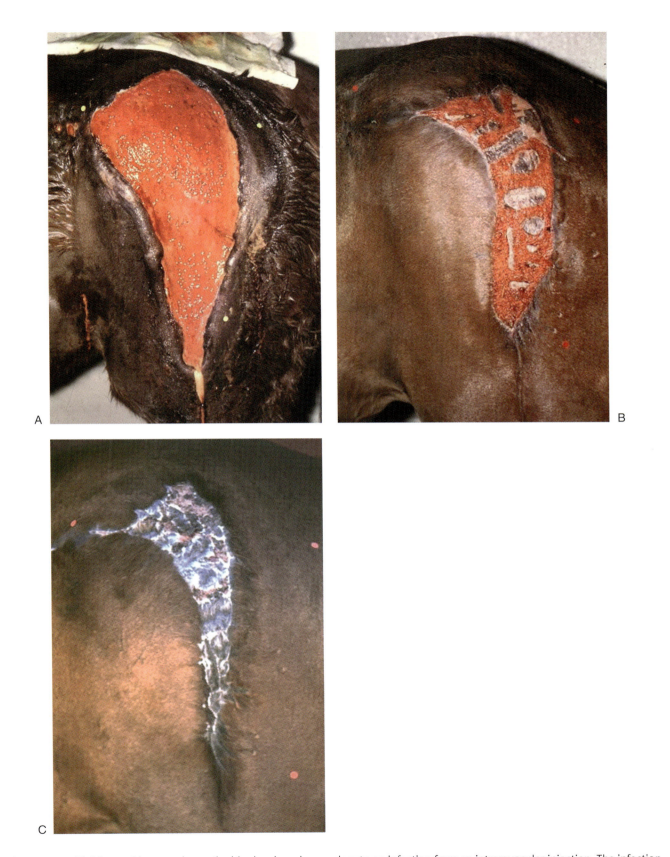

Figure 7.11. (A) A large skin wound over the hip developed secondary to an infection from an intramuscular injection. The infection has been eliminated and the wound has filled with healthy granulation tissue. (B) The wound has undergone considerable wound contraction and is much smaller. Tunnel grafts have recently been placed to assist healing. (C) The wound, which has undergone additional wound contraction and epithelialization from the skin grafts, is completely healed 6 months after it occurred. Considering the original wound size the blemish is very acceptable.

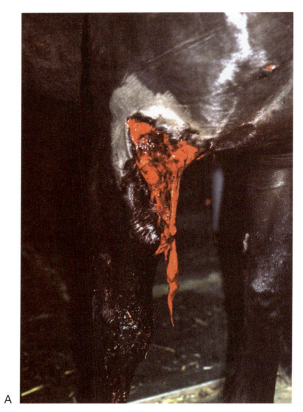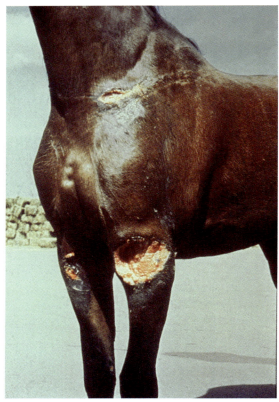

A   B

Figure 7.12. Typical lacerations of the proximal forearm. (A) This acute wound involves only the skin but suffers from considerable retraction of the skin edges. Primary closure might be attempted; however, the wound will likely dehisce because of excessive tension and motion in this area. (B) This wound involved the skin and extended partially into the extensor muscles of the forearm. The wound is granulating in but still shows a significant defect.

movement in the location of these wounds, the horse is quite sore and advances the limb carefully, even with superficial wounds. Horses with large muscle flaps develop considerable swelling of the carpal region in a couple of days. They do not advance the limb well because of pain upon carpal flexion. This can make it difficult to evaluate the amount of extensor function lost to injury. Bandaging the limb distal to the wound helps control and reduce swelling.

Most of these wounds heal very well by second intention (Figures 7.15a,b). Because of both skin retraction and skin loss, it is difficult to appose the wound edges without generating excessive tension. Any muscle or skin that is rolled out at the ventral border of the wound should be excised. The wound is treated with hydrotherapy twice daily, an ointment (e.g., Preparation H) is applied to the wound surface, and petroleum-based jelly is placed ventral to the wound to prevent serum scald. The limb distal to the wound can be bandaged and analgesics are given for a few days. It is important to actively encourage fibroplasia in those wounds with a muscle deficit. In the absence of a sufficient amount of granulation tissue, wound contraction occurs more slowly, and a permanent depression at the site of the healed wound is formed.

Closure of these forearm wounds is attempted in the following situations: (1) in very fresh wounds in which the tissues can be apposed without excessive tension, and (2) in wounds in which there is a large ventrally-based flap of skin and/or muscle. Large extensor muscle flaps (Figure 7.14a) should be sutured in an attempt to limit any loss of function by preserving as much muscle tissue as possible. The edge of the distal flap is the most susceptible to ischemia; its viability is estimated clinically by assessing the warmth of the tissue and bleeding when the flap is poked with a needle or its edges are trimmed. If the flap is cold and does not bleed when cut, it is not worth trying to save it. Often there is some warmth and bleeding, in which case the flap should be preserved despite uncertain long-term viability. While the edge of the distal flap may eventually die, closure of the wound will help preserve some viable tissue more distal in the flap.

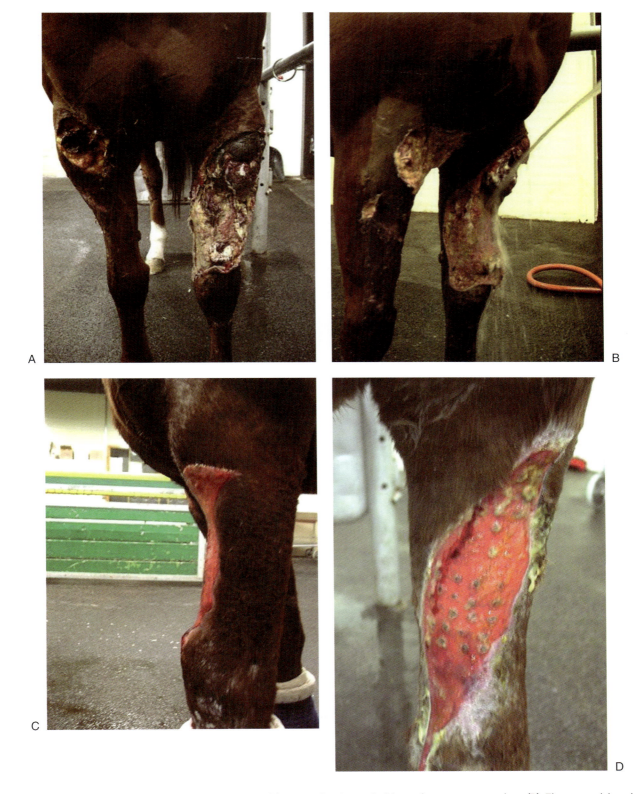

Figure 7.13. (A) Severe laceration of the forearm with extensive loss of skin and extensor muscles. (B) The wound has been debrided. Note the major loss of muscle tissue. Hydrotherapy, with water administered at medium pressure from a hose, is used to help debride the wound and stimulate granulation tissue formation. (C) The wound is granulating nicely but the loss of extensor muscle tissue is permanent and will generate a marked depression upon closure. (D) The wound has been pinch-grafted to enhance healing. The wound was completely healed 6 months after injury. The horse suffered from a reduced ability to flex and extend the leg but functioned well as a brood mare.

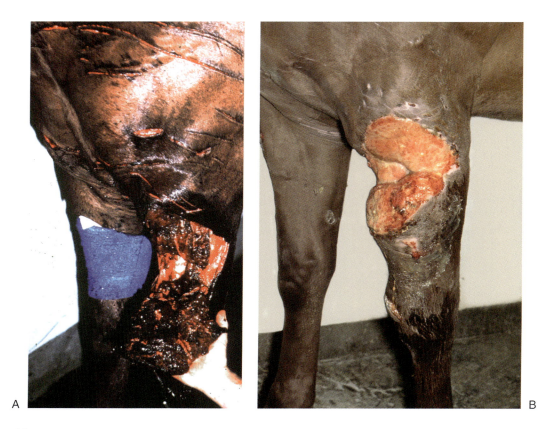

Figure 7.14. (A) Fresh laceration of the forearm resulting in a large ventrally based skin and muscle flap. Most of the extensor muscle bellies have been transected and are of questionable viability. Notice that the cortex of the radius is exposed (white area in the wound). (B) Despite primary closure and immobilization of the limb, a portion of the flap sloughed. The remaining wound healed by second intention but reduced extensor function ended this horse's athletic career.

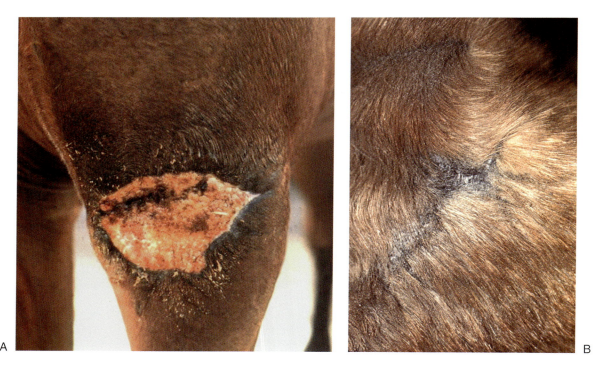

Figure 7.15. (A) Typical laceration of the proximal forearm that is healing by second intention. The defect has filled with granulation tissue. (B) Appearance of the laceration once completely healed. Cosmesis is very good because the defect filled with granulation tissue and contracted a maximum amount.

If the cortex of the radius is exposed, it will be ischemic and contaminated with bacteria, predisposing it to sequestrum formation (Figure 7.14a). In these cases, the bone should be aggressively cleaned with lavage delivered at 15 PSI[60] and in some cases the external cortex of the bone should be debrided ("partial decortication") with a power-operated burr or bone rasp, down to bleeding or oozing canaliculi on a thick cortex. If at all possible, the exposed bone should be covered with viable soft tissue. It is important to place Penrose drains that exit the skin distal to the wound prior to closure to ensure drainage of dead space.

Because of high tension and movement in this region, large synthetic suture material (#1 or #2) is recommended. If possible, a few interrupted sutures are placed in the subcutaneous tissue. The skin is closed with large suture material placed in a tension-relieving pattern. While the edges may not be completely apposed, sutures help hold the flap proximally, thus minimizing the wound area required to heal by second intention. Near-far-far-near sutures are very effective at apposing the skin edges in regions of high tension; quill sutures that make use of rubber tubing to dissipate the tension brought about by the suture may also be used. Skin necrosis can be caused by the sutures themselves or from the rubber stents, which should not be placed too close to the skin edges. Some sloughing of the tip of the flap commonly occurs after closure.

Post-operative care is directed at reducing the risk of dehiscence. The most critical objective is to protect the sutured wound from movement. The limb is wrapped with a full-limb modified Robert Jones bandage in which a full-length splint is applied to the caudal surface of the limb and the horse is cross-tied or tied to an overhead wire which allows it to walk back and forth but not lie down. The splint is changed every 3 to 4 days, under sedation if necessary. Splinting is continued for a minimum of 3 weeks, the sutures are removed, and the horse is kept cross-tied or on a wire for an additional 2 to 3 weeks. Unless there is extensive muscle loss, the prognosis for full return to function and for a cosmetic repair is very good.

Lacerations of the Pectoral Region

Wounds of the pectoral region are generally oriented in either a transverse or a sagittal plane. Laceration of the underlying musculature is usually minor with transverse wounds, but can be quite deep for those oriented sagittally. Retraction of the skin edges is usually minimal in transversely oriented wounds, compared to forearm injuries, and even less significant in sagittal lacerations. If the wounds are superficial and fresh they often can be successfully sutured, but they also heal quickly by second intention, and many clients prefer to have them managed in that fashion. Because most lacerations in the sagittal plane often extend deeper into the muscle and create greater tissue damage, they usually are left open; however, some can be successfully sutured (Figures 7.16a,b). Muscle loss leading to a cosmetic defect or loss of function is very rare. If a small flap of skin or muscle is found adjacent to the open wound, the everted tissue is excised. Drains are not usually necessary unless a portion of the wound is sutured, and exercise need not be restricted.

Lacerations of the Axilla

These lacerations are oriented in the sagittal plane between the pectoral muscles and the forearm (Figure 7.17a). The laceration is usually short (5 cm–10 cm), gaps open minimally, and involves a variable amount of muscle. Because of the depth of the wound, second intention healing is often favored. Although these often seem to be relatively minor wounds, they occasionally can result in some significant complications.

The most common complication is the development of subcutaneous emphysema (Figures 7.17b,c). This is thought to result from the wound opening acting as a one-way valve because of its location, with subsequent penetration of air into the normal tissue planes between the body and limb. Emphysema is first apparent in the immediate region of the wound but can quickly extend over the entire body, elevating the skin as much as 5 cm–7 cm off the underlying muscles. The trapped air can be absorbed within a few days after the wound stops acting as a one-way valve. With extensive emphysema, ischemia of the overlying skin or wound infection from bacteria migrating along the fascial planes are rare but may occur. As air dissects through tissue planes it can eventually penetrate the chest cavity; respiratory difficulty and sudden death secondary to pneumothorax have been seen by the author. Thus, a chest radiograph should be taken of horses that exhibit an elevated respiratory rate or dyspnea, to rule out pneumothorax.

Preventing subcutaneous emphysema is desired but not always possible. If the wound is fresh and can be sutured, subcutaneous emphysema will not develop. Managing open wounds is more difficult; the horse should be restricted to a stall and ideally cross-tied to limit the pumping action caused by walking. In this author's

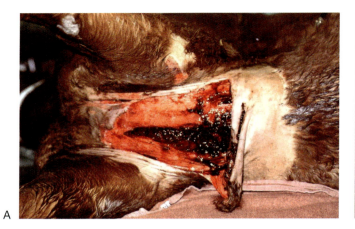
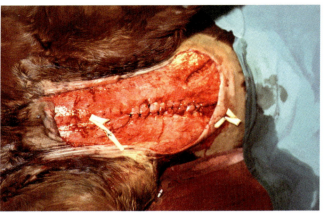

A

B

Figure 7.16. (A) Major skin degloving injury of the ventral pectoral region (head to the left). Note laceration of the pectoralis muscles in the sagittal plane. (B) The pectoral wound was closed after placement of a drain because the laceration was fresh and had sharp edges with minimal tissue trauma. The skin flap was non-viable and hence was excised.

experience, packing the wound opening with bandage material does not limit the extent of emphysema once it has developed. On the other hand, debridement of the wound opening in an effort to enlarge it and thus eliminate the valve effect has been successful. In cases managed this way, emphysema did not recur when the granulating wound closed.

If emphysema is extensive and progressive, subcutaneous air can be removed by locally inserting a hypodermic needle into the subcutaneous space and attaching it to a suction unit (Figure 7.17d). In horses suffering from involvement of the entire body, the needle will be placed in three to four sites on each side of the horse. Sedation is often unnecessary, but the puncture sites are surgically prepared and desensitized. The subcutaneous air can be "milked" toward the needle with the clinician's hands and removed by suction. This procedure can be repeated the following day if necessary, and seems to limit the extension and hasten the resolution of emphysema. If present, pneumothorax can be corrected by removal of the pleural air using a chest drain and suction. Repeat treatment might be necessary if leakage into the chest continues.

Lacerations of the Shoulder Region

Major lacerations of the cranial shoulder region are less common than those of the pectoral region or forearm. Most involve multiple short skin lacerations, often caused by several strands of barbed wire, and suffer minimal parting of the skin edges. Many can be successfully sutured, while some are so minor they heal easily by second intention with minimal or no care (Figure 7.1). Occasionally, avulsion injuries occur with loss of a large portion of the skin (Figures 7.18a,b); rarely is there significant injury to the underlying muscles. A wound in this area is capable of considerable contraction, obviating, in most cases, a grafting procedure. The point of the shoulder is an area of high motion such that initial box stall confinement is advised to encourage the development of an even bed of granulation tissue without cracks or fissures.

Lacerations of the Medial Thigh

These lacerations, usually caused by barbed wire, are primarily of the skin and may be multiple. Because the wounds are hidden from sight they initially may go undetected and hence often are presented when a few days old. Wound debridement in the standing horse is difficult because of the medial location. Surgical debridement with the horse under general anesthesia will hasten repair and should be considered in wounds requiring major debridement (Figure 7.19). Wound closure is rarely attempted because the edges are significantly retracted and because of tension and excess movement at this anatomic location. These wounds do well when allowed to heal by second intention.

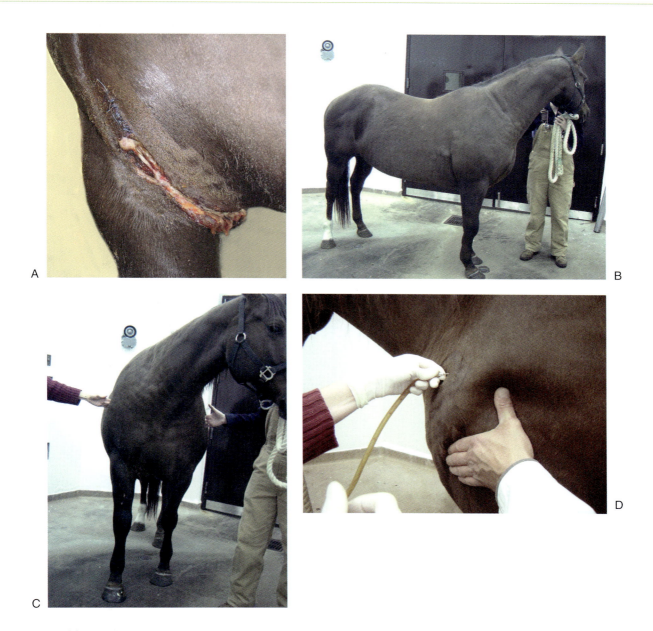

Figure 7.17. (A) Typical laceration of the axillary region caused by wire. There is minimal gaping of the wound edges and the wound is not excessively deep. Partial closure of the proximal portion was performed. (B) Severe subcutaneous emphysema developed a few days after injury. The emphysema was progressive and extended over the entire body. The horse's vital signs, including respiratory rate and sounds, were normal. (C) Notice how far the examiner's fingers can push the skin inward before contacting the musculature. (D) Much of the air was removed by suction via subcutaneously placed needles. The remaining subcutaneous air was naturally absorbed over the next few days.

In some cases only the skin is lacerated but a cleavage plane develops between the skin and medial thigh muscles. The dissection plane extends distal to the skin opening, forming a pocket which favors accumulation of exudate. Moreover, extension and flexion of the limb precludes skin adherence to the underlying musculature. A Penrose drain should be placed through a skin incision at the ventral aspect of the subcutaneous pocket to encourage drainage. Drains can be left in the wound until the cleavage plane has resolved and the ventral pocket has filled with granulation tissue. Exercise should be restricted to minimize movement between the skin and underlying muscles.

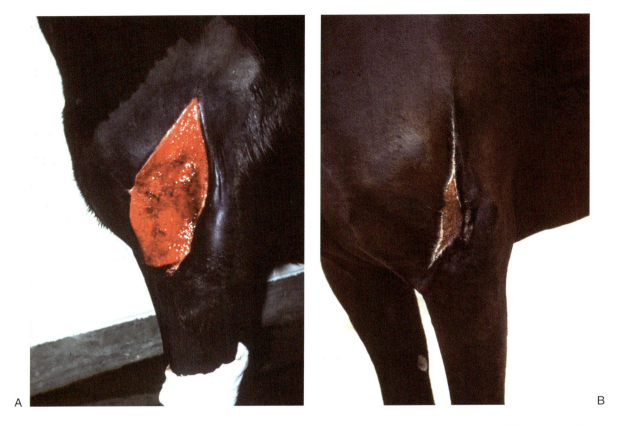

Figure 7.18. (A) Laceration of the lateral shoulder region with significant retraction of the skin edges. (B) The wound has almost completely healed by second intention with a minimal blemish.

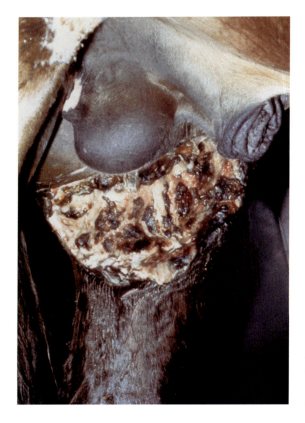

Figure 7.19. Laceration of the medial region of the thigh (caudal to the left) showing major retraction or skin loss. This wound requires debridement, and is located in an area of high motion. The wound was treated successfully by second intention healing.

Lacerations of the Lateral Chest Wall and Ventral Abdomen

Trauma in these locations more commonly leads to degloving type wounds with the production of skin and subcutaneous flaps. The flap usually has a broad base and hence remains viable, but often hangs away from the body surface (Figure 7.20). If the wound is suitable for closure and if the flap can be apposed without excessive tension, it may be sutured. An alternative is to excise the skin flap, if small, and allow the wound to heal by second intention. Even large wounds (approximately 20 cm–25 cm diameter) will develop minimal scarring with proper open wound management.

Some wounds are so large that flap preservation is required to avoid major delays in healing and to create a more cosmetic and functional surface (Figures 7.21a,b). Because these wounds cannot usually be protected or supported with a bandage, the major challenges are to provide a secure closure and eliminate dead space. It is crucial to use tension sutures of a material sufficient to withstand the forces placed on the closure. When

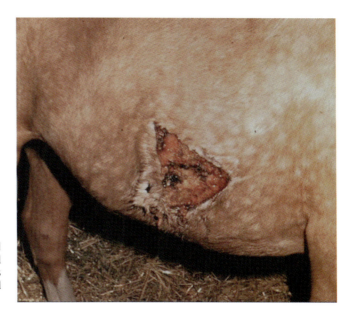

Figure 7.20. Skin flap of the lateral thoracic wall. This wound was partially closed by suturing the skin flap along its dorsal border and leaving the ventral area open to drain. A wound this size would easily heal by second intention, with a minimal blemish, if the skin flap was necrotic and had to be excised.

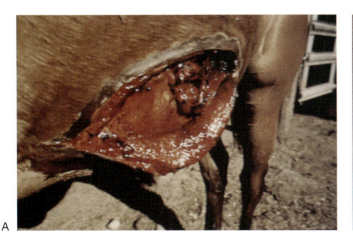

A

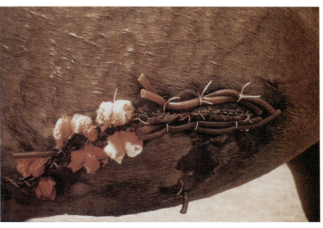

B

Figure 7.21. (A) Large skin flap caused by a sharp protruding object. The broad base of the flap provides a good blood supply but there is poor ventral drainage. With a flap this large every effort should be made to preserve it. (B) Rubber tubing and gauze were used to support the tension sutures. A drain was placed for ventral drainage. Courtesy of Dr. B Perce.

possible, the subcutaneous tissue should be closed separately with an interrupted suture pattern, for added security. Vertical mattress and near-far-far-near patterns are good for apposing tissues which suffer significant tension. The skin is closed with a combination of large tension sutures and interrupted appositional sutures, reinforced by quill sutures. Many objects can be used to disperse the pressure, including interrupted or continuous segments of rubber tubing, gauze rolls, or buttons (Figures 7.21a,b).

It is important to place these sutures well back from the wound edge and to avoid pulling them any tighter than necessary as this may encourage skin necrosis. A number of options are available when the skin edges cannot be adequately apposed. For example, additional undermining, especially of the region adjacent to the skin flap, may relieve tension sufficiently to allow closure. When undermining, it is important to elevate the subcutaneous tissue along with the skin to preserve cutaneous blood supply. The disadvantage of this technique is that it produces greater dead space and allows further retraction of the wound edges, should the latter dehisce. Tension can also be decreased by creating many small "mesh incisions" parallel to the skin edges on both sides of the wound.[2] If greater tension relief is required, a larger incision can be made parallel to the skin edge to create a bi-pedicle flap.[2] When this tension-relieving incision is placed ventrally it can double as a drainage port. Alternatively, the skin edges can be approximated and secured in this position with tension sutures. While the edges are not apposed, this reduces the wound area required to heal by second intention.

Closing dead space and providing ventral drainage is important. During closure, walking sutures have been proposed to help reduce dead space by attaching the subcutaneous tissue of the flap to the deeper tissues of the wound. The author has not found these sutures very helpful because they can pull out of large flaps. Moreover, they represent foreign bodies, which increase the susceptibility of the wound to infection. Instead, the author favors the placement of multiple large vertical mattress quill sutures through the skin and underlying musculature. When possible, the application of a bandage, including a stent bandage, will compress the dead space. Penrose drains should be preplaced in the depth of the wound prior to closure of the skin, and should exit below the sutured wound where they are secured by suturing them to the skin. The ventral exit hole should be sufficiently large to allow easy drainage. Drainage may be required for several days and both the drain and the exit site should be cleaned daily (see Chapter 2 for more information regarding management of drains).

Puncture Wounds

Puncture wounds can be caused by contact with any sharp object including nails, bolts, tree branches, and rails. They can occur on any part of the body but are seen primarily in areas with significant musculature such as the chest, shoulder, or thigh and are often caused by wood (Figures 7.22a,b).[61] These injuries are especially dangerous for a number of reasons: (1) they often seem innocuous because the skin opening can be small, and hence are not treated appropriately; 2) they are caused by objects that drive bacteria into the wound; (3) they may cause extensive damage to the deep musculature; (4) they may suffer from poor ventral drainage, and (5) they may penetrate the thoracic, abdominal, or a synovial cavity. Consequently, these wounds should not be closed primarily.

After surgical preparation, the wound should be explored with a flexible probe to determine both the depth and direction of penetration. This will help establish whether the wound is in proximity to a cavity or any major neurovascular structures or bones. A flexible plastic urinary catheter is preferred to a malleable metallic probe because wound tracts are often not completely linear and a plastic catheter is more likely to stay within the confines of the injury. If a foreign body is present it can sometimes be detected with the catheter tip. When the opening of the puncture is very small it should be enlarged to allow more complete probing; this will also facilitate lavage of the tract and subsequent drainage.

Radiographic and ultrasonographic examinations can be very helpful but should be performed prior to probing or lavage because these could produce artifacts via the introduction of air or fluid. Wooden foreign bodies will not be seen on a radiograph but placement of a metallic probe or a plastic catheter loaded with contrast material can yield useful information about the direction, depth, and limits of the tract.[61]

A contrast fistulogram may be performed but can be inconclusive in an acute situation because the tract is not "walled off" and contrast may leak into tissue planes. Wooden foreign bodies, on ultrasound examination, usually appear as linear hyperechoic shadows that are often surrounded by fluid.[62] If the presence of a foreign body is suspected following probing and the use of medical imaging techniques, and if the object is located close to the skin surface, the opening may be enlarged to allow its removal (Figures 7.23a–d).

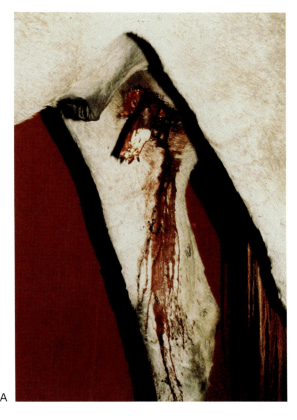

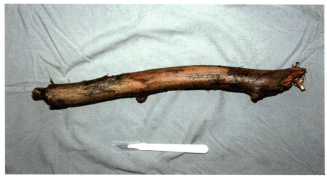

Figure 7.22. (A) Acute injury with a large piece of wood protruding from the medial aspect of the thigh (cranial to the left). The injury occurred while the horse was being ridden through an area of pasture containing freshly cut branches. (B) The wood was removed with the horse in a standing position to prevent further tissue damage or fragmentation of the branch by limb flexion upon recumbency. A single piece of wood was retrieved. Probing the wound after branch removal showed that the inserted tip of the branch came within 2 cm–3 cm of exiting the skin 2 cm–3 cm adjacent to the anus. There was excellent ventral drainage and recovery was rapid.

Wound lavage is important to reduce bacterial contamination and rid the wound of small debris. With a catheter placed into the depth of the wound, sterile saline or a dilute antiseptic solution can be used to flush. Fluid should not be injected under pressure because it may dissect along tissue planes. When lavage fluid does not easily exit the opening, signaling the aforementioned problem, flushing should be discontinued. Systemically delivered antibiotics are indicated due to the contamination, presence of deep tissue trauma, and likelihood of an anaerobic environment. Several antibiotics are effective but penicillin provides excellent coverage against Clostridial infections. The horse's tetanus vaccination status should also be verified. If the puncture wound suffers from poor drainage due to the presence of a significant ventral pocket, a Penrose drain should be placed though the most ventral aspect of the undermined tissue. Nonsteroidal anti-inflammatory drugs should be administered for a few days in an effort to reduce swelling and relieve pain to encourage exercise that may enhance drainage.

Puncture Wounds into a Synovial Cavity

If the puncture occurs close to a joint or tendon sheath, it is important to determine whether the synovial structure has been penetrated. Careful visual or digital (with a sterile glove) examination is sufficient in the case of a large opening. With smaller punctures, synovial fluid running from the wound freely or after limb flexion or application of direct pressure over the joint incriminates synovial cavity penetration. Conversely, if the synovial cavity is intact, the application of pressure will not elicit the escape of synovial fluid into the wound. It can

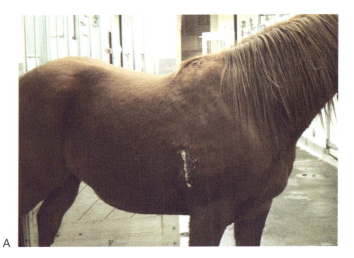

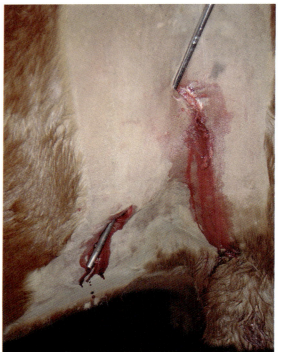
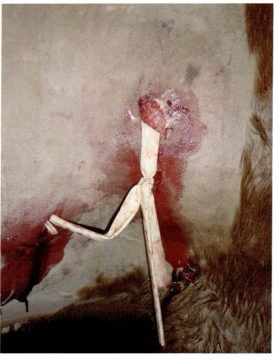

Figure 7.23. (A) A 1-week-old puncture wound of the lateral chest wall, draining purulent material. Probing with a gloved finger identified a piece of wood directly under the skin. This was easily removed by enlarging the hole and grasping the wood with forceps. (B) A Chambers mare catheter was used to determine the extent of the ventral pocket, which was subsequently opened to allow drainage. (C) A Penrose drain was placed and retained for several days to ensure adequate drainage.

be helpful to place a needle into the synovial cavity, at a site remote to the wound, to forcefully inject sterile fluid to see if it drains from the wound site. This should not be attempted if the needle must pass through contaminated tissue.

When the joint is inflamed secondary to infection, synovial fluid will contain a very high number of white blood cells ($>30 \times 10^9$/L), predominantly neutrophils ($>80\%$), and show a high protein concentration (>4.0 g/dL).[63] Sterile blue dye can be added to the sterile saline lavage solution for easier identification of joint leakage. If the joint is open, aggressive therapy including arthroscopic lavage and systemic antibiotics is recommended to prevent septic arthritis and its numerous sequelae. See Chapter 9 for a complete discussion of this topic.

Puncture Wounds of the Thoracic Cavity

Penetration of the thorax is uncommon but dangerous because of the potential for both pneumothorax and pleuritis. An elevated respiratory rate or dyspnea may be seen with acute pneumothorax, which can be identified radiographically (Figure 7.24). Pneumothorax of one pleural space can displace the mediastinum and subsequently compromise the function of the other lung.[64] This said, the author has seen horses with an open pneumothorax that did not suffer respiratory difficulty nor have elevated respiratory rates.

The wound must be carefully examined for foreign bodies, thoroughly debrided, lavaged, and if at all possible the thorax should be closed to prevent further contamination and lung collapse. Thoracoscopy has been recommended for a more thorough evaluation of the chest, but should be performed at a site remote from the wound.[64] Negative pressure can be re-established by removal of air via thoracocentesis. The pleural space can by drained or lavaged post-operatively, if necessary, via a thoracostomy tube. Larger wounds may require reconstructive procedures to allow closure. Muscle pedicle flaps from the longissimus dorsi and external abdominal oblique muscles have been described for this purpose.[65] If the wound cannot be closed it should be covered with a stent or thoracic bandage and allowed to heal by second intention. Systemic antibiotics are important as are nonsteroidal anti-inflammatory drugs because of the pleural pain. If septic pleuritis does not develop the prognosis for healing and return to function is quite good.

Puncture Wounds of the Peritoneal Cavity

Most punctures of the abdominal wall do not penetrate the peritoneal cavity, which could result in contamination of the abdomen or injury to its viscera. Any wound in the abdominal region should be examined carefully for the presence of foreign material. Careful probing of the wound may be accomplished with the horse standing, but a safer and more thorough exam can be conducted under general anesthesia. Abdominocentesis should be performed to verify cell count and protein concentration; elevations (white blood cells >5,000/μl; protein >2.5 g/dl) will be seen with peritoneal contamination. Small wounds that do not breach the peritoneum will heal best by second intention. If the wound is fresh with minimal contamination but penetrates the abdominal cavity, it should be thoroughly debrided and closed (Figures 7.25a–e).

As with wounds penetrating the thoracic cavity, systemic antibiotics and careful monitoring are required post-operatively. An exploratory midline celiotomy is indicated in wounds at greater risk of suffering from injury to the abdominal contents. This allows careful examination of the viscera and thorough lavage of the abdominal cavity prior to wound closure. It may not be possible to close some larger abdominal defects for lack of adequate tissue; placement of mesh in the abdominal wall is not indicated in open wounds because of the risk of infection. These wounds must thus be bandaged in a sterile fashion to prevent herniation and infection, with reconstruction of the defect (hernia) performed later.

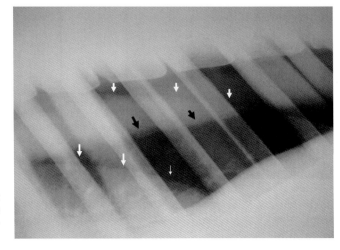

Figure 7.24. Bilateral pneumothorax caused by a penetrating wound to the chest. Notice the retracted dorsal border of the lung lobes which no longer fill the thoracic space and the abnormally clear ventral aortic margin.

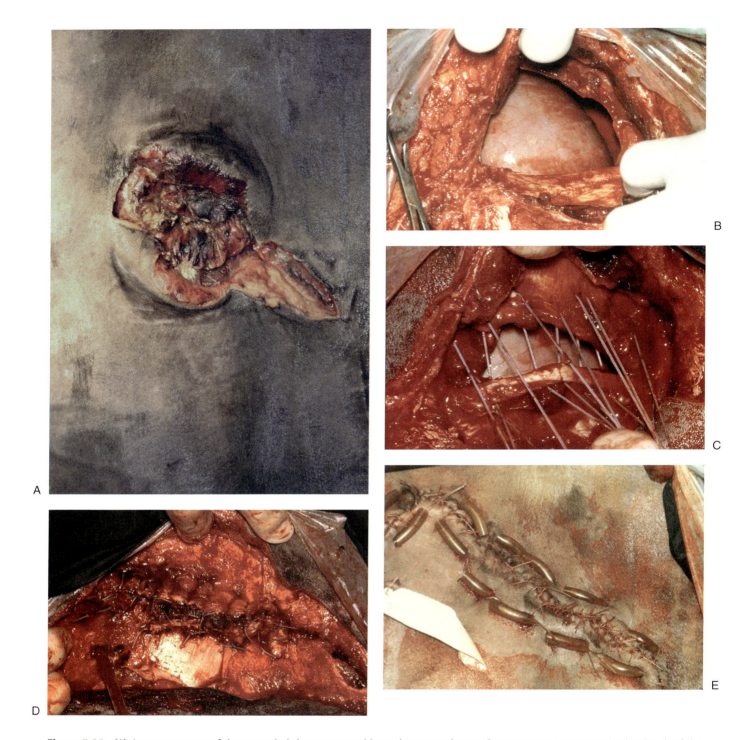

Figure 7.25. (A) Acute puncture of the ventral abdomen caused by a sharp metal post. Omentum was apparent in the depth of the wound. (B) The wound was debrided and the exposed omentum amputated. A 10 cm × 2.5 cm ring defect was present on the ventral midline. (C) The abdominal musculature was close in two layers. Note the preplacement of the sutures (#5 polyester) in the internal sheath of the rectus abdominus muscle. (D) A "relieving incision" of the rectus abdominus muscle and its external sheath (not shown) was required to close the abdominal defect without excessive tension. Note the tube placed into the abdominal cavity to facilitate post-operative drainage. (E) Horizontal mattress quill sutures with pieces of rubber tubing were used in the skin for additional support. The intra-abdominal drainage tube is secured with sutures placed through tape placed around the tube.

362

Chronic Draining Tracts

Chronic draining tracts are usually the result of either a bone sequestrum or a foreign body. Sequestra are uncommon in the upper body because of the superior muscle coverage compared to the extremities, while foreign bodies are frequently the cause of draining tracts. Wood is the most common foreign body but other objects including metal, plastic, or plant material have been identified.[61,66] Areas with a large muscle mass, especially the shoulder region, are most commonly involved, although foreign bodies can become imbedded at any site.

The most prominent clinical sign is drainage of large amounts of purulent material from a small skin opening (Figure 7.23a). There often is history of a previous puncture wound or laceration, which may have been caused by contact with a wooden fence. The drainage may occur through a portion of the original wound or may result from spontaneous rupture or lancing of an abscess at a distant site[61] (Figure 7.26a). Transitory healing followed by repeated episodes of drainage characterizes some cases, while most drain constantly. Because the wound is chronic and the foreign body has been "walled off," the horse is systemically normal and usually not lame despite the presence of a foreign body imbedded within the muscle.

Examination should include thorough probing of the wound, with either plain and contrast radiography or ultrasonography. In some cases all three are needed for an accurate diagnosis (Figures 7.26b,c). The author prefers a long flexible plastic catheter for probing, which follows the curved tract without puncturing its wall. While probing, one should ascertain the number of tracts; the tract direction; the relationship of the tract to bones, joints, or other vital structures; and if possible the tract length. Shallow foreign bodies may be balloted with the catheter tip, while deeper ones are beyond the reach of the catheter. This examination may provide sufficient information to allow removal of superficial foreign bodies while others may require further diagnostic procedures prior to surgery.

Ultrasonography and radiography should be performed prior to probing the tract to avoid the presence of artifacts created by the introduction of air during probing. Wooden objects on ultrasound examination are seen as linear hyperechoic zones surrounded by fluid (Figure 7.26c).[62] The size and number of foreign bodies, as well as their depth, can often be determined. Injection of saline or sterile water into the tract helps determine its course on ultrasound examination.[62] Wood will not be seen on radiographic examination unless it is located over the trachea, because its density is the same as that of muscle. However, radiographs may show air associated with the tract or from gas produced by bacteria. A positive contrast sonogram/fistulogram is often very helpful in identifying the number of foreign bodies and their location when these are situated deep within the musculature.

Water-soluble is preferred over oil-based contrast material because it is less viscous and penetrates the tract more completely. Contrast material should be injected under pressure for optimal tract identification. This is best accomplished using a catheter with an inflatable cuff at the tip (e.g., Foley). If the tract opening is too large to occlude, or the tract too shallow to fully insert the cuffed catheter tip, contrast material can alternatively be injected through a flexible polyethylene catheter placed in the depth of the wound. This will allow leakage of contrast material onto the skin, but useful information may yet be obtained. Foreign bodies are shown as linear, often rectangular, radiolucent zones in a tract otherwise filled with radio-opaque contrast material (Figure 7.26d). Because the foreign body prevents a portion of the tract from filling with contrast, these zones are referred to as "filling defects."

Removal of the foreign body will solve the problem of chronic drainage. Superficial foreign bodies are often identified during probing and removed by simply incising the overlying tissue. However, most are deeply imbedded and require a full work-up with ultrasound and radiology to determine the number and location of foreign bodies as well as the least traumatic approach for successful removal. Foreign bodies of chronic nature are usually encased within a fibrotic tract that is smaller than the diameter of the former. Hence, extraction cannot be achieved by simply grasping the foreign body with forceps, and enlargement of the fibrous tract is first necessary.

Removal can be accomplished by one of two approaches: either dissecting along the tract (Figures 7.26a–e) or approaching the foreign body through an incision distant to the draining tract. Injection of dilute methylene blue dye stains the tract and helps identify the lumen if it is transected during surgery. To reach the foreign body, the tract can either be incised along its length or a catheter can be placed into the lumen and dissection carried out along but not penetrating the tract. The author prefers the latter because it helps preserve the tract. Indeed, if the tract is accidentally transected the remaining part of the tract can sometimes no longer be

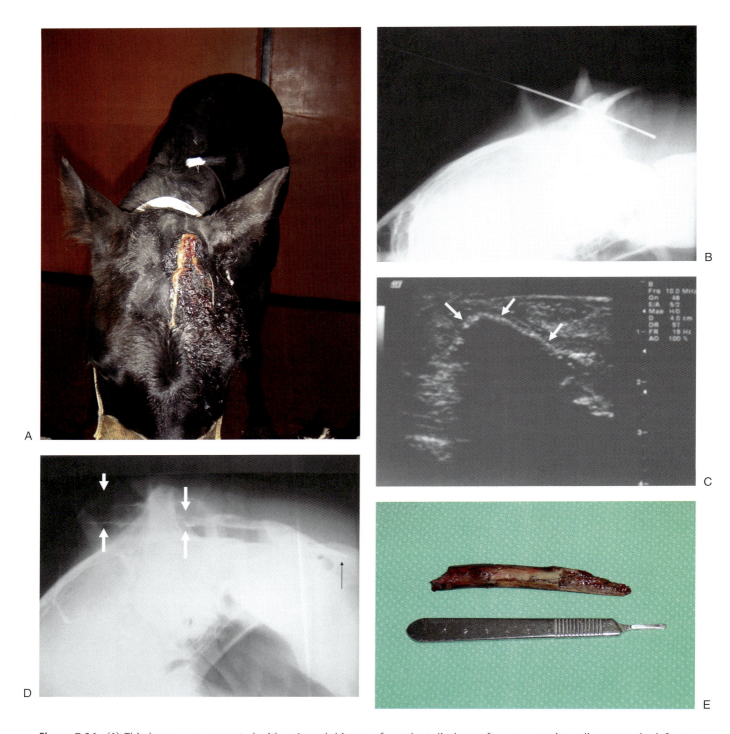

Figure 7.26. (A) This horse was presented with a 6-week history of purulent discharge from an opening adjacent to the left ear. Both digital exam and probing failed to identify a foreign body within the tract, which extended several inches caudally. (B) No abnormalities were seen on a plain radiograph with a metallic probe placed in the tract. (C) An ultrasonographic exam of the area immediately caudal to the opening shows a linear shadow indicative of a foreign body. (D) A contrast sinogram/fistulogram performed with barium shows a filling defect within the draining track. (E) A large wooden foreign body, located within one inch of the opening, was removed with forceps after enlarging the skin opening.

identified, despite staining, such that finding and removing the foreign body becomes very difficult or impossible.

In some horses, the least traumatic approach is to incise over the foreign body at a site distant from the tract. This applies in cases when the foreign body is located farther away from the tract opening than from the overlying skin (Figures 7.27a–c). Pre-operative contrast sinogram/fistulogram and ultrasonogram help determine the least traumatic approach for removal. Intra-operative ultrasonography can be helpful in locating the foreign body; alternatively, markers can be placed on the skin prior to surgery. Once the foreign body is accessible, the fibrous capsule overlying it is incised to allow extraction. With deeply-imbedded objects, access can be difficult and tissue retractors are often required.

Removal of the tract's inner "secretory" lining is not necessary but its lumen should be flushed and in some cases Penrose drains are placed to ensure patency required for drainage during healing. Systemic antibiotics are administered for a few days because new tissue planes were created surgically and contaminated with discharge. Healing will be prompt if all of the foreign body is removed.

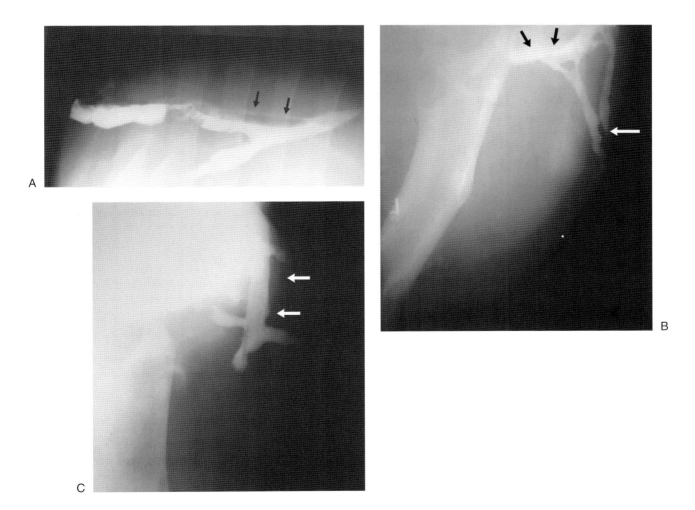

Figure 7.27. (A) A contrast sinogram/fistulogram, with a filling defect, of a long tract in the withers area. The wood was removed by incising directly over the filling defect rather than dissecting along the tract. (B) Notice the two tracts from the foreign body, present in the proximal lateral femoral area, that join prior to draining at the skin surface a few inches below the filling defect. The wood was further located by probing with needles, then removed by incising directly over it. (C) A filling defect in the proximal lateral femoral area, with a tract created by a puncture wound to the medial aspect of the limb. Ultrasonography was used to locate the piece of wood, which was removed by incising directly over it.

Abscesses, Hematomas, and Seromas

Hematomas usually develop secondary to blunt trauma to or overstretching of a muscle (Figure 7.28). The extent of the subsequent swelling depends on the size of the torn vessel and the ability of surrounding tissue to restrict enlargement. Seromas develop more commonly in the subcutaneous space as a result of shearing forces acting between the skin and underlying musculature (Figure 7.29). Abscesses can develop secondary to puncture of the skin or from hematogenous inoculation of traumatized tissue with bacteria (Figure 7.30).

These conditions differ in a number of ways. Hematomas and seromas usually arise quickly following trauma and reach their maximum size rapidly. In contrast, abscesses develop a few days after trauma and enlarge more slowly. Hematomas and seromas are usually soft, fluctuant swellings and are not hot or painful upon palpation. Abscesses are typically encapsulated and inflamed, hence they feel thicker-walled upon palpation and are painful to the touch.

Ultrasonography is helpful but not foolproof in distinguishing between these conditions. Seromas possess low cellularity and will appear as anechoic areas with fine loculations. Hematomas initially are echogenic; however, as the clot forms they take on the appearance of anechoic loculated fluid. The echogenicity of an abscess varies with the degree of cellularity and inspissation. Swirling of the fluid content can be seen upon ballottment of an abscess. Gas shadows produced by bacteria are sometimes visible in abscesses; however, an organized hematoma and an abscess share many features and cannot always be distinguished by ultrasonography.[62]

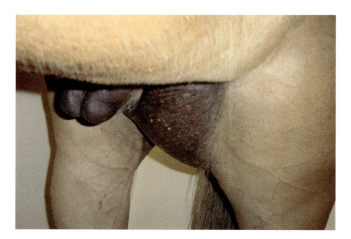

Figure 7.28. A large hematoma on the medial aspect of the thigh developed secondary to a fall with the limb in abduction. It caused marked pain, was hard and painful upon palpation, and persisted for several weeks.

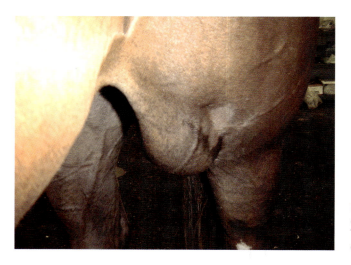

Figure 7.29. The stifle is a common place for a seroma to develop secondary to the horse injuring itself jumping a fence. The one in this figure was soft and fluctuant, but was not drained.

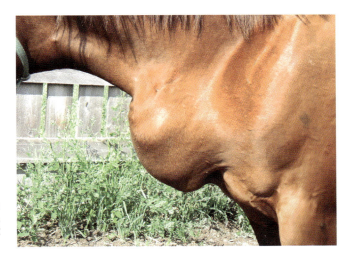

Figure 7.30. Large abscess in a breeding stallion thought to result from hematogenous inoculation of a chronic hematoma, itself the result of a kick. It resolved after lancing and placement of Penrose drains to ensure drainage.

Cytology of the fluid obtained by centesis will distinguish between these conditions, but is not routinely recommended because of the risk of inoculating a seroma or hematoma with bacteria. Centesis of the mass is done only when clinical and ultrasonographic findings cannot differentiate between an abscess and a hematoma. If centesis is performed, strict aseptic technique is mandatory.

Establishing good ventral drainage followed by lavage and occasionally the systemic administration of antibiotics is the treatment of choice for an abscess. In some cases, drains are placed to prevent premature closure of the cavity.

Management of hematomas and seromas is more controversial. The author prefers to allow natural resorption and would drain a seroma only if it was very large, in a location where it may be traumatized (e.g., hip) or is unsightly, and if the diagnosis was clear. The author believes hematomas should never be drained. While a conservative approach will limit the risk of iatrogenic infection or hemorrhage, disadvantages include a lengthy or incomplete resolution leading to a fibrotic blemish as well as the risk of hematogenous inoculation of bacteria leading to abscess formation (Figure 7.30).

While drainage of hematomas is not recommended by the author, if drainage is performed, large ventral incisions are preferred over repeated aspiration in an effort to reduce the likelihood of abscess formation. Whereas seromas drain easily, the clot from a hematoma will require more aggressive lavage or curettage. In both cases it is advisable to wait several days following development prior to establishing drainage. For seromas this interval allows healing so there is not continued leakage of serum, while with hematomas the delay reduces the risk of continued bleeding. Nonetheless, the larger the hematoma the greater the risk of post-drainage hemorrhage. The author has seen horses euthanized because hemorrhage following drainage could not be controlled.

Traumatic Abdominal Hernias

Rupture of the abdominal wall may occur following a major blow to the abdomen from a blunt object such as a foot or the top of a fence post. The injury most commonly seen is in the ventral abdomen, near the fold of the flank or between the flank and the pre-pubic tendon area (Figure 7.31), but can also occur on the ventral aspect of the abdomen (Figure 7.32a). The skin usually remains intact, likely because of its elasticity and mobility upon impact; however, rupture of the abdominal wall allows intestines to herniate into the subcutaneous space.

The defect in the abdominal wall is typically large (15 cm–20 cm in diameter) because of retraction of the ruptured muscles, which protects against bowel strangulation. Mild transient colic may develop initially, but usually subsides without treatment. A substantial swelling occurs immediately after herniation and may increase over the next few days from enlargement of the subcutaneous pocket. The swelling is soft and fluctuant, and in some cases the bowel may be felt under the skin. Within a few days edema develops and makes palpation

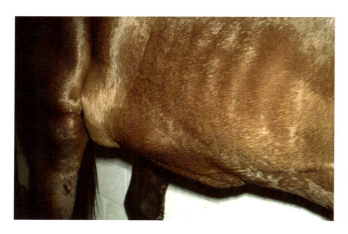

Figure 7.31. Typical swelling in the fold of the flank of a horse with a ventral body wall hernia caused by landing on a fence-post. The skin is intact but bowel has entered the subcutaneous space via an abdominal wall rupture located closer to the pelvic brim.

more difficult, but both auscultation and ultrasound examination confirm the presence of herniated bowel. External palpation of the hernial defect is often not possible because of the presence of herniated bowel and the fact that the defect is located deep (dorsal) to the swelling. With the horse anesthetized, the hernia is easily reduced and the location, size, and number of defects can be determined by palpation and ultrasonography. Rectal exam can be used to diagnose caudal abdominal wall defects in the standing horse.

It is important to differentiate a ventral hernia from other swellings produced by trauma to the caudal abdomen. Horses that get hung up over a fence can develop a seroma, a hematoma, or cellulitis, or in more chronic cases an abscess that look similar. It is imperative to not perform centesis on a hernia, because leakage of bowel contents can cause a serious infection and greatly complicate surgical repair.

Surgical repair of the defect is recommended because further trauma to the abdomen could injure the displaced intestines and because the horse is of limited use with the hernia. Placement of a prosthetic "patch" over the defect is preferred over attempts to suture the ruptured wall.[67,68] It is wise to postpone surgical repair following trauma unless bowel strangulation is suspected, because the ruptured wall will be edematous and will not withstand the forces applied to close the large defect. Furthermore, muscle layers will have retracted in different directions and to different degrees, making the limits of the defect difficult to determine. Moreover, placing a prosthetic patch over an acutely ruptured wall may result in herniation of bowel around the edge of the prosthesis with subsequent strangulation. The prosthetic repair is thus performed several months following injury once a strong fibrotic ring has formed at the hernia site.[67] Intestine is not usually injured when the rupture occurs and can remain in the subcutaneous space for several months with little risk of strangulation or adhesion formation.

Surgical repair is best done with the horse in dorsal recumbency. Strict adherence to aseptic technique is important to minimize the risks of infection of either the mesh or the abdominal cavity. Systemic broad-spectrum antibiotics are administered pre-operatively, and then continued for several days after surgery. Different prosthetic materials (meshes) are available, including non-absorbable and absorbable types. Although absorbable meshes are considerably more expensive, they are preferred because they minimize the risk of chronic infection of the implant. While various sites of mesh insertion have been described,[69] it is generally advocated to place the mesh retro-peritoneally to reduce the risk of bowel adhesion[67,68] (Figures 7.32b–f).

Either a single or double layer of mesh can be inserted; however, a double layer will likely result in a stronger repair with less sagging. The sheets of mesh can be placed together as a single layer (Figure 7.32d) or inserted separately in different tissue planes. The mesh is usually covered with a portion of the fibrous hernial flap when one is present (Figures 7.32c,f).

The skin incision can be made directly over the rupture site if that gives the best exposure; however, a curved incision adjacent to the defect is preferred (Figure 7.32b). If there is a fibrous hernial sac it is incised along one side (180°) and reflected (Figure 7.32c). The peritoneum and subperitoneal fat are separated from the fibrotic hernial ring and if possible sutured closed to isolate the mesh from the intestines (Figure 7.32c). The mesh will be inserted between the subperitoneal fat and the abdominal wall. A piece of mesh is cut such that it is larger than the defect and overlaps the fibrotic hernial ring by approximately 3 cm–5 cm (Figure 7.32d). If

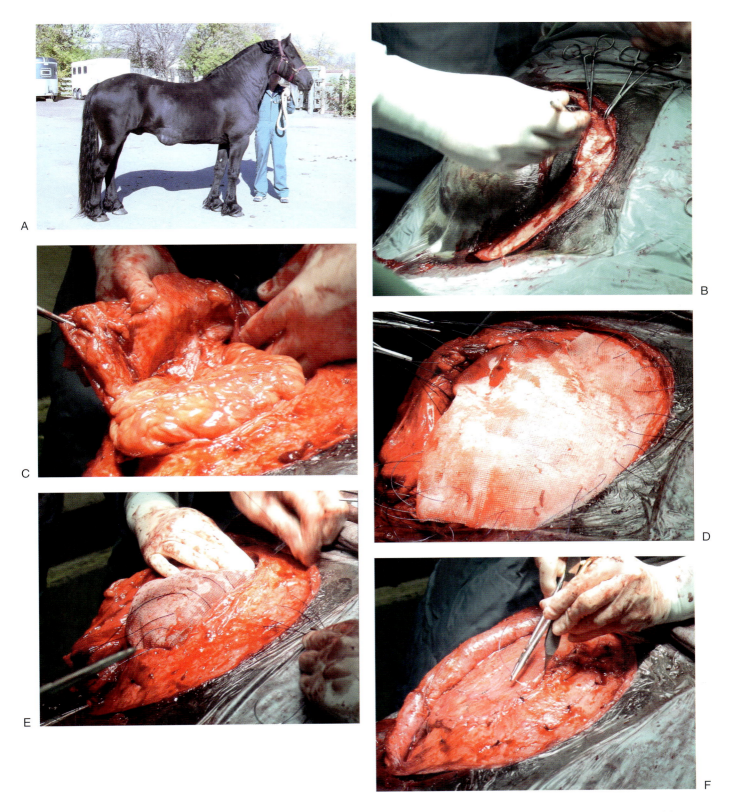

Figure 7.32. (A) Ventral hernia in a breeding stallion caused by landing on a sharp fencepost 2 years earlier. The skin had been breached but the subsequent infection resolved. (B) A curved incision adjacent to the defect was made to expose the hernial ring to place a meshed prosthesis. (C) The fibrous hernial sac (held by instrument and right hand) was incised in a curved manner and reflected; the adhered and adjacent subperitoneal fat was dissected free and the peritoneum closed so the mesh could be placed retro-peritoneally. (D) Two stacked layers of polypropylene mesh are used for the repair. The mesh was cut large enough to overlap the edge of the hernial ring where preplaced mattress sutures secured it to the abdominal wall. (E) The mattress sutures on the far side were placed and pulled tightly to secure the mesh along one side. The mattress sutures on the near side were placed but not tied until later. (F) The excessive portion of the fibrous hernial sac was removed to create a flat surface when sutured over the mesh. The mattress sutures that secured the mesh extended through the abdominal wall adjacent to the fascial flap.

a single layer of mesh is used, its edges are folded over to provide greater holding strength for the sutures; however, this is not necessary when two layers of mesh are used (Figure 7.32d).

The mesh is removed from the defect and large (#1 or #2) mattress sutures, composed of the same material as the mesh, are preplaced in the mesh along its periphery. It is important to pull the mesh snuggly across the defect to minimize sagging. If the mesh is placed into position and secured along one side first, any "extra" mesh can be pulled out during placement of the sutures on the opposite side (Figures 7.32d,e). Numerous pre-placed mattress sutures are positioned close together and traverse the entire thickness of the body wall to enhance security and strength of the repair.

The reflected fibrous hernial sac is trimmed, laid over the mesh, and secured to the hernial ring, preferably with an absorbable monofilament suture (e.g., #1 polydioxanone) (Figure 7.32f). The subcutaneous tissue and skin are then closed, separately. Despite the presence of considerable dead space, drains are not recommended. The repair site is best dressed with a sterile plastic drape, and then covered with either a belly bandage or a stent bandage when possible. This protects the wound and will help eliminate dead space. Antibiotics and analgesics are administered for a few days and exercise is restricted for several weeks. Any seroma that forms at the surgical site should resorb spontaneously.

Conclusion

While several types of wounds can occur on the neck and body, most can be treated successfully. In many situations wound management may be prolonged, labor-intensive, and costly, but often the horse will eventually return to some level of activity. Research that advances our knowledge of wound healing mechanisms should allow us to manipulate wound healing to the benefit of our patients. Moreover, further scientific evaluation of commercially available wound healing products is indicated to help clinicians make the best decisions regarding treatment.

References

1. Barber SM: Management of neck and head injuries. Vet Clin North Am Equine Pract 2005;21:191
2. Bailey JV: Principles of reconstructive and plastic surgery. In JA Auer and JA Stick, eds. *Equine surgery* (3rd edition). Philadelphia: WB Saunders, 2006, p.254
3. Hendrickson D: Factors that affect equine wound repair. Vet Clin North Am Equine Pract 2005;21:33
4. Wilson DA: Principles of early wound management. Vet Clin North Am Equine Pract 2005;21:45
5. Stashak TS: Wounds of the Body. In Stashak TS, ed. *Equine wound management*. Philadelphia: Lea and Febiger, 1991, p.145
6. Baines SJ: Surgical Drains. In D Fowler and JM Williams, eds. *Manual of canine and feline wound management and reconstruction*. Cheltenham UK: British Small Animal Veterinary Association, 1999, p.47
7. Cruse PJE, Foord R: A five-year prospective study of 23,649 wounds. Arch Surgery 1973;107:206
8. Swaim SF: Drains. In S Swaim, ed. *Surgery of traumatized skin: management and reconstruction in the dog and cat*. Philadelphia: WB Saunders, 1980, p.157
9. Wilmink JM, Van Weeren PR: Second intention repair in the horse and pony and management of exuberant granulation tissue. Vet Clin North Am Equine Pract 2005;21:15
10. Woollen N, DeBowes RM, Leiplod HW, et al: A comparison of four types of therapy for the treatment of full-thickness skin wounds of the horse. Proceedings Am Assoc Eq Pract 1987, p.569
11. Bigbie RB, Schumacher J, Swaim SF, et al: Effects of amnion and live yeast cell derivative on second intention healing in horses. Am J Vet Res 1991;52:1376
12. Knighton DR, Silver LA, Hunt TK: Regulation of wound healing angiogenesis—effect of oxygen gradients and inspired oxygen concentration. Surgery 1981;90:262
13. Barber SM: Second intention wound healing in the horse: The effect of bandages and topical corticosteroids. Proceedings Am Assoc Eq Pract 1989, p.107
14. Barber SM: Diseases of the Guttural Pouches. In PT Colohan, AM Merritt, JN Moore, IG Mayhew, eds. *Equine medicine and surgery* (5th edition). Philadelphia: Mosby, 1999, p.502
15. Hare WCD: Equine respiratory system. In R Getty, ed. *Sisson and Grossman's the anatomy of domestic animals* (5th edition). Philadelphia: WB Saunders, 1975, p.511
16. Scott EA: Ruptured trachea in the horse: a method of surgical reconstruction. Vet Med/Small Anim Clin 1978;73:485
17. Caron JP, Townsend HGG: Tracheal perforation and widespread subcutaneous emphysema in a horse. Can Vet J 1984;25:339

18. Fubini SL, Todhunter RJ, Vivrette SL, et al: Tracheal rupture in two horses. J Am Vet Med Assoc 1990;187:69
19. Kirker-Head CA, Jakob TP: Surgical repair of ruptured trachea in a horse. J Am Vet Med Assoc 1990;196:1635
20. Freeman DE: Trachea. In J Beech, ed. *Equine respiratory disorders*. Malvern: Lea and Febiger, 1991, p.389
21. Shappell KK, Stick JA, Derksen FJ, et al: Permanent tracheostomy in equidae: 47 cases (1981–1986). J Am Vet Med Assoc 1988;192:939
22. McClure SR, Taylor TS, Honnas CM, et al: Permanent tracheostomy in standing horses: Technique and results. Vet Surgery 1995;24:231
23. Robertson JT, Spurlock GH: Tracheal reconstruction in a foal. J Am Vet Med Assoc 1986;189:313
24. Yovich JV, Stashak TS: Surgical repair of a collapsed trachea caused by a lipoma in a horse. Vet Surgery 1984;13:217
25. Tate LP, Koch DB, Sembrat RF, et al: Tracheal reconstruction by resection and end-to-end anastomosis in the horse. J Am Vet Med Assoc 1981;178:253
26. Siger L, Hawkins JF, Andrews FM, et al: Tracheal stenosis and collapse in horses. Compend Contin Educ Pract Vet 1998;20:628
27. Charlton C, Tulleners E: Transendoscopic contact neodymium: yttrium aluminum garnet laser excision of tracheal lesions in two horses. J Am Vet Med Assoc 1991;199:241
28. Adams SB, Fessler JF: Tracheotomy. In Adams SB, Fessler JF, eds. *Atlas of equine surgery*. Philadelphia: WB Saunders, 2000, p.185
29. Randall RW, Myers VS: Partial tracheal stenosis in a horse. Vet Med/Small Anim Clin 1973;68:264
30. Tessier GJ, Neuwirth LA, Merritt AM: Peritracheal abscess as the cause of tracheal compression and severe respiratory distress in a horse. Equine Vet Educ 1996;8:127
31. Rigg DL, Ramey DW, Reinertson EL: Tracheal compression secondary to abscessation of cranial mediastinal lymph nodes in a horse. J Am Vet Med Assoc 1985;186;283
32. Fingland RB, Rings DM, Vertweber JG: The etiology and surgical management of trachea collapse in calves. Vet Surgery 1990;19:371
33. Stick JA: Esophagus. In JA Auer and JA Stick, eds. *Equine surgery (3rd edition)*. Philadelphia: WB Saunders, 2005, p.351
34. Dechant JE, MacDonald DG, Crawford WH, et al: Pleuritis associated with perforation of an isolated oesophageal ulcer in a horse. Equine Vet J 1998;30:170
35. Risnes I, Mair TS: Traumatic oesophageal rupture in a horse complicated by subsequent rupture of the common carotid artery. Eq Vet Educ 2003;15:120
36. Read EK, Barber SM, Wilson DG, et al: Oesophageal rupture in a Quarter Horse mare: unique features of liquid enteral hyperalimentation and fistula management. Eq Vet Educ 2002;14:126
37. Craig DR, Shivy DR, Pankowski RL, et al: Esophageal disorders in 61 horses: Results of non-surgical and surgical management. Vet Surgery 1989;18:432
38. Peacock EE: Esophagus. In Peacock EE, ed. *Wound repair (3rd edition)*. Philadelphia: WB Saunders, 1984, p.451
39. Stick JA, Krehbiel JD, Kunze DJ, et al: Esophageal healing in the pony: Comparison of sutured vs non sutured esophagotomy. Am J Vet Res 1981;42:1506
40. Todhunter RJ, Stick JA, Slocombe RF: Comparison of three feeding techniques after esophageal mucosal resection and anastomosis in the horse. Cornell Vet 1986;76:16
41. Todhunter RJ, Stick JA, Trotter GW, et al: Medical management of esophageal stricture in seven horses. J Am Vet Med Assoc 1984;185;93
42. Stick JA, Slocombe RF, Derksen FJ, et al: Esophagostomy in the pony: Comparison of surgical techniques and form of feed. Am J Vet Res 1983;44:2123
43. Stick JA, Derksen FJ, Scott EA: Equine cervical esophagostomy: Complications associated with duration and location of feeding tubes. Am J Vet Res 1981;42:727
44. Wingfield Digby NJ, Burguez PN: Traumatic oesophageal rupture in the horse. Eq Vet J 1982;14:169
45. De Moor A, Wouters L, Mouens Y, et al: Surgical treatment of a traumatic oesophageal rupture in a foal. Eq Vet J 1979;11:26
46. Lunn DP, Peel JE: Successful treatment of traumatic oesophageal rupture with severe cellulitis in a mare. Vet Rec 1985;116:544
47. Hackett RP, Dyer RM, Hoffer RE: Surgical correction of esophageal diverticulum in a horse. J Am Vet Med Assoc 1978;173:998
48. Murray RC, Gaughan EM: Pulsion diverticulum of the cranial cervical esophagus in a horse. Can Vet J 1993;34:365
49. Tillotson K, Traub-Dargatz JL, Twedt D: Balloon dilation of an oesophageal stricture in a one-month-old Appaloosa colt. Equine Vet Educ 2003;15:67
50. Knottenbelt DC, Harrison LJ, Peacock PJ: Conservative treatment of oesophageal stricture in 5 foals. Vet Rec 1992;131:27
51. Suann CJ: Oesophageal resection and anastomosis as a treatment for oesophageal stricture in the horse. Equine Vet J 1982;14:163

52. Wagner PC, Rantanen NW: Myotomy as a treatment for esophageal stricture in a horse. Equine Pract 1980;2:40
53. Derksen FJ, Stick JA: Resection and anastomosis of esophageal stricture in a foal. Equine Pract 1983;5:17
54. Lowe JE: Esophageal anastomosis in a horse. A case report. Cornell Vet 1964;54:636
55. Craig D, Todhunter R: Surgical repair of an esophageal stricture in a horse. Vet Surgery 1987;16:251
56. Nixon AJ: Esophagomyotomy for relief of an intrathoracic esophageal stricture in a horse. J Am Med Vet Assoc 1983;183:794
57. Gideon L: Esophageal anastomosis in two foals. J Am Vet Med Assoc 1984;184:1146
58. Hoffer RE, Barber SM, Kallfelz FA, et al: Esophageal patch grafting as a treatment for esophageal stricture in a horse. J Am Vet Med Assoc 1977;171:350
59. Wilmink JM, van Weeren PR: Second intention repair in the horse and pony and management of exuberant granulation tissue. Vet Clin North Am Equine Pract 2005;21:15
60. Bhandari M, Anthony D, Schemitsch EH: The efficacy of low-pressure lavage with different irrigating solutions to remove adherent bacteria from bone. J Bone Joint Surgery 2001;83:412
61. Barber SM: An unusual location of foreign body in the horse. Can Vet J 1983;24:63
62. Wrigley RH: Ultrasonography of the tendons, ligaments, and joints. In TS Stashak, ed. *Adam's lameness in horses (5th edition)*. New York: Lippincott Williams and Wilkins, 2002, p.312
63. Schneider RK: Synovial and osseous infections. In JA Auer and JA Stick, eds. *Equine surgery (3rd edition)*. Philadelphia: WB Saunders, 2006, p.1121
64. Lugo J: Thoracic Diseases. In JA Auer and JA Stick, eds. *Equine surgery (3rd edition)*. Philadelphia: WB Saunders, 2006, p.616
65. Stone WC, Trostle SS, Gerros TC: Use of a primary muscle pedicle flap to repair a caudal thoracic wound in a horse. J Am Vet Med Assoc 1994;205:828
66. Stick JA: Management of sinus tracts and fistula. In JA Auer and JA Stick, eds. *Equine surgery (3rd edition)*. Philadelphia: WB Saunders, 2006, p.305
67. Adams SB, Fessler JF: Mesh repair of large body wall defects. In SB Adams and JF Fessler, eds. *Atlas of equine surgery*. Philadelphia: WB Saunders, 2000, p.401
68. Tulleners EP, Fretz PB: Prosthetic repair of abdominal wall defects in horses and food animals. J Am Vet Med Assoc 1983;182:258
69. Scott EA: Repair of incisional hernias in the horse. J Am Vet Med Assoc 1979;175:1203

8 Wounds of the Distal Extremities

8.1 Management of Wounds of the Distal Extremities

Jim Schumacher, DVM, MS, Diplomate ACVS, MRCVS, **and Ted S. Stashak**, DVM, MS, Diplomate ACVS

Introduction

Although there may be geographic differences in terms of type and incidence of wounds encountered, wounds of the distal limb (e.g., up to and including the carpus and tarsus) of horses are quite common and account for more than 60% of all wounds.[1] Geographic differences relate to how the horse is confined (e.g., paddock or pasture—barbed wire fences versus board, pipe, or plastic fences, etc.—or a stall and run) and the manner in which the horse is used (e.g., Western performance versus hunter/jumper).

Sharp objects such as sheet metal, broken glass, exposed nails or bolts, or barbed wire are usually responsible for lacerations and avulsion injuries, but serious wounds can result from smooth, high-tensile wire or from a rope. Protruding objects such as stubs of wood projecting from tree trunks or logs or nails and bolts that protrude from fences, buildings, or trailers are often the cause of penetrating wounds. If the penetrating object becomes embedded within tissue, a foreign-body reaction develops, usually resulting in a tract that drains persistently or intermittently.

The injury may be sustained by running into, brushing against, kicking at, or stepping on an object, or by becoming entangled in barbed or smooth wire or a rope (Figure 8.1). Horses that jump fences may sustain blunt trauma resulting in an abrasion or a penetrating wound, often in the pastern region. Blunt trauma to the dorsal surface of the carpus can occasionally cause a substantial hematoma or hygroma (Figure 8.2). Penetrating wounds from jumping injuries often occur just proximal to the coronet on the hind limbs or at the distal end of the antebrachium, and often a splinter of wood becomes embedded in the soft tissue (Figures 8.3a,b). Horses that become entangled in barbed wire may sustain a serious wound such as a degloving injury, which is

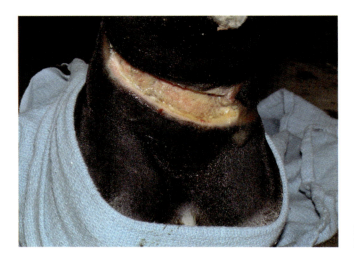

Figure 8.1. A full-thickness wound to the plantar pastern caused by a rope.

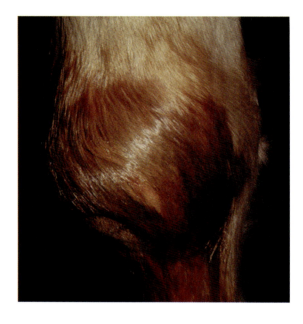

Figure 8.2. A hygroma, unresponsive to medical treatment, on the dorsal surface of the carpus.

particularly common in the metacarpal or metatarsal regions (Figure 8.4), or a laceration that extends into a synovial cavity (Figure 8.5) or through a heel bulb (Figure 8.6). The extensor or flexor tendons may also be injured. For more information regarding injuries to tendons and their sheaths, see Chapter 10.

Wounds in the distal aspect of the limb are often more difficult to suture than wounds of similar size on the body or proximal aspect of the limb because skin surrounding wounds in the distal aspect of the limb is more difficult to mobilize. Sutured wounds on the distal aspect of the limb are also more likely to dehisce.[1] Second-intention healing of wounds on the distal aspect of the limb proceeds more slowly than it does on wounds above the carpus and tarsus because unsutured wounds on the distal aspect of the limb expand more after injury and have a longer preparatory phase of healing, slower rate and earlier cessation of wound contraction, and slower rate of epithelialization compared with wounds above the carpus and tarsus.[2,3] Wounds of the distal aspect of the limb increase in size during the first 11–15 days following trauma, whereas those on the body change little in size.[2,4,5] Wounds in the flank epithelialize at a rate of 0.2 mm/day, compared with a rate as slow as 0.09 mm/day for wounds on the distal aspect of the limbs.[3]

The greatest difference in the healing rate of wounds on the body and those on the distal aspect of the limb is the greater contribution of contraction to the healing of wounds on the body.[6] Wounds that heal by

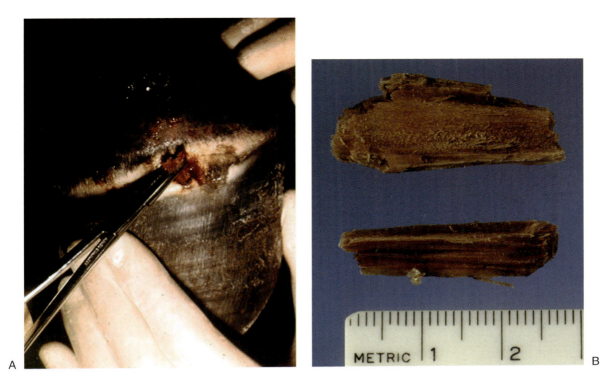

Figure 8.3. A case of persistent drainage from a wound at the coronet band. (A) Splinter of wood being removed. (B) Wood splinter after removal.

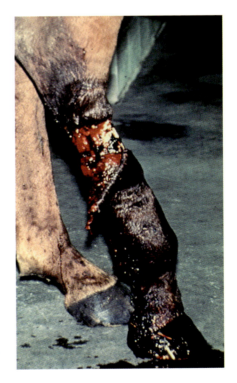

Figure 8.4. A degloving wound to the right hind limb. The metatarsal bone and the flexor tendons were exposed.

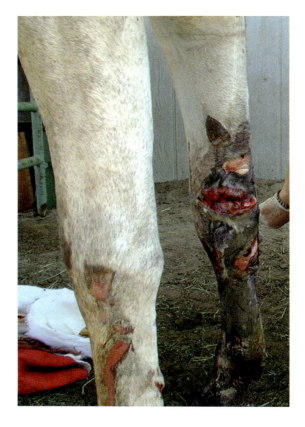

Figure 8.5. Acute laceration of the palmar carpal region that extended into the carpal canal.

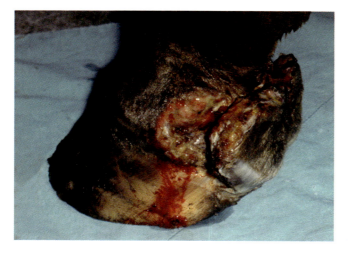

Figure 8.6. Chronically infected heel bulb laceration.

contraction are more cosmetic than those that heal by epithelialization; therefore, the appearance of healed, unsutured wounds of the body and proximal aspect of the limbs is much more cosmetic than the appearance of healed, unsutured wounds of similar size on the distal aspect of the limbs (Figure 8.7).

Horses have a propensity to develop exuberant granulation tissue compared to other species, and wounds on the distal aspect of the limbs that are healing by second intention have a tendency to develop exuberant granulation tissue compared with similar wounds proximal to the carpus and tarsus. Other factors besides location that promote exuberant production of granulation tissue in wounds of horses include chronic inflam-

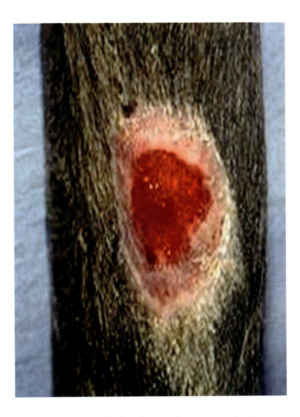

Figure 8.7. Wounds that heal to a large degree by epithelialization are less cosmetic than wounds that heal primarily by contraction because the epithelial scar is devoid of adnexa.

mation, motion, bandages and casts, and the size of the horse.[7,8] For more information regarding exuberant granulation tissue in the horse, see Treatment of Exuberant Granulation Tissue later in this chapter.

A wound to the distal aspect of the limb should be meticulously examined after it has been properly prepared, as outlined in Chapter 2, so that damage to a vital structure is not overlooked. A wound that appears to be relatively innocuous (Figure 8.8) may have suffered damage to vital structures deep within it, or it may contain a foreign body. Generally, primary closure is indicated for an acute, clean wound in which a vital structure has not been penetrated. For contaminated, contused wounds, delayed primary closure or delayed secondary closure is often selected. The decision to close the wound primarily or to delay closure—primary or secondary—or to allow it to heal by second intention can be made only after considering many factors (see Selection of Approaches to Wound Closure, Chapter 4). See Chapter 5 if reconstructive surgical techniques (e.g., skin mobilization) are needed.

Contaminated wounds and those that are so large that they cannot be apposed with sutures must heal by second intention. Without proper care, however, these wounds often develop exuberant granulation tissue, leading to an unsightly epithelial scar that is susceptible to re-injury (Figures 8.9a,b) or a fibrous granuloma (Figure 8.10) (see Treatment of Exuberant Granulation Tissue later in this chapter). See Chapter 11 if the wound is so large that skin grafting may be considered.

For purposes of discussion, this chapter has been separated into wounds (both open and closed) located from the fetlock to the carpus or tarsus, wounds of the pastern, avulsion injuries to the hoof capsule, penetrating wounds to the hoof, and wounds containing bone sequestra. Wounds to synovial cavities and treatment of horses with an avulsion injury accompanied by exposed bone are not discussed in depth in this chapter. For more information, see Chapter 9, which covers treatment of horses with wounds involving synovial structures, and Treatment of Exuberant Granulation Tissue later in this chapter, which covers treatment of horses with degloving injuries.

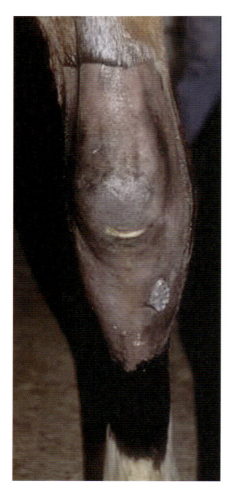

Figure 8.8. A harmless appearing wound over the tuber calcis that entered the calcaneal bursa, resulting in sepsis of that synovial structure.

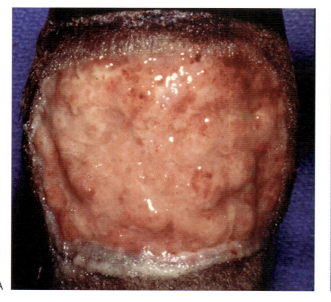

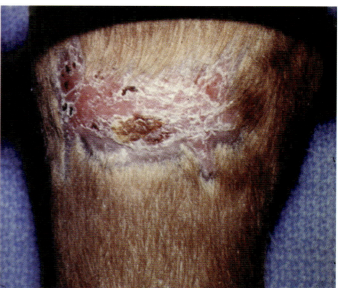

A

B

Figure 8.9. A wound that healed with an unsightly epithelial scar is susceptible to re-injury. (A) A square-shaped wound over the dorsal fetlock. (B) Healing after 75 days resulted in an unsightly epithelial scar susceptible to re-injury.

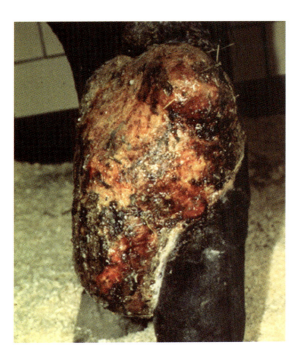

Figure 8.10. Extensive fibrous granuloma over the dorsal aspect of the hock.

Wound Categories

Wounds can be categorized as open or closed. Open wounds are those in which the entire thickness of the skin has been separated. They include incisions, which are wounds produced by a sharp object, either intentionally with a scalpel or accidentally by glass or sheet metal. The skin edge of an incision is cut cleanly, resulting in little damage to underlying tissue. The victim experiences little pain. Lacerations are the most common type of open wound and are characterized by an irregular cutaneous margin and extensive damage to underlying tissue. They are accompanied by bruising, which results in considerable pain. A laceration accompanied by loss of tissue is termed an avulsion. A puncture is another type of open wound; it is produced by a sharp object that perforates tissue. The perforating object may carry dirt, manure, and other debris to the depths of the wound and may enter a synovial cavity. Puncture wounds are easily trivialized, because their size belies their severity.

Closed wounds are those that do not involve the entire thickness of skin, including abrasions and contusions. An abrasion is a friction injury to the superficial layers of the skin and is characterized by oozing of serum and only a small amount of hemorrhage. Exposure of nerve endings results in considerable pain. A rope burn is an example of an abrasion. A contusion is a closed wound characterized by bleeding and destruction of tissue within and beneath undivided skin.

Wounds Involving the Fetlock, Metacarpus/Metatarsus, and Carpus/Tarsus

Causes

Lacerations involving the fetlock, metacarpus or metatarsus, and carpus or tarsus are commonly inflicted by barbed wire or other metal objects. The hind limb appears to be more prone than the forelimb to laceration in these areas. The soft tissues of the dorsal surface of the carpus are particularly prone to contusions and punctures, which are often incurred when the carpus strikes a fence or stall door, and these closed injuries and punctures often involve one of the many synovial structures found in the carpal region. Occasionally, a wire laceration on the palmar surface of the carpus will enter the carpal canal synovial sheath (Figure 8.5).

Closed Injuries

The most common type of closed injury to the distal portion of the limb is the carpal hygroma, which appears as a fluid-filled swelling over the dorsal surface of the carpus. Its usual cause is blunt force to the dorsum of the carpus or antebrachium, such as that which might occur when the horse jumps a fence or hits the stall door with a forelimb. A carpal hygroma forms from accumulation of fluid in an adventitious bursa in the subcutaneous tissue, usually from a subcutaneous hematoma that develops into a seroma.[9] A hygroma often resembles an abnormal accumulation of fluid in a tendon sheath of an extensor muscle, the cause of which is the same as that of a hygroma, such that differentiating the two conditions may be difficult.

Diagnosis

A carpal hygroma appears as a cyst-like, spherical fluctuant swelling containing serous fluid (Figure 8.2). The spherical appearance of a carpal hygroma helps distinguish it from a longitudinally oriented distended sheath of an extensor tendon and from a horizontally oriented distended carpal joint.

Carpal flexion may be restricted if the hygroma is large. Palpation of the swelling does not usually cause the horse to show signs of discomfort, unless the hygroma is infected, and usually the horse is lame only if the hygroma interferes mechanically with the gait or is infected. Although a carpal hygroma can typically be differentiated from a swollen sheath of an extensor tendon by inspection and palpation, ultrasonographic examination or contrast radiographic examination of the hygroma provides definitive diagnosis.

Treatment

The affected horse can usually be treated successfully by centesis and drainage of the hygroma, application of a pressure bandage, and confinement. A corticosteroid injected into the hygroma cavity at the same time the fluid is drained may be helpful in preventing reformation of fluid. If the hygroma fails to resolve in this manner, it can be drained through a distally located stab incision, through which the lining of the cavity is removed by using a large curette, with the horse standing, or by using an arthroscopically guided, motorized synovial resector, with the horse anesthetized. A Penrose drain tube inserted through the stab incision ensures that it remains open until production of fluid has subsided (Figure 8.11a). The limb is bandaged and held in extension with a splint for several weeks (Figure 8.11b). If the hygroma fails to resolve with these treatments, it can be excised under general anesthesia. After surgery, the limb is held in extension with a cast or splint for several weeks. The horse can begin walking exercise after about 1 month.

Prognosis

If the horse is chronically affected, treatment may not restore full range of carpal motion because fibrosis may limit carpal flexion. The owner should be warned that surgical treatment may worsen the condition if healing is disturbed by motion or infection.

Open Injuries

Diagnosis

The carpus, tarsus, metacarpus, or metatarsus may suffer a degloving injury, which by definition is a wound that exposes bone and often tendons as well. The injury may result from a circumferential laceration with detachment of skin from the limb (Figure 8.4) or from an avulsion injury that is accompanied by such an extensive loss of tissue that the wound cannot heal by second intention alone (Figure 3.4). A degloving wound caused by a laceration can be healed by primary, delayed primary, or secondary closure when no skin has been lost (Figure 8.12). A degloving wound with extensive loss of skin can usually be healed only by applying a free skin graft to the wound (see Chapter 11). A degloving injury may rarely be accompanied by vascular damage so severe that the hoof capsule may be lost (Figures 8.13a,b).

An avulsion injury to the carpus is particularly devastating because sheet grafting is difficult in view of the movement withstood in this region (Figures 8.14a,b). The carpus must be completely immobilized with a full-limb or sleeve cast for the graft to be accepted. Once the limb is no longer immobilized, after graft take, the graft and granulation tissue beneath the graft usually split transversely along the dorsal surface of the antebrachiocarpal and middle carpal joints, sometimes opening the sheath of the tendon of the extensor carpi radialis muscle.

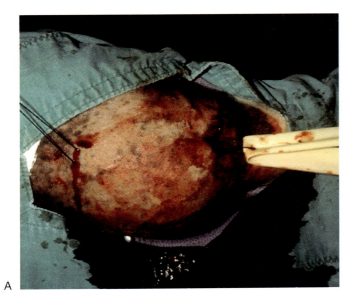
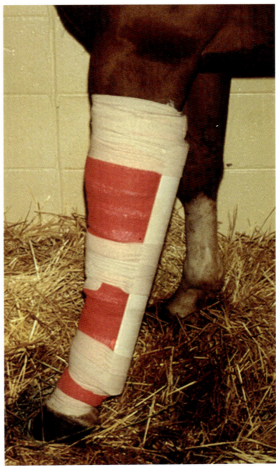

Figure 8.11. Same horse as in Figure 8.2, at surgery. (A) A Penrose drain tube is inserted through the stab incision at the distal extent of the hygroma. The drain ensures that the incision remains open until production of fluid has subsided, usually within 7 to 10 days. (B) The limb is bandaged and held in extension with a splint for several weeks.

Contraction of large wounds in people, dogs, and cats over the flexor surface of a joint often results in contracture of the associated joint and distortion of the limb.[10,11] Conversely, wound contraction in horses does not cause contracture and should be considered beneficial because it accelerates wound healing and decreases the size of the epithelial scar. Wounds healed by contraction are more cosmetic than those healed by epithelialization.

Wounds to the carpus, metacarpus, tarsus, or metatarsus frequently involve one or more of many tendons, tendon sheaths, bursae, or joint capsules found in these areas (Figures 8.2, 8.5, 8.8). Breach of a synovial structure can be confirmed by injecting sterile fluid into the synovial cavity suspected of being penetrated, at a site remote from the wound, and observing it egress the wound (see Figure 2.15). Sepsis of a synovial cavity can be determined by identifying an elevated concentration of neutrophils and protein in fluid aspirated from the cavity. For more information, see Chapter 9, which discusses lacerations associated with synovial structures.

Movement of an intact or severed tendon within a wound on a metacarpus or metatarsus often results in the formation of two separate granulation beds, one on the tendon and the other on tissue surrounding the tendon (Figures 2.3a,b, 8.15). Granulation tissue provides myofibroblasts that normally span the wound, causing it to contract, but this is prevented by the presence of two separate granulation beds. When movement of the tendon is restricted by immobilizing the limb, the granulation beds rapidly become confluent, resulting in prompt contraction of the wound.

The extensor tendons are frequently involved in lacerations located in carpal, tarsal, metacarpal, or metatarsal regions because of their superficial location in these regions. When the tendon of the extensor carpi radialis

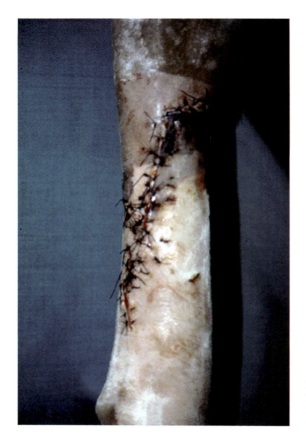

Figure 8.12. A degloving injury, similar to that seen in Figure 8.4, which was sutured within 4 hours of the injury. The limb is shown following cast removal; note that the skin at the proximal limits of the wound is discolored and had to be debrided at a later time.

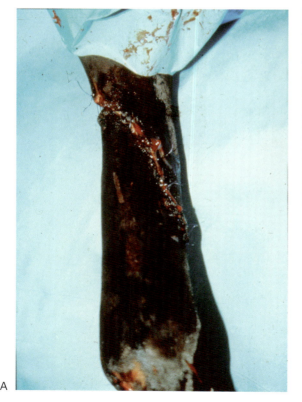

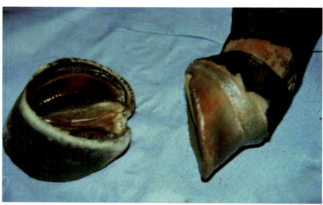

A

B

Figure 8.13 (A and B). This horse suffered a degloving injury to the metatarsus that so severely impaired the vascular supply to the foot that the hoof capsule was lost.

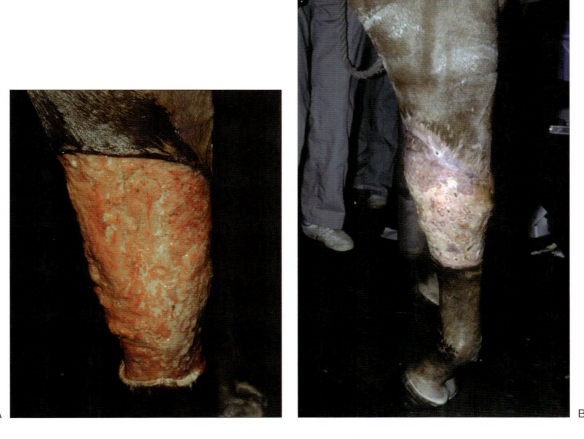

Figure 8.14. This horse suffered an extensive avulsion injury to the carpus. (A) Granulation tissue fills the wound. (B) The wound was covered with a free, split-thickness, meshed skin graft. A large portion of the graft was accepted.

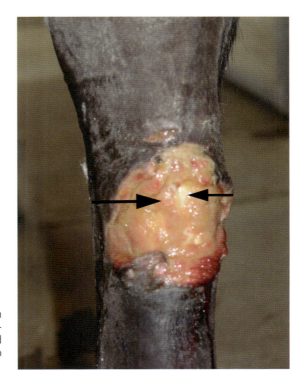

Figure 8.15. Movement of an intact or partially severed tendon within a wound on a metacarpus or metatarsus often results in two separate granulation beds, one on the tendon (between the left and right arrows) and the other on tissue surrounding the tendon. The arrows are pointing to the cleft created between the two granulation tissue beds.

muscle is lacerated, the horse is still able to extend the distal aspect of the limb because of the action of the common and lateral digital extensor muscles, but the carpus overflexes because resistance to the action of the flexor muscles is diminished.[12] Transection of the tendon of the common digital extensor muscle above or below the carpus seems to have no long-lasting detrimental effect on gait because the actions of the extensor carpi radialis and lateral digital extensor muscles and the extensor branch of the suspensory ligament compensate for loss of the action of this muscle.[13] Transection of the peroneus tertius tendon on the dorsal surface of the hock allows this joint to move independently of the stifle as a result of disruption of the reciprocal apparatus (Figure 8.16).

Whereas lacerations of the flexor tendons are typically associated with small wounds, those of the extensor tendons often are associated with large, avulsion wounds on the dorsal aspect of the metacarpus/metatarsus (Figure 8.17).[14] Extensor tendons of the hind limbs are lacerated far more frequently than those of the forelimbs,[15] and the tendon of the long digital extensor muscle is lacerated more frequently than the tendon of the lateral digital extensor muscle, although frequently, both tendons are lacerated.

Because the primary function of the extensor tendons of the distal aspect of the limb is not to support weight but to extend the digit during locomotion, laceration of one or more of the extensor tendons does not alter the conformation of the limb but may result instead in an inability of the horse to extend the toe, causing the fetlock to knuckle during locomotion. In contrast, the conformation of the limb is altered when a flexor tendon of the distal aspect of the limb is severed. See Chapter 10 for more information about diagnosis and treatment of horses with lacerations associated with tendons, paratendons, and tendon sheaths.

Lacerations to the dorsal, lateral, and medial surfaces of the metacarpus/metatarsus often expose large areas of bone, which are often devoid of periosteum (Figure 8.18). The extreme thickness of dorsal cortex of the diaphysis of the third metacarpal/metatarsal bone may predispose the outer third of the bone to develop a sequestrum, because trauma may deprive the bone of its periosteal blood supply leaving it dependent on medullary vessels traversing the cortex. Treatment for bone sequestrum is discussed later in this chapter. See Degloving Injuries, page 427, for additional information regarding treatment of horses with wounds of the distal portion of the limb that contain sequestered bone and for treatment of horses with large degloving wounds.

Occasionally, a foreign body becomes imbedded within the soft tissues on the palmar or plantar surface of the metacarpal or metatarsal region (Figures 2.16a–e). Although a foreign object can sometimes be identified by inserting a probe into the wound's tract, ultrasonographic examination or plain or contrast radiographic examination of the affected region is usually required to identify the foreign object (Figures 2.17a,b and 2.18a,b).

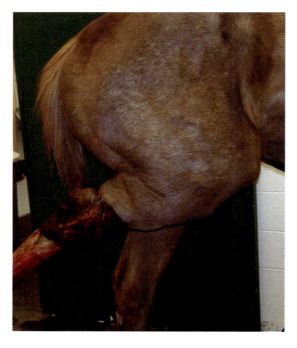

Figure 8.16. This horse sustained an avulsion injury to the dorsal surface of the hock that was complicated by laceration of the tendon of the peroneus tertius. Note that the hock is extended while the stifle is flexed.

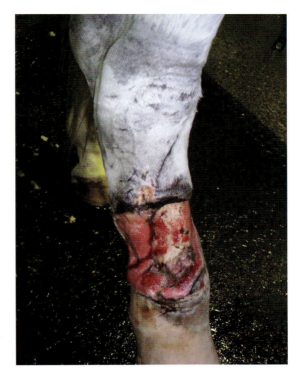

Figure 8.17. Large, degloving wounds on the dorsal surface of the meta-carpus/metatarsus often are associated with laceration of the long and lateral digital extensor tendons.

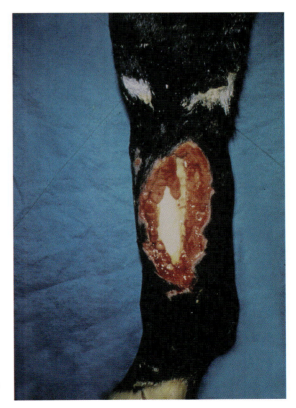

Figure 8.18. Laceration to the lateral surface of the metacarpus exposed a large area of bone. The upper layer of bone devoid of periosteum is ischemic and is likely to form a sequestrum.

Treatment

Sutured wounds of the carpus, tarsus, metacarpus, metatarsus, and fetlock are prone to dehisce because wounds in these regions rapidly become contaminated due to their proximity to the ground and because their blood supply is often attenuated. The risk of dehiscence caused by infection can be diminished by properly preparing the wound or by using delayed primary or delayed secondary closure. See Chapter 2 for a detailed account of techniques used to prepare wounds for suturing.

Wounds of the carpus, tarsus, metacarpus, metatarsus, and fetlock are often difficult to suture without tension because tissues in these regions are difficult to mobilize and these regions are highly mobile or contain highly mobile structures (e.g., tendons). Dehiscence of sutured wounds and excessive expansion of unsutured wounds can best be prevented by immobilizing the distal portion of the limb with a cast or with a splint applied over a bandage. Immobilizing the distal aspect of the limb with a short-limb cast or a splint may be helpful in preventing dehiscence of a sutured wound in a mobile region, such as the fetlock, especially if the wound is perpendicular or oblique to the limb's long axis. Enclosing a lacerated tarsus in a cast is difficult because of the reciprocal apparatus of the hind limb, but application of a full-limb cast or a bandage cast splint to a hind limb may sometimes be indicated. For more information regarding techniques for casting and bandage splinting, see Chapter 16.

The length of time for which the distal aspect of the limb is immobilized depends on the amount of tension exerted on the wound during closure. Wounds with a good blood supply that are sutured with minimal tension are immobilized for only 10–14 days, whereas wounds that are sutured under great tension or those with a blood supply marginal enough to delay healing should be immobilized for 17–21 days. A limb with a wound left unsutured to heal by second intention may require a considerably longer period (e.g., several months) of immobilization, especially if an extensor or flexor tendon has been transected.

Wounds closed under tension, especially those that have been excessively undermined, may dehisce because excessive stretching of the skin beyond its limits of maximal extensibility may obstruct blood flow through the dermal blood vessels, causing the sutured margin of the wound to necrose.[16] Techniques most commonly used to avoid excessive tension on the sutured laceration include undermining of the skin adjacent to the wound; presuturing the wound; applying tension sutures such as walking sutures or horizontal mattress, vertical mattress, or far-near tension sutures; and creating relaxing incisions.[17-21] For information regarding techniques used to relieve skin tension and for controlling wound contraction, see Chapter 5.

Horses with an infected wound containing a foreign body are usually presented with an intermittently or persistently draining tract within the wound. The wound fails to heal until the foreign object is removed (Figures 2.16a–e).[22] A foreign object provides a nidus for bacterial growth and its presence can cause infection when only a small quantity of bacteria contaminate the wound. Some foreign objects, such as those composed of wood, have a greater tendency than others, such as glass or metal, to potentiate infection.

Prognosis

When treated properly, a horse with a wound of the fetlock, metacarpus, metatarsus, carpus, or tarsus that does not extend into a supporting structure or synovial cavity has a good prognosis for an excellent cosmetic outcome and soundness. Treatment is difficult when a synovial cavity, tendon, or bone becomes infected, and the outcome is often disappointing. Horses that have incurred damage to a digital flexor tendon or its sheath have a guarded prognosis for return to soundness.[23]

The nature of the injury affects outcome. For example, cutaneous incisions, whether created accidentally or purposely, result in minimal trauma and negligible contamination. Lacerations caused by impact, whether clean or heavily contaminated, are more susceptible to infection than are incisional wounds, and they tend to heal poorly because of injury to the blood supply. Sutured wounds parallel to the long axis of the limb are more likely to heal without complication than are sutured wounds oriented transverse to the long axis of the limb. Sutured wounds aligned obliquely or transversely to the long axis of the limb are best protected from distractive forces by immobilization in a bandage splint or cast and commonly dehisce when protected by a bandage alone.

A deep wound to the dorsal surface of the metacarpal or metatarsal region is not usually career-ending, even if extensor tendons are injured, because extensor function is usually regained if the distal portion of the affected limb is immobilized for 4 to 6 weeks with a cast or a splint. Because extensor tendons do not support weight, a decrease in their mechanical strength is not critical to the outcome of the horse. A wound to palmar/plantar surface of the metacarpal/metatarsal region, however, is frequently career-ending or even life-threatening if the flexor tendons, suspensory ligament, or digital flexor tendon sheath is lacerated.

Infected wounds containing a foreign body generally heal without complication after the object has been removed. Antimicrobial therapy administered parenterally may temporarily decrease swelling and discharge from the wound,[24] but antimicrobial therapy alone is an ineffective treatment of a horse with a foreign object imbedded in a wound because drugs fail to contact bacteria harbored by the foreign object. Organic foreign objects, such as pieces of wood, provoke a greater inflammatory response, resulting in more discharge of exudate than do non-organic foreign objects, such as pieces of glass or metal. Bacterial culture of exudate from a draining sinus is not helpful in determining the organism associated with the foreign object because secondary pathogens rapidly colonize a draining sinus.

Wounds Involving the Pastern

Causes

The pastern is particularly susceptible to trauma because of its proximity to the ground. Lacerations of the pastern are commonly inflicted by barbed wire or other metal objects (Figures 8.6 and 8.19), and occasionally, the pastern is injured when it becomes entrapped between immovable objects such as the rails of a cattle guard or a wall and stall door. Entrapment injuries of the pastern are often accompanied by vascular trauma leading to ischemic necrosis of soft tissue and infection (Figure 8.20). The longer the horse is entrapped and the more it struggles to free itself the greater the vascular injury. Occasionally, a rope encircling the pastern causes a rope burn severe enough to result in loss of a partial- or full-thickness portion skin (Figure 8.1).

The coronary band of a hind limb sometimes incurs a penetrating wound when the horse jumps a barrier, and often a splinter of wood is imbedded within the wound (Figure 8.3). Lacerations of the pastern region frequently involve the coronary band and variable portions of the hoof capsule as well as structures deep to it. Lacerations to the coronary band may result in permanent defects in the hoof wall (see the section on laceration and avulsion wounds of the hoof capsule in this chapter). Because the pastern is close to the ground, a wound in this region quickly becomes contaminated with manure and dirt. A laceration incurred while the horse is at pasture may go unrecognized for days because it is hidden from view by grass.

The heel bulb is the region of the pastern most susceptible to injury. A heel bulb laceration, especially one caused by barbed wire, often extends in an arc from the quarter of the hoof wall to the depression between the heel bulbs (Figure 8.19), and occasionally the arc extends from one quarter to the other (Figure 8.6). In either case, the wound often gapes when the horse bears weight on the limb. The deeper the laceration, the greater the chances that one or more critical structures in the pastern or foot may be damaged. Lacerations of the pastern

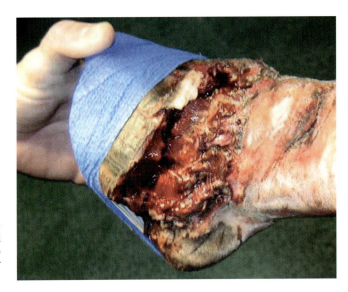

Figure 8.19. A heel bulb laceration often extends in an arc from the quarter of the hoof wall to the depression between the heel bulbs. A deep laceration, such as this one, is likely to extend into the distal interphalangeal joint, navicular bursa, or digital flexor tendon sheath.

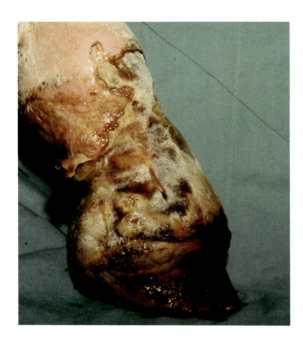

Figure 8.20. Vascular injury to the pastern that resulted from the limb becoming caught between the rails of a cattle guard. The hoof wall sloughed 2 weeks following the injury.

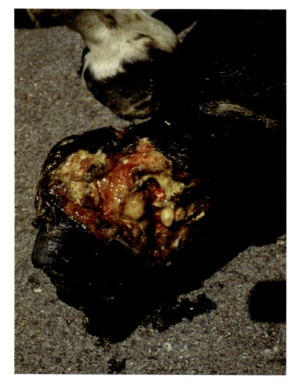

Figure 8.21. An extensive laceration of the pastern that entered the proximal and distal interphalangeal joints, transected the lateral collateral ligaments of both joints, and lacerated the collateral cartilage of the distal phalanx, as well as the coronary band.

that course deep to the hoof wall may involve one or more collateral ligaments, the capsule of the proximal or distal interphalangeal joint, the deep digital flexor tendon and its digital flexor tendon sheath, a collateral cartilage of the distal phalanx, and the navicular bone and its bursa and ligaments (Figure 8.21). Occasionally, a pastern laceration is accompanied by fracture of the middle or distal phalanx.

Rope burns are most commonly found on a pastern, usually that of a hind limb, and most commonly result from tangling of the limb in rope while the horse is picketed. A rope burn is a combination of abrasion and thermal damage caused by friction. A rope burn may be superficial partial-thickness (first-degree burn) or deep partial-thickness (second-degree burn), or it may extend through all layers (a full-thickness or third-degree burn) (Figure 8.1).

Diagnosis

Physical Examination

A horse with a pastern wound is frequently lame but the degree of lameness depends on the duration of the injury and the structures involved, and whether or not the wound has become infected. Generally, the deeper the laceration, the greater the lameness, but severance of a digital nerve may attenuate lameness. Even if a vital structure is not involved, the horse may be reluctant to fully bear weight on the injured limb, especially if the wound is infected.

Laceration of the digital artery and vein causes severe hemorrhage, sometimes resulting in cardiovascular shock. To avoid exacerbating hypotension caused by severe hemorrhage, the horse's cardiovascular status should be assessed prior to administering a sedative or tranquilizer to facilitate examination. Administration of a phenothiazine-derivative tranquilizer, in particular, should be avoided because it may cause severe hypotension in a horse suffering from hypovolemia. Hemorrhage from the digital vessels can usually be controlled by applying a pressure bandage for 1 or 2 hours, but if the wound requires immediate examination, the digital vessels are best ligated. Anesthetizing the ipsilateral palmar/plantar digital nerve at the level of the proximal sesamoid bones may aid ligation by preventing pain caused if the digital nerve, which courses next to the digital vessels, is disturbed during ligation.

Damage to deep structures may be difficult to recognize visually, and if so, the wound should be carefully palpated. To discriminatively inspect an acute laceration, the wound should be carefully palpated after the hair has been clipped and the wound irrigated with an antiseptic solution. Dilute (0.1%) povidone iodine solution may be superior to chlorhexidine diacetate solution for lavage of any laceration that might involve a synovial structure because chlorhexidine diacetate solution may damage synovial structures.[24]

Devitalized tissue should be excised, and gross contaminants removed using irrigation/cleansing. After donning a sterile glove, the depths of the wound are palpated to detect damage to deeper structures. Discerning damage to structures deep in the wound using digital palpation may be difficult if granulation tissue has already formed. For a more complete discussion of the approaches used for examining wounds, see Chapter 2.

Laxity and instability of the middle or distal interphalangeal joint indicate disruption of a collateral ligament, and a sucking noise may indicate that the proximal or distal interphalangeal joint has been opened. A puncture wound of the coronary band may appear deceptively unimportant, but it should be inspected closely for the presence of wood splinters (Figure 8.3). A laceration or puncture to the dorsal aspect of the coronary band may involve the dorsal pouch of the distal interphalangeal joint, which extends quite far proximal to the hoof capsule on the dorsal surface of the pastern (Figure 8.22).

The distal interphalangeal joint is the synovial structure most commonly involved in lacerations of the heel bulbs.[23] If the laceration extends completely through the collateral cartilage of the distal phalanx, the distal interphalangeal joint is likely to be breached because the collateral cartilage adjoins the capsule of this joint (Figure 8.23). If articular cartilage can be palpated or synovial fluid is seen, penetration of a joint capsule is certain. Discerning penetration of the digital flexor tendon sheath may be more difficult, but if a laceration in the deep digital flexor tendon can be palpated, penetration of the sheath is certain. A laceration over the palmar/plantar surface of the pastern is highly likely to have entered the digital flexor tendon sheath, which lies superficially in this region (Figure 8.24).

Determining the depth of a partial-thickness rope burn of the pastern may be difficult because swelling of the remaining skin may confound estimates of tissue loss. Depth of loss may best be estimated by the time required for the wound to epithelialize and the appearance of the wound after healing. Superficial partial-thickness rope burns epithelialize within 3 weeks, and pilation at the site of injury is good. Deep partial-thickness rope burns may take months to heal, and the site may remain scarred and hairless. A full-thickness rope burn of the palmar/plantar surface of the pastern may breach the digital flexor tendon sheath (Figure 8.1).

Imaging

The lacerated region should be examined radiographically to help ascertain the status of the bones and joints and to determine whether a foreign body is present (Figure 8.25). The proximity of the laceration to criti-

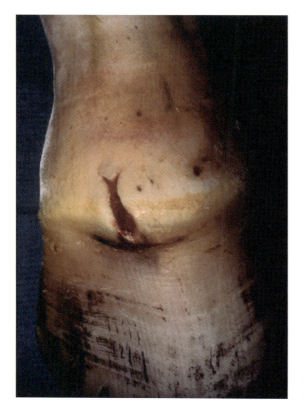

Figure 8.22. Wound to the coronary band that extended into the dorsal proximal pouch of the distal interphalangeal joint.

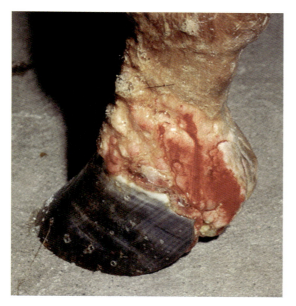

Figure 8.23. Extensive laceration of the pastern that extended through the collateral cartilage of the distal phalanx into the distal interphalangeal joint.

cal structures, such as the navicular apparatus, can be determined by examining radiographs of the pastern and foot taken following the insertion of a sterile probe into the depths of the wound. If a laceration of a collateral ligament of the distal interphalangeal joint is suspected, the region can be examined radiographically with the collateral ligament of the lacerated side stressed to determine if the bones of the joint are shifted abnormally relative to each other. To obtain a stress radiograph of the distal interphalangeal joint, mediolateral force is applied to the joint as the region is radiographed to determine if the middle and distal phalanges shift

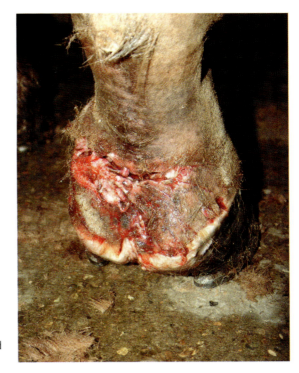

Figure 8.24. This wound over the palmar surface of the pastern entered the digital flexor tendon sheath, which lies superficially in this region.

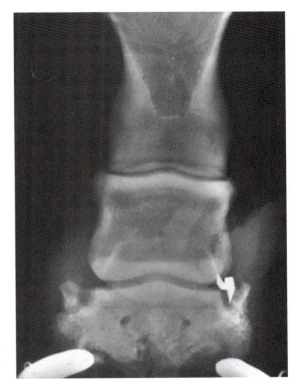

Figure 8.25. Radiographic examination of a deep wound to the pastern region might reveal the presence of a foreign body deep within the wound. This barb was not located by visual or digital inspection of the wound.

abnormally relative to each other. Force can be applied by standing the horse on a small block of wood placed under the hoof only on the side contralateral to the wound.

A contrast study may be helpful in the event that penetration of a synovial structure is suspected but cannot be confirmed by digital palpation. Air in the wound prevents accurate ultrasonographic examination of the injured pastern, but occasionally, ultrasonography may be valuable in detecting damage to ligaments or tendons. The structures involved in the laceration may sometimes be appreciated only during exploration and debridement of the wound under general anesthesia.

Treatment

Suturing a laceration in the pastern region and applying a short-limb or foot cast usually provides the best cosmetic and functional results. An acute laceration can be sutured without delay if the laceration is clean, tissue damage is minimal, and no synovial structure has been penetrated. In this case, systemic administration of an antimicrobial drug is often not necessary, but administration of a nonsteroidal, anti-inflammatory drug may be indicated to reduce pain and inflammation.

Closure of an acute wound and application of a cast should be delayed for 2 to 3 days following injury if the exposed tissue is grossly contaminated or severely traumatized, but performed before granulation tissue develops (delayed primary closure). The horse is best treated by secondary closure (closure delayed until granulation tissue has formed) if presented after the wound appears infected (Figure 8.6).

To prepare a contaminated or infected wound for suturing, skin surrounding the wound should be cleaned with an antiseptic soap, but application of soap to the wound itself should be avoided because detergent is cytotoxic and increases the wound's susceptibility to infection.[25] The wound is debrided; an antimicrobial solution, cream, or ointment is applied topically to the cleansed/irrigated wound to reduce the concentration of microorganisms within it; and the wound is bandaged. If the wound is infected and exudative or if it is difficult to debride, a debriding dressing (e.g., Kerlix AMD gauze, Covidien Animal Health/Kendall, Dublin, OH) can be applied for several days and changed daily. The bandage is usually changed daily or every other day to assess healing after the debridement dressing in discontinued. When the bandage is changed, the wound and surrounding skin and hoof wall are cleansed, and if necessary, the wound is again debrided.

The horse should receive broad-spectrum, antimicrobial therapy systemically, especially if a synovial structure has been penetrated. The duration of systemic administration of antimicrobial therapy is dictated by the horse's response to therapy. Administration of a nonsteroidal, anti-inflammatory drug to reduce pain and inflammation is usually indicated. When a synovial structure has been penetrated, closure of the wound and application of a cast should be delayed for several days, even if the wound is clean. Heavily contaminated or badly damaged tissue surrounding the open synovial structure should be debrided and synovial lavage should be executed through a needle or cannula inserted at a site remote to the wound, using 3L to 6L of sterile, physiological saline solution or a balanced electrolyte solution. Using arthroscopic equipment to lavage an infected synovial structure not only ensures thorough lavage but also allows direct examination of the structure, aiding in predicting prognosis (see Figure 2.19). After the wound has been debrided and the synovial structure lavaged, the wound is protected under a sterile bandage and the horse is confined to a dry area.

To aid resolution of synovial sepsis, an appropriate antimicrobial drug should be delivered to the infected tissue in a concentration greater than the minimum inhibitory concentration. Although broad-spectrum antimicrobial therapy should be administered systemically, vascular injury and thrombosis may limit drug delivery to the wound. Regional limb perfusion circumvents these limitations by delivering the antimicrobial drug, under pressure through the venous system, in a high concentration. For more information, see Chapter 9, which covers treatment of wounds involving synovial structures.

The wound is ready for delayed primary closure when it appears clean and contains little exudate, or it is ready for delayed secondary closure when healthy, pink, granulation tissue fills the wound (Figure 8.26a). If the horse remains or becomes severely lame, the wound should be reassessed to determine whether vital structures have been damaged. Provided that the horse is docile and the wound is uncomplicated, suturing can be done under sedation after desensitizing the pastern and foot using perineural anesthesia, but in most cases, the wound is best sutured under general anesthesia. The foot should be cleansed and trimmed, either before or after the horse is anesthetized, especially if a cast is to be applied. Lightly rasping the hoof wall distal to the wounded region reduces surface contamination. After the hoof has been scrubbed with antiseptic soap using a brush, a

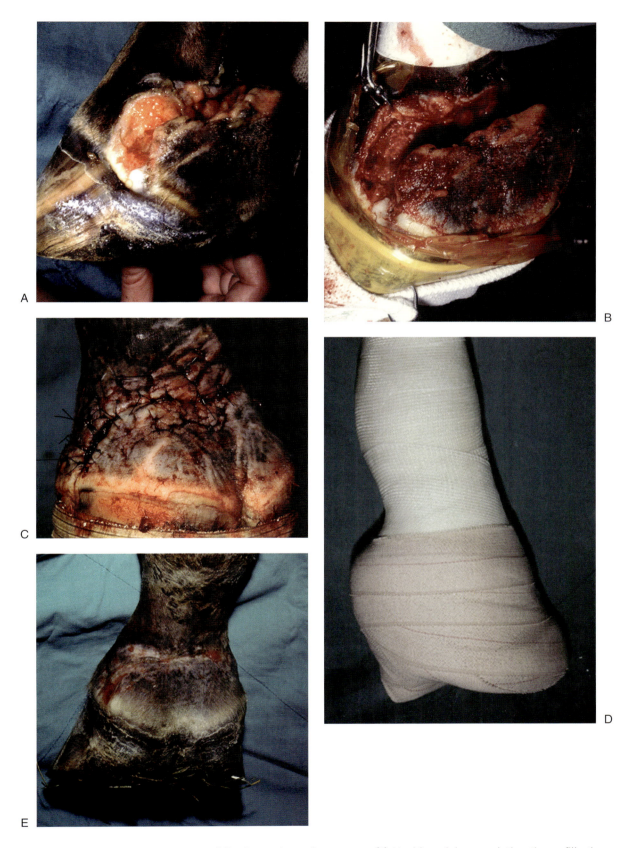

Figure 8.26. Same wound as in Figure 8.6, following 5 days of treatment. (A) Healthy, pink, granulation tissue fills the wound, indicating that it is ready for secondary closure. (B) Excessive granulation tissue has been excised from this wound. (C) A combination of vertical mattress tension and simple interrupted sutures were used to close this wound. (D) A short-limb cast. (E) Excellent healing was observed when the cast was removed after 2 weeks.

sterile glove is applied to the foot to protect the wound from contamination, and the wound is isolated with drapes. Applying a tourniquet proximal to the pastern may speed surgery by reducing hemorrhage and improving visibility.

Granulation tissue should be removed before the wound is sutured (Figure 8.26b) because this reduces the level of bacterial contamination, exposes the depth of the wound for examination, and enhances mobility of the wound margin for suturing. Care should be exercised to avoid damaging the digital vessels and unwounded portions of the coronary region during excision of the granulation tissue.[26]

After the wound has been debrided, it is closed with #0 or #1 sutures of monofilament nylon or polypropylene placed in a vertical mattress pattern (tension-relieving sutures) followed by apposition of the skin edges with 2-0 monofilament nylon or polypropylene placed in either a simple interrupted or an interrupted vertical mattress pattern (Figure 8.26c). The edges of a wound in the coronary band should be properly aligned to prevent or minimize the development of a defect in the hoof capsule. Sutures placed through the coronary band do not impair formation of the hoof capsule distal to the laceration. Sutures can be placed through the lacerated hoof capsule, if necessary, to stabilize a wound that extends into it. Thinning the wall with a rasp or burr prior to surgery eases placement of sutures through the hoof wall (see the section on laceration and avulsion wounds of the hoof capsule, below). The sutured wound is covered with a sterile, semi-occlusive dressing, which is maintained in position with sterile, elastic gauze. The distal portion of the limb or foot is then enclosed within a bandage or cast (Figures 8.26d,e).

Protecting an unsutured wound on the pastern with a bandage alone results in a substantially longer time to heal and a poorer cosmetic appearance, especially if the laceration involves a heel bulb, than does immobilization of the foot and pastern within a cast (Figure 8.27). Protecting the wound with a bandage can be more costly than protecting it with a cast, considering the quantity of bandage material that must be used over time. To minimize distractive forces on a sutured or unsutured laceration at a heel bulb, a cast that encompasses the foot and extends up to the mid-pastern region is usually sufficient, but to decrease distractive forces on a wound proximal to the bulbs of the heel, a cast that encompasses the foot and extends to the carpus or tarsus may be necessary.[26] Short-limb casts are more likely to result in cast sores than are casts applied to just the foot because foot casts do not incorporate the fetlock region, a frequent site of sores caused by short-limb casts.

The cast enhances healing of a laceration to the pastern by protecting the wound from the environment, limiting movement of wound edges and relieving tension on the wound, and providing a moist environment for epithelialization.[26] The time at which the cast is removed depends on the amount of tension required to close the wound or the deficit of tissue that must heal by second intention. The greater the tension on the sutured

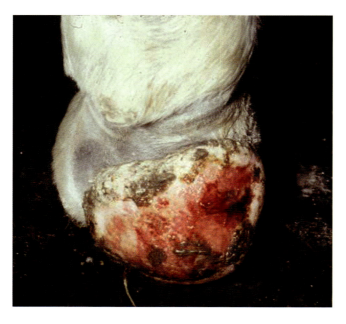

Figure 8.27. Failure to immobilize the distal portion of the limb of a horse that has incurred a heel bulb laceration is likely to result in movement, which in turn leads to production of exuberant granulation tissue.

wound or the larger the deficit of tissue, the longer the cast should be maintained. Leaving the cast for 14–21 days is usually sufficient to facilitate healing of most wounds to the pastern region.

Treatment of the horse with a recently acquired rope burn involves cleansing the wound, administering local and systemic anti-inflammatory drug therapy, and bandaging. Hair is clipped from the area in preparation for wound cleansing/irrigation. Skin surrounding the wound should be cleaned with an antiseptic soap, but application of soap to the wound itself should be avoided.

Cold hydrotherapy (using a hose), ice packs, or ice-water slurry is used to minimize edema. Ice-water slurries appear to deep-cool tissues more rapidly than ice or water alone, such that this is the authors' preferred approach. Cold therapy is applied for 30 minutes 2 to 3 times a day for 2 days. It can be accomplished by standing the horse in a cold stream (creek or river) of flowing water if hydrotherapy or ice is not available. In between cold treatments an antimicrobial ointment is applied to the wound and a topical anti-inflammatory drug such as dimethyl sulfoxide (DMSO) or diclofenac sodium (1%) cream (Surpass™, Idexx Laboratories, Westbrook, ME) should be applied liberally to the edematous tissues surrounding the wound (not in the wound) and proximal to it. Between treatments the wounded pastern is protected with a bandage to prevent further damage caused by excessive movement, wound contamination, and desiccation. The bandage should extend to the carpus or tarsus to prevent swelling of the limb and minimize movement of the wound. The horse should receive a nonsteroidal anti-inflammatory drug to attenuate pain and decrease swelling.

Prognosis

With proper treatment, a horse with a pastern laceration not involving a supporting structure or extending into a synovial structure has a good prognosis for a cosmetic outcome and return to soundness. When a synovial structure, tendon, or bone becomes infected, treatment is more problematic and the results are often poor. Horses that have incurred damage to a digital flexor tendon or its sheath have a guarded prognosis for return to soundness.[22] Infection of a collateral cartilage may result in lameness and development of one or more chronic draining sinuses at the coronary band (quittor). To prevent infection of a collateral cartilage, discolored portions of cartilage should be excised when the wound is debrided.

Healing of deep, partial- or full-thickness rope burns is usually protracted, and the wound often heals with a blemish that resembles a keloid. The degree of dermal destruction governs the time required for complete healing. The deeper the destruction into the dermis, the fewer the adnexa present to provide epithelial cells for epithelialization and the longer the time for healing. Full-thickness rope burns to the palmar/plantar surface of the pastern may require skin grafting.

Lacerations and Avulsion Wounds of the Hoof Capsule

Causes

Laceration and avulsion of a portion of the hoof capsule is a relatively uncommon injury that is most often caused by kicking at or stepping on a sharp object, but may occasionally occur when the foot becomes entrapped between two immovable objects.[26] The injury may result in permanent lameness, and in some cases may necessitate euthanasia of the horse. A portion of the hoof capsule may be totally avulsed or it may be partially avulsed so that it remains attached, to some degree, usually at the coronary band (Figure 8.28). The avulsion may involve critical structures deep to the hoof capsule, such as the distal phalanx or distal interphalangeal joint (Figures 8.29a–c).

Complications that may arise following injury to the hoof capsule include sepsis of exposed laminae, fracture or partial loss of the distal phalanx (Figure 8.29c), and sepsis of the distal interphalangeal joint or digital flexor tendon sheath (see Wounds Involving the Pastern, discussed earlier on page 389). Even in the absence of these complications, the horse may remain lame after the wound heals, simply in relation to the quantity of lost hoof capsule.

Diagnosis

Clinical Signs

The degree of lameness varies with the duration, extent, and location of the injury to the hoof capsule. Because of its close proximity to the ground, a wound in the hoof capsule quickly becomes contaminated with

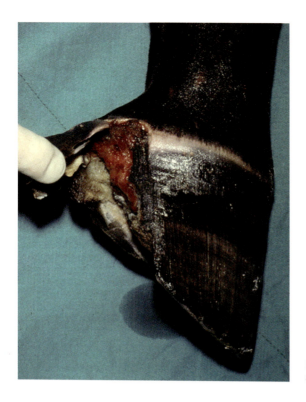

Figure 8.28. A partially avulsed portion of the hoof remains attached only at the coronary band.

manure and dirt, and if the horse is not treated properly and promptly, contamination results in infection. Migration of infection may cause surrounding epidermal and dermal laminae to separate (Figures 8.30a,b).[26] The horse may be severely lame if vital structures deep to the hoof capsule are involved in the injury.

The presence of a horny spur on the distal aspect of the pastern region, typically growing at a right or oblique angle to the pastern and possibly accompanied by abnormal growth of hoof distal to it, is an indication that the horse suffered partial avulsion of a portion of the hoof capsule and coronary band (Figures 8.31a,b).[26] Although the wound may be healed, the horse might frequently traumatize the avulsed and displaced portion of the coronary band, causing it to bleed. Palpation of the horny spur, particularly in an effort to push it proximad, usually causes the horse to show signs of discomfort.

Horses with an acute injury to the hoof wall, not involving critical structures deep to it, are usually only slightly to moderately lame, but palpation of the wound may cause the horse to show signs of considerable pain and may render the horse temporarily non–weight-bearing. Horses with extensive injury to the hoof capsule may refuse to bear weight on the affected limb. Lameness eventually subsides if the wound heals without complication. If lameness persists unabated, the wound should be physically and radiographically examined for evidence of a complication, such as a fracture of the distal phalanx or perforation of the capsule of the distal interphalangeal joint. An acute avulsion injury of the hoof capsule is obvious, but the involvement of deeper structures may be difficult to discern.

Before embarking on a meticulous examination of the wound, the wound and surrounding area should be cleaned. The hair should be clipped from a broad area surrounding the wound, and the hoof wall distal and adjacent to the wound should be rasped lightly to remove superficial contaminants. Only portions of the hoof wall that are attached firmly to the underlying dermal laminae should be rasped to avoid tearing laminar attachments. Skin surrounding the wound should be cleaned with an antiseptic soap, but application of soap to the wound itself should be avoided because detergent is cytotoxic and increases the wound's susceptibility to infection.[25]

The wound should be irrigated with a dilute antiseptic solution (e.g., povidone iodine [0.1%–0.2%] or chlorhexidine [0.5%]) using pressure lavage delivered at least at 7 PSI. For more information regarding the techniques of wound cleansing and irrigation, see Chapter 2. The wound should be palpated only after donning

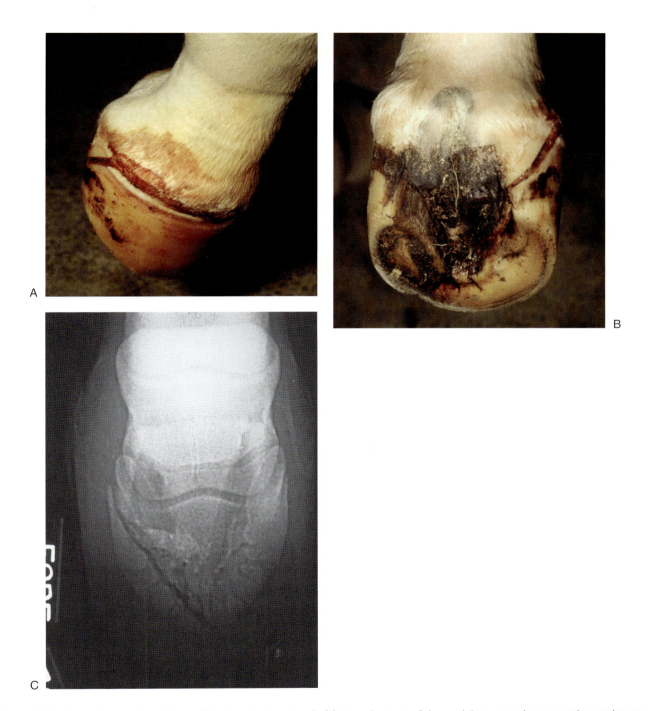

Figure 8.29. Extensive avulsion injury of the fore hoof and wall. (A) Dorsal extent of the avulsion; note the separation at the coronary band. (B) The injury resulted in separation of the collateral sulcus of the frog. (C) Dorsoproximal-palmarodistal oblique view of the distal phalanx identifying a lateral solar margin fracture.

sterile gloves. Manipulating the hoof and phalanges while palpating the wound may help to identify the extent of laminar separation, an open synovial structure, a fracture, or a lacerated supporting structure such as a collateral ligament or the deep digital flexor tendon.

Because fracture of the distal or middle phalanx may accompany a laceration to the hoof capsule, the foot should be examined radiographically after the wound has been grossly examined (Figure 8.29c). Contrast

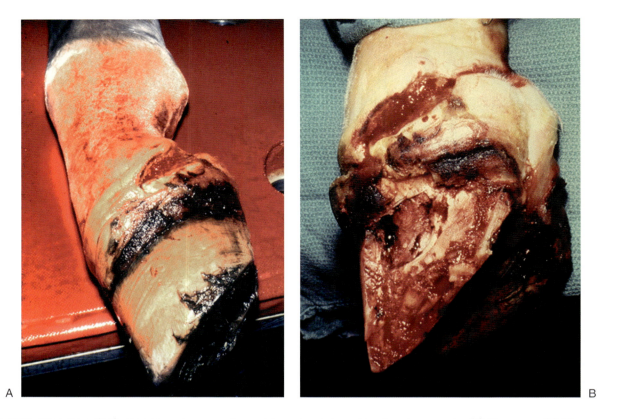

Figure 8.30. Migration of infection caused surrounding epidermal and dermal laminae to separate. (A) At surgery. (B) After removal of the undermined hoof wall.

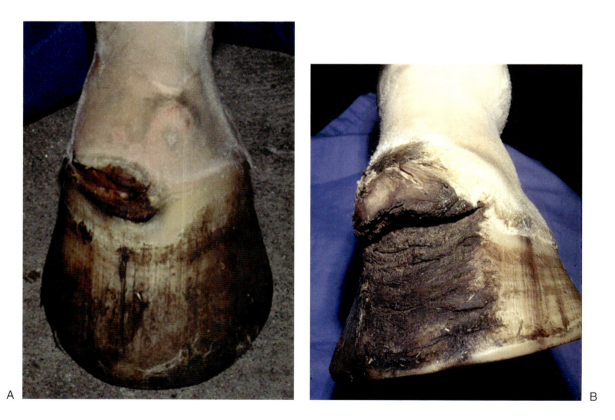

Figure 8.31. Partial avulsion of the dorsal hoof wall may cause lameness, and pushing the spur proximad often causes the horse to show signs of pain. (A) Small partial avulsion referred for surgery. (B) This large horn spur growing at a right angle to the pastern is accompanied by abnormal growth of hoof distal to it. This horse suffered partial avulsion of a portion of the hoof capsule and coronary band 1 year earlier. The horse was three out of five lame on this limb when the horn spur was not trimmed; the lameness would abate following trimming. Pushing the horn spur proximad caused the horse to show signs of discomfort.

radiographic studies of synovial structures associated with the foot region may be helpful in identifying a communication between the wound and a synovial structure.

Because healing of a complete avulsion injury or an incomplete avulsion injury with loss of the hoof capsule relies on epithelialization and reformation of the corium, rather than contraction, healing usually is protracted (3 to 5 months); thus, treatment can be costly, particularly if the horse has suffered a large avulsion injury (Figures 8.29 and 8.30). The wound should, therefore, be assessed carefully so that the owner can be apprised of the expense of treatment and the horse's prognosis for soundness or survival. If the distal or proximal interphalangeal joint is damaged, for example, degenerative joint disease is likely to develop and lead to permanent lameness, even if the horse receives proper treatment. Even after a wound is meticulously examined, predicting the horse's final outcome may be difficult. If a large portion of germinal tissue has been lost, or if infection has become established in a critical structure, the horse's initial response to therapy must be evaluated before outcome can be predicted.

Treatment

The selection of restraint required for repair depends on the nature and extent of the injury. An acute laceration or avulsion injury to the coronary band or hoof capsule can usually be sutured with the horse sedated after the foot is desensitized by administering regional anesthesia. The horse should be anesthetized if the laceration is extensive or involves the distal phalanx, a synovial cavity, or a supporting structure, such as a collateral ligament or the deep digital flexor tendon. The selection of treatment depends on whether the avulsion is partial or complete, whether the wound is fresh or chronic, and the extent of damage determined during exploration of the wound. If left to heal by second intention, a linear laceration to the coronary band usually results in a defect in the hoof horn distal to the coronet, whereas a partially avulsed segment of coronary band and hoof wall remains unstable, causing a hoof wall defect to develop. If the partially avulsed segment is U-shaped and involves the coronary band, it often becomes displaced proximad, producing a horny spur on the pastern that is susceptible to further trauma (Figure 8.31).

To prepare the horse for surgery, the hoof capsule surrounding the wound should be rasped to remove contaminants and the foot trimmed, if these procedures were not performed when the wound was initially evaluated. The wound and surrounding area should be cleaned as described previously, and the wound should be isolated with sterile drapes.

When suturing a partially avulsed segment of hoof and coronary band, a tourniquet is placed proximal to the foot to limit hemorrhage and aid visibility. One of two methods can be used to repair the avulsion: the hoof wall distal to the laceration in the coronet band can be retained and stabilized or the avulsed hoof wall can be removed. In both methods the coronet band is carefully sutured and the hoof is protected in a phalangeal cast.

In the first method, the hoof wall adjacent to the defect as well as the partially avulsed segment of hoof wall can be thinned with a motorized burr to ease placement of sutures through the hoof wall, and the defect in the hoof wall is debrided to provide a clean, vascular bed into which the partially avulsed segment of hoof is replaced. The thinned horn of the partially avulsed segment is sutured to the thinned hoof wall distal to the defect using #0, #1, or #2 polypropylene or nylon suture placed in a simple interrupted or vertical mattress pattern (Figure 8.32).

A partially avulsed segment of hoof can also be immobilized by anchoring several sheet metal screws (¼ in to ⅜ in) within the insensitive portion of the hoof on either side of the defect and lacing orthopedic wire across the segment and around the screw heads. The avulsed segment can also be held in place with a fiberglass patch attached to the hoof wall with screws. With the second method, the hoof wall distal to the separation of the coronary band is removed and the latter is carefully sutured, allowing healing distal to the coronary band to occur by second intention (Figure 8.33).[26] A small, partially avulsed portion of the hoof wall, without involvement of the coronary band, can be excised; the foot is then protected by a bandage or a foot cast until the wound has healed (Figure 8.34).

If the avulsion injury is associated with a fracture of the distal phalanx, in most cases the avulsed portion of the hoof capsule and the fracture fragment must be removed (Figures 8.35a,b). After removing the fracture fragment and avulsed portion of the hoof capsule, the foot is covered with an impermeable bandage. For more information on bandaging of the foot, see Chapter 16.

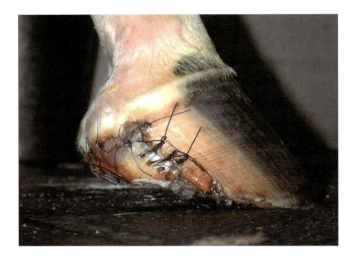

Figure 8.32. This laceration in the hoof capsule has been sutured.

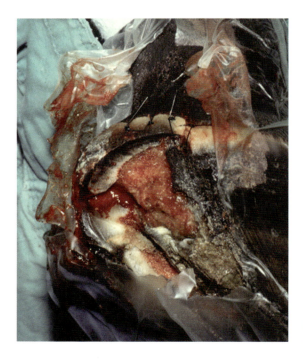

Figure 8.33. Same horse as in Figure 8.28 after excision of the avulsed hoof wall distal to the sutured coronary band.

In cases in which the wound resulting in proximal displacement of horn tissue is chronic, granulation tissue filling the defect in the hoof can be excised with a scalpel and the horny spur produced by the displaced coronary band can be contoured and thinned with the burr until it fits into the defect in the hoof wall. The coronary band is sutured with #0 polypropylene suture using a vertical mattress pattern (Figures 8.36a–c). Accurate approximation of the coronary band is important to ensure that hoof produced by it conforms as much as possible to the direction of hoof growth surrounding the wound so that a defect in the hoof wall does not develop.

If the proximally displaced section of coronary band and horn tissue cannot be replaced in the hoof wall defect, the horse is best treated by excision of the germinal tissue that produces the horny spur. This is especially the case if the horse is lame because of the injury but becomes sound after the painful, horny spur is trimmed (Figures 8.37a–c). Dermal papillae at the coronary band should be spared as much as possible during excision of the germinal tissue. The resulting wound proximal to the coronary band is left to heal by second intention.

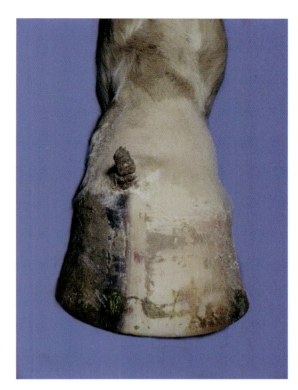

Figure 8.34. A small, partially avulsed portion of the dorsal hoof wall without involvement of the coronary band can be excised and protected by a bandage.

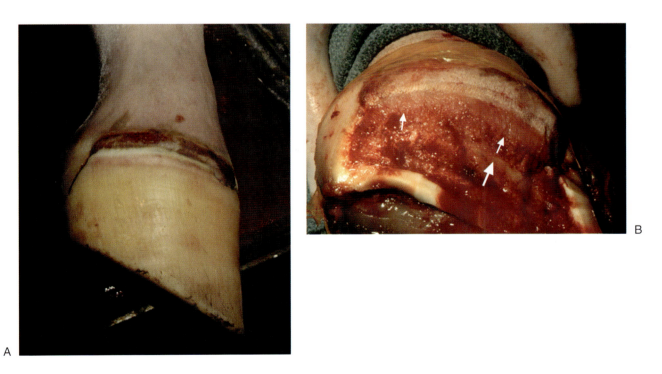

Figure 8.35. Same horse as in Figure 8.29. (A) The horse at surgery. (B) The avulsed hoof wall and fractured distal phalanx have been removed. Note the intact coronary papillae (small arrows) and the debrided border of the distal phalanx (large arrow).

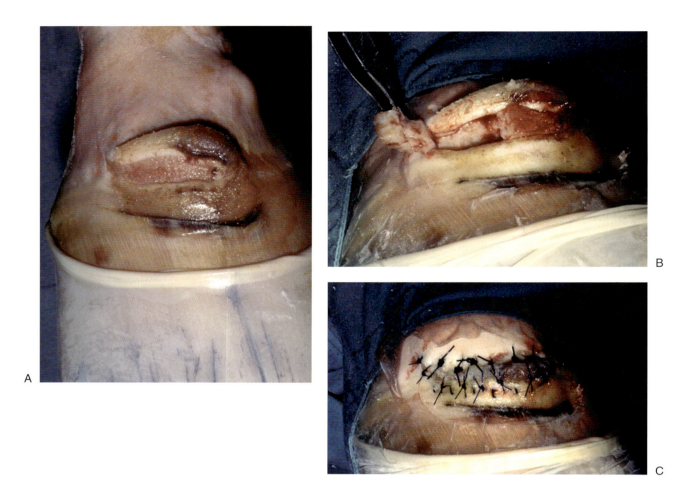

Figure 8.36. Same horse as in Figure 8.31a. (A) The hoof wall has been prepared for surgery by removing the cornified *stratum externum* from the outer hoof wall. (B) Granulation tissue filling the defect in the hoof was excised with a scalpel. (C) The coronary band is sutured with #0 polypropylene suture using a vertical mattress pattern. The foot was protected in a phalangeal cast for 3 weeks.

If the wound is large, island or sheet grafts can be used to shorten the healing time (Figure 8.37d). See Chapter 11 for more information regarding skin grafting.

After surgery is complete, an antimicrobial dressing (e.g., Iodosorb™, Oclassen Pharmaceuticals, Inc, San Rafael, CA), is applied to the wound. The foot should be immobilized with a phalangeal (short-limb; e.g., a cast that encompasses the foot and a portion of the pastern, Figure 8.38), usually for at least 3 weeks, because in the absence of a cast, the rigidity of the hoof capsule, combined with the constant loading and unloading of the hoof, results in considerable movement at the wound.[27,28] When the cast is removed at 3 to 4 weeks, the coronary band should be healed, and exposed laminae should be cornified, obviating the need for continued protection of the wound in most cases. If only the hoof capsule has been lacerated, a cast that encompasses just the foot can be applied (Figure 8.39).

Systemic administration of an antimicrobial drug after surgery is usually not necessary. If a large portion of the hoof capsule was lost, a full-support shoe (e.g., egg-bar combined with a heart-bar shoe, or an equine digital support system [EDSS] with a frog support pad and impression material) should be applied to the foot after the cast has been removed, and the region of the hoof wall distal to the defect should be removed (floated) to eliminate weight-bearing on that portion of the hoof wall (Figure 8.40). Some roughening and thickening of the hoof wall distal to the defect may be expected, in some cases, after healing,[27] but a hoof acrylic can be used to fill the cornified deficit in the hoof wall.

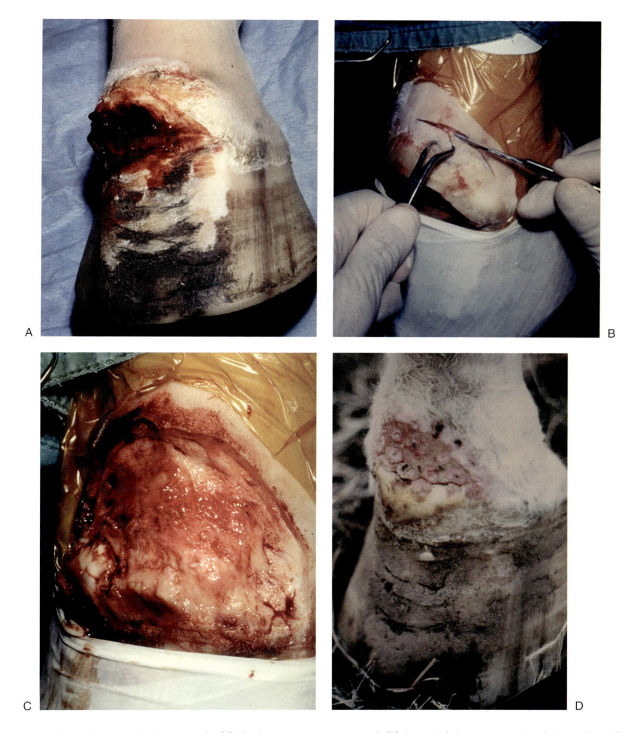

A

B

C

D

Figure 8.37. Same horse as in Figure 8.31b. (A) The horn spur was removed. (B) Germinal tissue was excised. Dermal papillae at the coronary band should be spared as much as possible during excision of the germinal tissue. (C) The wound bed after the germinal tissue was excised. The wound was bandaged and the horse was sent home with the recommendation that island grafts be inserted after a healthy bed of granulation tissue had developed. (D) The wound 4 weeks after surgery and 10 days after island skin grafting. This wound healed and there was no evidence of regrowth of horn spur 1 year after surgery. The horse was free of lameness.

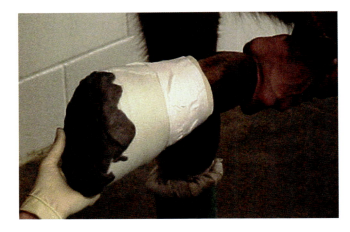

Figure 8.38. A phalangeal cast that encompasses the foot and a portion of the pastern.

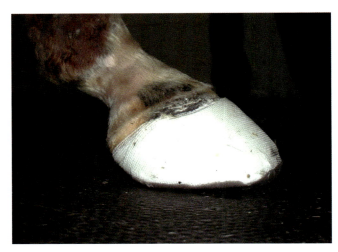

Figure 8.39. Same case as in Figure 8.32. A cast encompassing only the foot can be applied if just the hoof capsule has been lacerated.

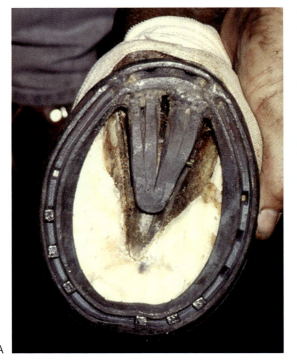

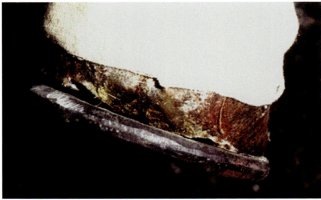

Figure 8.40. A complete support shoe is a combination of heart-bar and egg-bar shoes. (A) Solar view. (B) Side view. Note the quarter has been floated (does not contact the shoe) in the area beneath the avulsion injury.

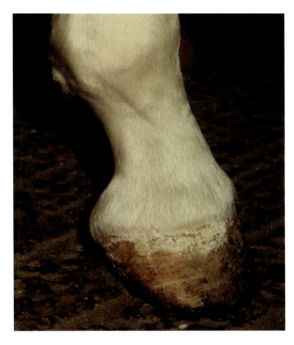

Figure 8.41. Same horse as in Figures 8.29 and 8.35, 6 months after surgery.

Prognosis

The time required for healing of an avulsion injury to the hoof and the prognosis for soundness depend on the extent of the injury and the method of treatment, but most avulsion injuries heal without complication if the horse is treated properly soon after the injury. Three to five months are usually needed for healing of a complete avulsion, (Figure 8.41), whereas incomplete avulsions that are reconstructed and sutured usually heal in 3 to 4 weeks. Even when healing is complete, soundness may not be appreciated for many months, and in some cases, up to 1 year. Partial loss of the distal phalanx, digital cushion, or a collateral cartilage does not appear to be a serious detriment to soundness. An avulsion injury that involves the coronary band may result in a permanent deformity of the hoof capsule (Figure 8.31b).

Predicting the horse's outcome is difficult at the onset of treatment because recovery is a lengthy process. If a portion of the wound remains unhealed or if a draining tract appears, infection of a deep structure, such as a collateral cartilage, should be suspected.

Penetrating Wounds to the Foot

Causes

The foot may be penetrated when the horse steps on or strikes a sharp object, such as a nail. A wound that penetrates only cornified tissue is considered to be superficial.[29] Wounds that penetrate germinal epithelium are considered to be deep and can be divided into three types, with each type affecting a particular region of the foot.[29] A type I deep puncture wound penetrates the solar corium, a type II wound penetrates the corium of the frog or one of its lateral sulci, and a type III wound penetrates the germinal epithelium of the coronary band.[29]

Structures that can be damaged by deep penetration include the distal phalanx, distal interphalangeal joint, deep digital flexor tendon, digital flexor tendon sheath, or a portion of the navicular apparatus (Figure 8.42).[29] A penetrating wound to the frog or a collateral sulcus of the frog (e.g., a type II wound) is more likely to jeopardize the horse's soundness, or even life, than is a penetrating wound to other regions of the foot because a penetration in this region is more likely to enter a synovial structure.[30] A deep, penetrating injury to the frog should be considered a potential threat to the horse's life.

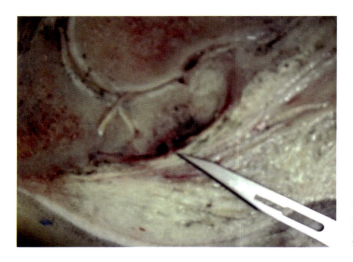

Figure 8.42. Saggital section of a foot of a horse that incurred damage to the navicular bone when a nail entered the frog. The scalpel blade points to a necrotic area on the flexor surface of the navicular bone.

Uncommonly, multiple synovial structures can be damaged when an object penetrates the solar surface of the foot. For instance, an object having penetrated the navicular bursa may also penetrate the impar ligament (*ligamentum impar* or *lig. sesamoideum distale impar*) which separates the bursa from the distal interphalangeal joint, resulting in infection of both the bursa and the distal interphalangeal joint. Or, an object that has penetrated the navicular bursa may also penetrate one of the collateral sesamoidean ligaments (suspensory ligaments or *lig. sesamoidean collateralia*) which lie in close proximity to the digital flexor tendon sheath, resulting in infection of both the bursa and the digital flexor tendon sheath.[29]

Diagnosis

Physical Examination

Injury to the sensitive tissue of the foot that results in infection is generally accompanied by swelling proximal to the foot. The swelling is most commonly restricted to the coronary band, and in some cases one heel bulb, but it may extend to the fetlock. The foot is often warmer than its contralateral counterpart, and the digital pulse is usually prominent, especially on the affected side of the foot. The digital flexor tendon sheath may be distended, even when it has not been penetrated.[31] A horse suffering from infection of the solar corium is usually moderately to severely lame, and the horse may load the affected foot asymmetrically to reduce pressure on the affected side. Exudate produced by infection of the solar corium may drain at the puncture site and/or at the ipsilateral heel bulb (Figure 8.43). Exudate produced by an infection in the white line may drain at the white line or at a cutaneous defect at the juncture of the coronary band and the hoof capsule. This condition is sometimes referred to as "gravel" (Figures 8.44a,b).[32] Proximal migration of sub-solar infection, caused by puncture of the sole, may cause a substantial portion of the epidermal and dermal laminae to separate.

A hoof tester may be useful in localizing the site of puncture causing infection of the corium of the sole or at the white line (Figure 8.44a), but if the wound is chronic, a larger area of the foot may be so sensitive to pressure that localizing the site using hoof testers is difficult. If infection is caused by a shoe nail that was accidentally driven into the sensitive corium, careful application of the hoof tester over each nail hole, after the shoe has been removed, may cause exudate to leak from the hole (Figure 8.44a).

A dark spot or defect in the sole should be explored to its depth to determine if it penetrates sensitive tissue. A previously unidentified puncture to the sole may become obvious after the foot is trimmed, whereas tracts left by penetration of the frog may be difficult to locate, even after the frog has been trimmed, because the soft horn of the frog collapses around the tract when the penetrating object is no longer present. After the foot is trimmed and desensitized, weight born on the affected foot or hoof tester application may cause enough pressure on infected tissue to allow trapped exudate to emerge from the sole (Figure 8.45).[32]

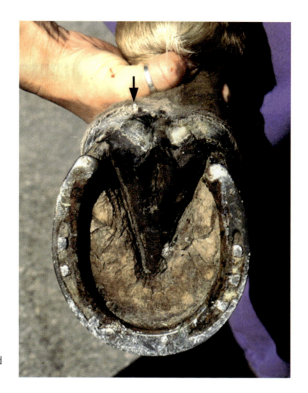

Figure 8.43. Exudate produced by infection of the solar corium caused swelling (black arrow) and drainage from the ipsilateral heel bulb.

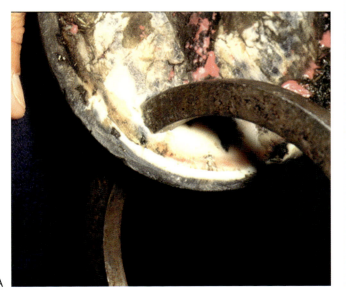

A

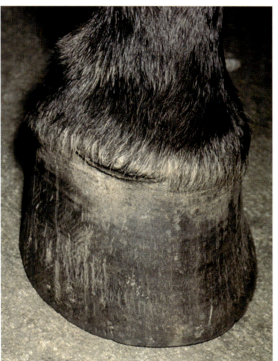

B

Figure 8.44. Penetrating wound at the white line. (A) Exudate produced from infection of the white line may cause drainage from this structure. In this case hoof tester pressure caused the exudate to exude from the puncture site. (B) Exudate produced by an infection in the white line has drained from this cutaneous defect at the juncture of the coronary band and the hoof capsule. This condition is sometimes referred to as "gravel."

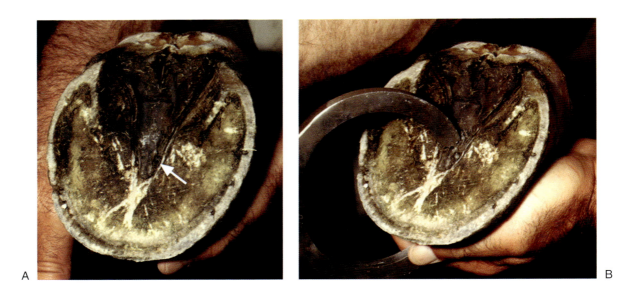

Figure 8.45. (a) A small hole at the apex of the frog became evident after the foot was trimmed (arrow). (b) Hoof tester application caused enough pressure to elicit a painful response and also allowed trapped exudate to emerge from the frog.

Imaging

A foreign body found penetrating the hoof capsule should be left in situ, and the foot examined radiographically so that the object's depth and direction of penetration can be determined, provided that the foot can be examined radiographically without delay (Figures 8.46a,b). If the foot cannot be immediately examined radiographically, the penetrating object should be removed to prevent more damage to the deep structures. The site of puncture should be marked, enabling it to be located at the time of radiographic examination so that a probe or a radiographic contrast medium can be inserted into the tract (Figures 8.46c and 8.47).

Nonmetallic foreign bodies in the foot, such as wood or glass, may not be identifiable during radiographic evaluation. If the penetrating object has been removed, the direction and depth of the wound can sometimes be evaluated radiographically after inserting a blunt, flexible probe into the tract (Figure 8.47).[29,32] The probe should be inserted carefully because forceful introduction may damage healthy tissue. Insertion of the probe is often facilitated by anesthetizing the palmar/plantar digital nerves at the level of the proximal sesamoid bones (e.g., an abaxial sesamoid nerve block) to desensitize the foot. Two projections taken at right angles to one another should be obtained so that the spatial relationship of the foreign body or probe to critical structures can be assessed.

Penetration of a synovial structure can be confirmed by injecting a sterile, balanced electrolyte solution into the synovial cavity at a site remote from the wound and observing it egress from the wound (see Figure 2.15). If penetration of a synovial structure is suspected but cannot be confirmed using this method, the foot can be examined radiographically after instilling contrast medium into the synovial structure with a hypodermic needle. Leakage of contrast medium from the synovial structure, seen on radiographs, indicates that the synovial structure has been penetrated.

The navicular bursa can be entered most easily by inserting an 18- or 20-gauge, 8.9 cm (3.5 in) disposable spinal needle midway between the bulbs of the heel, immediately proximal to the hoof capsule, with the foot and pastern flexed.[33] The spinal needle is advanced along the sagittal plane of the foot toward the intersection between the sagittal plane and the long axis of the navicular bone, which is assumed to be midway between the most dorsal and the most palmar/plantar aspect of the coronary band, about 1 cm distal to it. The needle is advanced until the tip contacts bone. Fluid is seldom obtained regardless of whether the bursa has been damaged. The foot should be examined radiographically immediately before the bursa is injected with contrast medium to confirm that the tip of the needle is against the navicular bone. An intact navicular bursa can be distended with 3 mL–5 mL of contrast medium before resistance to injection is encountered. Radiological identification of contrast medium within the bursa is evidence of a successful bursal injection, and leakage of contrast

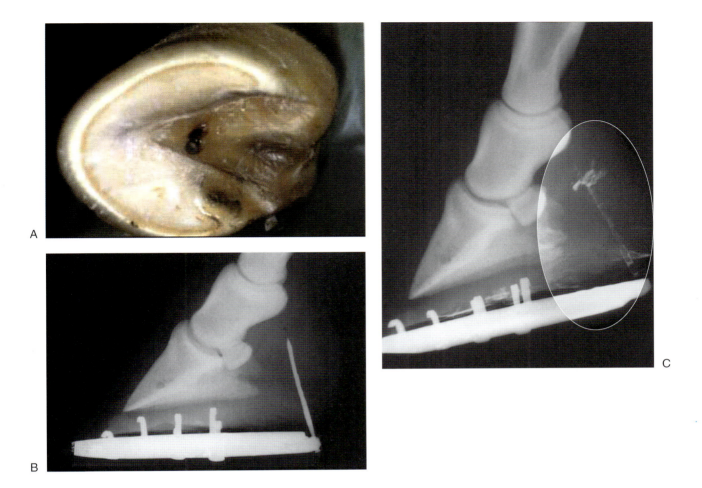

Figure 8.46. (A) A foreign body penetrating the bearing surface of the foot should be left in situ until the foot can be examined radiographically to determine the proximity of the foreign body to critical structures. (B) Radiograph revealed the depth and direction of the foreign body. The tip of the nail was close to the digital sheath. (C) Radiographic contrast medium injected into this tract (oval) revealed that the digital sheath had not been penetrated.

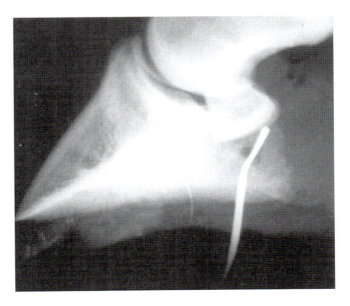

Figure 8.47. Inserting a blunt, flexible probe into a tract in the frog may help determine the direction and depth of the wound.

medium from the bursa, other than from site of centesis, indicates that the penetrating object has perforated the bursa.

The easiest method of entering the distal interphalangeal joint is to insert a 2.54 cm (1 in), 20- or 22-gauge hypodermic needle into the dorsal pouch of the joint.[33] The needle is inserted into the dorsal pouch through the coronary band, on the dorsal midline, at the junction of the hoof wall and skin, parallel to the bearing surface of the foot or perpendicular to the slope of the pastern until its point contacts the dorsal distal aspect of the middle phalanx. Synovial fluid usually appears in the needle hub. Centesis is most easily performed with the limb bearing weight (Figure 8.48a).

If a wound or infection precludes the use of the latter arthropuncture site, the distal interphalangeal joint can be entered from the lateral aspect of the joint by inserting the needle just proximal to the palpable, proximal edge of the collateral cartilage, approximately midway between the dorsal and palmar/plantar aspects of the middle phalanx (Fig 8.48b).[34] The needle is angled downward toward the distal end of the hoof wall on the contralateral side of the hoof. The depth of penetration is less than 2.5 cm. The procedure is most easily performed with the foot flexed, but the navicular bursa or digital tendon sheath is less likely to be inadvertently entered if the horse is bearing weight on the foot.

A reliable method of entering the digital synovial sheath is the palmar/plantar axial sesamoidean approach.[35] Using this approach, the needle is inserted through the palmar/plantar annular ligament of the fetlock. With the limb flexed, the needle is placed through the skin at the level of the midbody of the lateral proximal sesamoid bone 3 mm axial to the palpable palmar/plantar border of the lateral sesamoid bone and immediately axial to the palmar/plantar digital neurovascular bundle and advanced though the palmar/plantar annular ligament. The needle is inserted in a transverse plane and advanced to a depth of about 1.5 cm–2 cm at an angle to the sagittal plane, aiming toward the central intersesamoidean region.

Before instilling contrast media into a synovial structure, fluid should be obtained, if possible, for cytological examination and bacterial culture. A markedly elevated white blood cell count and high concentration of protein

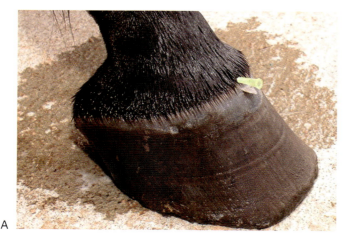

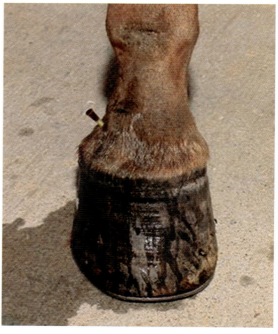

Figure 8.48. Arthropuncture of the distal interphalangeal joint. (A) Site for arthropuncture in the dorsal pouch through the coronary band, on the dorsal midline, at the junction of the hoof wall and skin. The needle is inserted parallel to the bearing surface of the foot or perpendicular to the slope of the pastern until its point contacts the dorsal distal aspect of the middle phalanx. Synovial fluid usually appears in the needle hub. (B) Lateral approach to arthropuncture of the joint by inserting the needle just proximal to the palpable, proximal edge of the collateral cartilage, approximately midway between the dorsal and palmar/plantar aspects of the middle phalanx.

in the fluid is suggestive of infection. For more information regarding laboratory findings associated with septic arthritis, see Chapter 9.

An alternative to injecting a synovial cavity with contrast material is to inject the contrast medium directly into a draining tract using a teat cannula or Foley catheter after which a radiograph is taken. Contrast medium entering a synovial structure confirms that it has been penetrated (Figure 8.49b).[32] The downside to this approach is that contrast medium is being injected into a contaminated or infected site, but this is of little consequence if appropriate treatment is to follow.

Confirmation of an injury to the solar corium or distal phalanx from a penetrating wound, without evidence of a draining tract, may be obtained with radiographic examination. If the solar corium has been penetrated, gas may be seen between the sole and solar corium (Figure 8.50). Injury to the distal phalanx may appear on radiographic examination as a spherical lucency or as a sequestrum (Figure 8.51).

Treatment

Horses with a superficial puncture wound to the sole or frog should be treated by removing undermined insensitive horn with a sharp hoof knife. The superficial margin of the wound should be beveled outward so that it does not close before the depth of the wound has healed (Figures 8.52a,b). Lameness caused by a superficial puncture wound usually resolves quickly after a route for escape of exudate has been established, and if debridement and drainage are adequate, the affected horse does not require systemic antimicrobial therapy. The foot should be covered with a bandage until the granulation tissue that develops in the wound becomes

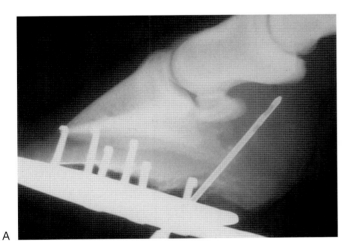

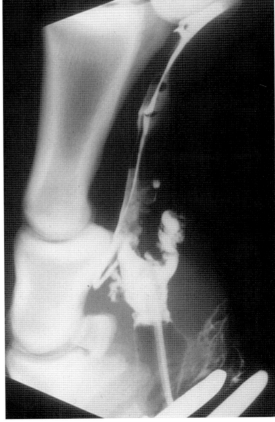

A

B

Figure 8.49. A sharp piece of wood was found to have penetrated the palmar one-third of the frog in this horse. (A) A teat cannula is inserted in the tract. (B) Injection of contrast medium revealed that the puncture wound extended into the digital sheath.

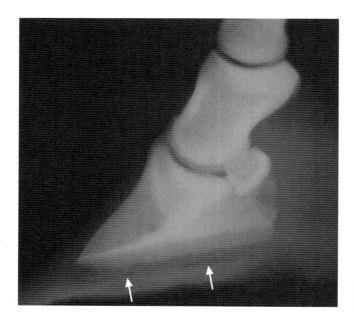

Figure 8.50. If the solar corium has been penetrated, gas (arrows) may be seen between it and the sole.

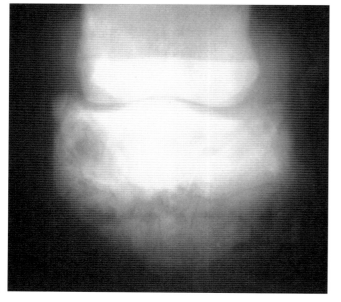

A

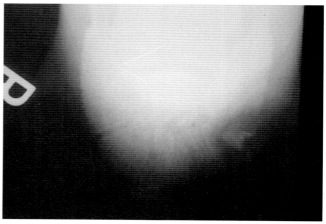

B

Figure 8.51 (A and B). Injury to the distal phalanx may appear on radiographic exam as a spherical lucency or a sequestrum.

cornified. If the defect is large or healing is protracted, a boiler plate (treatment plate) shoe can be applied to protect the sole (Figure 8.53).

Horses with penetration of the solar corium accompanied by septic osteitis of the distal phalanx (Figure 8.51) should be treated by curettage of the infected portion of bone, which is accessed through the sole by sharp enlargement of the penetrating wound or through a trephine hole created in the hoof wall adjacent to the infected portion of the phalanx. Horses are usually more comfortable after curettage if the distal phalanx is accessed through the hoof wall rather than through the sole. Only soft, infected bone that is easily detached with a curette is removed. Curettage can be performed with the horse standing after desensitizing the foot by anesthetizing the palmar/plantar digital nerves at the level of the proximal sesamoid bones (i.e., an abaxial sesamoid nerve

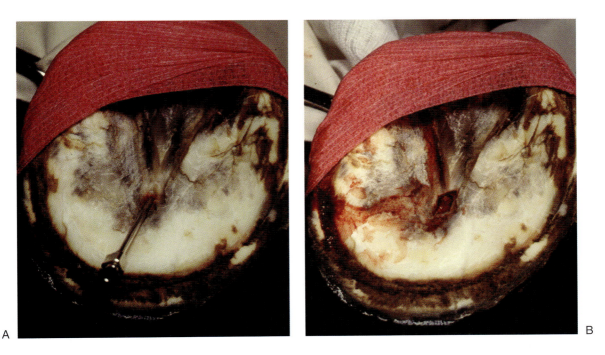

A   B

Figure 8.52. (A) Superficial puncture wound at the apex of the frog. (B) The superficial margin of the wound is beveled outward.

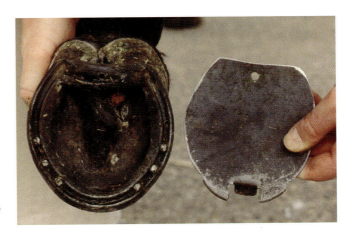

Figure 8.53. A boiler plate shoe can be applied to protect the sole.

block) or by anesthetizing the palmar/plantar and palmar/plantar metacarpal/metatarsal nerves at the level of the distal end of the splint bone (i.e., a low, four-point nerve block). A tourniquet applied to the fetlock region controls hemorrhage and increases visibility. Diseased bone should be submitted to a laboratory for bacterial culture and antimicrobial sensitivity testing of isolated bacteria. Culture of infected tissue usually produces growth of a variety of Gram-positive and Gram-negative bacteria, the most common being coliforms.[31] Regional limb perfusion with a broad-spectrum antimicrobial drug, used in conjunction with systemic administration of the drug, may be indicated.

With the street-nail procedure, a section of the frog, digital cushion, and deep digital flexor tendon are sharply excised to expose the flexor surface of the navicular bone (Figures 8.54a,b). Discolored areas of the digital cushion and deep digital flexor tendon are sharply excised, and those on the flexor surface of the navicular bone

Horses with a deep puncture wound to the frog or one of its lateral sulci (i.e., a type II wound) that enters the navicular bursa are best treated while anesthetized. The extent of damage can be assessed and diseased tissue removed after exposing the navicular bone using the "street-nail" procedure or arthroscopically.

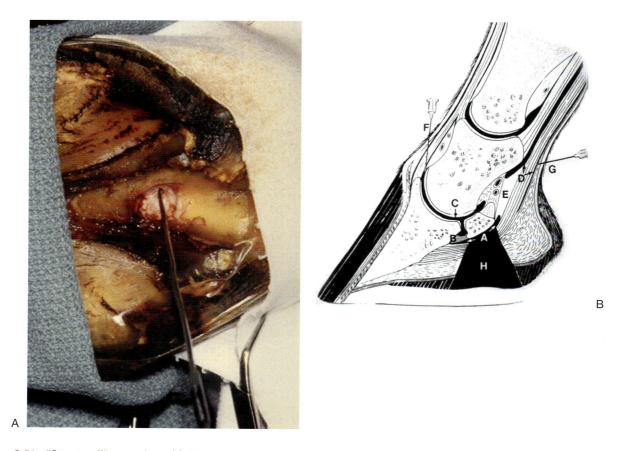

Figure 8.54. "Street nail" procedure. (A) Sharp dissection of the frog exposes the digital cushion and the wound tract. Excision is continued through the deep digital flexor tendon to enter the navicular bursa. (B) Saggital illustration defining the path of dissection through the frog to the navicular bone.

are removed by curettage (Figure 8.42). Diseased tissue is submitted to a laboratory for bacterial culture and antimicrobial sensitivity testing of isolated bacteria. Communication between the distal interphalangeal joint and navicular bursa, through the impar ligament, can be determined by instilling a sterile, isotonic electrolyte solution, under pressure, into the distal interphalangeal joint, as described earlier. Exit of fluid through the navicular bursa is evidence of communication. Communication between the digital flexor tendon sheath and the navicular bursa, through one of the collateral sesamoidean ligaments, can be determined by instilling a sterile, isotonic electrolyte solution, under pressure, into the digital flexor tendon sheath, as described earlier.

The navicular bursa can also be examined, and diseased tissue excised, using endoscopy.[36] The arthroscope is inserted proximal to the lateral collateral cartilage on the abaxial border of the deep digital flexor tendon, axial to the digital neurovascular bundle. The digital flexor tendon sheath and the palmar/plantar pouch of the distal interphalangeal joint can also be examined through this portal. Instruments used to excise diseased tissue are introduced on the contralateral side of the pastern or through the wound on the solar surface of the foot. An endoscopic approach to examine the navicular bursa and bone and to treat disease encountered is less invasive. Postoperative care of the horse is simpler, and the results are better than treatment using the street-nail procedure.[36]

The selection of antimicrobial drugs administered to horses with deep wounds to the foot, with or without involvement of a synovial cavity or the distal phalanx, is guided by results of antimicrobial sensitivity testing of bacterial isolates. Until the definitive results are known, the horse should receive broad-spectrum antimicrobial therapy, such as a combination of penicillin or another β-lactam antibiotic and an aminoglycoside. Regional limb perfusion with an antimicrobial drug, used in conjunction with systemic administration of an antimicrobial drug, may be indicated. The horse should receive analgesic therapy, usually with phenylbutazone or flunixin meglumine. Relieving pain in the affected hoof decreases the likelihood of the contralateral limb developing laminitis. The horse should receive appropriate prophylaxis against tetanus.

Prognosis

Sepsis of the navicular bursa leads to serious sequelae, making it the most frequent reason for euthanizing a horse that has suffered a perforating wound to the foot.[30] A horse with a puncture wound that extends into the navicular bursa has a more favorable prognosis for soundness and for survival if a hind limb, rather than a fore limb, is affected and if it receives surgical treatment within a week after the injury.[29,30] Systemic antimicrobial therapy alone is incapable of eliminating infection of the navicular bursa. Chronic infection of one or more of the synovial structures of the foot, erosion of articular cartilage, septic osteitis, or fibrous adhesions between the deep digital flexor tendon and the navicular bone may be responsible for unremitting pain resulting in failure of the horse to return to soundness.[30] The navicular bone may suffer a pathological fracture, or the deep digital flexor tendon may rupture, even after infection has resolved.[30]

Horses that are lame because of a penetrating injury to the foot that does not involve a synovial structure or the distal phalanx, such as a puncture wound to the solar corium, are likely to regain soundness, provided they are properly treated for the injury.

Wounds Containing Sequestered Bone

Causes

Wounds on the distal aspect of the limb are often characterized by extensive crushing or avulsion of soft tissue, exposure of bone (degloving injury), vascular compromise, and severe contamination, making second intention healing or free skin grafting the only options. The regions most susceptible to degloving and crushing injury are the metacarpal and metatarsal regions because they contain little soft tissue and are exposed to trauma more often than are other regions of the body. When underlying bone is injured, with or without loss of skin, new bone may proliferate (Figure 8.55) or the superficial layers of the cortex may die from ischemia and form

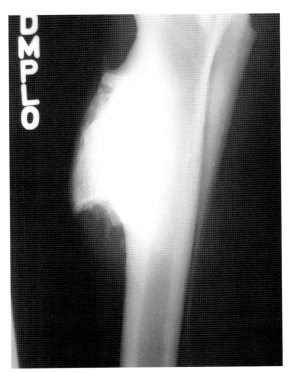

Figure 8.55. Injury to the periosteum may result in formation of new bone.

a sequestrum. Occasionally, continuous pressure, such as that which may develop beneath a cast or an encircling wire, can lead not only to ischemic necrosis of soft tissues but also to formation of proliferative new bone or a bone sequestrum.[26]

Wounds on the distal aspect of the limb expand for approximately 11–15 days after wounding as the result of distractive forces applied across the wound during the inflammatory and cellular debridement stages of healing.[2,4,5] These distractive forces are countered by myofibroblasts that are formed when granulation tissue develops within the wound; therefore, the quicker a granulation bed is formed, the faster the wound begins to contract. Degloving wounds in which bone devoid of periosteum is exposed contract in a tardy fashion as a result of the slow development of granulation tissue.[37]

Periosteum may be avulsed from the bone at the time of injury, or infection may cause the periosteum to separate from the bone.[38,39] Loss of periosteal blood supply leaves the bone dependent on endosteal vessels traversing the cortex, resulting in ischemic necrosis of the superficial portion of the cortex.[39,40] Small areas of dead bone may be re-vascularized by vessels in advancing granulation tissue, or the exposed bone may be re-vascularized by endosteal vessels of cortical bone deep to the dead bone.[37] Dead cortical bone too thick to re-vascularize becomes sequestered by granulation tissue produced from viable bone. The body's attempts to extrude or absorb the dead bone result in a persistent sinus tract and excessive production of exudate. Ischemia caused by loss of periosteal blood supply alone, however, may not be sufficient to provoke formation of a sequestrum[39]; in these, bacterial infection of the bone seems to be necessary as well. Because the periosteum of young horses plays a greater role in cortical circulation, they may be more likely to form a sequestrum than are mature horses,[41,42] and horses are more likely than ponies to develop a sequestrum, perhaps in relation to their greater susceptibility to develop infection at the wound.[1]

Diagnosis

Physical Examination

Clinical signs most often produced by a sequestrum include soft-tissue swelling over the affected bone, palpation of which may cause the horse to show signs of discomfort, a mild lameness on the affected limb, and a draining tract found in granulation tissue or in the epithelial scar of a wound that appears to have otherwise healed.[42] A probe introduced into the tract may strike bone, and occasionally, a sequestrum may be visible in the depths of a defect in the granulation tissue. Clinical signs either fail to resolve or only temporarily resolve when the horse receives anti-inflammatory and antimicrobial therapy.[42] Bone sequestration must be differentiated from other causes of chronic drainage from a sinus within the wound, such as a foreign body or communication of the wound with a synovial structure.

Imaging

Radiographically, a sequestrum appears as a sclerotic segment of bone surrounded by a radiolucent zone of osteolysis (Figure 8.56).[39,40] The sequestrum and zone of osteolysis are surrounded by an envelope of sclerotic bone, termed an involucrum. The opening in the involucrum, through which exudate drains, is termed a cloaca. Extensive periosteal reaction is frequently observed on adjacent, normal bone, and young horses generally develop a more extensive periosteal reaction than do adult horses because of the greater osteoblastic activity.[23,41] A triangular area of new bone that develops adjacent to the cortex from elevation of the periosteum ("Codman's triangle") is sometimes observed at the proximal and distal extents of the involucrum.[39] The bone sequestrum contains no new periosteal bone, which aids in its identification.

Exposed bone beneath a fresh wound should be examined radiographically about 10–14 days after injury to determine if a bone sequestrum is developing. Radiographic signs of a sequestrum cannot be detected for at least 7 days following injury but are usually evident within several weeks of injury (Fig 8.56).[39,40] An early radiographic sign that a sequestrum is forming, often seen 10–12 days after injury, is the presence of one or more radiolucent lines within the outer third of the bone cortex.[39,40] During subsequent radiographic examination, these fine radiolucent lines may be seen to have enlarged and coalesced into one radiolucent band, which separates viable and nonviable bone.[39] These early radiographic signs of formation of a sequestration sometimes vanish, and the sequestrum fails to form.[39]

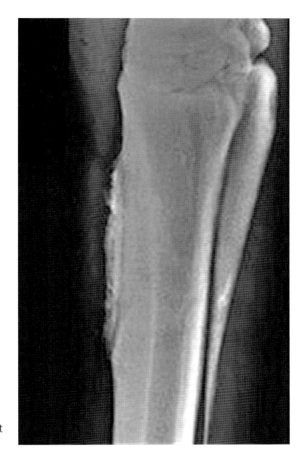

Figure 8.56. A sequestrum is seen radiographically as a sclerotic segment of bone surrounded by a radiolucent zone of osteolysis.

Treatment

Because bacterial infection of the bone contributes to the formation of a sequestrum, efforts should be made to prevent exposed bone from becoming infected.[1,38,43] To prevent septic osteitis, the horse should receive parenteral, broad-spectrum, antimicrobial therapy soon after injury. Regional limb perfusion with an antimicrobial drug, used in conjunction with systemic administration of an antimicrobial drug, may be indicated. A hydrogel dressing should be applied to the exposed bone to prevent desiccation, and the wounded portion of the limb should be bandaged to protect it from contamination and to absorb exudate. Nonsteroidal anti-inflammatory drugs have been reported to have an adverse effect on the incidence of infection by negatively affecting migration of leukocytes, and so they should be used to relieve swelling and pain only when indicated.[44,45]

Because the loss of periosteum may cause ischemia of the outer third of the cortex, superficial ostectomy performed at the time of wound debridement to remove ischemic bone may prevent a sequestrum from forming or at least minimize its extent. A shallow portion of exposed bone is excised with an osteotome[46] or a bone rasp or an air drill[47] until either punctuate hemorrhage or a yellow, serum-like fluid exudes from the cortex (see Figures 2.22 and 2.23). Hemorrhage exudes if the horse's bone is immature (e.g., newly formed proliferative exostosis), and serum-like fluid exudes if the horse's bone is mature. Granulation tissue grows directly from viable, exposed bone; therefore, exposing fresh, bleeding bone may speed proliferation of granulation tissue from the bone.[48] Drilling small holes in exposed bone may promote healing by allowing osteogenic factors from the medullary cavity access to the wound.[49] For more information regarding techniques to promote granulation tissue formation over exposed bone, see Degloving Injuries later in this chapter.

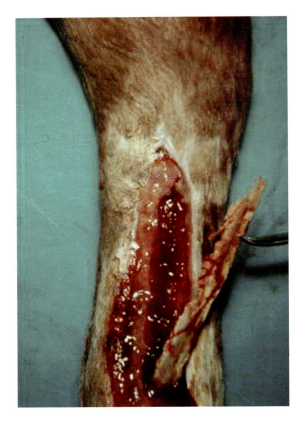

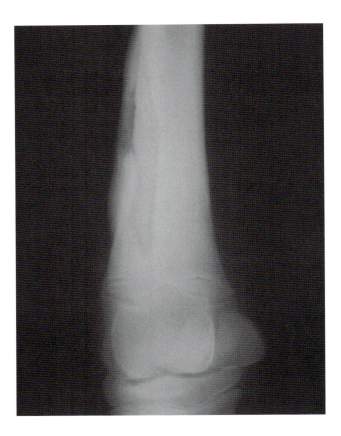

Figure 8.57. This sequestrum, which is not covered by granulation tissue, is being removed in the standing horse.

Figure 8.58. Radiograph identifying a large sequestrum embedded in bone.

Removing the sequestrum is the most effective treatment, but occasionally a sequestrum is shed spontaneously and rarely a small sequestrum may be reabsorbed. The horse may respond initially to parenterally administered antimicrobial therapy by a decrease in swelling and discharge from the wound,[42] but treating an affected horse with antimicrobial therapy alone is ineffective because the lack of blood supply to the sequestrum isolates bacteria harbored by the sequestrum from antimicrobial drugs. Culture of exudate from the draining sinus, or even from around the sequestrum, is unlikely to be helpful in determining the organism involved in formation of a sequestrum because secondary pathogens rapidly colonize an open wound or sinus.

Often, a sequestrum can be removed easily with the horse standing, provided that at least one edge of the sequestrum is not covered with granulation tissue (Figure 8.57). A sequestrum covered by tissue or embedded in the marrow cavity is best removed with the horse anesthetized (Figure 8.58). The sequestrum should be removed as soon as its separation from viable bone is radiographically apparent. Large sequestra embedded in the marrow cavity may have to be divided to remove them through the cloaca (Figures 8.59a–c). In these cases, a limb cast should be applied prior to recovering the horse from anesthesia to reduce stress concentration at the cloaca, thereby decreasing the risk of a complete fracture.

Primary closure of the wound may be possible if the wound from which the sequestrum was removed is small,[41] but if a large amount of soft tissue was avulsed, the wound must heal by second intention or skin grafting. Broad-spectrum perioperative antimicrobial treatment should be administered in cases in which primary closure is planned. See Chapter 2 for more information regarding the use of perioperative antimicrobial drugs. At surgery, separate gloves and instruments should be used to retrieve the sequestrum and to remove the membrane of the involucrum by curettage. After the sequestrum has been removed and the involucrum curetted, the latter is irrigated with a dilute antiseptic solution (e.g., 0.1%–0.2% povidone iodine), after which new sterile gloves are donned and sterile instruments are used to close the wound. Proliferative bone, if present, can be removed prior to closing the wound (Figures 8.60a–g).

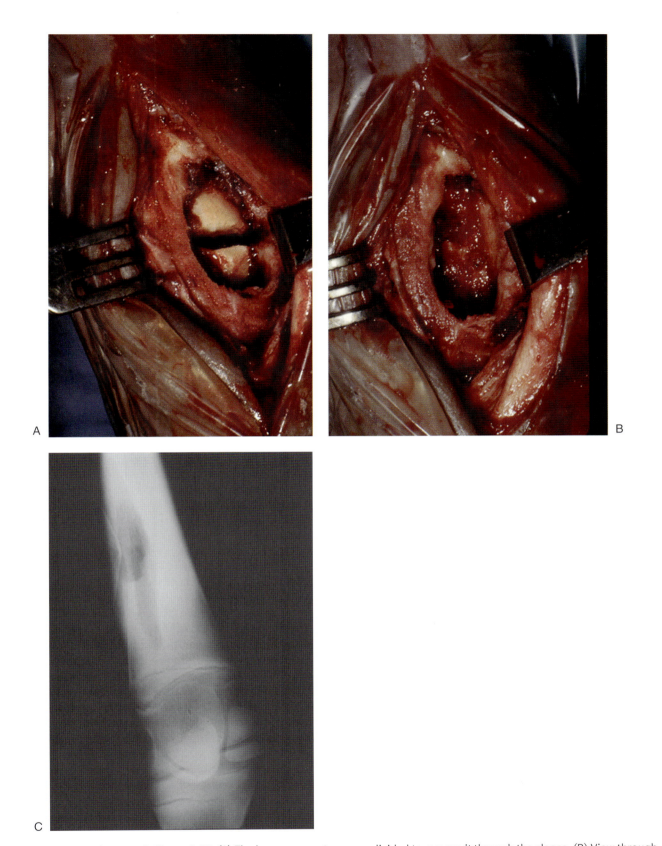

Figure 8.59. Same horse as in Figure 8.58. (A) The larger sequestrum was divided to remove it through the cloaca. (B) View through the cloaca of the involucrum prior to debridement of its lining of granulation tissue. (C) Postoperative radiograph documents removal of the sequestrum seen in Figure 8.58. A limb cast should be applied prior to recovering the horse from anesthesia to reduce stress concentration at the cloaca, thereby decreasing the risk of a complete fracture.

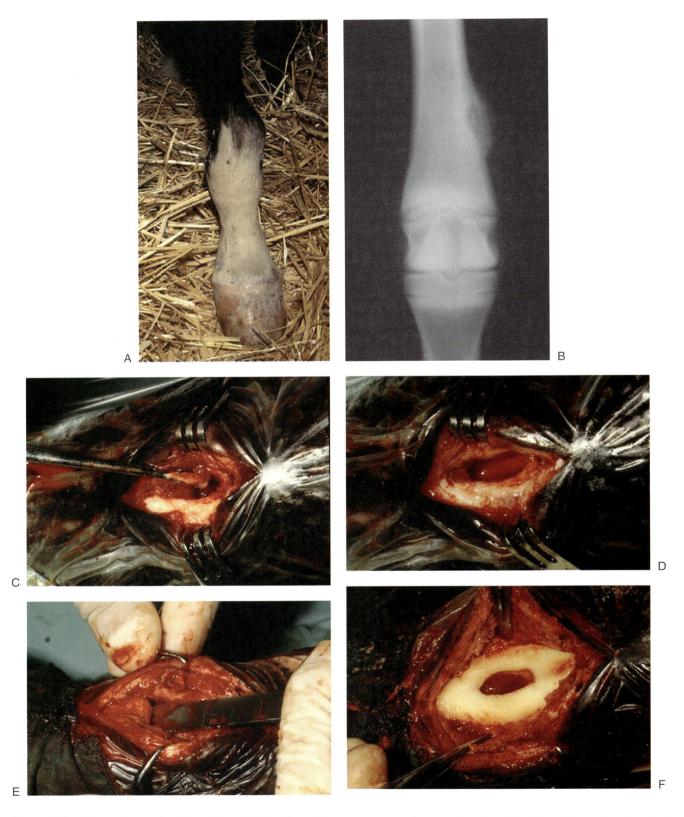

Figure 8.60. (A) Swelling on the lateral distal third of the left fore metacarpus in a yearling. Exudate drained from a tract located in the center of the swelling. (B) Radiographic evidence of a sequestrum. (C) The sequestrum was removed at surgery. (D) After sequestrectomy and curettage of the granulation tissue lining the involucrum, the wound was irrigated with a dilute antiseptic solution. Gloves and instruments were discarded and new ones were used to extend the incision in the skin overlying the proliferative bone. (E) Proliferative bone being removed with an osteotome. (F) Proliferative bone removed. Sharp periostectomy over the proliferative bone was performed with a #15 Bard Parker scalpel blade, after which a drain was inserted and the wound sutured. A pressure bandage was applied. The drain was removed 24 hours later. (G) (next page) One year follow-up; good cosmesis achieved.

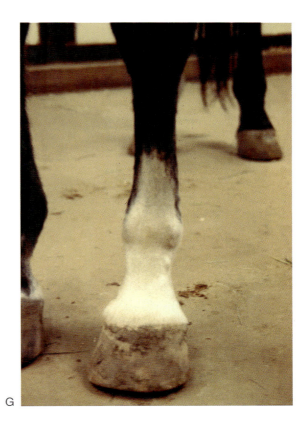

Figure 8.60. *Continued*

G

Large avulsion wounds with exposed bone must granulate to heal. Without granulation tissue to cover the exposed bone, the wound cannot contract, epithelium cannot migrate, and a free skin graft cannot be accepted. Therefore, formation of granulation tissue in the wound should be encouraged, at least initially. See Degloving Injuries later in this chapter for more information regarding methods to accelerate the formation of granulation tissue over exposed bone.

Prognosis

Extrusion, resorption, or removal of the sequestrum usually resolves associated wound infection and concomitant lameness. Granulation tissue rapidly fills the void in the wound, allowing contraction and epithelialization to proceed unimpeded.

Conclusion

The distal portion of the limb contains many critical synovial and supporting structures, injury to any one of which can result in permanent loss of function and even death. A horse with an injury to the distal portion of the limb that involves a critical structure may be able return to full function when treated appropriately, but appropriate treatment requires early and accurate assessment of the wound. Identifying which structures have been damaged requires careful physical examination and various imaging techniques and may necessitate surgical exploration of the wound. This chapter has attempted to provide helpful information about common injuries of the distal portion of the limb to enable the reader to accurately assess injuries in this region and select the most appropriate treatment to achieve the best possible outcome.

References

1. Wilmink JM, van Herten J, van Weeren PR, et al: Retrospective study of primary intention healing and sequestrum formation in horses compared to ponies under clinical circumstances. Equine Vet J 2002;34:270

2. Jacobs KA, Leach DH, Fretz PB, et al: Comparative aspects of the healing of excisional wounds on the leg and body of horses. Vet Surg 1984;13:83

3. Stashak TS: Principles of wound healing. In Ted Stashak, ed. *Equine wound management (1st edition)*. Philadelphia: Lea and Febiger, 1991, p.1

4. Bertone AL, Sullins KE, Stashak TS, et al: Effect of wound location and the use of topical collagen gel on exuberant granulation tissue formation and wound healing in the horse and pony. Am J Vet Res 1985;46:1438

5. Schumacher J, Brumbaugh GW, Honnas CM, et al: Kinetics of healing of grafted and non-grafted wounds on the distal portion of the forelimbs of horses. Am J Vet Res 1992;53:1568

6. Wilmink JM, Stolk PWTH, Van Weeren PR, et al: Differences in second-intention wound healing between horses and ponies: macroscopic aspects. Equine Vet J 1999;31:53

7. Bertone AL: Management of exuberant granulation tissue. Vet Clin N Am Equine Pract 1989;5:551

8. Wilmink JM, Van Weeren PR: Treatment of exuberant granulation tissue. Clin Tech Equine Pract 2004;3:141

9. Garvican E, Clegg P: Clinical aspects of the equine carpal joints. UK Vet 2007;12:1

10. Peacock EE: Collagenolysis and the biochemistry of wound healing. In Erle Peacock, ed. *Wound repair (3rd edition)*. Philadelphia: WB Saunders, 1984, p.102

11. Rudolph R, Vande Berg J, Ehrlich HP: Wound contraction and scar contracture. In: I. Kelman Cohen, Robert Diegelmann, and William Lindblad, eds. *Wound healing: biochemical and clinical aspects (1st edition)*. Philadelphia: WB Saunders Co, 1992, p.96

12. Adams OR: Lameness. In OR Adams, ed. *Lameness in horses (3rd edition)*. Philadelphia: Lea and Febiger, 1974, p.198

13. Booth TM, Abbot J, Clements A, et al: Treatment of septic common digital extensor tenosynovitis by complete resection in seven horses. Vet Surg 2004;33:107

14. Baxter GM: Retrospective study of lower limb wounds involving tendons, tendon sheaths, or joints. Proc Am Assoc Equine Pract 1987;33:715

15. Belknap JK, Baxter GM, Nickels FA: Extensor tendon lacerations in horses: 50 cases (1982–1988). J Am Vet Med Assoc 1993;203:428

16. Swaim SF: Management of skin tension in dermal surgery. Compend Contin Edu Pract Vet 1980;2:758

17. Stashak TS: Principles of reconstructive surgery. In Ted Stashak, ed. *Equine wound management (1st edition)*. Philadelphia: Lea and Febiger, 1991, p.70

18. Bigbie RB, Shealy P, Moll D: Presuturing as an aid in the closure of skin defects created by surgical excision. Pro Am Assoc Equine Pract 1990;36:613

19. Liang M, Briggs P, Heckler FR, et al: Presuturing—A new technique for closing large skin defects: clinical and experimental studies. Plast Reconstr Surg 1988;81:694

20. Scardino M, Swaim SF, Henderson RA: Enhancing wound closure on the limbs. Compend Contin Educ Pract Vet 1996;18:919

21. Bailey JV, Jacobs KA: The mesh expansion method of suturing wounds on the legs of horses. Vet Surg 1983;12:78

22. Lawrence WT: Clinical management of nonhealing wounds. In I. Kelman Cohen, Robert Diegelmann, and William Lindblad, eds. *Wound healing: biochemical and clinical aspects (1st edition)*. Philadelphia: WB Saunders Co, 1992, p.541

23. Janicek JC, Dabareiner RM, Honnas CM, et al: Heel bulb laceration in horses: 101 cases (1988–1994). J Am Vet Med Assoc 2005;226:418

24. Wilson DG, Cooley AL, Mac Williams PS, et al: Effects of 0.05% chlorhexidine lavage on the tarsocrural joints of horses. Vet Surg 1994;23:442

25. Edlich RF, Schmolka IR, Prusak MP, et al: The molecular basis for toxicity of surfactants in surgical wounds. J Surg Res 1973;14:277

26. Stashak TS. Wound management and reconstructive surgery of problems associated with the distal limb. In Ted Stashak, ed. *Equine wound management (1st edition)*. Philadelphia: Lea and Febiger, 1991, p.163

27. Markel MD, Richardson GL, Peterson PR, et al: Surgical reconstruction of chronic coronary band avulsions in three horses. J Am Vet Med Assoc 1987;190:687

28. Riggs CM, Proudman CJ, Hughes I, et al: Management of traumatic, partial hoof avulsion in two horses. Equine Vet Educ 1995;7:140

29. Richardson GL, Pascoe JR, Meagher D: Puncture wounds of the foot in horses: Diagnosis and treatment. Compend Contin Educ Pract Vet 1986;8:379

30. Steckel RR, Fessler JF, Huston LC: Deep puncture wounds of the equine hoof: A review of 50 cases. Proc Am Assoc Equine Pract 1989;35:167

31. DeBowes RM, Yovich JV: Penetrating wounds, abscesses, gravel, and bruising of the equine foot. Vet Clin N Am Equine Pract 1989;5:179
32. Stashak TS: Penetrating wounds of the foot. In Ted Stashak, ed. *Adams' lameness in horses (5th edition)*. Philadelphia: Lippincott William and Wilkins, 2002, p.703
33. Moyer W, Schumacher J, Schumacher J: *A guide to equine joint injections and regional anesthesia (4th edition)*. Yardly, PA: Veterinary Learning Systems, 2007; p.14
34. Vazquez de Mercado R, Stover SM, Taylor, KT, et al: Lateral approach for arthrocentesis of the distal interphalangeal joint in horses. J Am Vet Med Assoc 1998;212:1413
35. Hassel DM, Stover SM, Yarbrough TB, et al: Palmar-plantar axial sesamoidean approach to the digital flexor tendon sheath in horses. J Am Vet Med Assoc 2000;217:1343
36. Wright IM, Phillips TJ, Walmsley JP: Endoscopy of the navicular bursa: A new technique for the treatment of contaminated and septic bursae. Equine Vet J 1999;31:5
37. Brown, PW: The fate of exposed bone. Am J Surg 1979;137:464
38. Jann HW, Peyton LC, Fackelman GE: The pathogenesis and treatment of traumatically induced sequestra in horses. Compend Contin Educ Pract Vet 1987;9:182
39. Moens Y, Verschooten F, De Moor A, et al: Bone sequestration as a consequence of limb wounds in the horse. Vet Radiol 1980;21:40
40. Butler JA, Colles CM, Dyson SJ, et al: The metacarpus and metatarsus. *Clinical radiology of the horse (2nd edition)*. Oxford: Blackwell Science, 1993, p.122
41. Caron JP, Barber SM, Doige CE, et al: The radiographic and histologic appearance of controlled surgical manipulation of the equine periosteum. Vet Surg 1987;16:13
42. Clem MF, DeBowes RM, Yovich JV, et al: Osseous sequestration in the horse. A review of 68 cases. Vet Surg 1988; 17:2
43. Wilmink JM, van Weeren PR: Differences in wound healing between horses and ponies: application of research results to the clinical approach of equine wounds. Clin Tech Equine Pract 2004;3:123
44. Kahn LH, Styrt BA: Necrotizing soft tissue infections reported with nonsteroidal anti-inflammatory drugs. Ann Pharmacother 1997;31:1034
45. Sedgwick AD, Lees P, Dawson J, et al: Cellular aspects of inflammation. Vet Rec 1987;120:529
46. Booth LC, Feeney DA: Superficial osteitis and sequestrum formation as a result of skin avulsion in the horse. Vet Surg 1982;11:2
47. Stashak TS: Wound Infection: contributing factors and selected techniques for prevention. Proc Am Assoc of Equine Pract 2006;52:270
48. Lees MF, Fretz PB, Bailey JV, et al: Second-intention wound healing. Compend Contin Educ Pract Vet 1989;11:857
49. Hanson R: Management of avulsion wounds with exposed bone. Clin Tech Equine Pract 2004;3:123

8.2 Degloving Injuries

R. Reid Hanson, DVM, Diplomate ACVS and ACVECC

Introduction

Horses are subject to trauma in relation to their locale, use, and character. Wire fences, sheet metal, or other sharp objects in the environment, as well as entrapment between two immovable objects or during transport, are often the cause of injury. The wounds are commonly associated with extensive soft tissue loss, crush injury, and harsh contamination, which necessitate open wound management and second intention healing. One of the most difficult of these wounds to heal is the degloving injury that exposes bone by avulsion of the skin and subcutaneous tissues overlying it.

Exposed bone is defined as bone denuded of periosteum, which in an open wound can delay second intention healing indirectly and directly.[1] The rigid nature of bone indirectly inhibits contraction of granulation tissue and can prolong the inflammatory phase of repair.[1] Prolonged periods may be required for extensive wounds of the distal extremity with denuded bone and tendon to become covered with a healthy, uniform bed of granulation tissue.[2] Desiccation of the superficial layers of exposed bone can lead to sequestrum formation, which is one of the most common causes for delayed healing of wounds of the distal limb of horses.[3] Rapid coverage of exposed bone with granulation tissue can decrease healing time and prevent desiccation of exposed bone and subsequent sequestrum formation. Exposed bone in distal limb wounds (Figure 8.61) can result in extensive periosteal new bone growth that can lead to increased wound size and result in an enlarged limb, even after healing is complete.[4] Cortical fenestration, curettage, and scraping of exposed bone have been reported in horses, humans, and dogs as a means of promoting granulation tissue formation to enhance second intention healing or provide a vascular bed for skin grafting procedures.[4–7] In one study, drilling holes in the bone produced a greater amount of clot than did scraping the bone. This clot provided an early coverage for the bone and protected it from desiccation. The ingrowth of fibroblasts and capillaries from the bone surface and surrounding tissue into the clot to form granulation tissue was a desired effect.[8]

Skin grafting procedures are commonly used in the management of distal limb wounds in horses.[9] Skin grafts can be applied to fresh wounds that are vascular enough to produce granulation tissue, but graft survival is poor over areas of exposed bone because revascularization of the graft is slow or absent.[10] A healthy and uniform bed of granulation tissue must form over exposed bone before skin grafting procedures can be used.[11]

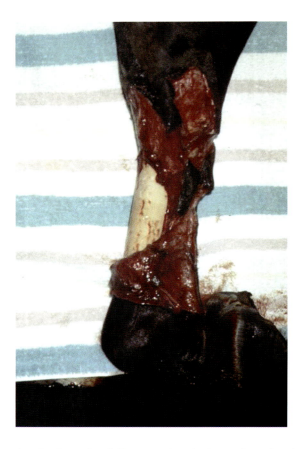

Figure 8.61. Degloving injury, with extensive loss of soft tissue and periosteum along the dorsal surface of the third metatarsal bone. Larger wounds with exposed bone take longer to form a granulation bed, which subsequently delays wound contraction. Reprinted from *Clinical Techniques in Equine Practice*, Vol 3, R. Reid Hanson, Management of avulsion wounds with exposed bone, p. 189, (2004), with permission from Elsevier Saunders.

Numerous studies have been performed to evaluate various aspects of wound healing at the distal aspect of the limb in horses.[2,4,12–20] Most have used models of full-thickness cutaneous wounds of variable size without excision of any appreciable amount of subcutaneous tissue or periosteum. To the author's knowledge, only two studies of wounds of the distal extremity of horses have examined the impact of denuded bone on wound healing.[4,7]

This chapter will review the healing of distal limb wounds and complications related to degloving injuries which expose the underlying bone. Therapies to promote wound healing and control granulation tissue, as well as bandaging methods, will be reviewed. Grafting techniques which could facilitate the healing of distal limb wounds are discussed in Chapter 11.

Healing of Distal Limb Wounds

Vascularity and Granulation

The ability of a tissue to produce granulation tissue is directly related to its vascularity.[3] Tissue with an abundant blood supply, such as muscle, can rapidly produce granulation tissue. Tissue with a poor vascular supply, such as bone, produces granulation tissue slowly, resulting in delayed wound healing.[3] As healthy granulation tissue develops, there is a rapid decrease in total wound area.[4,17] The use of pressure bandages may control the amount of limb edema (Figure 8.62). Exuberant granulation tissue can enlarge a wound by "pushing" its edges apart. For injuries associated with exposed bone, excessive periosteal new bone growth may contribute to a prolonged period of wound expansion.[4]

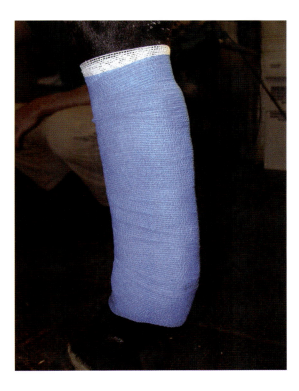

Figure 8.62. Pressure bandage with comfortable absorptive dressing provides protection from wound contamination and assists in wound debridement, absorption of exudate, and reduction in limb swelling. Reprinted from *Clinical Techniques in Equine Practice*, Vol 3, R. Reid Hanson, Management of avulsion wounds with exposed bone, p. 189, (2004), with permission from Elsevier Saunders.

Wound Contraction

Wound contraction is the inward or central movement of the wound edges due to "pulling" forces generated within the wound and is one of the major means of wound closure in second intention healing. Fibroblasts and myofibroblasts are the major cell types that contribute to wound contraction. Reorganization of collagen by fibroblast cell membrane movement causes wound contraction by condensing or "piling up" the collagen into a smaller unit.[21] Skin, which is attached to the granulation tissue, is subsequently moved toward the center of the wound. The exact role of the myofibroblast is poorly understood because it has been shown that rat wounds lacking myofibroblasts can contract.[22] Myofibroblasts may play a passive role by counteracting tensile forces on the skin during wound healing.[21]

Second Intention Healing

Second intention healing of wounds located at the distal aspect of the limb of horses can be lengthy and complicated. Wounds of the distal extremity in horses heal less quickly than those of the trunk because of comparatively slower rates of epithelialization and contraction.[4] There are also differences in wound healing between horses and ponies.[4,12,13] Similar wounds on the dorsal aspect of the metatarsal region heal more slowly in horses, compared to ponies, because wound contraction in ponies occurs to a greater extent than it does in horses.[4,12]

Histological analyses of these wounds showed a prolonged inflammatory phase in the horse, as well as less organization of the myofibroblasts, compared to ponies.[4,12] The higher TGF-β concentrations present in the wounded tissues of ponies may explain the more intense inflammatory response and greater degree of wound contraction.[23] The slower rates of epithelialization have been attributed to inhibition of cell mitotic and migratory activity by exuberant granulation tissue.[12] As a result of this finding, authors have investigated whether intramuscular administration of recombinant equine growth hormone (10 ug/kg daily for 7 days, then 20 ug/kg daily for 49 days) would increase the epithelialization rate by increasing the mitotic and migratory activity of the epithelium. Their finding, however, discovered that the use of equine growth hormone does not appear to have any beneficial clinical effect on healing of equine limb wounds.[24]

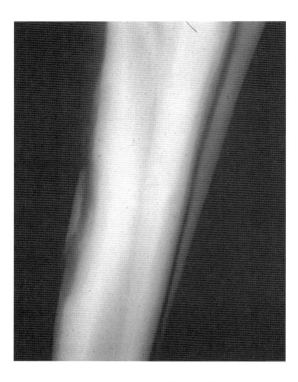

Figure 8.63. Lateral medial radiograph of the third metatarsal bone (MT3) with sequestrum formation of the dorsal aspect of MT3 secondary to a degloving injury 26 days earlier. The sequestrum incites an inflammatory response with accumulation of exudate and eventual wound drainage. Reprinted from *Clinical Techniques in Equine Practice*, Vol 3, R. Reid Hanson, Management of avulsion wounds with exposed bone, p. 190, (2004), with permission from Elsevier Saunders.

Sequestra Formation

Sequestra development can be a sequel to trauma and is a common cause of delayed healing of wounds of the distal limbs of horses.[1] Sequestra can result from any insult that interrupts the blood supply to bone. Periosteal trauma may lead to local vascular stasis by reducing venous outflow.[3] Afferent vessels from the periosteum and medullary cavity provide blood flow to the compact portion of long bones. Haversion canals, which are connected by Volkmann canals, contain the capillaries which provide nutrition to compact bone. Outflow, or efferent flow, occurs at the periosteal and endosteal levels. The blood supply in the cortex of equine long bones is sensitive to trauma because the dense mineralized matrix of the bone cortex prevents rapid collateralization of vessels following injury.[25] Ischemia of the superficial layers of the cortex leads to necrosis of the affected area (Figure 8.63).[1] The necrotic portion of bone incites an inflammatory response with accumulation of exudate and can lead to the formation of a draining tract in wounds where the skin has healed over the area.[3] Most reports suggest that infection is required for sequestrum formation, while others counter this hypothesis.[3] Sequestra can delay wound healing by serving as foci of continued inflammation and/or infection, which postpone the ensuing phases of repair.

Impediments to Wound Healing

A rapid reduction in wound area due to contraction and epithelialization, following an initial period of wound expansion, has been reported in several studies.[4,7] Exuberant granulation tissue can decrease the rate of wound contraction and epithelialization by providing a physical barrier that impedes movement of the wound margins and advancing epithelium (Figure 8.64).[26] Persistent swelling, associated with wound inflammation, increases the total circumference of the limb, thereby increasing the surface area of each wound. A large amount of periosteal new bone growth beneath the wound may also contribute to increased total wound area measurements.

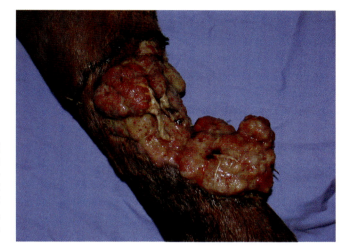

Figure 8.64. Exuberant granulation tissue in a wound located on the dorsal aspect of the metatarsus. Exuberant granulation tissue can decrease the rate of wound contraction and epithelialization by providing a physical barrier that impedes movement of the wound margins and advancing epithelium. Reprinted from *Clinical Techniques in Equine Practice*, Vol 3, R. Reid Hanson, Management of avulsion wounds with exposed bone, p. 190, (2004), with permission from Elsevier Saunders.

Healing of Degloving Wounds

Trauma to the distal aspect of the limb is frequently complicated by exposed or denuded bone.[27] Exposed cortical bone, denuded of periosteum, is subject to desiccation of the superficial layers of the cortex, which may result in infectious superficial osteitis and sequestrum formation.[1,6] The presence of denuded bone in wounds can delay healing by prolonging the inflammatory and repair phases of wound healing. Exposed bone within a wound can delay healing directly if the bone becomes infected, or indirectly because its rigid structure and the limited blood supply available at its cortical surface can impede the formation of granulation tissue and wound contraction.

Distal limb avulsion wounds with exposed bone increase in size for 14–21 days. Wound expansion is due primarily to the distraction forces applied across the wound during the inflammatory and debridement stages of repair and the absence of a granulation bed in the center of the wound to counteract tensile forces exerted on the wound margins by the surrounding skin. Wounds with little or no exposed bone expand for a shorter period because less time is required for granulation tissue to fill the wound. Larger wounds with exposed bone take longer to form a granulation bed, which subsequently delays wound contraction (Figure 8.61).

Complications Associated with Denuded Bone

Injuries involving bones in horses stimulate more periosteal new bone growth than similar wounds in other species and ponies.[4] Periosteal insults from blunt trauma, tendon/joint capsule strain, surgical manipulation, or laceration/degloving injuries may result in extensive periosteal exostosis.[4,28] More extensive periosteal reaction in young versus adult horses has been attributed to a greater osteoblastic activity of the periosteum in the young horse.[28] The extensive periosteal new bone growth seen in adult horses is poorly understood. A species-related delay in collagen lysis may be a contributing factor.[4] The more extensive periosteal new bone formation in horses compared to ponies is believed to result from a slower onset and longer duration of the periosteal response as well as prolonged extensive limb swelling related to the inefficient resolution of the inflammatory response to injury.[4] Bone sequestration is associated with wound drainage, the formation of unhealthy granulation tissue, and inadequate wound contraction and epithelialization (Figures 8.65a,b). Discoloration of exposed bone is not a reliable indicator of sequestrum formation.[1]

Methods to Stimulate the Growth of Granulation Tissue

Despite the frequent presence of exposed bone associated with trauma to the distal aspect of the limb of horses, there has been little investigation into methods of stimulating coverage by granulation tissue. Granulation tissue plays a very important role in second intention healing because it provides a barrier to infection and mechanical trauma for the underlying tissues. Moreover, healthy granulation tissue provides a moist surface

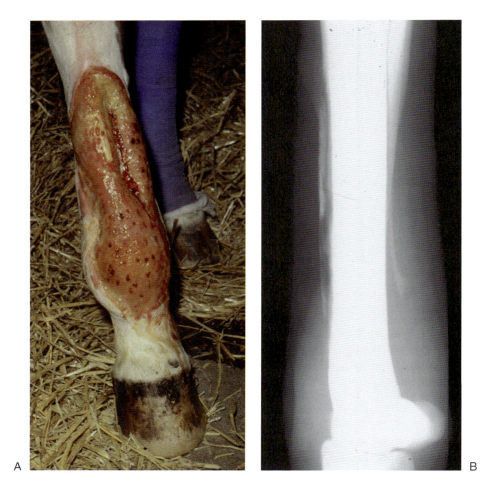

Figure 8.65. (A) Degloving injury of 3 months duration involving the dorsal metatarsus. Note the linear defect in the granulation tissue which was associated with wound drainage, unhealthy granulation tissue, as well as inadequate wound contraction. These signs are typical of sequestrum formation. The dark spots in the granulation tissue, particularly overlying the fetlock region, are pinch grafts that have been accepted. (B) Lateral radiograph of the third metatarsal bone revealing a linear sequestrum with involucrum formation along the dorsal surface of the bone. Courtesy of Dr. T. Stashak.

for epithelialization. Therefore, the delay in wound healing related to exposed bone has incited the search for different methods to promote granulation tissue coverage of bone in other species.

In humans, head trauma, thermal injury, and surgical oncology often lead to exposed bone of the cranium.[6,29] In these cases the outer cortex of the exposed portion of the cranium is fenestrated with drill holes, burrs, or laser to expose the medullary cavity from which granulation tissue grows to cover the exposed bone.[5,6] Likewise, exposed cortices of long bones in humans have been fenestrated with drill holes to promote granulation tissue formation.[4] It appears that the drill holes promote healing by allowing osteogenic factors from the medullary cavity access to the wound, or they may enhance healing of bone and soft tissue by a nonspecific response known as "the regional acceleratory phenomenon."[30] Cortical fenestration (Figure 8.66) combined with drugs that promote local fibroplasia may accelerate granulation tissue coverage, though further investigation is needed to verify this hypothesis.

Drilling 1.6 mm holes in the cortex of the second metacarpal bone in experimentally created wounds in dogs resulted in clot formation over the bone that promoted the development of granulation tissue and may have protected the bone's outer layers from desiccation.[8] The effects of 3.2 mm cortical fenestrations were evaluated in experimentally created wounds at the distal aspect of the limb of horses.[7] Fenestrated wounds were covered with granulation tissue earlier than were control wounds, because of the formation of granulation tissue directly from the cortical fenestration sites (Figure 8.67); however, fenestration had no significant effect on sequestrum formation. If the wounds are not large (<6 cm × 6 cm), it may be difficult to distinguish a significant

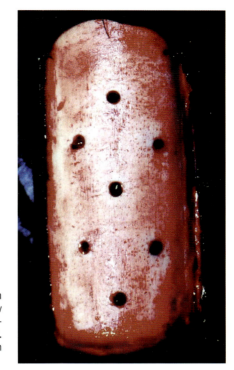

Figure 8.66. Cortical fenestration of the dorsal aspect of the third metatarsal bone in a diamond shaped pattern using a 3.2 mm drill. The cortical fenestration sites allow for the rapid formation of granulation tissue within the drill sites and over the associated exposed bone. Reprinted from *Clinical Techniques in Equine Practice*, Vol 3, R. Reid Hanson, Management of avulsion wounds with exposed bone, p. 192, (2004), with permission from Elsevier Saunders.

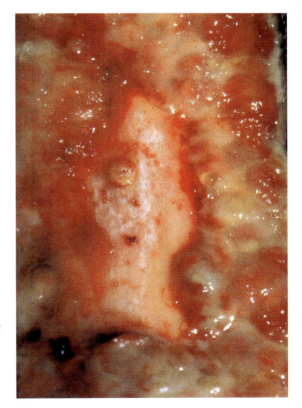

Figure 8.67. Granulation tissue production from cortical fenestration sites as well as the cortical bone in an 11-day-old degloving injury of dorsal metacarpus. Wounds > 6 cm × 6 cm in diameter can obtain a significant contribution of granulation tissue from cortical fenestration sites. Reprinted from *Clinical Techniques in Equine Practice*, Vol 3, R. Reid Hanson, Management of avulsion wounds with exposed bone, p. 192, (2004), with permission from Elsevier Saunders.

additive contribution from the granulation tissue growing directly from the cortical fenestration sites alone. Cortical fenestration may also be beneficial if it is used with other methods of promoting fibroplasia in larger wounds because there may be an additive effect.[7]

Management of Degloving Injuries

Wound Preparation and Evaluation

Because exposed bone stripped of its periosteum is very susceptible to infection, it is important to use aseptic techniques when cleansing and bandaging the wound. In one study, less *S. aureus* adhered to periosteum than to cortical bone, cut cortical bone, and endosteal surfaces.[31] The surrounding skin should be clipped and cleaned carefully to reveal the full extent of the wound. The wound should be flushed with sterile saline to which a diluted antiseptic solution (e.g., 0.5% chlorhexidine or 0.1%–0.2% povidone iodine) is added, using low pressure (10–14 PSI) lavage with a 19-gauge needle (or catheter) and a 35 ml syringe. Any obvious debris must be removed.

Following lavage, the wound should be explored digitally with sterile gloves to establish the extent of injury and degree of periosteal damage. Injury to adjacent synovial structures, tendons, and ligaments should be noted. Examination of the wound should also aim to determine the presence of any bony fragments or palpable foreign bodies. For a more in-depth discussion of wound preparation, see Chapter 2.

Bone distortion suggests a concurrent fracture, and open fractures carry a poor prognosis. In these cases, radiography is indicated to assess the amount of bone involved, including the possibility of partial, complete, or non-displaced fractures and the possibility of joint involvement. If there is no fracture, the limb should be bandaged as described later. When there is the possibility of a fracture, tendon laceration, or joint involvement, a splint should be incorporated into the bandage as described later. For more information regarding bandage splinting, see Chapter 16.

Surgical Management

Surgical debridement remains the technique of choice for removal of devitalized tissues. Proper debridement removes tissues heavily contaminated by dirt and bacteria and also those which impede wound healing. Debridement of small, relatively clean wounds can be done under local anesthesia in the standing horse. Larger chronic/infected wounds are often best handled with the patient under general anesthesia (Figures 8.68a,b).

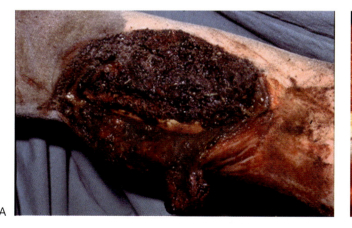
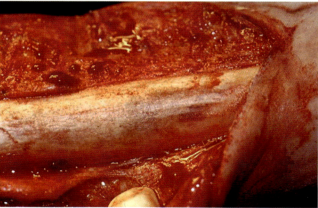

A

B

Figure 8.68. (A) Contaminated degloving wound with exposed bone present on the distal lateral aspect of the third metatarsus. Dried, necrotic tissue along with soiled debris is present in the wound. (B) Wound after surgical debridement. Surgical debridement remains the technique of choice for removal of devitalized tissues. Proper debridement removes tissues heavily contaminated by dirt and bacteria and also those which impede wound healing. The wound was sharply debrided until only healthy tissue remained. Courtesy of Dr. S. Barber.

The wound is sharply debrided until only healthy tissue remains. See chapters 2 and 4 for more information regarding preparation of a wound to reduce the chances of infection.

If a flap of skin is available, its base and a portion of degloved skin can often be sutured using a far-near, near-far pattern with a monofilament suture.[27] The part of the wound (<6 cm × 6 cm) that cannot be covered by the skin flap is allowed to heal by second intention or the cortex can be drilled to facilitate the formation of granulation tissue over the wound. To achieve this, a 3.2 mm drill is used to make full-thickness drill holes into the medullary portion of the bone. The drill holes should be placed in a diamond shaped pattern allowing 12 mm–15 mm of separation between each drill hole. A bone rasp or curette, although not as effective in stimulating the formation of granulation tissue, can be used in areas where full-thickness drilling of the bone is contraindicated.

Open Wound Management

Systemic Treatments and Antimicrobial Therapy

Following wounding, the horse should receive tetanus prophylaxis and should initially be treated with systemic antibiotics. Nonsteroidal anti-inflammatory drugs may be administered to decrease pain and inflammation. Systemic antibiotics are indicated during the initial exudative response to injury. An initial course of 5 days of intramuscularly administered procaine penicillin can be followed by a prolonged course of trimethoprim sulfur oral powders or paste. This regimen would be recommended for large avulsion wounds with exposed bone and for bone injuries in which the cortical surface is fenestrated.

If the wound is severely contaminated or if a synovial cavity has been penetrated, intravenous and regional perfusion of broad-spectrum antibiotics should be initiated (Figures 8.69, 12.1–12.4). One study evaluating synovial fluid concentrations and pharmacokinetics of amikacin in the equine limb distal to the carpus following intraosseous and intravenous regional perfusion found that both techniques produced mean peak concentrations ranging from 5 to 50 times that of peak serum concentrations required for therapeutic efficacy.[32] See chapters 9 and 12 for more information regarding this.

Antibiotic impregnated polymethylmethacrylate (PMMA) or plaster of paris (POP) beads have been used for the local delivery of biologically active antimicrobials (Figure 12.6). Each method results in the local delivery of a high concentration of a single or multiple antibiotics. Approximately 80% of gentamicin was released in

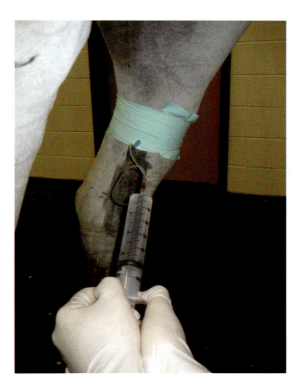

Figure 8.69. Intravenous regional limb perfusion of the left hind limb. Intravenous regional limb perfusion can provide concentrations of antibiotic 5 to 50 times the peak serum concentrations recommended for therapeutic efficiency.

the first 48 hours in a POP in vitro model while 63% and 79% of gentamicin or metronidazole, respectively, were released from PMMA during the first 24 hours of another in vitro model. Plaster of paris-impregnated beads inhibited the growth of *E. coli* during the 14-day period of the study. The drugs retain their bactericidal activity after ethylene oxide sterilization and storage at room temperature for up to 2 months with PMMA and 5 months with POP. Antibiotic elution is directly related to the amount of antibiotic incorporated into the cement.[33,34] While antibiotic beads may be effective in the short-term management of wounds, they are no substitute for thorough and meticulous debridement at the initial stages of treatment. For more information regarding the treatment of synovial wounds and infected wounds, see chapters 9 and 12, respectively.

Wound Dressings and Topical Agents to Promote Healing

Clean Wounds. Rapid coverage by granulation tissue of extensive wounds of the distal limb prevents desiccation of the exposed tissue.[2] Prior to the formation of granulation tissue, hydrogel dressings are comfortable and supportive, provide protection from further wound contamination, assist in wound debridement, absorb some wound fluid within their polymer matrix, and reduce limb swelling.[32,35–37] These dressings are particularly useful for rehydrating necrotic tissue and enhancing autolytic debridement. Hydrogels (CarraDres™, Carrington Laboratories, Irving, TX) should only be applied to wounds that appear clean and healthy. The dressing is applied to the wound bed, followed by application of a conformable absorptive bandage dressing. A firm cotton bandage is applied as a tertiary layer to provide warmth and support.

Contaminated Wounds. Debridement dressings can be used to accelerate the transition from a heavily contaminated to a clean status. Application of a finely threaded and widely meshed, woven, cotton gauze dressing bandage or an antiseptic gauze dressing (Xeroform™ petroleum gauze, Covidien Animal Health/Kendall, Dublin, OH; Kerlix™ antimicrobial dressing, Covidien Animal Health/Kendall, Dublin, OH) in a wet-to-dry fashion is most commonly used when wound fluids have a high viscosity or when the wound surface is dehydrated and scabs have formed. This approach facilitates wound debridement and drainage and reduces the bacterial load. It is also an excellent dressing for packing deep contaminated wounds associated with the body or upper limbs. When the dressing dries, fibrin adheres it to the wound's surface, achieving debridement. If further debridement is needed, another wet-to-dry dressing is applied. Usually one to three applications of the wet-to-dry dressing are all that are needed to effectively debride most wounds.

Calcium alginate dressings (EquineGinate™, Carrington Laboratories, Irving, TX), which can absorb 20–30 times their weight in wound fluid, are useful in moderate to heavily exudative wounds during the transition from the debridement to repair phases of healing, or in wounds with substantial tissue loss such as degloving injuries. Calcium alginate dressings should be used only in heavily exuding wounds and applied no more than once, or at most, twice because they require moisture to function properly. They are not indicated for dry sloughing wounds or those covered with hard necrotic tissue. See Chapter 3 for more information regarding wound dressings.

During the exudative period an antiseptic or antibiotic such as Betadine ointment (The Purdue Frederick Company, Stamford, CT) or silver sulfadiazine (Par Pharmaceutical, Inc., Spring Valley, NY) may be applied to the wound, because neither delays wound healing. While furacin (Phoenix Pharmaceuticals, Inc., St. Joseph, MO) is an effective antimicrobial against Gram-positive and Gram-negative organisms, it has little effect against *Pseudomonas* spp. Moreover, it has been shown to decrease epithelialization in laboratory animals and humans by 24% and to delay wound contraction in horses.[38] Therefore, the author does not advocate its use in the management of wounds in horses. Silver sulfadiazine has a wide antimicrobial spectrum including *Pseudomonas* spp and fungi. Contrary to what has been noted in other species, it does not decrease the rate of wound contraction in horses.[39]

Honey has many useful properties including a broad-spectrum antimicrobial activity, anti-inflammatory actions, and stimulation of new tissue growth.[40] The stimulatory effect of honey on wound healing may in part be related to the up-regulation of inflammatory cytokines (tumor necrosis factor alpha [TNF-α], interleukin-1 beta [IL-1β], and interleukin-6 [IL-6]) within monocytes.[41] Sugardine is obtained by adding granular sugar to a povidone iodine solution until a workable paste consistency is reached. It is a hypertonic agent that, via osmosis, draws exudate from the wound. A 10% povidone iodine ointment has not been associated with a delay in wound healing.[39]

Neither Betadine ointment nor a topical antibiotic should be applied to the wound concurrently with honey, sugar, silver-coated dressing, or Kerlix AMD (Kerlix™ antimicrobial dressing, Covidien Animal Health/Kendall, Dublin, OH). Gentamicin sulfate has a narrow antimicrobial spectrum but may be applied to wounds with

Gram-negative bacteria, particularly *Pseudomonas aeruginosa.* Application of a 0.1% oil-in-water cream base slowed epithelialization and wound contraction in dogs.[42] Cefazolin is an effective antimicrobial against Gram-positive and some Gram-negative organisms. The powder form provides an appropriate tissue concentration for a longer period than does the solution, which can be used to treat established infections. For more information regarding wound dressings and topical medications, see Chapter 3.

Equine bandages are composed of a primary and secondary layer, as well as a tertiary layer that maintains the dressing in place. The primary bandage (wound dressing) should be selected according to the condition of the wound and the current phase of repair. Depending upon clinician preference the primary dressing is covered with conforming gauze (Kling gauze™, Johnson and Johnson, Inc., New Brunswick, NJ), which is applied circumferentially around the limb to assist in securing the dressing. The principal purpose of the secondary layer is to absorb harmful agents such as serum, blood, exudate, bacteria, and other necrotic debris from a wound (SteriRoll™, The Franklin-Williams Company, Lexington, KY). This layer should be thick enough to collect absorbed moisture, pad the wound against trauma, and splint the wound to prevent excessive motion.

Materials used in the secondary layer are conforming gauze and cotton pads, which must be carefully applied to conform to the shape of the limb. The tertiary layer is usually composed of materials stiffer than those used for the secondary layer. The purpose of this outer layer is to hold the previous layers in place, prevent contamination and trauma, provide pressure to minimize swelling of the limb which will reduce tension at the wound edges, and decrease the range of motion.

The final layer should be porous yet waterproof. Elastic self adhesive bandages (Vet Wrap™, 3M Company, St. Paul, MN) are frequently used as the tertiary layer. The tertiary layer must be applied with constant pressure that is gradually increased as the bandage is wrapped in a distal-to-proximal direction. The most proximal and distal aspects of the cotton pad (secondary layer) are initially left uncovered to avoid pressure points that may affect circulation with intact skin. As a final step, the proximal and distal ends of the bandage are covered with an adhesive bandage (Elasticon™, Johnson and Johnson, Inc., New Brunswick, NJ) that adheres to the outer layer and the skin. This prevents penetration of foreign bodies such as shavings and dirt between the skin and bandages, which may cause skin sores and wound contamination. For more information regarding techniques of bandaging, see Chapter 16.

General Care. Phenylbutazone is continued at 4.4 mg/kg every other day during the initial 5-day period. Alternate-day bandage changes are continued until the wound is covered by a healthy bed of granulation tissue. After early formation of granulation tissue, non-adherent, semi-occlusive bandages provide absorption of exudate and keep the wound surface moist, which favors maximal epithelial migration. A hydrogel-based sheet or gauze dressing provides for early, rapid contraction and exudate absorption (CarraDres™ and CarraGauze™ Carrington Laboratories, Irving, TX). Once granulation tissue has filled the wound bed, bandaging and protection from contamination may no longer be necessary if the horse is housed in a clean environment and there are economic constraints. Indeed, a healthy bed of granulation tissue provides resistance to infection due to improved vascular dynamics and the subsequently superior oxygen delivery.

Control of Granulation Tissue. Ketanserin gel (Vulketan gel™, Janssen Animal Health, Beerse, Belgium) is effective in preventing exuberant granulation tissue formation in equine lower limb wounds. Ketanserin is thought to antagonize the serotonin-induced suppression of wound macrophages and thus allow a strong and effective inflammatory response to occur within wounds. This should translate into a superior control of infection and a better orchestration of the later phase of repair when the cytokines and growth factors released by the activated macrophages play an important role. Ketanserin is 2 to 5 times more likely to result in successful closure by reducing infection and proud flesh formation than antiseptics or desloughing agents.[43]

Silicone gel dressings (Cicacare™, Smith and Nephew, Largo, FL) have been effective in controlling hypertrophic and keloidal scarring in human burn patients by apparently exerting pressure on the microvasculature of the scar and altering levels of various growth factors, notably pro-fibrotic TGF-β.[44] The anoxic fibroblasts are then thought to undergo apoptosis rather than proliferating and secreting extracellular matrix components, which normally contribute to scarring. Silicone gel dressings greatly surpassed a conventional non-adherent absorbent dressing in preventing the formation of exuberant granulation tissue in experimental wounds located on the distal limbs of horses. Contraction and epithelialization progressed faster in the first 2 weeks of repair, possibly as a result of healthier granulation tissue. Furthermore, tissue quality exceeded that of wounds treated conventionally, which may translate into superior tissue strength.[45,46]

Topical administration of antibiotics is warranted if surface infection seems to delay wound healing or if infection spreads to surrounding tissues.[26,37,47] Topically administered gentamicin ointment can significantly suppress bacterial counts in wounds. Triple antibiotic (bacitracin, neomycin, polymixin) and silver sulfadiazine ointments promote healing and do not appear to suppress epithelialization, while nitrofurazone ointment significantly suppresses epithelialization and wound contraction.[48]

Products that promote angiogenesis, fibroblast migration or proliferation, and/or collagen deposition promote the formation of granulation tissue. Topically applied platelet-derived growth factor (PDGF) and TGF-β have been shown to increase fibroblast number and collagen content in experimentally created wounds in laboratory animals.[49] Acemannan, a water soluble polysaccharide, enhances the release of IL-1 from macrophages, which in turn stimulates angiogenesis.[8] Live yeast cell derivative, a component of hemorrhoid medication, has been used to increase collagen synthesis and thus granulation tissue formation in wounds of horses.[15]

Occlusive dressings have likewise been shown to enhance the formation of granulation tissue in humans and horses,[2,14] possibly by lowering the ambient oxygen tension and reducing the local tissue pH.[14] In an equine study evaluating the effects of a flexible hydroactive dressing in a clinical setting, rapid and uniform fibroplasia occurred in wounds that are notoriously difficult to cover with granulation tissue.[2,35] The use of occlusive dressings should be discontinued once granulation tissue fills the wound bed, prior to it becoming exuberant.

Surgical resection is a simple and effective method to control exuberant granulation tissue. The procedure is performed with the horse standing because granulation tissue is not innervated (Figure 8.70).[26] Strips of granulation tissue can be shaved from the wound bed in a distal to proximal direction to produce a flat surface level with or slightly (~2 mm) below the surrounding wound edges. The epithelial margin should be preserved to allow continued healing. A pressure bandage is usually necessary to control hemorrhage after excision.[9] In lower limb wounds of horses this technique has been successful in enhancing second intention healing that was delayed because of protruding granulation tissue. This technique is preferred for the removal of exuberant granulation tissue over other methods such as application of caustic drugs because it is easy to perform, provides tissue for histological evaluation (if needed), and preserves the epithelial margin for continued healing. As with any alternate technique, healing by contraction and epithelialization must subsequently be supported or excessive granulation will recur.

Corticosteroids may be applied topically to curb the early formation of exuberant granulation tissue, hence facilitating epithelialization and wound repair.[50] The ability of some corticosteroids to suppress the formation of exuberant granulation tissue in the early phases of healing may be related to their ability to selectively

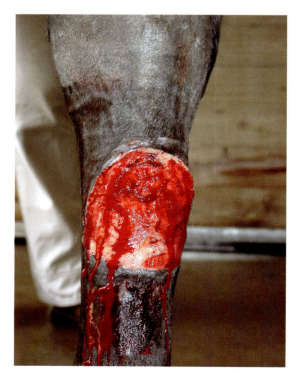

Figure 8.70. Fully granulated wound on the dorsal surface of the third metatarsus. Surgical resection of granulation tissue, as in this case, is a simple and effective method to control exuberant granulation tissue. Shaving the wound bed in a distal to proximal direction allows for better visualization of the wound margins during debridement. Reprinted from *Clinical Techniques in Equine Practice*, Vol 3, R. Reid Hanson, Management of avulsion wounds with exposed bone, p. 194, (2004), with permission from Elsevier Saunders.

decrease the release of pro-fibrotic TGF-β from monocytes and macrophages, therefore inhibiting lysosomal activity and fibroblastic proliferation.[51] Corticosteroids are generally applied at the earliest signs of formation of exuberant granulation tissue; one or two applications are all that are needed to achieve the desired effect. Continued applications are not recommended because this may exert negative effects on wound contraction, epithelialization, and angiogenesis.[52] Corticosteroids should not be applied to an infected wound because they inhibit the inflammatory response required to eliminate micro-organisms. More information on the treatment of exuberant granulation tissue is provided later in this chapter.

Immobilization of the Wound

Bandaging Methods

One of the most challenging areas to bandage on a horse is the hock. The conformation and the combination of forces that allow flexion and extension (e.g., reciprocal apparatus) impose some important considerations when applying a bandage to this region. Horses are reluctant to accept any restriction to movement in this region and frequently disrupt the bandages as a result of exaggerated flexion. The primary and secondary layers should be applied, avoiding excessive pressure over the point of the hock (calcaneal tuberosity), using the same technique as for the carpus. For the tertiary layer, a figure-8 bandage is applied starting with circumferential wraps around the distal aspect of the tibia and continuing down with figure-8 wraps below and above the hock. Applying a length of 10 cm wide, low-stretch adhesive tape (Elasticon™, Johnson and Johnson, Inc., New Brunswick, NJ) longitudinally along the plantar aspect and incorporating it at the proximal and distal end of the bandage assists in preventing slippage of the bandage (Figure 16.7a–c).

In addition the author uses a thick cotton bandage as a secondary layer on the distal aspect of the limb from the coronary band to the most proximal aspect of the metatarsus (Figure 16.8b). This also helps to prevent slippage of the hock bandage, and by decreasing the range of motion of the fetlock, restricts movement of the hock. A rigid bandage or splint applied to the distal limb with the fetlock in partial flexion greatly decreases the range of motion of the hock, thereby increasing longevity of the bandage and allowing optimal wound healing. For more information regarding bandage application and splinting techniques, see Chapter 16.

Casting

Application of a cast to a lower-limb wound provides maximal immobilization. Wounds over joints and/or tendons may require immobilization because continued movement disrupts healing. Frequently the hock or carpus is involved in these types of compound injuries. When the limb is mechanically stable, the wound should be bandaged for a few days prior to applying a cast to allow superior wound debridement and permit dissipation of edema, which will ensure a better-fitting cast. Casts minimize the formation of exuberant granulation tissue by reducing motion. Casts should be maintained no longer than necessary over lower-limb wounds for reasons similar to those mentioned for bandages and to minimize the development of cast sores. Generally casts over wounds should be changed every 3 to 10 days but this will depend on the nature and location of the wound and the temperament of the horse. Skin grafts can be used after cast removal to facilitate wound coverage. A splint bandage is continued during this period.[53] For more information regarding splint bandage and cast application, see Chapter 16.

Management of Sequestra

Removal of bony sequestra, either naturally or surgically, is required for a wound to heal completely. Radiographs will identify the presence of the developing sequestrum 2 to 4 weeks after trauma (Figures 8.63 and 8.65b). Once its presence has been confirmed the sequestrum is located and removed by excising the overlying granulation tissue and the area is curetted to eliminate any residually infected tissue from within the involucrum (Figure 8.71). It is unwise to try to dislodge a developing sequestrum by chiseling the bone surface, which could increase the risk of fracture during surgery or recovery. After removal of sequestra, the horse should be recovered from general anesthesia wearing a rigid splint to avoid possible complications such as fracture.[53] Many sequestra, however, can be removed under local anesthesia and sedation while the horse is standing (Figure 8.72a,b). Regular follow-up radiographs should be taken at 2–3 week intervals. For

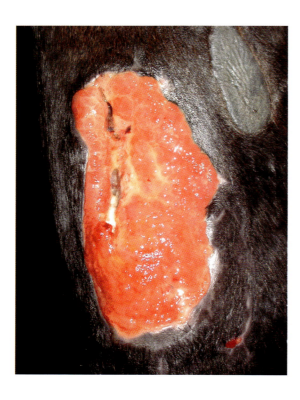

Figure 8.71. Sequestrum formation of the distal medial radius beneath a central area of the wound devoid of granulation tissue. The sequestrum was located and removed by excising overlying granulation tissue and the area was curetted to eliminate any residual infected tissue. Reprinted from *Clinical Techniques in Equine Practice*, Vol 3, R. Reid Hanson, Management of avulsion wounds with exposed bone, p. 195, (2004), with permission from Elsevier Saunders.

more information regarding management of sequestra, see Management of Wounds of the Distal Extremities, in the first section of this chapter.

Skin Grafting

The goals of managing wounds of the distal extremities in horses are to protect the wounds from further trauma and heal the wounds in the most efficient, cost-effective manner possible. This may require application of a skin graft after a suitable bed of granulation tissue has formed. Skin grafts may be applied to fresh wounds that are vascular enough to rapidly produce granulation tissue or on wounds with clean, healthy appearing beds of granulation tissue. Survival of grafts over exposed bone is poor because vascularization occurs slowly. Skin grafting is usually employed following a period of open wound management and after granulation tissue formation. The granulation tissue bed to be grafted should appear red to pink, smooth, and free of any defects. For more information regarding the methods used for skin grafting, see Chapter 11.

Conclusion

Regardless of the methods used to heal wounds over exposed bone, the formation of healthy granulation tissue in the wound is required. Wound healing over exposed bone relies upon the same cellular and humoral elements that contribute to healing of other superficial wounds. The inflammatory, debridement, and repair phases work in concert to prepare the wound bed for granulation tissue formation, contraction, epithelialization, and maturation, but the presence of exposed bone in wounds may directly or indirectly delay healing.

Wounds that expose bone that are fenestrated with 3.2 mm drill holes are covered with granulation tissue earlier than control wounds, because of the formation of granulation tissue directly from the cortical fenestration sites. Cortical fenestration may also be beneficial if it is used with other methods of promoting fibroplasia in larger wounds because there may be an additive effect. Prior to the formation of granulation tissue, hydrogel dressings are comfortable and supportive, provide protection from further wound contamination, assist in

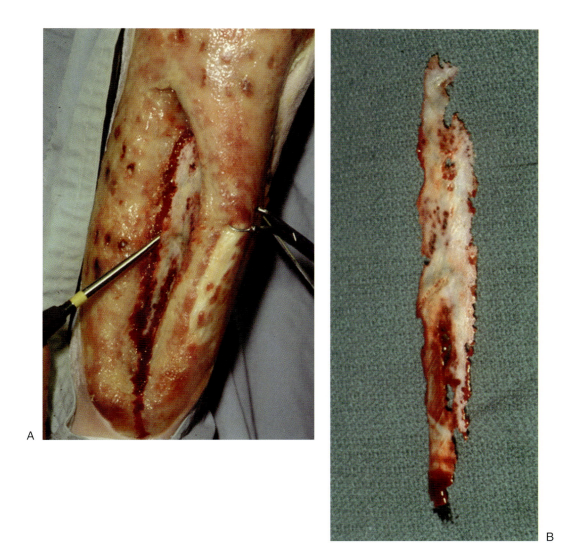

Figure 8.72. Same horse as in Figure 8.77. (A) Sequestra was removed on the standing horse following local anesthesia and sedation. A periosteal elevator was used to elevate the sequestrum from the associated involucrum. (B) Excised sequestra. Courtesy of Dr. T. Stashak.

wound debridement, absorb some wound fluid within their polymer matrix, and reduce limb swelling. Debridement dressings can be used to accelerate the transition from a heavily contaminated to a clean status. This approach facilitates wound debridement and drainage and reduces the bacterial load. This chapter has attempted to provide the reader with the most current methods to enhance the healing of degloving wounds in the horse.

References

1. Clem MF, DeBowes RM, Yovich JV, et al: Osseous sequestration in the horse: a review of 68 cases Vet Surg 1988;17:2
2. Blackford JT, Wan PY, Latimer FG, et al: Treatment of distal extremity lacerations using a flexible hydroactive occlusive dressing. Proc Am Assoc Equine Pract 1993;39:215
3. Gift LJ, DeBowes RM: Wounds associated with osseous sequestration and penetrating foreign bodies. Vet Clin N Am Equine Pract 1989;5:695
4. Wilmink JA, Stolk PW, VanWeeren PR, et al: Differences in second-intention wound healing between horses and ponies: macroscopic aspects. Equine Vet J 1999;31:53

5. Bailin PL, Wheeland RG: Carbon dioxide (CO_2) laser perforation of exposed cranial bone to stimulate granulation tissue. Plast Reconstr Surg 1985;75:898

6. Latenser J, Snow SN, Mohs FE, et al: Power drills to fenestrate exposed bone to stimulate wound healing. J Dermatol Surg Oncol 1991;17:265

7. Johnson RJ: The effects of cortical fenestration on second intention healing of wounds over exposed bone of the distal aspect of the limb of horses. Masters Thesis, Auburn University July 11, 2000.

8. Lee AH, Swaim SF, Newton JC: Wound healing over denuded bone. J Am Anim Hosp Assoc 1987;23:75

9. Schumacher J, Hanselka DV: Skin grafting of the horse. Vet Clin N Am Equine Pract 1989;5:591

10. McGregor IA: Free skin grafts. In Ian McGregor ed. *Fundamental techniques of plastic surgery and their surgical applications (8th edition)*. New York: Churchill Livingstone, 1989, p.39

11. Schumacher J: Skin grafting, In Jorge Auer and John Stick, eds. *Equine surgery (3rd edition)*. St. Louis: Saunders Elsevier, 2006, p.269

12. Wilmink JA, VanWeeren PR, Stolk PW, et al: Differences in second-intention wound healing between horses and ponies: histological aspects. Equine Vet J 1999;31:61

13. Bertone AL, Sullins KE, Stashak TS, et al: Effect of wound location and the use of topical collagen gel on exuberant granulation tissue formation and wound healing in the horse and pony. Am J Vet Res 1985;46:1438

14. Howard RD, Stashak TS, Baxter GM: Evaluation of occlusive dressings for management of full-thickness excisional wounds on the distal portion of the limbs of horses. Am J Vet Res 1993;54:2150

15. Bigbie RB, Schumacher J, Swaim SF, et al: Effects of amnion and live yeast cell derivative on second-intention healing in horses. Am J Vet Res 1991;52:1376

16. Butt TD, Bailey JV, Dowling PM, et al: Comparison of 2 techniques for regional antibiotic delivery to the equine forelimb: intraosseous perfusion vs. intravenous perfusion. Can Vet J 2001;42:617

17. Ford TS, Schumacher J, Brumbaugh GW, et al: Effects of split-thickness and full-thickness skin grafts on secondary graft contraction in horses. Am J Vet Res 1992;53:1572

18. Fretz PB: Low energy laser irradiation treatment for second intention wound healing in horses. Can Vet J 1992;33:650

19. Madison JB, Gronwall RR: Influence of wound shape on wound contraction in the horse. Am J Vet Res 1992;53:1575

20. Schumacher J, Brumbaugh GW, Honnas CM, et al: Kinetics of healing of grafted and non-grafted wounds on the distal portion of the forelimbs of horses. Am J Vet Res 1992;53:1568

21. Rudolph R, Vandeberg J, Ehrlich HP: Wound contraction and scar contracture. In Kelman Cohen, Robert Diegelmann, and William Lindblad, eds. *Wound healing: biochemical and clinical aspects (1st edition)*. Philadelphia: Saunders, 1992, p.96

22. Ehrlich HP, Keefer KA, Myers RL, et al: Vanadate and the absence of myofibroblasts in wound contracture. Arch Surg 1999;134:494

23. Van Den Boom R, Wilmink JM, O'Kane S, et al: Transforming growth factor-β levels during second intention healing are related to the different course of wound contraction in horses and ponies. Wound Repair Regen 2002;10:188

24. Dart AJ, Cries L, Jeffcott LB, et al: The effect of equine recombinant growth hormone on second intention wound healing in horses. Vet Surg 2002;31:314

25. Markel MD, Lopez MJ: Bone biology and fracture healing. In Jorge Auer and John Stick, ed. *Equine surgery (3rd edition)*. St. Louis: Saunders Elsevier, 2006, p.991

26. Stashak TS: Principles of wound healing. In Ted Stashak, ed. *Equine wound management (1st edition)*. Philadelphia: Lea and Febiger, 1991, p.1

27. Stashak TS: Wound management and reconstructive surgery of problems associated with the distal limbs. In Ted Stashak, ed. *Equine wound management (1st edition)*. Philadelphia: Lea and Febiger, 1991, p.163

28. Caron JP, Barber SM, Doige CE, et al: The radiographic and histologic appearance of controlled surgical manipulation of the equine periosteum. Vet Surg 1987;16:13

29. Bradley DM, Swaim SF, Stuart SW: An animal model for research on wound healing over exposed bone. Vet Comp Orthop Traumatol 1998;11:131

30. Specht TE, Colahan PT: Osteostixis for incomplete cortical fracture of the third metacarpal bone: Results in 11 horses. Vet Surg 1990;19:34

31. Bauer SM, Santschi EM, Fialkowski J, et al: Quantification of *staphylococcus aureus* adhesion to equine bone surfaces passivated with plasmalyte™ and hyperimmune plasma. Vet Surg 2004;33:376

32. Scheuch, BC, Van Hoogmoed LM, Wilson DW, et al: Comparison of intraosseous or intravenous infusion for delivery of amikacin sulfate to the tibial tarsal joint of horses. Am J Vet Res 2002:63;374

33. Ramos JR, Howard RD, Pleasant RS, et al: Elution of metronidazole and gentamicin from polymethylmethacrylate beads. Vet Surg 2003:32;251

34. Santschi EM, McGarvey L: In vitro elution of gentamicin from plaster of paris beads. Vet Surg 2003:32;128

35. Swaim SF, Hanson RR, Coates JR: Pressure wounds in animals. Compend Contin Educ Pract Vet 1996;18:203

36. Campbell BG: Current concepts and materials in wound bandaging. Proc N Am Vet Conf 2004;18:1217

37. Bertone AL: Second-intention healing. Vet Clin N Am Equine Pract 1989;5:539
38. Farstvedt E, Stashak TS, Othic A: Update on topical wound medications. Clin Tech in Eq Pract 2004:3;164
39. Berry DB, Sullins KE: Effects of topical application of antimicrobials and bandaging on healing and granulation tissue formation in wounds of the distal aspect of the limbs in horses. Am J Vet Res 2003:64;88
40. Kingsley A: The use of honey on the treatment of infected wounds: case studies. Brit J Nurs 2001;10:S13 (suppl 22)
41. Tonks AJ, Cooper RA, Jones KP, et al: Honey stimulates inflammatory cytokine production from monocytes. Cytokine 2003:21;242
42. Swaim SF: Topical wound medications: A review. J Am Vet Med Assoc 1987:190;188
43. Engelen M, Besche B, Lefay MP, et al: Effects of ketanserin on hypergranulation tissue formation, infection, and healing on equine lower limb wounds. Can Vet J 2004:45;144
44. Rickets CH, Martin L, Faria DT, et al: Cytokine mRNA changes during the treatment of hypertrophic scars with silicone and non silicone gel dressings. Dermatol Surg 1996:22;955
45. Ducharme-Desjarlais M, Celeste CJ, Lepault E, et al: Effect of a silicone-containing dressing on exuberant granulation tissue formation and wound repair in the horse. Am J Vet Res 2005;66:1133
46. Theoret L: Wound repair in the horse: Problems and proposed innovate solutions. Clin Tech in Eq Pract 2004:3;134
47. Baxter GM: Wound healing and delayed wound closure in the lower limb of the horse. Equine Pract 1988;10:23
48. Woolen N, DeBowes RM, Leipold HW, et al: A comparison of four types of therapy for the treatment of full thickness skin wounds of the horse, in Proc Am Assoc Equine Pract 1987;33:569
49. Hosgood G: Wound healing: the role of platelet-derived growth factor and transforming growth factor beta. Vet Surg 1993;22:490
50. Stashak TS: Selected factors that affect wound healing. In Ted Stashak, ed. *Equine wound management (1st edition)*. Philadelphia: Lea and Febiger, 1991, p.19
51. Beck LS, Deguzman L, Lee WP, et al: TGF-beta 1 accelerates wound healing: reversal of steroid-impaired healing in rats and rabbits. Growth Factors 1991:5;295
52. Hashimoto I, Nakanishi H, Shono Y, et al: Angiostatic effects of corticosteroid on wound healing on the rabbit ear. J Med Invest 2002:49;61
53. Knottenbelt DC. *Handbook of equine wound management (1st edition)*. London: Saunders, 2003, p.95

8.3 Treatment of Exuberant Granulation Tissue

Christine L. Theoret, DMV, PhD, Diplomate ACVS, **and Jacintha M. Wilmink,** DVM, PhD, Diplomate RNVA

Introduction

The development of exuberant granulation tissue (EGT) in the horse has long been an enigma, but despite research to unravel this phenomenon, there is currently no universally accepted treatment protocol. Several studies have focused on EGT over the last decade. The findings and interpretations of these investigations have been united in this chapter. They appear to complement one another and have shed light on one of the most common complications disturbing the repair of limb wounds in horses. The etiology of EGT appears to be multifactorial, involving environmental, biochemical, immunological, and genetic factors. New insights on the physiology/pathology, predisposing factors, prevention, and treatment of EGT are described and discussed herein.

Physiology and Pathology

Fibroplasia and the Development of Exuberant Granulation Tissue

Fibroplasia, or the formation of granulation tissue, is an essential phase of wound healing. Apart from the nuisance of becoming exuberant, granulation tissue has many important functions, which change continuously during the healing process. It fills in the wound gap, forms a barrier against external contaminants, provides myofibroblasts for wound contraction, and forms the bed over which epithelium can migrate.

Granulation tissue provides several cell types that have important functions during healing. Endothelial cells form capillaries and blood vessels through which both oxygen and nutrients are transported to sustain cell metabolism and through which leukocytes can migrate into the wound site. Leukocytes clear the wound of contaminating agents and debris. Furthermore, they recruit additional inflammatory and mesenchymal cells and initiate the healing process. Fibroblasts form the extracellular matrix (ECM) needed to support cell division, growth, and migration. The composition of ECM gradually changes as it is remodeled through the simultaneous synthesis and degradation of components. Ideally, proliferation of granulation tissue decreases as soon as the wound is filled in, and contraction and epithelialization ensue. However, in many limb wounds of horses, proliferation continues for an indefinite period, resulting in the formation of EGT.

Exuberant granulation tissue is typically irregular and unhealthy in appearance, with many grooves and clefts, and protrudes over the wound margins. It is seen often in limb wounds but rarely in body wounds. Exuberant granulation tissue is characterized histologically by chronic inflammation and remains of fibrin deposits which have not been cleared by the acute inflammatory response. Histologically, the tissue has an immature, chaotic appearance due to its disorganized cellular population (Figures 8.73a,b).[1,2] Within wounds suffering from EGT, cellular proliferation remains active, contraction is delayed, and the protruding granulation tissue may physically impede epithelial migration and/or may inhibit epithelial cell mitosis.[2,3]

Fibroblast Phenotype and Function

The fibroblast, the major cell type in granulation tissue and EGT, changes its phenotype during healing. Fibroblast phenotype and function are closely related. When healing is uncomplicated, phenotypes reflect the various needs of the wound as healing progresses, and they succeed one another as the wound matures.

This process depends on many factors in the wound environment. Initially, fibroblasts have a migratory phenotype, allowing them to move from the surrounding tissues into the wound bed. Migration depends on many chemoattractive agents in the wound that are generated by the injury and released by platelets and macrophages at the wound border.[4] Once at its ultimate destination, the fibroblast phenotype changes into a proliferative and synthetic form. The number of fibroblasts increases and ECM is produced.

Fibroblast proliferation is strongly enhanced by low oxygen tension (hypoxia),[5] while the synthesis of ECM is stimulated by several cytokines, such as transforming growth factor beta (TGF-β), either released by inflammatory cells or by the fibroblasts themselves. Thereafter, fibroblasts can differentiate into myofibroblasts, the phenotype which contains smooth muscle actin filaments and can bring the wound edges together via the contractile force exerted by these filaments.[6] Both differentiation into myofibroblasts and the generation of contractile forces are also strongly stimulated by TGF-β but inhibited by many other mediators produced during chronic inflammation.

Once wound contraction ceases, fibroblasts and myofibroblasts disappear from the wound by apoptosis (i.e., fragmentation followed by phagocytosis by macrophages and activated fibroblasts) and the cellularity of the repair tissue diminishes.[7,8] Apoptosis, a form of programmed cell death, is thus critical to the transition from

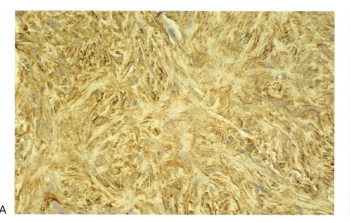
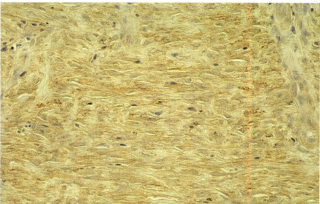

A   B

Figure 8.73. Exuberant granulation tissue, when viewed histologically, shows (A) a high number of chaotically arranged cells and capillaries and looks very immature in contrast to (B) the regularly arranged cells and parallel capillaries of more differentiated and contracting granulation tissue. Smooth muscle actin staining. Reprinted with permission.[57]

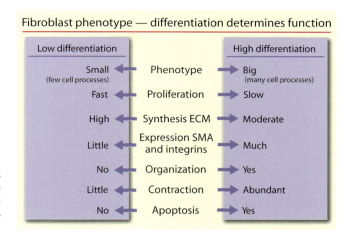

Figure 8.74 Fibroblast phenotype—differentiation determines function in an exclusive way; fibroblasts able to contract have different phenotypic features and are more differentiated than those exhibiting a proliferating phenotype. Reference of all facts with exception of apoptosis;[13] apoptosis[43]

one phase of repair (proliferation and contraction) to the next (remodeling). It has been postulated that myofibroblasts represent the terminal differentiation state of fibroblasts following which apoptosis can occur. Apoptosis seems induced by anoxic circumstances,[9,10,11] whereas hypoxia, via the expression of hypoxia-inducible factor (HIF)-1α, can exert anti-apoptotic effects and thus encourage fibroplasia.[12]

It has been observed that the development of EGT in a wound coincides with a disordered succession of fibroblast phenotypes. Specifically, the proliferative and synthetic phenotypes predominate in EGT while differentiation into functional myofibroblasts is delayed. This is consistent with the microscopic observation in limb wounds that persistent mitotic activity accompanies chaotically arranged myofibroblasts, which is not conducive to contraction,[1,2] and the clinical observation that the presence of EGT is often coupled with poor wound contraction. Confirmation of this phenomenon was established in vitro, where the proliferative rate appeared inversely proportional to the contraction capacity of fibroblasts because rapidly proliferating fibroblasts produced lower contractile forces (Figure 8.74).[13] Indeed, as myofibroblasts represent the terminal differentiation state of fibroblasts, tardy progression to the contractile phenotype also implies that apoptosis will be impaired and high cellularity will be maintained, favoring the development of EGT.

Because EGT occurs primarily in poorly contracting limb wounds as opposed to quickly contracting body wounds, it was hypothesized that fibroblasts from diverse anatomical origins might possess inherently different characteristics responsible for the variable succession of phenotypes. However, it was found that the elevated mitotic activity in limb wounds is not based on innate differences in growth characteristics between limb and trunk fibroblasts because those of limb origin grow significantly more slowly than those of trunk origin, at least in vitro.[13,14] Additionally, the inadequate wound contraction seen in limb wounds is not based on limited inherent contractile capacity of limb fibroblasts; fibroblasts from limbs contracted more than those from trunk origin, at least in vitro.[13]

In summary, it appears that the different phenotypes and functions attributed to either limb or trunk fibroblasts, as well as the contrasting modes of repair characterizing limb and body wounds, are not based on distinct intrinsic cellular characteristics but instead must be the result of other factors. The extracellular environment's biochemical, molecular, and physical components govern the fibroblast phenotype, whereas the phenotype will determine the fibroblast's response to environmental signals.[6]

Factors Affecting the Formation of Exuberant Granulation Tissue

While the exact causes have not yet been established, research has revealed a number of factors that may contribute to the excessive development of granulation tissue during wound repair in the horse. Some of these factors cannot be controlled or can be only partially controlled while others may be prevented or eliminated to a large extent.

Physiological Factors

Inflammatory Response

An inefficient inflammatory response to injury is hypothesized as determining fibroblast phenotype and function and thus playing an important role in the development of EGT in limb wounds of horses (Figure 8.75).[15] It is known that following trauma the acute inflammatory response in limb wounds of horses is weaker during the first 3 weeks and levels of TGF-β are lower during the first 10 days compared to those which occur in ponies.[2,16,17] TGF-β1 not only stimulates production of ECM but also favors the differentiation of fibroblasts into myofibroblasts, which encourages contraction. Inferior initial TGF-β levels may delay this differentiation, resulting in the presence of fewer myofibroblasts in favor of the rapidly proliferating and synthesizing phenotypes. A reduced number of myofibroblasts means that wound contraction is delayed and inefficient, whereas fibroblast proliferation and ECM synthesis continue (Figure 8.75).

The weak acute inflammatory response was shown to be followed by a persistent or chronic inflammatory response,[2] due in part to the continued presence of contaminants and non-viable tissue not resolved by the initial, weak response. Additionally, delayed contraction means that the surface area of an open wound remains larger, thus perpetuating the inflammatory response because leukocytes only disappear after epithelium migrates over the surface. The significant presence of leukocytes in exposed granulation tissue may explain up-regulated synthesis of cytokines in the absence of epithelium,[18] and may lower wound oxygen tension as a result of the high oxygen consumption by leukocytes. Persistence of mediators such as TGF-β, platelet-derived growth factor (PDGF), and fibroblast growth factor (FGF) induce fibrosis, whereas prostaglandin (PG)E$_1$, PGE$_2$, and interferon (IFN)γ inhibit wound contraction, while yet others such as tumor necrosis factor (TNF)α, interleukin (IL)-1 and IL-6 do both (Figure 8.75).[19,20] Lower oxygen tension further stimulates fibroblast proliferation and ECM production.[5] It is thus likely that the persistent inflammation found in limb wounds of horses both enhances the formation of EGT and inhibits wound contraction, phenomena which are often seen simultaneously in the clinical setting. This hypothesis is reinforced by the fact that corticosteroids, potent anti-inflammatory drugs, decrease EGT formation in the wounds of horses.[21]

In summary, the combination of an inefficient, weak, acute inflammatory response and the ensuing chronic inflammation in limb wounds of horses delays the differentiation of fibroblasts into myofibroblasts, reducing wound contraction and favoring fibroblast proliferation and protein synthesis. This results in a fast increase in tissue volume by proliferation rather than a decrease in tissue volume by contraction (Figure 8.76). The chronic inflammation inherent to second intention healing in limb wounds of horses, while often unrecognized clinically because of the mild symptoms, is thus no doubt a very important trigger of EGT formation.[15] The interaction between inflammation, subsequent formation of EGT, and lack of wound contraction establishes a vicious cycle because these physiological phenomena stimulate one another.

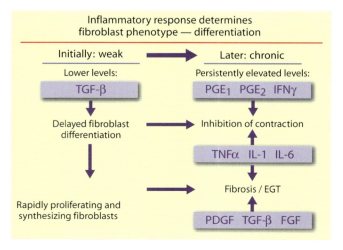

Figure 8.75. Fibroblast phenotype and differentiation is influenced by several cytokines present during the acute and chronic inflammatory response to wounding. Both the inefficient, weak acute inflammatory response and the ensuing chronic inflammation in limb wounds of horses delay the differentiation of fibroblasts into myofibroblasts, ultimately reducing wound contraction and favoring fibroblast proliferation.

Clinical consequences of differences
in fibroblast phenotype — differentiation

Low differentiation	High differentiation
↓	↓
Increase in tissue volume	Decrease in tissue volume

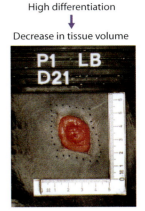

Figure 8.76. Experimental wounds, initially of the same size, 21 days after creation on the limb of a horse (left) or on the buttock of a pony (right), which show the clinical consequences of differences in fibroblast phenotype and differentiation. Delayed differentiation of fibroblasts in limb wounds favors their proliferation but inhibits wound contraction, which results in an increase in tissue volume. In contrast, the faster differentiation of fibroblasts into myofibroblasts in buttock wounds and ensuing contraction reduces tissue volume.

Local Cytokine Profile

The aforementioned development of chronic inflammation in limb wounds of horses substantiates several studies reporting that the local cytokine profile in limb wounds is rich in fibrogenic mediators which encourage migration, proliferation, and synthesis, but inhibit ECM turnover.[16,22,23,24] One of these mediators, TGF-β1, stimulates fibroblast proliferation and the production of ECM proteins such as fibronectin and collagen,[25] while inhibiting the degradation of ECM.[26,27] It is thus noteworthy that the expression of TGF-β1 persists in limb wounds throughout the proliferative phase of repair, whereas it quickly returns to baseline values in thoracic wounds after the initial inflammatory phase.[16,23] Lasting production of TGF-β1 may partially be the work of the wound fibroblast, which also expresses more TGF-β receptors;[28,29] the signaling components are thus in place to stimulate cellular proliferation and encourage the synthesis of ECM components.

The persistent expression of TGF-β1 can be explained, at least in part, by factors characterizing limb wounds in horses: absence of epithelium, presence of tightly-fixed surrounding skin, and local tissue hypoxia. It has been shown that synthesis of pro-fibrotic cytokines is up-regulated in the absence of an epithelial cover, as mentioned before.[18] Persistent mechanical tension in a wound also plays a role because mechanical unloading of fibroblasts is required to desensitize cytokine receptors, abrogating cytokine responsiveness, which favors apoptosis.[30] Consequently, relief of mechanical stress is necessary for a wound to progress from granulation tissue to scar via apoptosis.[30] Additionally, the secretion of TGF-β1 by fibroblasts is strongly stimulated by low oxygen tension (see below).[31] While not yet verified, hypoxia is likely present in granulation tissue of limb wounds, because microvessel occlusion is found significantly more often in this location than in wounds of the body.[32]

Collagen Synthesis, Deposition, and Lysis

It has been assumed for some time that aberrant collagen metabolism plays a role in the formation of EGT. Theoretically, either abundant synthesis or impaired lysis may lead to excessive collagen deposition. The horse forms collagen speedily in response to wounding, indicating a prompt and excessive connective tissue response compared to other species.[33] As described above, protracted expression of TGF-β1 in limb wounds may give rise to excessive formation of collagen and other ECM proteins.[16,23] Furthermore, a recent study comparing mRNA levels for type-I collagen, collagenase (MMP-1), and tissue inhibitor of metalloproteinase (TIMP)-1 found more type-1 collagen mRNA in limb wounds, no difference in expression of MMP-1 mRNA between limb and thoracic wounds, and greater TIMP-1 mRNA levels in limb wounds than in thoracic wounds both 1 and 4 weeks after injury.[24] Because TIMP-1 inhibits collagen lysis, high levels present 4 weeks post-wounding might favor accumulation of ECM, as is commonly seen in wounds located on the lower limb. The authors deduced that an imbalance between collagen synthesis and degradation is likely correlated to the development of EGT and that agents inhibiting collagen synthesis or stimulating the activity of MMPs, in particular collagenase, may represent novel treatment options. However, because an imbalance between synthesis and degradation of a single ECM component is not likely to be the sole basis of EGT formation, the effect of influencing only collagen metabolism might be limited. Indeed, an attempt to accelerate collagen maturation to prevent the excessive formation of granulation tissue, by use of a preformed collagen gel, yielded no positive effects.[34] It is more likely that stimulation of the entire synthetic machinery, including fibroblast proliferation and their production of ECM components, by certain mediators such as TGF-β1, play a role in EGT formation. As such, specifically targeting fibroblast function may hold more potential.

Wound Oxygenation

Hypoxia within the granulation tissue is thought to contribute to the development of EGT since the lumens of microvessels populating limb wounds have been shown to be occluded significantly more often than those within thoracic wounds,[32] possibly as a result of endothelial cell hypertrophy.[11] Hypoxia is known to stimulate both proliferation of fibroblasts[35] and synthesis of ECM components by these cells.[36] Indeed, low oxygen tension stimulates fibroblasts to secrete PDGF and up to 9-fold more TGF-β1.[31] Thus, hypoxia, via TGF-β and PDGF, enhances collagen production by activating the synthesis and transcription of the α1(I) procollagen gene[36,37] and hinders fibrinolysis, collagen degradation, and matrix remodeling by decreasing the synthesis of MMPs[38] such as collagenase as well as plasminogen activator (PA).[39,40]

Apoptotic Process

As mentioned previously, a deficient apoptotic process may contribute to the persistent mitotic activity present in limb wounds. It was recently found that the balance of apoptotic signals is altered against apoptosis in limb versus body wounds.[32] Persisting TGF-β1 levels in limb wounds may play a role because this particular cytokine appears to have an anti-apoptotic effect on fibroblasts.[41,42] Furthermore, in addition to encouraging the synthesis of fibrogenic cytokines, the absence of an epithelial cover such as afflicts EGT debilitates apoptosis because many of the signals which favor cell elimination by this process are normally released by the epithelial cell.[43] Apoptosis signals also participate in decreasing collagen deposition, not only by reducing fibroblast numbers but also by activating collagenase.[43]

If the signal to down-regulate fibroblast and myofibroblast activity is delayed beyond a specific point in time, then apoptosis is permanently impaired.[43] This may explain why wounds chronically affected with EGT are unlikely to resolve spontaneously; indeed, the impairment of apoptosis will limit the elimination of unwanted cells and subsequent transition to the next phase of repair.

General Clinical Factors

Wound Location

The likelihood that a wound will develop EGT depends upon its anatomical location. Wounds of the body heal quickly and without the formation of EGT in contrast to limb wounds, which heal slowly and are prone to excessive fibroplasia. The exact location of the wound on the limb further influences healing and formation of EGT; wounds over the dorsal aspect of the metacarpo/metatarsophalangeal (fetlock) joint heal more slowly than similar wounds located over the dorsal metatacarpus/metatarsus.[34,44] Additionally, limb wounds located on the extensor and flexor surfaces of joints as well as in the heel bulb region appear prone to the development of EGT.

These clinical differences are assumed to relate to movement, which tears the granulation tissue and causes grooves and clefts and incites further inflammation and cell proliferation (Figure 8.77). The movement of partially lacerated or frayed tendons may exert a similar influence. Indeed, restricting movement by applying a cast or splint can favor healing and reduce EGT formation in these wounds, despite the fact that the local environment created by the cast would normally favor the formation of EGT.[45]

Another factor enhancing the formation of EGT in the distal limb is the relative lack of tissue coverage of the underlying bone, and subsequently a reduced vascular bed and limited collateral circulation. Following trauma, this would result in slightly lower oxygen tension in the healing wound. As mentioned before, a hypoxic environment stimulates the proliferation of fibroblasts and the synthesis of cytokines such as PDGF and TGF-β, increasing the production of collagen and other ECM components.[31] Conversely, thick and well-vascularized

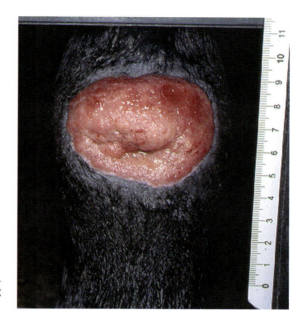

Figure 8.77. A 3-week-old wound at the dorsal surface of the fetlock joint. The groove in the granulation tissue is probably caused by tearing during flexion, which predisposes to EGT formation.

musculature covers most structures of the trunk, such that perfusion of a wound is not usually disturbed by injury.

Breed

Formation of EGT is influenced by the breed; however, not in an exclusive manner. Horses and ponies both can develop EGT, although to differing extents.[1] Ponies tend to form EGT with lesser frequency and quantity, and it disappears spontaneously after the wound is left uncovered. In contrast, horses form more EGT, which does not disappear and must be surgically excised. This inconsistent predilection could act as a confounding factor which would explain the conflicting conclusions of past investigations of whether ponies heal with or without EGT.[21,34,45] It also substantiates the clinical impression that wounds of ponies require less trimming, whereas wounds of horses are more reliably plagued with EGT.

Infection- and Inflammation-related Factors

Many factors in the wound can stimulate the overproduction of granulation tissue; most of them are infection- and/or inflammation-related. A generalized wound infection may not result in EGT but might arrest healing, resulting in an indolent wound. On the other hand, local infection related to the presence of bony sequestra; necrotic segments of tendons, ligaments, or other tissue; and/or foreign bodies triggers a chronic inflammatory response leading to the aforementioned cycle, especially when the condition is long-standing. Similarly, wound contamination with dirt or bacteria strongly attracts leukocytes, leading to chronic inflammation. The presence of an abundant periosteal reaction can also provoke the formation of EGT, probably as a result of chronic inflammation, although bacterial interference may also contribute.

This emphasizes the importance of a thorough examination of a wound with EGT in an effort to identify or exclude infection- and inflammation-related factors. In the event that no specific causal factor can be incriminated, it may well be that the inherent chronic inflammatory response commonly occurring in limb wounds of horses is the trigger for the formation of EGT. This may in fact be the most common cause of EGT, which is often not recognized because the symptoms may be limited to irregularity of the wound surface accompanied by the limited presence of purulent exudate. These clinical symptoms as well as bacterial cultures do not indicate a wound infection. However, the wound usually improves dramatically by reducing surface contamination in combination with a single local application of corticosteroids, a fact which substantiates the involvement of chronic inflammation.

Specific Clinical Factors

Bandages and Casts

Bandages and casts applied to full-thickness distal limb wounds have been shown to promote the formation of EGT.[21,28,32,44,45,46] This effect is thought to result from the following phenomena:

- An increase in the oxygen gradient between tissue and wound surface, which stimulates angiogenesis[47]
- A reduction in oxygen tension in the wound tissues, which enhances fibroblast proliferation[5]
- The creation of a moist, warm and acidic environment, which favors cellular migration and proliferation.

Furthermore, some dressings can irritate the wound, causing exudate to accumulate at its surface. All of these features prompt the formation of EGT.[48] In this respect, management practices can explain, at least partially, why EGT is more often seen in limb wounds because these are usually bandaged while body wounds are not. Interestingly, it appears that bandaged body wounds also form EGT, albeit to a lesser degree.[1] It is thus likely that EGT would form more often in body wounds if these were routinely bandaged. In conclusion, the influence of occlusion may contribute to the effect of location on EGT formation.

The use of pressure bandages in view of restraining excessive fibroplasia is counterproductive. These bandages may effectively suppress the swelling of young edematous granulation tissue, but generally do not impair its formation.

The precise effect of bandages on the development of EGT is dependent on the type of dressing contacting the wound surface. For example, dressings made of equine amnion significantly reduced the formation of EGT and accelerated healing when compared to synthetic non-adherent control dressings (Release®, Johnson and Johnson, New Brunswick, NJ).[49] However, such an effect could not be confirmed in a later study, in which amnion was compared with a non-adherent gauze pad (Telfa™, Covidien Animal Health/Kendall, Dublin, OH).[50]

Interestingly, these studies not only provide information about the effect of equine amnion but also about the effect of the control dressings, one of which is more beneficial to healing than the other. Synthetic fully occlusive dressings (BioDres®, DVM Pharmaceuticals Inc., Miami, FL) stimulate the formation of EGT, thus increasing the need to trim granulation tissue,[50] possibly by favoring bacterial proliferation and encouraging inflammation in response to excess accumulation of wound exudate. In contrast, synthetic non-adherent occlusive silicone gel dressings (CicaCare®, Smith & Nephew, Hull, UK), prevented the formation of EGT in horse limb wounds when compared to a non-adherent, permeable control dressing (Melolite®, Smith & Nephew, Hull, UK).[10]

The silicone gel dressings caused more frequent occlusion of microvessels, which, it was postulated, might generate anoxia within the underlying granulation tissue, forcing fibroblasts to undergo apoptosis rather than proliferate and secrete further ECM components. Furthermore, while this remains to be proven, application of a silicone dressing may relieve mechanical tension in the wound, abrogating cellular responsiveness to TGF-β, which would encourage apoptosis. Indeed, the silicone dressing decreased the expression of an apoptosis inhibitor, although more apoptosis could not be confirmed quantitatively in this particular study.[10]

The fact that bandages and casts have been shown to promote the formation of EGT does not prohibit their use in wound management. To the contrary, bandages exert many positive influences on healing, which should be used. They keep the wound clean and prevent contamination and irritation by environmental factors such as dirt and straw, all of which induce inflammation. They facilitate administration of local wound therapies, stimulate more rapid formation of granulation tissue, which is initially required, accelerate epithelialization due to the moist environment, encourage the development of a more cosmetic scar,[45] reduce the risk for sarcoid transformation of the wound, and prevent trauma. Additionally, casts restrict movement in highly mobile regions, thus reducing disruption of the healing process. All of these functions limit the development of EGT. Therefore, both bandages and casts are important components of second intention healing, since the aim to support the overall healing process largely exceeds the need to prevent EGT.

Iatrogenic Factors

The way in which a wound is managed in the early stages has a dramatic effect on the time required for healing as well as the formation of EGT. Application of non-physiological materials, including powders and strong chemicals (e.g., full-strength antiseptics) as well as some antibiotics, may adversely affect wound healing.

Additionally, application of caustic substances—including copper sulfate, nitric acid, acetic/malic acid mixtures, silver nitrate, triple dye, supersaturated potassium permanganate, hypochlorite (Dakin's solution), lye, and many other home remedies—in an effort to prevent or treat EGT also seriously delays repair. These caustics induce necrosis not only of the granulation tissue but also of the migrating and proliferating epithelium.[48,51,52]

Cryogenic surgery applied to granulating wounds similarly delays healing.[45] Indeed, the resultant necrosis encourages a chronic inflammatory response and the release of many mediators which inhibit wound contraction and overstimulate cellular proliferation as described before. Healing by both epithelialization and wound contraction is arrested and the stimulus for formation of granulation tissue accrued, leading to a recurrence of EGT. Therefore, cautery of any type delays healing and promotes more EGT. When wounds treated in this way eventually heal, they are frequently characterized by unacceptable scarring.[52] The aforementioned problem is still encountered in some equine practices, because many owners manage a wound themselves prior to consulting a veterinarian.

Differential Diagnoses

Exuberant granulation tissue can be confused with tumors, in particular equine sarcoids (Figures 8.78a,b). First, an equine wound can transform into a sarcoid, which is a serious cause of wound healing failure (for more information, see Chapter 14). Sarcoid transformation can occur at any wound site but there are remarkable differences in the type of sarcoid that develops. In distal limb wounds, the sarcoid is invariably fibroblastic in nature, which explains the confusion with EGT. Transformation can occur very soon after wounding, and also

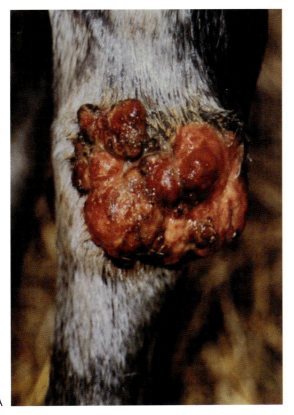
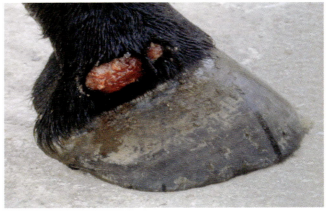

Figure 8.78. (A) A wire wound on the dorsal surface of the tarsus of a 5-year-old Andalusian mare, which failed to heal. Biopsy confirmed pure sarcoid in the upper area and a mixture of sarcoid and EGT in the lower regions of the wound site. (B) Five-week-old wound in the pastern region of a thoroughbred-cross gelding. The horse was admitted because the wound remained exuberant. Tissue was excised and examined histologically to diagnose a pure fibroblastic sarcoid. Courtesy of Dr. D. Knottenbelt. Reprinted with permission.[57]

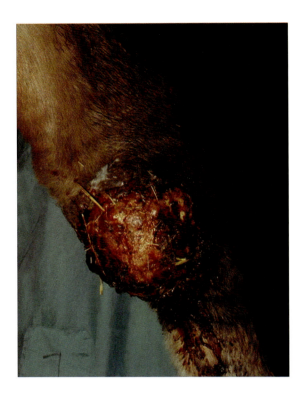

Figure 8.79. Wound on the dorsal surface of the tarsus which was treated for 6 months without resolution. Histology of biopsied tissue confirmed transformation to a squamous cell carcinoma. Courtesy of Dr. T.S. Stashak.

in very young foals.[52] Horses with sarcoids at other sites appear to be particularly prone to sarcoid transformation of wounds, as are those in close contact with other horses bearing sarcoids. Transformation is also more likely in uncovered wounds in summer months, when flies are abundant; as such the likelihood of transformation depends on geographical region. Although uncommon, chronic granulating wounds can also transform into a squamous cell carcinoma (Figure 8.79). Second, tumors such as sarcoids, some hemangiomas, and squamous cell carcinomas can develop independently of an apparent wound and adopt the aspect of granulation tissue during growth.

Therefore, in wounds showing particularly complicated healing or frequent recurrence of EGT, excised tissue or a biopsy should be obtained for histological examination and definitive diagnosis. This is critical because the current best practice for managing EGT is contraindicated in the management of most sarcoid lesions or other tumors.[52]

Prevention of Exuberant Granulation Tissue

Exclusion of Infection- and Inflammation-related Factors

The likelihood of EGT formation can be reduced by excluding causal factors, particularly those that are infection- and inflammation-related. The wound should be carefully examined for bony sequestra, necrotic segments of tendon or ligament, foreign bodies, etc. Irritating and caustic substances should not be applied to the wound surface, which must be kept clean. Despite harboring a microclimate conducive to cellular proliferation and ECM synthesis, bandages play an important role in preventing additional contamination and trauma, protecting exposed bone and tendons from dessication and contamination and reducing motion, thus decreasing the impetus for EGT formation.

Use of Bandages

Because bandages favor fibroplasia it may be desirable in some situations to limit the development of EGT by leaving the wound unbandaged. This should occur once the wound has filled in with healthy appearing granulation tissue. This approach is reasonable when less labor-intensive treatment is preferred; for example, when costs must be limited, the horse is difficult to treat, or the cosmetic result is of less importance. In some cases it may even be acceptable to leave the granulating wound temporarily unbandaged until the granulation bed is flat and wound contraction begins. This approach will also reduce the risk of developing EGT. The wound can subsequently be bandaged with a semi-occlusive dressing to encourage epithelialization. This "alternating approach" may hold some appeal in cases in which EGT frequently recurs; however, in most clinical cases bandaging is maintained in an uninterrupted manner until complete healing for practical reasons.

The fact that bandages favor the development of EGT, which itself delays healing, has led to the practice of controlling EGT formation by omitting bandaging once a wound has filled with granulation tissue. This approach was partly inspired by evidence that unbandaged experimental wounds in ponies healed faster and without EGT, although with more scarring, than did bandaged wounds in which healing was delayed by interfering EGT.[45]

Other studies have since determined that this may not be so straightforward. Healing of unbandaged and bandaged wounds in horses was of similar duration when interfering EGT was excised upon formation such that it did not negatively impact healing.[46] Moreover, another study showed that healing of unbandaged experimental wounds in horses was slower than that occurring in bandaged wounds, despite the less frequent formation of EGT, probably because the unbandaged wounds became more contaminated and dessicated during the study.[44]

In conclusion, the fact that bandages favor the formation of EGT, which can subsequently delay healing, must not be taken to mean that healing can be stimulated by leaving off bandages. When managed correctly, EGT does not delay healing and bandages mainly bear advantages depending on the type of dressing contacting the wound surface. Furthermore, the extensiveness of many traumatic wounds dealt with in the clinical setting often makes bandaging obligatory, in contrast with wounds created for experimental purposes that can harmlessly be left unbandaged.

Skin Grafts

Skin grafts exert a significant inhibitory effect on the formation of EGT; proliferation of endothelial cells as well as fibroblast proliferative and synthetic activities are repressed. It is proposed that the inhibitory effect of grafts on fibroblast proliferation and collagen synthesis may be regulated by a soluble epithelial-derived product which potentiates apoptosis of underlying cells.[43,53] A vascularized skin flap also favors fibroblast and vascular cell apoptosis and rapid remodeling of the underlying granulation tissue. This is likely the result of reduced TGF-β1 expression along with increased ECM degradation due to an altered balance between MMPs and their inhibitor TIMP-1, as well as increased inducible nitric oxide synthase (iNOS) expression generating free radicals.[54] Additionally, the ability of the graft to reduce the size of the exposed wound area and thus the inflammatory response will contribute to its inhibitory effect on the development of EGT. It is recommended that the graft be obtained from a site which normally heals well and in which contraction is prominent (e.g., lateral cervical, abdominal, or pectoral regions).[55]

Treatment of Exuberant Granulation Tissue

The treatment of EGT depends, to a certain extent, upon the age of the wound and the nature of the granulation tissue. This section describes the situations most often encountered clinically.

Protruding Young Edematous Granulation Tissue

Young edematous granulation tissue protruding just above the wound margins generally does not require special treatment. Swelling can usually be limited by moderate pressure applied by a bandage; increased swelling is noted upon bandage change. Protrusion of the tissue increases when the wound is left uncovered for a short time (Figure 8.80). Frequently, the edematous swelling disappears when wound contraction begins. The tissue may be characterized as EGT when the protrusion feels firm and takes on a granular appearance. As soon as firm tissue protrudes over the wound margins, it should be treated.

Exuberant Granulation Tissue in General

Most limb wounds will form EGT to some degree during the process of wound healing. It is important to determine whether the periosteum was injured upon exposure of cortical bone or if partial or complete rupture

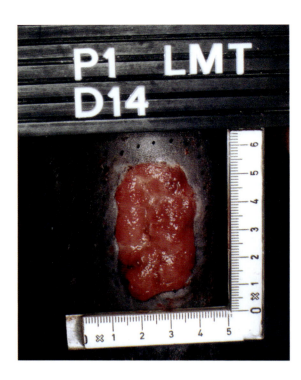

Figure 8.80. Example of a 2-week-old wound on a pony limb showing edematous, protruding granulation tissue which does not yet qualify as EGT. Such increase of the swelling can be seen upon bandage change. Reprinted with permission.[57]

of a tendon or ligament has occurred. Bone sequestra, necrotic parts of tendons or ligaments, foreign bodies, or dirt can induce and maintain chronic inflammation, which favors the development of EGT; therefore, these factors should be resolved. Careful and thorough examination of the wound is important.

Clefts that have formed within the new granulation tissue should be palpated with both flexible and rigid sterile probes to identify draining tracts. Complementary diagnostic modalities such as radiographic or ultra-sonographic examination may be required; for example, in the case of exposed cortical bone, radiographs should be taken to rule out the possibility of a bone sequestrum. When the wound is located near or over a joint, movement is likely the grounds for the excess formation of granulation tissue. Immobilization, via the application of a cast, can be helpful when the granulation tissue is freshly exuberant and appears healthy. However, in cases in which the EGT is due to chronic inflammation and requires repeated treatment, a bandage splint is preferred.

When no underlying inciting cause can be found, the most probable cause for the formation of EGT is the inherent chronic inflammatory response, characteristic of limb wounds of horses. Reduction of surface contamination followed by a single topical application of corticosteroids will halt the aforementioned vicious cycle and allow healing to ensue.

In most cases, treatment of EGT is straightforward and surgical excision appears to be the best choice.[15] This should be done as soon as the granulation tissue protrudes above the wound margins. Excision can be performed in the standing horse and anesthesia of the wound is not necessary because granulation tissue is not innervated. Care must be taken to preserve the newly migrating epithelium at the wound periphery. The goal of surgical excision is to remove excess and nonviable tissue, as well as gross contaminants and, consequently, a large number of leukocytes present in the superficial layer of the granulation tissue. This will diminish the stimulus for chronic inflammation (Figures 8.81a–c).[15]

Dramatic improvement of the health of the wound surface is usually achieved when excision is preceded by aseptic preparation of the wound site and followed by sterile bandaging and a short period of topical anti-bacterial or antiseptic therapy to further reduce surface contamination (Figs 8.81a–c). Indeed, repair gets a new impulse: wound contraction is "jump-started" and epithelialization takes place. This said, resection may have to be repeated a few times.

The use of silicone gel dressings to prevent recurrence of EGT in horses has recently been validated.[10] The dressing should be applied following surgical excision of EGT and maintained until wound contraction and

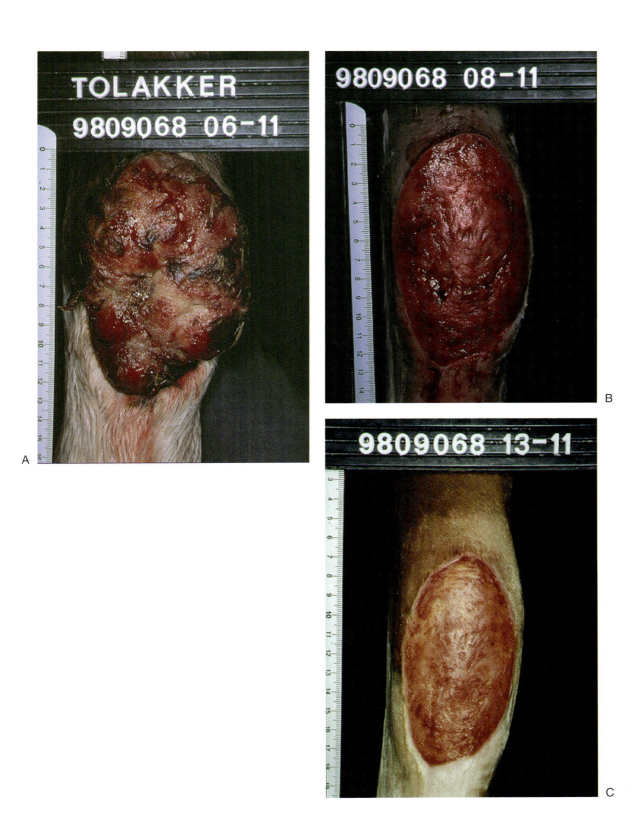

Figure 8.81. (A) Wound on the plantar surface of the metatarsus of a 3-year-old mare. Exuberant granulation tissue had been present for a couple of weeks and healing had ceased. (B) Two days after surgical excision of EGT, dramatic improvement of the wound bed can be observed. (C) Excision was followed by short-term topical antibacterial treatment supplemented with one topical application of corticosteroids the day before the picture was taken. Wound contraction has occurred and epithelialization has begun, thus diminishing the risk for recurrence of EGT. Reprinted with permission.[57]

epithelialization are well under way, after which the silicone dressing can be replaced by a non-adherent pad. The silicone dressing is reusable, which offsets its initial high cost. Washing it gently under tap water with mild liquid detergent, as recommended by the manufacturer, does not alter its exceptional adherence to the wound surface.

Topical application of corticosteroids to arrest the formation of EGT remains controversial. There is evidence that some corticosteroids may selectively reduce the release of fibrogenic TGF-β1 and -β2 from monocytes and macrophages, counteracting fibroblast proliferation and ECM formation. Additionally, corticosteroids decrease the overall inflammatory response and levels of other inflammatory mediators that induce fibrosis. This makes corticosteroid use rational in the treatment of newly formed EGT. On the other hand, corticosteroids have been shown to exert a negative influence on angiogenesis and subsequent wound contraction and epithelialization.[56] Therefore, if corticosteroids are used, one or two applications at the first signs of excessive fibroplasia are often all that are needed.

The use of caustic agents or cryogenic surgery is not recommended because these induce necrosis, stimulate chronic inflammation, decrease contraction, damage the new epithelial border, and inhibit healing by promoting proliferation of the granulation tissue.

Recurrent Exuberant Granulation Tissue

Although a cause may not be identified, in some cases EGT may recur despite several excisions and topical treatment to reduce accompanying chronic inflammation. In these cases it may be wise to temporarily remove all bandages in an effort to diminish the stimulus for fibroplasia (Figure 8.82). In large wounds, it is advantageous to resume bandaging once the wound is flat and contracting, in view of encouraging epithelialization. If exuberant-appearing granulation tissue recurs despite the aforementioned approach, one must suspect tumor transformation of the wound. Histological examination of a tissue sample should be performed in such cases to determine the appropriate therapy.

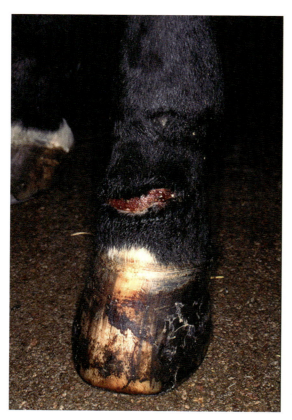

Figure 8.82. Wound at the dorsal aspect of the pastern joint, in which EGT recurred after a number of surgical excisions. The bandages were left off for 1 week before this photograph was taken and the stimulus for proliferation appeared to have decreased. Subsequently, the wound did not form more EGT. Reprinted with permission.[57]

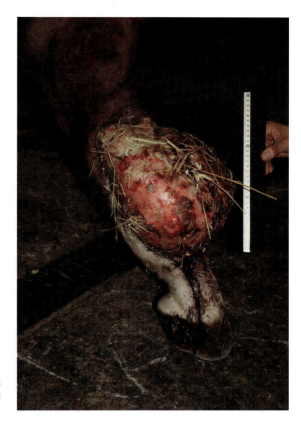

Figure 8.83. A wound with marked and chronic EGT. Treatment of such a wound is more challenging. Surgical excision of EGT followed by skin grafting is the best approach to get these wounds to heal.

Exuberant Granulation Tissue after Skin Grafting

Exuberant granulation tissue can be seen following skin grafting. In these cases, surgical excision is not advisable because of the risk of damage to the newly-grafted tissue. Early on, further development of EGT can be limited by intermittent use of corticosteroids. Generally the corticosteroid is topically applied only once or twice and should not be used for a longer period because growth of the grafts will be disturbed. As soon as epithelialization around the graft sites occurs, the development of EGT should be naturally controlled.

Chronic Exuberant Granulation Tissue

Chronic cases of EGT having formed large lumps are unfortunately known to most practitioners (Figure 8.83). At this stage, the exuberant tissue is usually very fibrous, is nourished via larger blood vessels, and in some cases may be partially innervated. In these wounds, the impetus for healing has disappeared and is unlikely to be recovered, even after excision. Intensive therapy is thus often required. Surgical excision of EGT followed by skin grafting is the best approach to get these wounds to heal at an optimum rate and with an acceptable outcome.[48]

Debulking of the wound can be performed in the standing, sedated patient; however, general anesthesia is often preferred because of the more violent reactions in these patients during excision, possibly as a result of partial reinnervation of the tissue. Following excision of the exuberant fibrous tissue, a pressure bandage is applied to control hemorrhage. Although excision can reportedly be followed immediately by skin grafting, in most cases it is preferable to apply a bandage for a few days until hemorrhage is controlled and a new, healthy bed of granulation tissue begins (for more information on skin grafting, see Chapter 11).

Conclusion

The formation of EGT is a frequent complication in wounds healing by second intention on the limbs of horses. Among a large number of contributing factors, the presence of chronic inflammation is foremost and often goes unrecognized because of the mild symptoms. The stimulus for formation of EGT is reduced when prevention and treatment of chronic inflammation are combined with surgical excision of the protruding tissue. Transition from the fibroblastic phase into the phases of wound contraction and epithelialization will occur smoothly, and usually obviate the recurrence of EGT.

Many agents have been used to treat or prevent EGT formation; however, the best therapy at this time remains surgical excision of the protruding tissue. The limited and indicated application of a corticosteroid and the use of silicone gel dressings as well as skin grafting are useful options for EGT prevention.

New treatments to prevent EGT are currently being sought via fundamental research in equine wound healing. Innovative therapies consisting of specialized interactive dressings combined with engineered reconstitution of tissues via cell-based therapy, scaffold-based therapy, and/or bioactive molecule-based therapy can be expected in the future.

References

1. Wilmink JM, Stolk PWT, van Weeren PR, et al: Differences in second-intention wound healing between horses and ponies: macroscopical aspects. Equine Vet J 1999;31:53
2. Wilmink JM, van Weeren PR, Stolk PWT, et al: Differences in second-intention wound healing between horses and ponies: histological aspects. Equine Vet J 1999;31:61
3. Shakespeare V, Shakespeare P: Effects of granulation-tissue–conditioned medium on the growth of human keratinocytes in-vitro. Br J Plastic Surg 1991;44:219
4. Moulin V: Growth factors in skin wound healing. Eur J Cell Biol 1995;68:1
5. Kirsner RS, Eaglstein WH: The wound healing process. Dermatol Clin 1993;11:629
6. Clark RAF: Regulation of fibroplasia in cutaneous wound repair. Am J Med Sci 1993;306:42
7. Stadelmann WK, Digenis AG, Tobin GR: Physiology and healing dynamics of chronic cutaneous wounds. Am J Surg 1998;176:26
8. Studzinski DM, Benjamins JA. Cyclic AMP differentiation of the oligodendroglial cell line N20.1 switches staurosporine-induced cell death from necrosis to apoptosis. J Neurosci Res 2001;66:691
9. Kischer CW, Shetlar MR, Shetlar CL: Alteration of hypertrophic scars induced by mechanical pressure. Arch Dermatol 1975;111:60
10. Ducharme-Desjarlais M, Lepault E, Céleste C, et al: Determination of the effect of a silicone dressing (CicaCare®) on second intention healing of full-thickness wounds of the distal limb of horses. Am J Vet Res 2005;66:1133
11. Dubuc V, Lepault E, Theoret CL: Endothelial cell hypertrophy is associated with microvascular occlusion in limb wounds of horses. Can J Vet Res 2006;70:206
12. Suzuki H, Tomida A, Tsuruo T: Dephosphorylated hypoxia-inducible factor 1alpha as a mediator of p53-dependent apoptosis during hypoxia. Oncogene 2001;20:5779
13. Wilmink JM, Nederbragt H, van Weeren PR, et al: Differences in wound contraction between horses and ponies: the in vitro contraction capacity of fibroblasts. Equine Vet J 2001;33:499
14. Bacon Miller C, Wilson DA, Keegan KG, et al: Growth characteristics of fibroblasts isolated from the trunk and distal aspect of the limbs of horses and ponies. Vet Surg 2000;29:1
15. Wilmink JM, van Weeren PR: The ins and outs of exuberant granulation tissue. North American Veterinary Conference Proceedings 2003, p.270
16. Van Den Boom R, Wilmink JM, O'Kane S, et al: Transforming growth factor-β levels during second intention healing are related to the different course of wound contraction in horses and ponies. Wound Rep Regen 2002;10:188
17. Wilmink JM, Veenman JN, van den Boom R, et al: Differences in polymorphonucleocyte function and local inflammatory response between horses and ponies. Equine Vet J 2003;35:561
18. LePoole IC, Boyce ST: Keratinocytes suppress TGF-β1 expression by fibroblasts in cultured skin substitutes. Br J Derm 1999;140:409
19. Ehrlich HP, Wyler DJ: Fibroblast contraction of collagen lattices in vitro: inhibition by chronic inflammatory cell mediators. J Cell Physiol 1983;116:345
20. Kovacs EJ: Fibrogenic cytokines: the role of immune mediators in the development of scar tissue. Immunol Today 1991;12:17
21. Barber SM: Second intention wound healing in the horse: the effect of bandages and topical corticosteroids. North American Veterinary Conference Proceedings 1990, p.107
22. Cochrane CA: Models in vivo of wound healing in the horse and the role of growth factors. Vet Derm 1997;8:259
23. Theoret CL, Barber SM, Moyana TN, et al: Expression of transforming growth factor β1, β3, and basic fibroblast factor in full-thickness skin wounds of equine limbs and thorax. Vet Surg 2001;30:269
24. Schwartz AJ, Wilson DA, Keegan KG, et al: Factors regulating collagen synthesis and degradation during second-intention healing of wounds in the thoracic region and the distal aspect of the forelimb of horses. Am J Vet Res 2002;63:1564

25. Ignotz RA, Massague J: Transforming growth factor-β stimulates the expression of fibronectin and collagen and their incorporation into the extracellular matrix. J Biol Chem 1986;261:4337

26. Laiho M, Sakesela O, Andreasen PA, et al: Enhanced production and extracellular deposition of the endothelial-type plasminogen activator inhibitor in cultured human lung fibroblasts by transforming growth factor-beta. J Cell Biol 1986;103:2403

27. Quaglino D, Nanney LB, Ditesheim JA, et al: Transforming growth factor-β stimulates wound healing and modulates extracellular matrix gene expression in pig skin: incisional wound model. J Invest Dermatol 1991; 97:34

28. Theoret CL, Barber SM, Moyana TN, et al: Preliminary observations on expression of transforming growth factors β1 and β3 in equine full-thickness skin wounds healing normally or with exuberant granulation tissue. Vet Surg 2002;31:266

29. De Martin I, Theoret CL: Spatial and temporal expression of types I and II receptors for transforming growth factor β in normal equine skin and dermal wounds. Vet Surg 2004;33:70

30. Grinnell F, Zhu M, Carlson MA, et al: Release of mechanical tension triggers apoptosis of human fibroblasts in a model of regressing granulation tissue. Exp Cell Res 1999;248:608

31. Falanga V, Qian SW, Danielpour D, et al: Hypoxia upregulates the synthesis of TGF-beta 1 by human dermal fibroblasts. J Invest Dermatol 1991;97:634

32. Lepault E, Céleste C, Doré M, et al: Comparative study on microvascular occlusion and apoptosis in body and limb wounds in the horse. Wound Rep Regen 2005;13:520

33. Chvapil M, Pfister T, Escalada S, et al: Dynamics of the healing of skin wounds in the horse as compared with the rat. Exp Mol Pathol 1979;30:349

34. Bertone AL, Sullins KE, Stashak TS, et al: Effect of wound location and the use of topical collagen gel on exuberant granulation tissue formation and wound healing in the horse and pony. Am J Vet Res 1985;46:1438

35. Siddiqui A, Galiano RD, Connors D, et al: Differential effects of oxygen on human dermal fibroblasts: acute versus chronic hypoxia. Wound Rep Regen 1996;4:211

36. Falanga V, Zhou L, Yufit T: Low oxygen tension stimulates collagen synthesis and COLIA1 transcription through the action of TGF-beta1. J Cell Physiol 2002;191:42

37. Falanga V, Martin TA, Takagi H, et al: Low oxygen tension increases mRNA levels of alpha 1 (I) procollagen in human dermal fibroblasts. J Cell Physiol 1993;157:408

38. Saed GM, Zhang W, Diamond MP: Effect of hypoxia on stimulatory effect of TGF-β1 on MMP-2 and MMP-9 activities in mouse fibroblasts. J Soc Gynecol Investig 2000;7:348

39. Idell S, Swieb C, Boggaram J, et al: Mechanisms of fibrin formation and lysis by human lung fibroblasts: Influence of TGF-beta and TNF-alpha. Am J Physiol 1992;263:487

40. Holmdahl L, Eriksson E, Eriksson B, et al: Depression of peritoneal fibrinolysis during operation is a local response to trauma. Surg 1998;123:539

41. Chodon T, Sugihara T, Igawa HH, et al: Keloid-derived fibroblasts are refractory to Fas-mediated apoptosis and neutralization of autocrine transforming growth factor–beta1 can abrogate this resistance. Am J Path 2000;157:1661

42. Jelaska A, Korn JH: Role of apoptosis and transforming growth factor beta1 in fibroblast selection and activation in systemic sclerosis. Arthritis Rheum 2000;43:2230

43. Greenhalgh DG: The role of apoptosis in wound healing. Int J Biochem Cell B 1998;30:1019

44. Woollen N, RM DeBowes, Liepold HW, et al: A comparison of four types of therapy for the treatment of full thickness wounds of the horse. North American Veterinary Conference Proceedings 1987, p.569

45. Fretz PB, Martin GS, Jacobs KA, et al: Treatment of exuberant granulation tissue in the horse: Evaluation of four methods. Vet Surg 1983;12:137

46. Berry DB, Sullins KE: Effects of topical application of antimicrobials and bandaging on healing and granulation tissue formation in wounds of the distal aspect of the limbs in horses. Am J Vet Res 2003;64:88

47. Knighton DR, Silver IA, Hunt TK: Regulation of wound-healing angiogenesis. Effect of oxygen gradients and inspired oxygen concentration. Surg 1981;90:262

48. Bertone AL: Management of exuberant granulation tissue. Vet Clin North Am Equine Pract 1989;5:551

49. Bigbie RB, Schumacher J, Swaim SF, et al: Effects of amnion and live yeast cell derivative on second-intention healing in horses. Am J Vet Res 1991;52:1376.

50. Howard RD, Stashak TS, Baxter GM: Evaluation of occlusive dressings for management of full-thickness excisional wounds on the distal portion of the limbs of horses. Am J Vet Res 1993;54:2150

51. Stashak TS: Principles of wound management and selection of approaches to wound closure: second intention healing. In Ted S. Stashak, ed. *Equine wound management (1st edition)*. Philadelphia: Lea and Febiger, 1991, p.45

52. Knottenbelt DC: Equine wound management: are there significant differences in healing at different sites on the body? Vet Derm 1997;8:273

53. Desmoulière A, Redard M, Darby I, et al: Apoptosis mediates the decrease in cellularity during the transition between granulation tissue and scar. Am J Path 1995;146:56

54. Darby IA, Bisucci T, Pittet B, et al: Skin flap–induced regression of granulation tissue correlates with reduced growth factor and increased metalloproteinase expression. J Pathol 2002;197:117

55. Knottenbelt DC: Skin grafting. In Derek Knottenbelt, ed. *Handbook of equine wound management.* London: WB Saunders Co, 2003, p.79

56. Hashimoto I, Nakanishi H, Shono Y, et al: Angiostatic effects of corticosteroid on wound healing of the rabbit ear. J Med Invest 2002;49:61

57. Wilmink JM, van Weeren PR: Treatment of exuberant granulation tissue. Clin Tech Equine Pract 2004;3:141

9 | Diagnosis and Management of Wounds Involving Synovial Structures

Gary M. Baxter, VMD, MS, Diplomate ACVS

Introduction

Wounds that enter synovial structures (joints, tendon sheaths, and bursae), particularly of the distal limbs, are common in horses. These injuries are due to a variety of causes and occur in all shapes and sizes. Regardless of the cause or size, if left untreated, these wounds can result in infection within the synovial cavity leading to permanent disability of the horse. Prompt recognition of synovial involvement together with appropriate treatment for the infection will prevent many of the negative consequences of these wounds. The objectives of this chapter are to:

- Make the reader aware of the most common synovial structures involved upon wounding
- Review the basic anatomy and physiology of synovial structures
- Review the pathogenesis of synovial infections
- List the bacteria that cause many of these infections
- Provide methods that can be used to document synovial involvement
- Describe treatment methods for both acute (<6–8 hours old) and chronic (>6–8 hours old) synovial wounds
- Update the reader on the use of local delivery of antimicrobials to synovial structures

Throughout this chapter, general approaches to management of these wounds will be emphasized because similar principles apply whether the wound involves a joint, a tendon sheath, or a bursa.

Location of Injuries

Although synovial infections associated with a laceration or puncture wound can involve any joint, tendon sheath, or bursa in the horse, the synovial cavities of the distal limb (distal to and including the carpus and tarsus) are most commonly involved.[1-4] Synovial structures that are often penetrated include: the navicular bursa, distal and proximal interphalangeal joints, digital tendon sheath, metacarpo/metatarsophalangeal joint, carpal and tarsocrural joints, calcaneal, bicipital and infraspinatus bursae, and tarsal and carpal sheaths.[4-11] Although most traumatic injuries involve a single synovial structure, large wounds—particularly of the foot, shoulder, and tarsal regions—may contaminate multiple synovial structures.

If treated appropriately, acute synovial wounds (<6–8 hours old) only contaminate the synovial structure without developing a true infection.[1-3] However, a synovial infection can develop quickly in the absence of proper treatment and any wound affecting a synovial structure that is >6–8 hours old should be considered to have an established synovial infection (chronic injuries). Chronic injuries should be viewed as potentially career-limiting because pathologic changes secondary to the synovial infection can lead to permanent disabilities in performance horses. In many cases, the severity of these wounds is magnified because of the delay in diagnosis and treatment of the infection.

Synovial Anatomy and Physiology

Joints

Synovial structures (joints, tendon sheaths, and bursae) surround joints and tendons in specific locations to allow normal limb flexion and freedom of movement. Joints are closed, sterile spaces of variable size and shape located around opposing bony surfaces. The bone ends within joints are covered with hyaline cartilage and are usually stabilized by a combination of collateral ligaments, joint capsule, tendons, and muscle, depending on their location. The synovial capsule of joints is lined by an inner synovial membrane that is highly vascular and functions as an exchange site for nutrients and waste products between the synovial fluid and the systemic circulation.[12] This synovial lining also has several absorptive and secretory functions that help maintain the normal synovial environment.[12] This is especially important in joints because the synovial fluid is vital to maintain the overall health of the articular cartilage. The outer fibrous joint capsule is attached to bone and/or soft tissue structures on the perimeter of the joint and serves to protect the joint cavity from injury.

All synovial cavities contain lubricating substances (i.e., hyaluronan) within synovial fluid that permit movement of opposing bone and/or soft tissue structures.[12] The fibrous synovial layer and annular ligament/retinaculum closely approximate the skin in many synovial cavities and are often damaged upon traumatic laceration. Although it is possible for a wound to penetrate the outer fibrous capsule without penetrating through the inner synovial membrane, this is uncommon with most traumatic injuries in horses. Secondary complications of joint infections in horses include articular cartilage damage leading to osteoarthritis and lameness, fibrosis of the joint capsule causing reduced range of motion, and osteomyelitis leading to chronic infection.[2]

Tendon Sheaths and Bursae

Tendon sheaths and bursae serve to protect and promote normal gliding motion of tendons in several areas of a horse's limb.[5,7-10] A bursa is usually located between a tendon and an adjacent bone in a high motion area; examples are the navicular and the bicipital bursae. In contrast to joints, the bone surfaces within these structures are covered with fibrocartilage rather than hyaline cartilage. Tendon sheaths are also located in high motion areas such as the palmar/plantar regions of metacarpo/metatarsophalangeal joints and serve a very similar function to bursae. Annular ligaments and retinaculi (adjacent to many sheaths and bursae) enclose the synovial cavity and form an inelastic canal for tendons to glide through.[5]

Anatomically, the inner synovial and outer fibrous membrane of tendon sheaths and bursae are similar to those of joints, except that most have one or more annular ligaments and/or retinaculi that function to stabilize the tendon.[5,8,9] Damage to these supporting structures can result in "subluxation" of the tendon from the synovial cavity; this occurs most commonly in the calcaneal bursa.[2,13] The synovial fluid within a tendon sheath or bursa is also very similar to that within joints and possesses many of the same properties and functions. Lubrication of the synovial surfaces within tendon sheaths and bursae is possibly even more critical to pain-free movement than within joints due to the high mobility within these synovial cavities.[5,8] Secondary complications of tendon sheath and bursae infections related to wounds in horses include adhesion or scar tissue formation within the sheath, leading to restricted movement and lameness, tendonitis, and osteomyelitis of the adjacent bone.

Pathogenesis of Synovial Infections

Lacerations or puncture wounds into synovial structures often directly introduce bacteria and contaminants (e.g., hair, dander, dirt, etc.) into the synovial space. Initially the synovial structure may only be contaminated with bacteria. Provided that appropriate treatment is performed at this point, infectious arthritis/tenosynovitis/bursitis may be avoided with minimal to no secondary damage.[1,2] Therefore, early diagnosis and treatment of open joint, tendon sheath, and bursal injuries is very important to successfully managing and returning horses to pre-injury athletic performance.

The size of the bacterial inoculum required to produce a synovial infection varies according to the type and virulence of the bacteria; the specific joint, tendon sheath, or bursa involved (apparently proportional to the size of the synovial cavity); the severity of the concurrent soft tissue trauma; the immune response of the animal; and whether foreign material is present.[3,14,15] Experimentally, 1.5×10^5 and 1.6×10^6 colony-forming units (CFU) of *Staphylococcus aureus* were used as infective doses in the tarsocrural joints of normal horses.[16] In a separate study, as few as 33 CFU of *Staphylococcus aureus* were determined to represent a subinfective dose in the middle carpal joint of horses.[17] The results of these studies indicate that a very small bacterial inoculum is capable of causing synovial infections under appropriate conditions.

Upon bacterial colonization of the synovial membrane, an inflammatory response ensues in attempt to re-sterilize the synovial structure.[15] The inflammatory cascade promotes the release of a multitude of cytokines, proteolytic enzymes, and other inflammatory mediators from a variety of cell types within the synovial cavity. These inflammatory mediators serve to increase vascular permeability within the synovium, attract neutrophils and monocytes to the synovial space, degrade hyaluronan within the synovial fluid, and promote the formation of fibrin.[15] Reactive oxygen metabolites and proteolytic enzymes derived from infiltrating neutrophils, chondrocytes, synoviocytes, monocytes, macrophages, and the bacteria themselves may all contribute to the degradation of hyaluronan and depletion of articular cartilage proteoglycans observed in infectious arthritis.[18,19] The end result is often the formation of a fibrinocellular clot, referred to as pannus, which is similar to the bio-slime found on the surface of bone in osteomyelitis.[14]

Pannus impedes treatment of synovial sepsis by protecting foreign debris and devitalized tissue, serving as a bacterial growth medium and impeding drug delivery to the site of infection.[14] Although pannus is a term used primarily to describe what occurs in joint infection, a similar yet possibly more substantial process occurs with tendon sheath and bursal infections. Fibrin formation is often abundant within infected tendon sheaths and bursae and should be removed because it serves as a scaffold for secondary fibrous tissue/adhesion formation within these structures.

The longer the duration of the infection, the greater the likelihood of permanent damage to the synovial structure. Alterations in synovial fluid usually occur early during infection, often before clinical signs are present, and can impede synovial membrane function in all synovial cavities, as well as interfere with chondrocyte nutrition within joints.[15,20] The prolonged inflammatory response in chronic infections can contribute to synovial hyperplasia and hypertrophy, vascular proliferation, thrombosis of synovial vessels, pannus formation, and fibrosis of the joint capsule.[14,15] Additionally, prolonged infection in a joint may contribute to abnormalities in the articular cartilage resulting in the loss of proteoglycans and exposure of the cartilage to mechanical damage and enzymatic breakdown.[15,18] Irreversible cartilage damage is the end stage of infectious arthritis and contributes to impaired joint function, permanent lameness, and a poor outcome (Figure 9.1).

Chronic infection within tendon sheaths and bursae can lead to fibrosis of the synovial lining, tendonitis with superficial fraying of the tendon, adhesion formation, development of fibrotic masses within the sheath, and secondary osteomyelitis of bone within the synovial cavity.[2,5,8] Chronic navicular bursal infections commonly invade the navicular bone, and chronic infections within the digital sheath can erode through the inner lining of the sheath to involve the proximal sesamoid bones. Finally, secondary infection within the tendon itself (septic core lesions) that courses through the tendon sheath or bursa is also possible but uncommon in horses.[21,22]

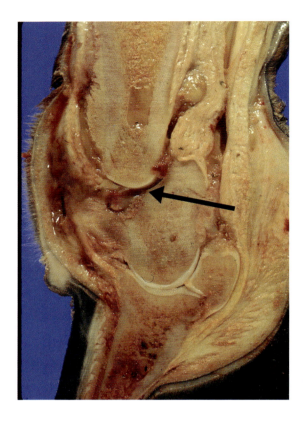

Figure 9.1. This postmortem saggital section of the phalanges demonstrates the damage that can occur with chronic infection of the proximal interphalangeal joint secondary to a wound. There was complete loss of the articular cartilage from all joint surfaces, and bone lysis was present within the middle phalanx (arrow).

Imaging

Radiography (Plain and Contrast)

Radiography is crucial in chronic synovial wounds to rule out secondary bone involvement (osteomyelitis) that may be present with chronic infections (Figure 9.2). Periosteal proliferation, multifocal areas of osteolysis, collapsing joint space with subchondral bone erosion, as well as periarticular osteophytes may be present depending on the duration of the infection.[2,23] Routine radiographs of the injured site also may reveal evidence of gas within the synovial space, confirming its communication with the wound, and will be useful to document concurrent bone and/or osteochondral damage. Nevertheless, many acute synovial injuries are characterized by soft tissue swelling in the absence of bone abnormalities. Suspected involvement of synovial structures can often be confirmed using contrast radiography or fistulography (Figures 9.3a,b).

Ultrasonography

Ultrasonography is most useful in identifying the character of the synovial fluid, damage to soft tissue support structures, gas accumulation within the synovial space, and radiographically unapparent foreign bodies and osseous abnormalities.[5,9,24] Septic synovial fluid typically shows increased echogenicity and is heterogenous because of the presence of fibrin clots and cellular debris.[5,7] Secondary tendon injuries (e.g., tears, fraying, and adhesions) associated with the synovial wound/infection can also usually be documented ultrasonographically.[25,26] Osseous abnormalities (e.g., fractures, destructive lesions), particularly those associated with synovial structures of the upper limb, can be identified with complete ultrasound examination.[9,25,26] Although contrast radiography can be a valuable tool to identify foreign bodies in a wound tract, sheath, or bursa, foreign bodies that become buried within the synovium or reside at the extremity of the synovial structure can be difficult to image. Ultrasound can be very helpful in these cases (Figures 9.4a,b).

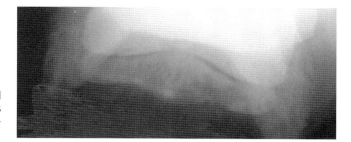

Figure 9.2. This skyline radiograph is from a horse that had sustained a puncture wound to the foot approximately 6 weeks earlier. Severe lysis of the navicular bone was evident, consistent with chronic infection of the navicular bursa.

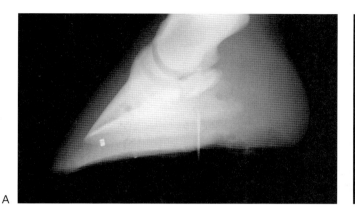

A

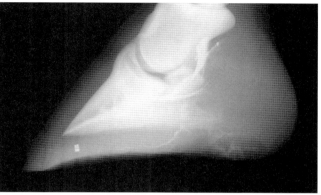

B

Figure 9.3. This horse sustained a puncture wound to the foot a few hours earlier. (A) Lateral radiograph of the foot after placing a small metallic cannula into the wound suggested penetration of the navicular bursa. (B) The radiograph was repeated after injecting contrast material through the cannula, which outlined the navicular bursa and confirmed the diagnosis.

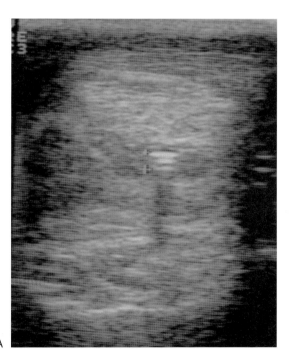

A

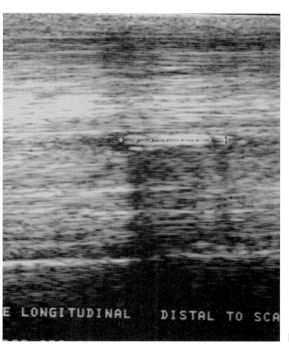

B

Figure 9.4. (A) This transverse ultrasound image, in the mid-metacarpal region, identified a hyperechoic density (cursor) located at the distal extent of the carpal canal sheath between the carpal check ligament and deep digital flexor tendon. (B) A longitudinal ultrasound image of the same area also identified a hyperechoic density (cursor) consistent with a foreign body. Ultrasound was very useful in this case to identify a piece of wood that was not identified using contrast radiography. Reprinted from Proceeding of the American Association of Equine Practitioners, 52, Stashak TS, Wound infection: contributing factors and selected techniques for prevention, pp. 270–280, Copyright (2006), with permission from American Association of Equine Practitioners.

MRI and CT

The advanced imaging techniques MRI and CT have become more available for use in horses to document both soft tissue and bone abnormalities that are not readily apparent with radiography or ultrasonography. However, these techniques are usually unnecessary in horses with acute synovial injuries, and many chronic infections have obvious abnormalities detected with radiographs and ultrasound. In addition, synovial injuries in horses are often emergency situations, making more advanced imaging techniques impractical in many cases.

Synoviocentesis

Aspiration of synovial fluid for gross examination and cytology is one of the first diagnostic steps used to document a synovial infection. However, many acute synovial wounds may not have synovial distention, making this difficult. In these cases, assessment of communication between the wound and the synovial cavity can be made by injecting sterile fluid into the synovial structure at a site remote from the wound and watching for fluid exiting the wound (Figure 9.5).[27,28]

Knowledge of the multiple joint/synovial pouches that can be used for synoviocentesis of joints, tendon sheaths, and bursae is helpful to decide where to place the needle distant from the wound. If synovial distention is present, the needle can usually be placed in the most distended site of the synovial cavity for both synoviocentesis and injection of sterile saline, if needed. In general, synoviocentesis of tendon sheaths and bursae is usually more difficult than for most joints. Swelling, edema and cellulitis associated with traumatic wounds can further complicate synoviocentesis because routine anatomic landmarks may be difficult to palpate. Ultrasound-guided synoviocentesis may be necessary in some cases, particularly in synovial cavities in the proximal region of the limb such as the bicipital or infraspinatus bursae.[9]

In most cases, the wound should be cleaned and explored before performing synoviocentesis. Clipping the hair is not necessary for synoviocentesis but is usually performed to better evaluate the wound. Skin preparation of the synoviocentesis site with a minimum 5-minute antiseptic scrub (povidone-iodine or chlorhexidine) is recommended. Alcohol should not be used in or around the wound. Samples of synovial fluid should be

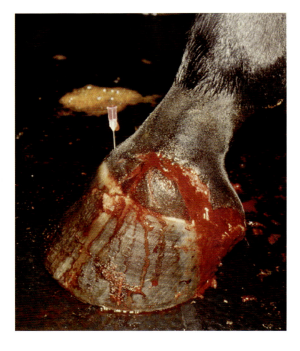

Figure 9.5. A sterile needle was placed into the distal interphalangeal (coffin) joint, in a site remote to the wound, to inject sterile fluid into the synovial structure and document that it had been breeched. Reprinted from Proceeding of the American Association of Equine Practitioners, 52, Stashak TS, Wound infection: contributing factors and selected techniques for prevention, pp. 270–280, Copyright (2006), with permission from American Association of Equine Practitioners.

obtained for gross and cytological examination (EDTA tube) as well as for culture and sensitivity. Synovial fluid that is cloudy, turbid, and discolored (brown to sanguineous) with poor viscosity on gross evaluation is suggestive of infection.

Cytological Evaluation

Cytological evaluation of synovial fluid is considered critical in the diagnosis of synovial infections. However, low white blood cell (WBC) count and total protein concentrations inconsistent with infection in acute synovial wounds do not necessarily indicate lack of synovial involvement. Synovial fluid WBC counts >30,000 cells/μl and total protein concentrations >3.5–4 g/dl are considered to be highly consistent with infection.[2,14,27] Many synovial infections have WBC counts >100,000 cells/μl in synovial fluid and the severity of clinical signs often correlates with the WBC count.

Infections within tendon sheaths and bursae may result in more variable changes in synovial fluid WBC and total protein values (generally lower than in joints), but still fall into the previously stated guidelines (average values of 34,750 cells/μl and 5 g/dl total protein in one study of infectious tenosynovitis).[4,29] In one study of synovial infections, the average WBC count and total protein concentration were 76,500 cells/μl (range 1,100–380,000) and 5 g/dl (range 2.5–9.8) respectively.[4] In this study there were no significant differences in these parameters between joint and tendon sheath infections. The majority of the WBC were neutrophils (average was 83.7%) and bacteria were observed on direct smears of the fluid in 24% of the samples.[4] Other synovial fluid parameters which suggest infection but are used less frequently include pH, glucose concentration, and mucin clot formation.

Culture Methods

Identification of the causative organism(s) is extremely helpful in the management of synovial infections. Positive cultures and sensitivity patterns not only direct antimicrobial therapy but may also help determine the likelihood of successful therapy. Infections caused by highly resistant and virulent bacteria are usually more difficult to treat than those associated with more commonly isolated bacteria. Direct culturing of synovial fluid is commonly performed, with variable results, but remains the most frequently used technique to document infection. While several studies have reported more than 70% success in identifying the causative organism of synovial infections via culturing of synovial fluid,[4,29,30] culturing the synovial membrane has been advocated to increase the probability of obtaining a positive culture. However, a clinical study in horses and an experimental study in dogs both showed that synovial fluid yielded more positive cultures than did synovial membrane.[30,31] It may be beneficial to place synovial fluid into blood culture media (BBL Septi-chek™, Becton Dickinson and Co, Cockeysville, MD) for 24 hours to increase the probability of bacterial isolation.[31] In dogs, synovial fluid incubated in blood culture media was significantly more reliable in growing bacteria than was direct culturing of synovial fluid and synovial membrane biopsies.[31] However, blood culture media is rarely used by the author because it delays results by another 24 hours. In addition, gram staining can provide early information as to the cause of the infection (especially with anaerobic bacteria),[32] and results of the gram stain correlate well with the eventually cultured organism(s).[30,33]

With wounds that involve synovial structures, the likelihood of having a positive culture may vary widely depending on the duration and severity of the injury. In injuries only a few hours old, identifying bacteria within synovial fluid may be less likely than in more chronic injuries with established synovial infection.[2] Isolation of bacteria in synovial infections should be possible in many horses with wounds, but a negative culture does not preclude synovial contamination or infection. Direct culture of synovial fluid is attempted initially by the author. If fluid cannot be obtained and endoscopic exploration of the synovial cavity is performed, samples of fibrin, synovial membrane, or infected bone are obtained at surgery and submitted for both aerobic and anaerobic culture and sensitivity.

Causative Bacteria

Synovial infections due to wounds may be monomicrobial or polymicrobial depending on the type of wound as well as the cause and duration of the injury. In the author's experience, the most common presentation will be a horse with a wound involving a synovial structure of the distal limb that is >24 hours old and most likely contaminated by multiple bacteria. Chronic synovial infections are often polymicrobial with environmental bacteria such as Gram-negative enterics, streptococci, and staphylococci commonly associated with these types of infections.[4,14,34] Anaerobes and resistant strains of *Staphylococcus aureus* may be identified but are far less common than in bone infections or synovial infections secondary to intra-articular treatment in horses.[32] Aerobic and anaerobic bacterial culture and sensitivity of the involved synovial cavity are highly recommended because of the variety of bacteria that may be contributing to the infection. Negative results on synovial fluid culture are not uncommon and do not indicate the absence of infection. Reasons for difficulty in obtaining bacterial growth are: sequestration of bacteria in the synovial membrane or within neutrophils or fibrin, intrinsic bactericidal properties of septic synovial effusions, as well as previous administration of antimicrobials.[5,27] Placing synovial fluid from horses being treated with antimicrobials into antimicrobial removal devices has been recommended to improve the success of subsequent culturing but this is not performed routinely by the author.[27]

Acute Synovial Wounds (Less than 6 to 8 Hours Old)

Lacerations or puncture wounds into synovial structures often directly introduce bacteria and other contaminants into the synovial space. Initially the synovial structure may only be contaminated with bacteria and the goal of treatment should be to prevent the development of an established synovial infection, thereby minimizing performance-limiting complications. In one clinical study of open joint injuries, horses treated within 24 hours had a significantly lower risk of developing infectious arthritis and increased chance of survival compared to horses treated after 24 hours.[35] Nonetheless, of the horses treated within 24 hours, 53% developed infection and only 65% survived, suggesting that still earlier intervention of open synovial injuries is needed to improve treatment success. An improved prognosis associated with early treatment of synovial wounds was also found in a similar study,[36] but not in a recent study which evaluated horses with septic calcaneal bursitis.[13]

In the author's opinion, wounds involving synovial structures that are treated appropriately within 6 to 8 hours of injury rarely develop an established synovial infection. Two caveats of treating these injuries within this timeframe are: (1) early recognition of synovial structure involvement and (2) encouraging horse owners/trainers to seek veterinary assistance within this short time frame. Although equine veterinarians have minimal control over the latter, they should strive for early diagnosis of synovial involvement.

Clinical Findings and Diagnosis

Horses with acute synovial injuries may or may not be lame at the walk depending on the severity and duration of the injury. Clinical signs consistent with synovial infection are not commonly apparent within 6 to 8 hours, but there may be soft tissue swelling, heat, and pain associated with the injury itself.[27] In many of these cases, additional diagnostic procedures are necessary to document synovial involvement. However, physical examination and most diagnostic tests used to evaluate a synovial wound have a limited ability to predict the presence of foreign material within the synovial cavity. In a clinical study of contaminated and infected synovial cavities, 40% of synovial cavities examined endoscopically contained foreign material while the presence of foreign material had been predicted in only 15% based on pre-operative diagnostics.[37]

Treatment

Once synovial involvement is documented, treatment should include parenteral broad-spectrum antimicrobials, some form of synovial lavage, drainage or endoscopic exploration, intrasynovial antimicrobials, wound debridement ± closure, and regional IV perfusion of antimicrobials when possible. The primary goal of these treatments is to prevent the development of a synovial infection to decrease the overall cost of treatment and greatly improve the success. Broad-spectrum antimicrobials are recommended for all acute synovial injuries until the results of culture and sensitivity are known.[38,39] The combination of penicillin and gentamicin is used most commonly but combinations of penicillin and amikacin, penicillin and ceftiofur, and penicillin and enrofloxacin may also be employed (Table 9.1).

Table 9.1. Systemic antimicrobials used to treat horses with synovial wounds and infections.

Antimicrobial	Dosage	Combinations and indications
Penicillin	22,000–44,000 IU/kg q 6–12 hours IV or IM	Combined with aminoglycoside, ceftiofur, or enrofloxacin (Gram-positive infections).
Ampicillin	22 mg/kg IV q 8 hours	Combined with aminoglycoside.
Cefazolin	10 mg/kg q 8 hours IV or IM	Can be used alone; usually combined with gentamicin or amikacin.
Gentamicin	6.6 mg/kg q 24 hours IV or IM	Combined with penicillin, cephalosporin, or ampicillin (Gram-negative infections).
Amikacin	15–25 mg/kg q 24 hours IV or IM (divided 8–12 h for foals)	Combined with penicillin, cephalosporin, or ampicillin (Gram-negative infections).
Ceftiofur	2.2 mg/kg q 12 hours	Can be used alone or combined with penicillin or aminoglycoside (Staphylococcus infections).
Enrofloxacin	7 mg/kg q 24 hours IV or PO	Not recommended for foals (resistant Gram-negative infections; poor for anaerobes).
Doxycycline	10 mg/kg PO q 12 hours	Used as follow-up to parenteral antimicrobials.
Trimethoprim-sulfonamides	30 mg/kg q 12 hours PO	Used as follow-up to parenteral antimicrobials.
Vancomycin	7.5 mg/kg IV q 8 hours	Methicillin-resistant staphylococcal and enterococcal infections.

In acute synovial injuries, the technique of synovial lavage (through-and-through with needles or cannulas or a rigid endoscope) is thought to be less crucial than in chronic injuries with established synovial infections. However, many wounds with synovial involvement have foreign material within the synovial cavity which can be visualized and removed best by endoscopy.[37,40] The type of sterile fluid used for lavage is less critical than the volume, and the author no longer uses DMSO in lavage solutions because it does not appear to generate clinical improvement in most horses. Intrasynovial antimicrobials (250 mg–500 mg of amikacin and/or 300 mg timentin) should be placed into the synovial structure following lavage.[2,14,38] Regional IV perfusion of antimicrobials is advocated by the author as another effective method to prevent the establishment of a synovial infection (see Local Antimicrobial Therapy, discussed later on page 480, for more details). Regional IV perfusion is recommended over intraosseous delivery because it is less invasive and easier to perform and it achieves comparable synovial fluid and soft tissue concentrations of antimicrobials.[41,42]

Probably the most difficult decision to make in horses with acute synovial injuries is whether or not to perform primary closure of the wound and synovial structure. Trapping bacteria within the synovial space without appropriate drainage would most likely cause a synovial infection, defeating the primary goal of early treatment of these injuries. However, primary closure of the wound will often greatly decrease the healing time and cost of treatment, and may reduce the likelihood of iatrogenic synovial infections (Figure 9.6).

If wound closure is considered, endoscopic/arthroscopic evaluation of the synovial cavity is preferred to ensure thorough lavage and removal of all debris from the joint, tendon sheath, or bursa prior to wound closure.[2,37] Wounds located in high-motion areas such as the dorsal surface of the metacarpo/metatarsophalangeal joint or the palmar/plantar surface of the pastern and fetlock regions often undergo prolonged healing by second intention. Synovial wounds in these areas should be closed if possible and immobilized with a fiberglass cast, bandage cast, or bandage and splint to prevent wound dehiscence. Casts should be maintained for a

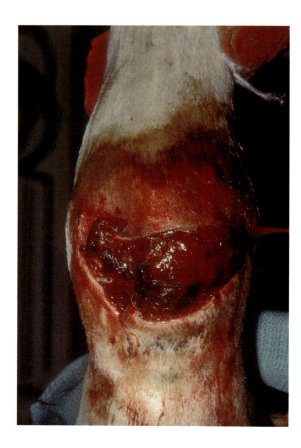

Figure 9.6. This recent(<4 hours duration) laceration that transected the dorsal surface of the metatarsophalangeal joint is an ideal candidate for closure and casting due to its location in a very mobile area. Delayed closure would be difficult while managing this because an open wound would potentially lead to wound healing complications.

minimum of 2 to 3 weeks to ensure adequate healing. Casting is usually unnecessary if the wound is not closed. However, the author does not feel that casting (pastern, half-limb, or sleeve) interferes with postoperative patient assessment, and can speed both wound and joint capsule healing in many types of wounds.

In many cases the decision to close the wound is a moot point due to the surrounding soft tissue damage, size of the wound, or loss of skin (Figure 9.7). If primary wound closure is possible, it is the author's opinion that it can be performed safely without risking subsequent synovial infection provided all of the treatment procedures previously described are performed concurrently (parenteral broad-spectrum antimicrobials, endoscopic lavage, intrasynovial antimicrobials, and regional IV perfusion of antimicrobials).[2,37] If in doubt, it is probably best to leave the wound to heal by second intention.

Alternatively, delayed primary or secondary closure of the wound may be performed in 2 to 4 days.[1] This will permit a greater time to re-sterilize the synovial structure with administration of appropriate antimicrobials prior to wound closure. Although delaying repair for a few days will likely make it more difficult to close the wound due to granulation tissue formation and skin retraction, wound closure can usually be accomplished by removal (debulking) of the granulation tissue, limited undermining of the skin edges, and use of skin tension suturing techniques. Therefore, the author recommends primary closure of acute and some chronic synovial wounds whenever possible.

The decision to close chronic wounds is often based on size, location, and the severity of the infection. It is usually unnecessary to close small puncture-type wounds but larger wounds in high-motion areas may be best closed to minimize wound healing complications. However, the final decision is often based on the clinical (lameness, drainage, swelling, etc.) and laboratory (synovial WBC count and total protein concentration) findings related to the severity of the infection.

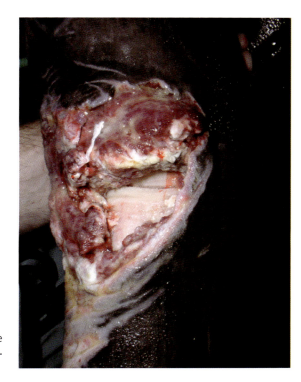

Figure 9.7. This wound involving the tarsometatarsal joint would be impossible to close due to the loss of skin and macerated wound margins. Second intention healing should work well in this location.

Chronic Synovial Wounds (More than 6 to 8 Hours Old)

Unfortunately, many horses with synovial wounds do not develop signs of infection for several days following injury, delaying veterinary care, possible referral, and appropriate treatment. This time frame often coincides with the wound becoming sealed with a fibrin plug and/or in some cases discontinuing antimicrobial therapy. The synovial fluid can no longer drain through the wound, resulting in distention of the synovial structure, pain, swelling, and lameness. The infection also becomes trapped within the synovial structure without the benefit of antimicrobial therapy, leading to acute signs of synovial infection and prompting further treatment (Figure 9.8). In general, synovial wounds greater than 6 to 8 hours old (chronic injuries) should be considered to have an established synovial infection and treated accordingly.

Clinical Findings and Diagnosis

Adult horses with infected synovial structures are usually presented because of severe (four to five out of five) lameness.[1,2,4,9] Joint, tendon sheath, or bursal effusion is usually present together with concurrent soft tissue edema, swelling, and heat with severe infections.[2,27] Most horses exhibit signs of severe pain upon manipulation and flexion of the affected synovial structure. Those with concurrent open wounds will often have a yellowish to clear, sticky fluid, consistent with synovial fluid, exiting the wound (Figure 9.9).

The majority of these are puncture-type wounds located in close proximity to the involved synovial structure.[27,37] Heat and pain upon direct pressure are detectable over the involved synovial structure, and synovial fluid can sometimes be expressed through the wound by applying pressure to the opposite side of the joint or tendon sheath. Fever is not a consistent clinical finding in adult horses with synovial infections secondary to lacerations, such that its absence cannot be used to rule out a possible infection.

In one study, approximately 50% of adult horses and foals with synovial infections were febrile at initial examination.[4] However, this study included foals with hematogenous sources of synovial infection, which often are febrile; thus overestimating the percentage of animals with synovial wounds that are likely to exhibit a fever. Complete blood counts and fibrinogen concentrations usually have limited diagnostic value in adult horses

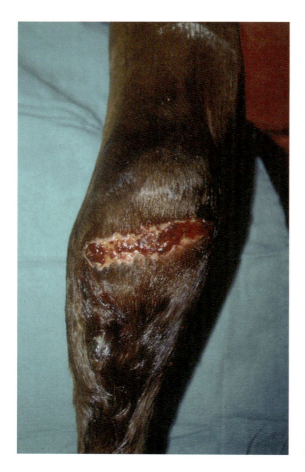

Figure 9.8. This horse sustained a laceration to the caudal surface of the calcaneus 2 to 3 weeks earlier. The wound closed by second intention but infection was trapped within the calcaneal bursa, causing the horse to become severely lame.

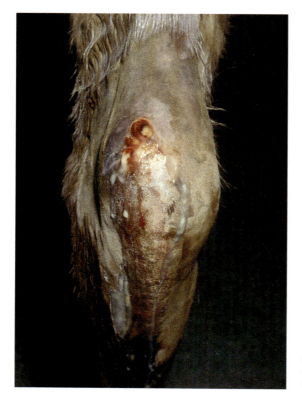

Figure 9.9. This puncture wound on the medial surface of the calcaneus was draining an abundant quantity of yellowish, sticky fluid, consistent with infection within the calcaneal bursa.

with synovial wounds. These laboratory indices are most useful in horses with chronic osteomyelitis, especially foals with hematogenous bone infections.

Treatment

Systemic Antimicrobials

Systemic antimicrobials are the cornerstone of therapy for synovial infections in horses. In an experimental infectious arthritis study, increasing the dose of antimicrobials from once daily to twice daily, regardless of the method of joint drainage, significantly decreased the isolation rate of S. aureus at the end of the study.[16] Increasing the dose of antimicrobials was the only treatment that significantly decreased the number of positive cultures at the end of the study.[16]

However, systemically administered antimicrobials are rarely used alone to treat horses with severe or chronic synovial infections. Broad-spectrum antimicrobials are recommended for all chronic synovial injuries until results of culture and sensitivity are known (Table 9.1). The combination of penicillin and gentamicin is used most commonly, but the combinations of penicillin and amikacin, penicillin and ceftiofur, or penicillin and enrofloxacin may also be employed. First-generation cephalosporins may be substituted for penicillin.

Despite their low cost and ease of administration, trimethoprim-sulfonamides should not be used routinely to treat horses with chronic synovial injuries until culture and sensitivity results are known because of the high bacterial resistance to this drug.[34] Oral trimethoprim-sulfonamides, and more recently doxycycline, are often used as follow-up therapy after the infection has been controlled with parenteral antimicrobials.[2,14,33]

Parenteral (IV) antimicrobials are recommended for a minimum of 5 to 7 days before changing to an oral drug. Antimicrobials are usually continued for approximately 2 to 3 weeks, depending on the severity of the infection, the response to therapy, and the specific drainage technique(s) employed.[2,14,28,43] The author usually prefers 7 days of parenteral therapy followed by 7 to 10 days of oral antimicrobials to treat most synovial wounds. However, if concurrent osteomyelitis is present, antimicrobials should be continued for an additional 2 to 3 weeks or longer, depending on the response to treatment.

Other antimicrobials that are used less frequently to treat horses with synovial wounds include metronidazole, rifampin, enrofloxacin, chloramphenicol, vancomycin, and tobramycin. Metronidazole is indicated for anaerobic infections that are resistant to penicillin.[5] Rifampin is used rarely by the author but may be beneficial in treating staphylococcal infections. It should always be combined with another antimicrobial to decrease the development of bacterial resistance.[33] Enrofloxacin is a fluoroquinolone antimicrobial that has a very broad spectrum of activity and is useful in the treatment of aminoglycoside-resistant Gram-negative bacteria.[44] Enrofloxacin may cause articular cartilage damage in young animals and therefore should be avoided in foals.[44] Chloramphenicol is an effective antimicrobial but presents a risk to human health by causing aplastic anemia and should therefore be used sparingly and with the necessary precautions. Vancomycin and tobramycin are rarely used parenterally because of the expense but may be beneficial to treat refractory infections through local delivery.[14,38,45-47] Indeed, vancomycin at 7.5 mg/kg IV every 8 hours has recently been reported to successfully treat methicillin-resistant staphylococcal and enterococcal infections in horses.[48]

Intrasynovial Antimicrobials

In recent years, intrasynovially administered antimicrobials have become the standard of care to treat infectious synovitis in horses. Initial studies which evaluated intra-articularly administered gentamicin (150 mg) demonstrated that its concentration within synovial fluid remained well above the minimum inhibitor concentration (MIC) values for many common equine bacterial pathogens for 24 hours following intra-articular injection and the use of intra-articular gentamicin significantly reduced the isolation of E. coli from infected joints when compared to intra-articular buffered gentamicin or IV gentamicin.[49] Intrasynovial administration of antimicrobials is also thought to result in significantly higher intrasynovial antimicrobial concentrations and comparable subchondral bone concentrations compared to IV regional limb perfusion.[50]

Currently, amikacin (250 mg–500 mg) has replaced gentamicin as the preferred intrasynovial antimicrobial because of its increased spectrum of activity against equine pathogens.[2,4,38] Other antimicrobials that may be used intrasynovially (depending on the offending bacteria) include gentamicin (200 mg–500 mg), cefazolin (500 mg), penicillin ($2–5 \times 10^6$ IU), ceftiofur (150 mg–500 mg), and timentin (300 mg–400 mg).[2,4,14,38,51]

Antimicrobials used less frequently intrasynovially include enrofloxacin, methicillin, oxacillin, and imipenem-cilastatin.[38] The dose and frequency of administration of these antimicrobials is empirical but should probably not exceed one-half of the systemic dose of the drug and should not be repeated more than every 24 hours.[2,38] If repeat intrasynovial administration of antimicrobials is considered necessary, the author prefers an every-other-day treatment regimen with a total of no more than two to three doses (Table 9.2).

There have been two clinical reports and one research report of using continuous infusion of antimicrobials into synovial structures to help treat synovial infections.[52–54] The research report targeted the tarsocrural joint and delivered gentamicin for 5 days, resulting in gentamicin levels 100 times greater than the MIC required to kill most equine pathogens.[52] However, there were complications associated with the catheter system. Two recent clinical reports used a Joint Infusion System[53] (Mila International, Florence, KY) and the On-Q Painbuster post-op pain relief system[54] (I-Flow Corporation, Lake Forest, CA). The two systems were similar in design and included tubing that was placed into the synovial cavity, flow control tubing to adjust delivery, and a balloon reservoir that contained the antimicrobial drug. The infusion systems were used in a variety of synovial cavities in both foals and adults, and results appeared to be comparable to those obtained with other techniques.[53,54]

The majority of synovial infections treated with the infusion systems appeared to be very chronic and refractory to standard treatments. Mean duration of constant antimicrobial infusion was 4.5 days (range 3 to 8 days)[54] and 6.1 days (range 3 to 14 days)[53] in the two different studies. As with any catheter system used in horses, there were a few malfunctions but these appeared to be infrequent. A major advantage of this technique would be the ability to maintain high synovial fluid antimicrobial concentrations within joints where IV regional perfusion could not be performed, such as the stifle, without the need to repeat intrasynovial injections. The main disadvantage would be the cost of the infusion system and the additional surgery time needed to place the catheter. The infusion systems appeared very safe; there was no evidence of morbidity associated with their use.

Synovial Lavage/Drainage

Methods of synovial lavage/drainage include through-and-through lavage, closed suction drainage, endoscopy with or without synovectomy, arthrotomy, and either passive or active egress drainage. The goals of synovial lavage/drainage are to remove potentially damaging inflammatory mediators, bacteria, and debris

Table 9.2. Concentration-dependent antimicrobials used for local delivery (intrasynovial, regional perfusion, impregnated beads) in horses with synovial infections.

Antimicrobial	Dosage	Methods of delivery
Cefazolin	1 g	All modes of local delivery.
Ceftazidime/Ceftriaxone	2 g (100 mg/hour)	Intrasynovial continuous infusion.
Na penicillin/ampicillin	1/4–1/2 systemic dose	Intrasynovial or regional perfusion.
Gentamicin	0.5–1 g	All modes of local delivery.
	1.8 mg/kg/day	Intrasynovial continuous infusion.
Amikacin	0.5–1 g	All modes of local delivery. (Used most often by author.)
	5.5 mg/kg/day 2–3 g (100 mg/hour)	Intrasynovial continuous infusion.
Ceftiofur	150 mg–1 g	Intrasynovial or regional perfusion.
Ticarcillin plus clavulanate	300–400 mg	All modes of local delivery.
Tobramycin	0.5–2 g	PMMA or other impregnated beads.
Vancomycin	300 mg	Regional perfusion, PMMA or other impregnated beads.
Enrofloxacin	500 mg	All modes of local delivery.

(dirt, hair, etc.) from the synovial structure, debride osseous lesions if present using endoscopy/arthroscopy, and decrease intrasynovial distention and pain. The method(s) used depend(s) on the characteristics of the infection (location, presence of an open wound, duration, severity, etc.), value of the horse, and clinician preferences. Endoscopy is the recommended approach, whenever possible, to completely evaluate the synovial structure.[37,55] However, one single method of synovial drainage may not be used universally, and each case should be evaluated individually as to the most appropriate method. Regardless of the drainage/lavage technique used, it should be combined with appropriate systemic, intrasynovial, and local antimicrobial therapy to achieve the best success.

Through-and-Through Lavage/Drainage. Through-and-through lavage is the easiest, least expensive, and thus most commonly used method to drain synovial structures.[27] It is most appropriate for acute and less severe infections not afflicted by abundant fibrin deposits. Any type of sterile fluid may be used for lavage including a 10% DMSO solution, because the volume of fluid lavaged through the synovial structure is more important than the specific type of fluid used. Most synovial structures can be lavaged adequately using large needles (14 gauge),[43] but a more thorough lavage can be accomplished using ingress and egress arthroscopic cannulas (without attaching the camera).[1,2] The disadvantages of through-and-through lavage are the inability to assess articular cartilage damage, debride osseous lesions if present, remove fibrin or foreign material, and thoroughly lavage the entire synovial structure. Needle lavage is usually neither appropriate nor successful in chronic or severe synovial infections in which fibrin and foreign material are likely to be present within the synovial space.

Closed Suction Lavage/Drainage. Closed suction drainage for the treatment of infectious arthritis of the tarsocrural joint has been reported in the horse.[56] Fenestrated, latex drains (Jackson-Pratt Hubless, American Hospital Supply Co., Chicago, IL) were placed through the dorsal surface of the joint and tunneled subcutaneously proximal to the joint following arthroscopic exploration and partial synovectomy. The drains were attached to 60 ml syringes that maintained constant negative pressure within the joint, keeping the joint decompressed. Closed suction drainage can also be used in the stifle, carpus, and fetlock joints, and in the digital flexor tendon sheath, but drains function poorly in smaller joint cavities.[43] Concurrent use of ingress drains to instill fluid into a synovial structure is not recommended because of the potential to develop superinfection of the synovial cavity.[56] The advantages of closed suction drainage include the removal of damaging enzymes and bacteria from the synovial space, maintenance of synovial decompression, and the ability to close synovial lacerations at the initial surgery. Disadvantages include the technical difficulties of managing the drains, risk of secondary infections, and the relatively short duration of synovial drainage. This technique is rarely used by the author.

Endoscopic Lavage/Drainage. Endoscopic lavage of infected joints, tendon sheaths, and bursae has essentially replaced through-and-through needle lavage in severe and chronic synovial infections.[2,5,9,37,55] However, endoscopy may not be possible in all open joint/tendon sheath/bursae injuries because the size of the wound may preclude adequate synovial distention. Endoscopy permits more thorough lavage, identification, and removal of foreign material and fibrin, debridement of osseous or tendinous lesions if present, assessment of cartilage and osseous damage, and performance of a synovectomy if needed (Figure 9.10).[2,37,55] Endoscopy also aids in determining the severity of the infection and thus the prognosis based on abnormalities within the synovial structure.

Endoscopic exploration of the entire synovial space should be performed to maximize the benefit of the procedure. Partial synovectomy may be performed but is most often limited to the contaminated or infected synovium associated with the wound. The decision to perform a more complete synovectomy should be based on the duration of the infection and the appearance of the synovium at the time of endoscopy. Endoscopic lavage and debridement is the preferred method of synovial drainage in all horses presenting wounds with synovial involvement but especially in wounds >24 hours old.[2,23,55] This is especially true for puncture wounds to the navicular bursa where, in the author's opinion, endoscopy has replaced the more invasive street nail procedure to manage wounds involving this region.[55]

Arthrotomy/Ventral Drainage. Following synovial lavage, continued synovial drainage after surgery may be beneficial in some horses with chronic synovial wounds. However, in a recent study of horses with contaminated or infected synovial cavities, as many wounds as possible were closed at the time of endoscopy with very good results.[37] Post-operative synovial drainage can usually be accomplished by leaving the wound to heal by second intention, partially closing the wound, or enlarging the wound if it is very small (Figure 9.11). However, if the

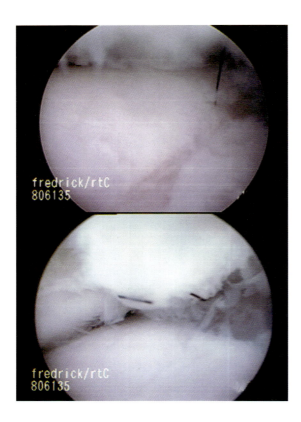

Figure 9.10. An arthroscopic view of the distal interphalangeal (coffin) joint that had sustained a penetrating wound 24 hours earlier. Note the pieces of hair and debris in the joint. These foreign bodies would not have been identified and it is unlikely they would have been removed by lavage alone without arthroscopic visualization. Reprinted from Clinical Techniques in Equine Practice, 3, Baxter GM, Management of wounds involving synovial structures in horses pp. 204–214, Copyright (2004), with permission from Elsevier Inc.

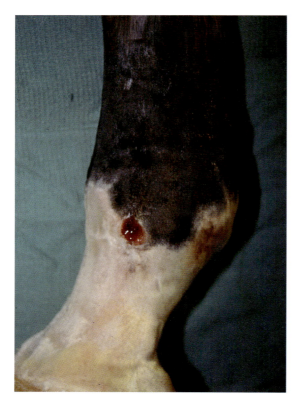

Figure 9.11. This small chronic wound that involved the metacarpophalangeal joint was left open after performing through-and-through lavage of the joint. In the author's opinion there is no advantage to closing acute or chronic synovial wounds such as these.

wound is located in an area that would not provide drainage, a separate incision in the most dependent region of the synovial structure may be necessary.

Alternatively, endoscopic portals may be enlarged to provide continued drainage. In one experimental study, the use of a tarsocrural joint arthrotomy was more effective in eliminating joint infection than were arthroscopy and partial synovectomy, but was associated with a higher risk of ascending contamination of the joint and wound healing complications.[16,57] In a clinical study, very good success was reported using open drainage of joint and tendon sheath infections with few problems with wound healing or secondary infections.[58] The decision of whether to provide additional drainage in horses with chronic synovial wounds will depend on the location of the original wound as well as the duration and severity of the infection. Additional drainage of the synovial cavity is unnecessary in most cases, provided that a thorough endoscopic lavage and exploration has been performed and that systemic, intrasynovial, and local antimicrobial therapies have all been employed.[2,37]

Ingress-Egress and Egress Drainage. Egress drainage resembles ventral drainage except that some type of drain (e.g., Penrose) is placed within the synovial cavity in an effort to ensure more prolonged drainage of the structure. Similar to arthrotomy/ventral drainage, this technique is rarely used by the author if a thorough endoscopic examination of the synovial cavity has been performed. Ingress-egress drainage is used most commonly in tendon sheaths or bursae that course up and down the limb (e.g., digital tendon sheath and calcaneal bursa). A fenestrated drain is usually placed proximad-to-distad within the synovial cavity and often exits the most dependent portion of the synovial structure. This permits passive drainage around the drain as well as active lavage of the synovial cavity as often as is considered necessary (Figure 9.12).

The main advantage of this technique is the ability to perform repeated lavage of the synovial cavity with minimal morbidity to the patient and without the need for general anesthesia. The major disadvantages are the risk of superinfection through the egress portals and the propensity for the fenestrated drain to become plugged with fibrin. Fibrin formation can be prevented by flushing the drain with heparin prior to placement and at regular intervals while it remains within the synovial cavity. In the past, the author used a single ingress-egress fenestrated drain to successfully treat synovial infections of tendon sheaths and bursae secondary to wounds, without the development of superinfection. Lavage is usually performed once daily and the drain is maintained for 2 to 4 days, depending on the severity of the infection and the response to treatment.

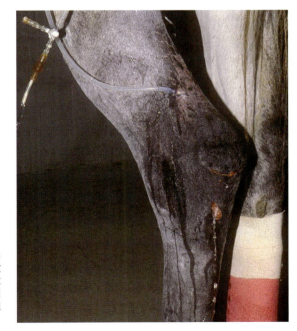

Figure 9.12. A fenestrated drain was placed through the calcaneal bursa in this horse to facilitate active lavage of the synovial cavity following surgery. The primary wound was sutured at the initial surgery to prevent wound healing complications. This type of system has also been reported as a method to provide continuous antimicrobial infusion to synovial structures if attached to a balloon reservoir.[54]

Local Antimicrobial Therapy

Additional methods to deliver high concentrations of antimicrobials locally to sites of synovial and bone infection in horses include intravenous (IV) and intraosseous (IO) regional limb perfusion as well as placement of antimicrobial impregnated polymethylmethacrylate (PMMA) or biodegradable polymers. Any of these methods may be used to treat synovial infections, but IV regional perfusion of antimicrobials is preferred by the author because it is easier to perform, less invasive, and equally effective compared to IO perfusion. Regional IV antimicrobial perfusion is recommended in all horses with wounds that involve a synovial structure either to prevent the development of synovial infection in acute injuries or to treat an established synovial infection in horses with chronic wounds.

Regional Limb Perfusion. This technique involves infusion of antimicrobials into either a superficial vein or the medullary cavity of bone to achieve high concentrations of the drug within the selected bone, soft tissues, and/or synovial structure (Figures 12.1–4).[41,42,51,59–62] In the initial studies, 1 gram of gentamicin was diluted with sterile fluid to a volume of approximately 60 ml and this was infused into the medullary cavity of the metacarpus over 30 minutes.[59,60] High concentrations of the drug (100 times that of serum) were found in the synovial fluid and membrane of the antebrachiocarpal joint, and it appeared that IO bone perfusion was more effective at eliminating infection (based on bacterial cultures) from the joint than was gentamicin given IV.

Several additional studies have since confirmed that regional IV or IO perfusion of gentamicin and amikacin results in high concentrations of drug within the synovial fluid and bone of the perfused site.[41,51,61] One study documented significantly greater synovial fluid concentrations of amikacin within the tarsocrural joint following IV regional perfusion compared with IO perfusion.[41] Currently, the author prefers IV regional perfusion over IO perfusion whenever possible. Exceptions may include horses with severe soft tissue swelling of the affected limb, preventing access to a peripheral vein; IO perfusion may be performed more easily in these horses.

The dose of antimicrobial used for regional perfusion is empirical but generally does not exceed one-half of the recommended systemic dose of the antimicrobial and is usually diluted to a volume of 30 ml–60 ml. In most cases the total dose of antimicrobial should not exceed 1 gram and less than this may be equally effective.[14,38] Amikacin (0.5 g–1 g) is used most commonly by the author but any concentration-dependent bactericidal antimicrobial may be used (gentamicin, ceftiofur, penicillin, cefazolin, timentin, enrofloxacin, vancomycin, etc.). However, a recent study found that 250 mg of amikacin used for intravenous perfusion was inadequate to obtain effective tissue concentrations of the drug and that enrofloxacin caused vasculitis in three of seven horses following IV perfusion.[63] Nonetheless, concentrations above MIC were maintained for 24–36 hours in bone and synovial fluid when enrofloxacin was delivered at 1.5 mg/kg.[63]

A bored-out 4.5 mm or 5.5 mm bone screw with a Luer-lock head and a small syringe simplify the IO perfusion procedure compared to the more complicated instruments used in the initial studies.[27,61] In addition, the male end of an extension set fits securely into a 4 mm hole in the bone and can also be used as a simple and effective method for IO perfusion. However, IV perfusion of antimicrobials into a superficial vein has potentially superior efficacy to IO perfusion and can be performed with minimal instrumentation (19–25 gauge butterfly catheter and 30 ml–60 ml syringe (Figure 9.13).[2,41,62] With both procedures, a tourniquet is placed above the site

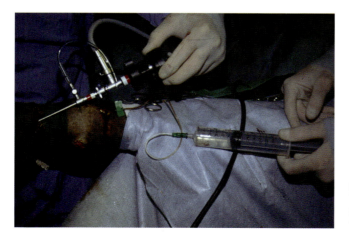

Figure 9.13. This intraoperative photograph demonstrates IV regional limb perfusion using a butterfly catheter and 60 mL syringe. The lateral palmar vein in the abaxial sesamoid region is the preferred site by the author to perform distal limb perfusion. Endoscopy of the navicular bursa was also performed in this horse.

of perfusion in the distal limb, or both above and below the proposed perfusion site if it is located more proximally on the limb, such as at the carpus or tarsus. The infusion is performed over a 1–10 minute period and the tourniquet is maintained for 20–30 minutes more to prevent systemic absorption of the drug.

Antimicrobial-impregnated PMMA. The use of antimicrobial-impregnated PMMA (Surgical Simplex P™, Howmedica, Rutherford, NJ) has been advocated for the prevention and treatment of synovial and bone infections in horses.[14,38,45,64] PMMA is a high-density plastic formed by combining a fluid monomer and powdered polymer; upon addition, an antimicrobial will become suspended in the cement as it hardens.[45,64] The cement can be placed into the surgical wound while still doughy, such as is done with plate luting or hip arthroplasty, or PMMA can be shaped into beads that are strung on a wire or piece of suture material or shaped into larger cylindrical implants (Figure 12.6).[14,38,45] The cement is allowed to harden and the implants are placed into the wound. The antimicrobials are released from the PMMA by diffusion because the tissue fluids surrounding the PMMA implant create a concentration gradient for elution of the antimicrobial from the implant. Elution is bimodal with the greatest quantity of drug released during the first few days followed by a gradual decrease.[45] The specific elution rates depend on the selected antimicrobial, the dose used, and the characteristics of the wound.[14,64]

The primary advantage of antimicrobial-impregnated PMMA is the prolonged generation of high, local concentrations of antimicrobials (up to 200 times that achieved through systemic administration) at the site of infection.[45] In horses, expensive, highly effective antimicrobials (such as amikacin, tobramycin, timentin, vancomycin) can be used locally without the need for systemic administration. Antimicrobials used with PMMA should be bactericidal, heat stable, and available in powdered form if possible (Figure 9.14).[38,45,64] Gentamicin, tobramycin, amikacin, cefazolin, and timentin are the most common antimicrobials incorporated into PMMA, but amoxicillin, metronidazole, enrofloxacin, imipenem, vancomycin, and ceftiofur may also be used.[14,38,45,65,66] The quantity of antimicrobial used is empirical but a rule of thumb is 5% to 10% of the weight of PMMA: 0.5 g–2 g for every 10–20 g of PMMA cement.[14,38] While the amount of antimicrobial eluted from the PMMA is proportional to the amount placed in it, an excessive quantity (particularly liquid antimicrobials) can prolong or inhibit the set-up time and the quality or strength of the PMMA.

To achieve the greatest drug concentration and thus the greatest success with antimicrobial-impregnated PMMA, wound closure is logical and considered necessary by some surgeons.[67] Irrigation-suction drainage should not be employed because the irrigation fluid will wash away the high concentrations of antimicrobials.[67]

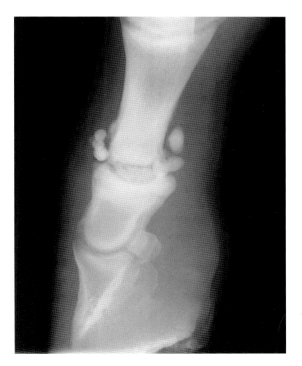

Figure 9.14. This lateral radiograph is of a 6-month-old foal that developed osteomyelitis of the middle and proximal phalanges secondary to a pastern wound. PMMA beads containing amikacin were placed into the wound and the proximal interphalangeal joint. The limb was immobilized in a cast and the joint eventually ankylosed.

The PMMA is usually removed in human patients, but this is not necessary in all cases in horses.[14,38,45] Biodegradable polymers (polylactic acid, plaster of paris, collagen sponges, and high amylase starch implants) are being investigated for local antimicrobial delivery and their use may obviate some of the potential problems associated with the non-absorbable PMMA polymer.[65,68–71]

In horses, antimicrobial impregnated PMMA may be most effective at treating soft tissue infections associated with open fractures or in prevention of osteomyelitis and implant infection in long bone fractures.[38,45] Antimicrobial impregnated PMMA is not used routinely in horses with chronic synovial wounds unless other methods have failed to resolve the infection, osteomyelitis is present, or if highly resistant bacteria have been isolated from the wound or synovial cavity (Figure 9.14). The author has not placed PMMA beads within high-motion synovial cavities because of the risk of iatrogenic damage to the articular cartilage and synovium that these beads have been reported to cause.[72]

Wound Closure

In the past, most clinicians did not consider closing synovial wounds with established infection for fear of trapping the infection within a closed compartment. Synovial drainage and decompression were considered the standard treatment and arthrotomies were recommended to drain closed infected joints. More recently, the pendulum appears to be swinging in the opposite direction as better methods to treat the synovial infection have been developed (endoscopic exploration, regional perfusion, continuous antimicrobial infusion, etc.). Currently, many synovial wounds can be closed at the time of endoscopy/lavage without the risk of continued infection, and arthrotomies to treat synovial sepsis are being performed infrequently.

A recent study of horses with contaminated or infected synovial cavities reported that many of the wounds (48 of 121 cases) were closed at the time of endoscopy with very good results.[37] Another recent study found no appreciable difference in the degree of joint or tendon sheath distention between horses in which the synovial structure was closed as opposed to left open, although resolution of synovial infection was not confirmed via culturing.[54]

The author agrees with the results of these studies and attempts to close wounds associated with synovial structures whenever possible (Figures 9.15a,b). This said, not all synovial wounds with an established infection are suitable for closure such that good surgical judgment must be used when making this decision. Clean, acute wounds in which the synovial cavity has been evaluated endoscopically or arthroscopically are best suited for wound closure. Conversely, chronic wounds with established infection, secondary cellulitis, osteomyelitis, and marked pannus within the synovial cavity may not be suitable for closure. However, in some cases the risks of continued infection must be weighed against the complications of wound healing (i.e., high-motion area) when deciding whether of not to close a wound.

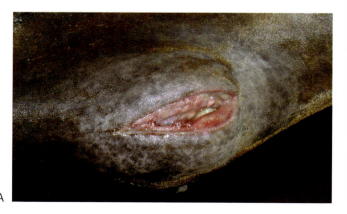
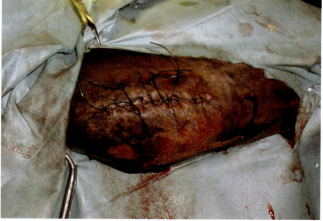

A   B

Figure 9.15. (A) This chronic laceration involved the lateral aspect of the calcaneal bursa. (B) The bursa was lavaged and the wound was debrided and closed in an effort to prevent wound healing complications because of its location in such a high motion area. A bandage-sleeve cast was placed for immobilization and the wound healed with no complications.

Adjunctive Therapy

Annular Ligament/Retinacula Release Procedures

The annular ligament on the palmar/plantar surface of the digital sheaths and retinaculi within the tarsal and carpal sheaths create an inelastic canal through which the associated tendons glide.[5,9] With chronic infection, this inelastic canal can become smaller due to swelling of the synovial lining, pannus formation, and secondary tendonitis. Movement of the tendon through this narrowed canal can lead to pain and lameness, contributing to patient morbidity. Transection of the annular ligament and carpal and tarsal retinaculi can be performed in horses with chronic infectious tenosynovitis to help alleviate constriction within the affected tendon sheath.[5,7,8] However, these procedures are usually reserved for horses with chronic, established infections that have not responded to previous treatment.[5] They can be performed using either open or endoscopic approaches and rarely contribute to permanent disability of the horse.

Nonsteroidal Anti-Inflammatory Drugs (NSAIDs)

The anti-inflammatory and analgesic benefits of NSAIDs in horses with acute or chronic synovial injuries greatly outweigh the potential risks of these drugs. Phenylbutazone, the most commonly used NSAID, decreases the production of inflammatory mediators, particularly prostaglandin E_2, preventing articular cartilage damage and joint pain.[27,28] The analgesic effects of NSAIDs help improve ambulation and joint motion, thereby improving articular cartilage nutrition and inhibiting periarticular fibrosis. In addition, maintaining some movement within tendon sheaths and bursae is considered beneficial to prevent the formation of fibrous adhesions between the tendons and the synovium.

Phenylbutazone is most commonly used at 4.4 mg/kg orally every 12 hours initially, and then the dose is gradually decreased within 48 hours to no more than 4.4 mg/kg daily as the clinical signs improve. In the author's opinion, the risk of phenylbutazone or any other NSAID complicating the clinical assessment of a patient with synovial infection is minimal, provided that it is used at a dose of no greater than 4.4 mg/kg daily.

Local and Systemic Synovial Therapy

The use of intrasynovial medications to help prevent secondary synovitis and osteoarthritis in horses with synovial infections is controversial. Corticosteroids and polysulfated glycosaminoglycan (PSGAG) have been associated with an increased risk of infection following intrasynovial injection;[17] and therefore, may worsen the infectious process. Hyaluronan, administered intrasynovially, has anti-inflammatory capabilities and may be beneficial during the early treatment of infection, but the inflammatory response present within most infected synovial structures may degrade the drug before it can exert its beneficial effects. In horses with persistent synovial inflammation, corticosteroids alone or combined with hyaluronan may be used as local anti-inflammatory agents, with minimal risk, after the infection has resolved (2 to 3 weeks after clinical signs have subsided).

IV hyaluronan (Legend, Bayer Pharmaceutical) may be the most beneficial adjunctive medication to use for synovial infections. The IV route of administration eliminates the potential complications of intrasynovial use while helping to decrease the inflammation within the synovium early in the course of treatment.[73] Similarly, IM PSGAG (Adequan, Luitpold Pharmaceutical, Shirley, NY) is thought to have anti-inflammatory activity, and may also decrease the inflammatory response in infected synovial structures. Intrathecal hyaluronan may be beneficial, especially in tendon sheath and bursal infections early in the treatment period (within 2 weeks) to help prevent adhesion formation within the synovial cavity.[74] However, the author does not routinely use intrasynovial hyaluronan or other joint medications within infected synovial cavities for a minimum of 2 weeks after resolution of the infection.

Rest and Physical Therapy

In most cases, horses with synovial wounds will benefit from stall confinement in the early postoperative period. Confinement is necessary to prevent wound dehiscence, improve wound healing, and minimize damage to the less resilient articular cartilage in infected joints. External support using bandages, splints, or casts is necessary to decrease soft tissue swelling, edema, and pain, and to immobilize the wound. The duration of confinement will vary depending on the location of the wound, the synovial structure that is involved, the severity of the synovial infection, and whether the wound is closed or left to heal by second intention.

In general, it appears that passive motion and other forms of physical therapy are begun earlier postoperatively and are used more aggressively in people than in horses. Passive manipulation of joints undergoing elective arthroscopic surgery is often recommended at the time of suture removal in horses to reduce adhesion formation and prevent periarticular fibrosis. This often will include periods of hand walking to regain joint flexibility and to improve cartilage health. Similarly, physical therapy (passive manipulation and hand walking) should be instituted in horses with synovial wounds as soon as the infection is resolved and the wound is considered to be healing adequately. Hand walking is considered essential in horses with tendon sheath and bursae wounds to reduce the risk of adhesion formation. However, this must be adjusted on a case-by-case basis because complete healing of the external wound should be given priority over prevention of adhesion formation, especially in high-motion areas.

Complications

The most significant complication when managing synovial wounds is the inability to resolve the infection and re-sterilize the synovial cavity. The continued infection damages the articular cartilage and subchondral bone in joints and can lead to bone and tendon damage in tendon sheaths and bursae (Figure 9.16). In addition, the chronic inflammatory response contributes to fibrosis within the synovial capsule, leading to a reduced range of motion, fibrous adhesions within the synovial space, and permanent enlargement of the synovial cavity. In most cases, the wound can be managed successfully if the synovial infection can be resolved. Therefore, the treatment approach in most synovial wounds in horses should be to resolve the synovial infection first and deal with the wound second. However, wound healing complications are common in horses and wounds involving synovial structures should be approached no differently than wounds elsewhere on the limb. Complete or partial wound closure should be performed whenever possible and the limb immobilized when indicated. Synovial fistulae may develop in a small percentage of wounds that are left to heal by second intention or those that dehisce, due to the continuous flow of synovial fluid exiting the wound (Figure 9.17). Most will resolve with time and adequate immobilization, but occasionally delayed closure of the fistula will be necessary.

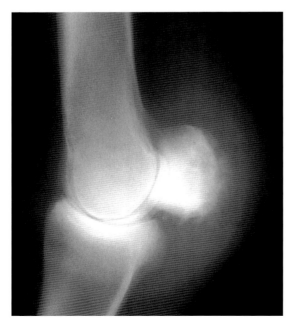

Figure 9.16. This lateral radiograph of a horse with chronic infection of the digital tendon sheath revealed periosteal reaction and lysis of the abaxial surfaces of both proximal sesamoid bones. The long-standing infection eroded through the soft tissues of the tendon sheath, causing secondary infection within the sesamoid bones.

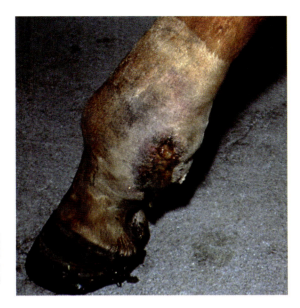

Figure 9.17. This horse developed a synovial fistula within the digital tendon sheath secondary to a small laceration in this region. Synovial fluid can be seen exiting the wound. Synovial fistulae tend to occur more commonly within tendon sheaths and bursae than within joints in horses.

Prognosis

Factors likely to affect the prognosis of horses with acute and chronic synovial wounds include the intended use of the horse, the specific synovial structure(s) involved, the duration of the infection before treatment, and whether a concurrent osseous or tendinous lesion was present.[13,27,37,55] In general, the more quickly synovial involvement can be identified and treated, the better the prognosis. Additionally, the absence of secondary osseous or tendinous injuries should improve the prognosis regardless of the location of the injury.[13,27,37]

Early studies of horses with synovial wounds and infections reported survival rates ranging from 54%–85%.[4,35,29,56] The percentage of horses returning to their intended use following treatment of synovial infections ranged from 33%–77%.[4,35,29,56] In a recent retrospective case series of 121 horses with contaminated or infected synovial cavities treated with endoscopy, 90% of the horses survived and 81% of the horses returned to their preoperative level of performance.[37] A recent study evaluating septic calcaneal bursitis in 24 horses reported a 67% survival rate with 81% of those horses returning to full performance.[13] Additionally, 13 of 16 horses returned to their intended use following treatment of infectious synovitis with a constant rate infusion system.[54]

Horses with wounds involving the navicular bursa and distal interphalangeal joint represent the most difficult challenge to return to performance.[55,75] Nonetheless, 10 of 16 horses with septic navicular bursitis returned to their pre-injury performance level following endoscopic lavage and debridement.[55] Based on the results of these recent studies and the clinical impression of the author, endoscopic exploration/lavage of synovial wounds combined with systemic, intrasynovial, and IV regional perfusion of antimicrobials has increased our ability to successfully treat the majority of affected horses.

Conclusion

Wounds involving synovial structures (joints, tendon sheaths, or bursae) are very common in horses. Synovial structures of the distal limb (distal to and including the carpus and tarsus) are most commonly involved, although any synovial space can be affected. Acute injuries will usually have bacterial contamination of synovia without a true synovial infection, and if treated promptly will have a very good outcome. More chronic injuries will often have an established synovial infection and should be treated aggressively to minimize the impact of the secondary infection. The prognosis for horses with more chronic wounds depends on the duration of the infection, the specific synovial structure involved, whether a concurrent osseous or tendon injury is present, and the intended use of the horse.

The causative bacteria in synovial wounds varies but environmental Gram negatives are highly probable and should be considered when selecting the most appropriate antimicrobial(s) to either prevent or treat these infections. Endoscopic exploration of the affected synovial structure is the treatment of choice in nearly all cases, but particularly in chronic synovial wounds. Endoscopy/arthroscopy permits removal of foreign debris if present, contaminating bacteria, and inflammatory exudate, and helps to restore the normal synovial environment more quickly than synovial lavage alone. Systemic, intrasynovial, and IV regional antimicrobial therapy are considered the standard of care for most synovial wounds, and have improved our success in resolving most synovial infections. Wound debridement and closure should be considered whenever possible in synovial wounds, especially after a complete endoscopic exploration of the synovial cavity has been combined with local and systemic antimicrobials. Endoscopic surgery should permit thorough cleansing of the synovial cavity and a closed wound minimizes the risk of further contamination.[37]

If the wound is closed, casting or splinting to immobilize the wound in high-motion regions such as the fetlock, pastern, tarsus, or carpus should be used if it is considered necessary for optimal wound healing. Wounds that are left to heal by second intention should be bandaged (with or without splinting) to permit frequent wound treatment and are usually not placed under a cast. The prognosis is variable depending on the characteristics of the synovial infection, but should be very good in horses with a single affected synovial cavity and without secondary osseous or tendinous injuries.

References

1. Baxter GM: Management of wounds. In P Colahan, I Mayhew, A Merritt, and J Moore, eds. *Equine medicine and surgery vol II (5th edition)*. Philadelphia: Mosby, 1999, p.1808
2. Baxter GM: Treatment of wounds involving synovial structures. Clin Tech Equine Pract 2005;3:204
3. Stashak T: Wound infection: Contributing factors and selected techniques for prevention. Proc Am Assoc Equine Pract 2006;52:270
4. Schneider RK, Bramlage LR, Moore RM, et al: A retrospective study of 192 horses affected with septic arthritis/tenosynovitis. Equine Vet J 1992;24:436
5. Janicek JC, Hunt RJ: Septic tarsal sheath tenosynovitis. Comp Contin Educ Pract Vet 2006;2:94
6. Hand DR, Watkins JP, Honnas CM, et al: Osteomyelitis of the sustentaculum tali in horses: 10 cases (1992–1998). J Am Vet Med Assoc 2001;219:341
7. Santschi EM, Adams SB, Fessler JF, et al: Treatment of bacterial tarsal tenosynovitis and osteitis of the sustentaculum tali of the calcaneus in five horses. Equine Vet J 1997;29:244
8. Frees KE, Lillich JD, Gaughan EM, et al: Tenoscopic-assisted treatment of open digital tendon sheath injuries in horses: 20 cases (1992–2001). J Am Vet Med Assoc 2002;220:1823
9. Whitcomb MB, Le Jeune SS, MacDonald MM, et al: Disorders of the infraspinatus tendon and bursa in three horses. J Am Vet Med Assoc 2006;229:549
10. Vastista NJ, Pascoe JR, Wright IM, et al: Infection of the intertubercular bursa in horses: four cases (1978–1991). J Am Vet Med Assoc 1996;208:1434
11. Tudor RA, Bowman KF, Redding RW, et al: Endoscopic treatment of suspected infectious intertubercular bursitis in a horse. J Am Vet Med Assoc 1998;213:1584
12. Todhunter RJ: Anatomy and physiology of synovial joints. In CW McIlwraith and G Trotter, eds. *Joint disease in the horse*, (1st edition). Philadelphia: WB Saunders, 1996, p.1
13. Post EM, Singer ER, Clegg PD, et al: Retrospective study of 24 cases of septic calcaneal bursitis in the horse. Equine Vet J 2003;35:662
14. Goodrich LR, Nixon AJ: Treatment options for osteomyelitis. Equine Vet J 2004;16:340
15. MacDonald MH: The pathophysiology of equine synovial infections. Proc Am Coll Vet Surg 1995;5:43
16. Bertone AL, McIlwraith CW, Jones RL et al: Comparison of various treatments for experimentally induced equine infectious arthritis. Am J Vet Res 1987;48:519
17. Gustafson SB, McIlwraith CW, Jones RL: Comparison of the effect of polysulfated glycosaminoglycan, corticosteroids, and sodium hyaluronate in the potentiation of a subinfective dose of *Staphylococcus aureus* in the midcarpal joint of horses. Am J Vet Res 1989;50:2014
18. Hardy J, Bertone AL, Malemud CJ: Effect of synovial membrane infection in vitro on equine synoviocytes and chondrocytes. Am J Vet Res 1998;59:293
19. Speirs S, May SA, Harrison LJ, et al: Proteolytic enzymes in equine joints with infectious arthritis. Equine Vet J 1994;26:48
20. Tulamo RM, Bramlage LR, Gabel AA: The influence of corticosteroids on sequential clinical and synovial fluid parameters in joints with acute infectious arthritis in the horse. Equine Vet J 1989;21:332

21. Kidd JA, Dyson SJ, Barr AR: Septic flexor tendon core lesions in five horses. Equine Vet J 2002;34:213
22. Platt D, Wright IM. Chronic tenosynovitis of the carpal extensor tendon sheaths in 15 horses. Equine Vet J 1997;29:11
23. Gibbs C: Radiological signs of bone infection and neoplasia. Equine Vet Educ 1994;6:103
24. Stashak TS: Current concepts in wound management in horses. Proc North Am Vet Conf 2003;17:231
25. Reef VB. Musculoskeletal ultrasonography. In V Reef, ed. *Equine diagnostic ultrasound (1st edition)*. Philadelphia: WB Saunders, 1998, p.39
26. Reimer JM: Synovial structures. In J Reimer, ed. *Atlas of equine ultrasonography (1st edition)*. St Louis: CV Mosby Co, 1998, p.66
27. Baxter GM: Instrumentation and techniques for treating orthopedic infections in horses. Vet Clin North Am Equine Pract 1996;12:303
28. Gaughan EM: Wounds of the tendon sheaths and joints in horses. Compend Contin Educ Pract Vet 1994;16:517
29. Honnas CM, Schumacher J, Cohen ND, et al: Septic tenosynovitis in horses: 25 cases (1983–1989). J Am Vet Med Assoc 1991;199:1616
30. Madison JB, Sommer M, Spencer PA: Relations among synovial membrane histopathologic findings, synovial fluid cytologic findings, and bacterial culture results in horses with suspected infectious arthritis: 64 cases (1979–1987). J Am Vet Med Assoc 1991;198:1655
31. Montgomery RD, Long IR, Milton JL, et al: Comparison of aerobic culturette, synovial membrane biopsy, and blood culture medium in the detection of canine bacterial arthritis. Vet Surg 1989;18:300
32. Moore RM: Diagnosis and treatment of obligate anaerobic bacterial infections in horses. Compend Contin Educ Pract Vet 1993;15:989
33. Brown MP: Antimicrobial selection and advances. Proc Am Coll Vet Surg 1995;5:40
34. Moore RM, Schneider RK, Kowalski J, et al: Antimicrobial susceptibility of bacterial isolates from 233 horses with musculoskeletal infection during 1979–1989. Equine Vet J 1992;24:450
35. Gibson KT, McIlwraith CW, Turner AS, et al: Open joint injuries in horses: 58 cases (1980–1986). J Am Vet Med Assoc 1989;194:398
36. Baxter GM: Retrospective study of lower limb wounds involving tendons, tendon sheaths, or joints in horses. Proc Am Assoc Equine Pract 1987;33:715
37. Wright IM, Smith MR, Humphrey DJ, et al: Endoscopic surgery in the treatment of contaminated and infected synovial cavities. Equine Vet J 2003;35:613
38. Schneider RK: Orthopedic infections. In JA Auer and JA Stick, eds. *Equine surgery (2nd edition)*. Philadelphia: WB Saunders, 1999, p.727
39. Orsini JA, Elce Y, Kraus B: Management of severely infected wounds in the equine patient. Clin Tech Equine Pract 2004;3:225
40. Cauvin ERJ, Tapprest J, Munroe GA, et al: Endoscopic examination of the tarsal sheath of the lateral digital flexor tendon in horses. Equine Vet J 1999;31:219
41. Scheuch BC, Van Hoogmoed LM, Wilson WD, et al: Comparison of intraosseous to intravenous infusion for delivery of amikacin sulfate to the tibiotarsal joint of horses. Am J Vet Res 2002;63:374
42. Palmar SE, Hogan PM: How to perform regional limb perfusion in the standing horse. Proc Am Assoc Equine Pract 1999;45:124
43. Ross MW: Clinical management of synovial infection. Proc Am Coll Vet Surg 1995;5:45
44. Hughes KJ, Hodgson JL, Hodgson DR: Use of fluoroquinolone antimicrobial agents in equine practice. Equine Vet Educ 2002;14:240
45. Sayegh AI, Moore RM: Polymethylmethacrylate beads for treating orthopedic infections. Compend Contin Educ Pract Vet 2003;25:788
46. Trostle S, Peavey CL, King DS, et al: Treatment of methicillin-resistant Staphylococcus epidermidis infection following repair of an ulnar fracture and humeroradial joint luxation in a horse. J Am Vet Med Assoc 2001;218:554
47. Rubio-Martinez LM, Lopez-Sanroman J, Cruz AM, et al: Evaluation of safety and pharmacokinetics of vancomycin after intravenous regional limb perfusion in horses. Am J Vet Res 2005;66:2107
48. Orsini JA, Snooks-Parsons C, Stine L, et al: Vancomycin for the treatment of methicillin-resistant staphylococcal and enterococcal infections in 15 horses. Can J Vet Res 2005;69:278
49. Lloyd KCK, Stover SM, Pascoe JR, et al: Synovial fluid pH, cytologic characteristics, and gentamicin concentration after intra-articular administration of the drug in an experimental model of infectious arthritis in horses. Am J Vet Res 1990;51:1363
50. Werner LA, Hardy J, Bertone A: Bone gentamicin concentration after intra-articular injection or regional perfusion in the horse. Vet Surg 2003;32:559
51. Mills ML, Rush BR, St Jean G, et al: Determination of synovial fluid and serum concentrations, and morphologic effects of intraarticular ceftiofur sodium in horses. Vet Surg 2005;29:398
52. Lescun TB, Adams SB, Wu CC, et al: Continuous infusion of gentamicin into tarsocrural joints of horses. Am J Vet Res 2000;61:407

53. Lescun TB, Vasey JR, Ward MP, et al: Treatment with continuous intrasynovial antimicrobial infusion for septic synovitis in horses: 31 cases (2000–2003). J Am Vet Med Assoc 2006;228:1922

54. Meagher DT, Latimer FG, Sutter WW, et al: Evaluation of a balloon constant rate infusion system for treatment of septic arthritis, septic tenosynovitis, and contaminated synovial wounds: 23 cases (2002–2005). J Am Vet Med Assoc 2006;228:1930

55. Wright IM, Phillips TJ, Walmsley JP: Endoscopy of the navicular bursa: A new technique for the treatment of contaminated and septic bursae. Equine Vet J 1999;31:5

56. Ross MW, Orsini JA, Richardson DW, et al: Closed suction drainage in the treatment of infectious arthritis of the equine tarsocrural joint. Vet Surg 1991;20:21

57. Bertone AL, Davis DM, Cox HU, et al: Arthrotomy versus arthroscopy and partial synovectomy for the treatment of experimentally induced infectious arthritis in horses. Am J Vet Res 1992;53:585

58. Schneider RK, Bramlage LR, Mecklenburg LM, et al: Open drainage, intra-articular and systemic antibiotics in the treatment of septic arthritis/tenosynovitis in horses. Equine Vet J 1992;24:443

59. Whitehair KL, Bowersock TL, Blevins WE, et al: Regional limb perfusion for antibiotic treatment of experimentally induced septic arthritis. Vet Surg 1992;21:367

60. Whitehair KL, Blevins WE, Fessler JF, et al: Regional perfusion of the equine carpus for antibiotic delivery. Vet Surg 1992;21:279

61. Mattson S, Boure L, Pearce S, et al: Intraosseous gentamicin perfusion of the distal metacarpus in standing horses. Vet Surg 2004;33:180

62. Pille F, DeBaere S, Ceelen L, et al: Synovial fluid and plasma concentration of ceftiofur after regional intravenous perfusion in the horse. Vet Surg 2005;34:610

63. Parra-Sanchez A, Jugo J, Boothe DM, et al: Pharmacokinetics and pharmacodynamics of enrofloxacin and low dose for amikacin administered via regional intravenous limb perfusion in standing horses. Am J Vet Res 2006;67:1687

64. Swalec Tobias KM, Schneider RK, Besser TE: Use of antimicrobial-impregnated polymethylmethacrylate. J Am Vet Med Assoc 1996;208:841

65. Santschi EM, McGarvey L: In vitro elution of gentamicin from plaster of Paris beads. Vet Surg 2003;32:128

66. Ramos JR, Howard RD, Pleasant RS, et al: Elution of metronidazole and gentamicin from polymethylmethacrylate beads. Vet Surg 2003;32:251

67. Klemm KW: Antibiotic bead chains. Clin Orthop Relat Res 1993;295:63

68. Summerhays GE: Treatment of traumatically induced synovial sepsis in horses with gentamicin-impregnated collagen sponges. Vet Rec 2000;147:184

69. Cook VL, Bertone AL, Kowalski JJ, et al: Biodegradable drug delivery systems for gentamicin release and treatment of synovial membrane infection. Vet Surg 1999;28:233

70. Ivester KM, Adams SB, Moore GE, et al: Gentamicin concentrations in synovial fluid obtained from the tarsocrural joints of horses after implantation of gentamicin-impregnated collagen sponges. Am J Vet Res 2006;67:1519

71. Huneault LM, Lussier B, Dubreuil P, et al: Prevention and treatment of experimental osteomyelitis with ciprofloxacin-loaded high amylase starch implants. J Ortho Res 2004;22:1351

72. Farnsworth KD, White NA, Robertson J: The effect of implanting gentamicin impregnated polymethylmethacrylate beads in the tarsocrural joint of the horse. Vet Surg 2001;30:126

73. Kawcak CE, Frisbie DD, Trotter GW, et al: Effects of intravenous administration of sodium hyaluronate on carpal joints in exercising horses after arthroscopic surgery and osteochondral fragmentation. Am J Vet Res 1997;58:1132

74. Gaughan EM, Nixon AJ, Krook LP, et al: Effects of sodium hyaluronate on tendon healing and adhesion formation in horses. Am J Vet Res 1991;52:764

75. Honnas CM, Welch RD, Ford TS, et al: Septic arthritis of the distal interphalangeal joint in 12 horses. Vet Surg 1992;21:261

10 Tendon and Paratendon Lacerations

Henry Jann, DVM, MS, Diplomate ACVS, **and Ted S. Stashak**, DVM, MS, Diplomate ACVS

Introduction

One of the most career-compromising and life-threatening musculoskeletal injuries that can occur in a horse is the traumatic division of a tendon. This is particularly true with severance of a flexor tendon. Many advances in the management of these injuries have been made in recent years in an effort to improve the prognosis for return to performance. Successful management of tendon lacerations requires an understanding of tendon anatomy and healing. An accurate diagnosis of the involved structure or structures as well as and the development of a sound therapeutic plan are foremost in restoring limb function.

The aim of this chapter is to review tendon anatomy and healing and the approach to clinical diagnoses as well as treatment strategies in hopes of providing the reader with adequate information to successfully manage wounds associated with tendons and paratendinous structures.

Tendon

Function

Tendons possess great tensile strength and low extensibility and are highly innervated, well vascularized structures which have the ability to store, conserve, amplify, and transmit energy. In mechanical terms, tendons are force transmitters, allowing the musculoskeletal system to perform an amazing spectrum of activities ranging from the most precise and delicate manipulations to supporting incredible feats of speed, stamina, and strength. Other mechanical functions ascribed to tendons include the ability to store elastic energy and act as a dynamic amplifier and force attenuator during rapid and unexpected movement.[1] The biomechanical property that allows tendons to perform these functions is elasticity, a result of collagen fibrils which are longitudinally arranged in a helical configuration and fiber bundles which are packed into a zigzag pattern of tightly crimped fiber bundles.[2]

Anatomy

Several structures of surgical importance contribute to the ability of tendons to perform their functions as transmitters and modulators of biomechanical force. Annular ligaments or retinacula are strong fibrous bands that act to maintain the tendon in its correct position, parallel to the long axis of bones and joints, when tensile force is applied. Tendon sheaths surround tendons where they cross joints to reduce friction in areas where tensile force changes direction (Figure 10.1). Tendon sheaths provide a gliding surface to ensure smooth and effortless locomotion. The tendon sheath is composed of two distinct layers: an outer parietal layer and an inner visceral layer (Figure 10.2). The outer layer provides structural durability while the inner layer produces synovial fluid to lubricate the gliding tendon. The mesotendon is contained within the visceral layer of the sheath, which carries the extrinsic blood supply to the tendon. In some locations the mesotendon is replaced by a band of highly elastic connective tissue called the vinculum, which serves the same purpose.

Tendon sheaths usually have a sickle fold at the proximal extremity to accommodate tendon gliding (Figure 10.3). When tendons traverse anatomic regions in which the tensile force does not change directions during locomotion, such as the diaphysial region of the metacarpal/metatarsal bones, they are covered by paratendon (Figure 10.4). A paratendon is a highly vascular and extremely elastic layer of connective tissue that provides gliding function and structural support for extrinsic vascular components.[3]

Tendons receive their blood supply in several ways: vessels originating from muscle or bone insertions, mesotendon- or vinculum-derived vessels in the tendon sheath, and vessels in the paratendon. Muscle and bone

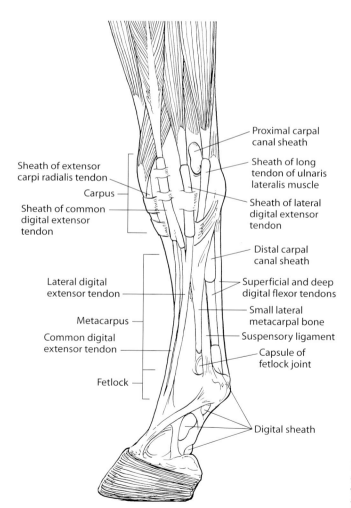

Sheath of extensor carpi radialis tendon

Carpus

Sheath of common digital extensor tendon

Lateral digital extensor tendon

Metacarpus

Common digital extensor tendon

Fetlock

Proximal carpal canal sheath

Sheath of long tendon of ulnaris lateralis muscle

Sheath of lateral digital extensor tendon

Distal carpal canal sheath

Superficial and deep digital flexor tendons

Small lateral metacarpal bone

Suspensory ligament

Capsule of fetlock joint

Digital sheath

Figure 10.1. Lateral view of sheathed and non-sheathed tendons of the fore limb. Note that tendon sheaths surround tendons where they cross joints to reduce friction in areas where tensile force changes direction.

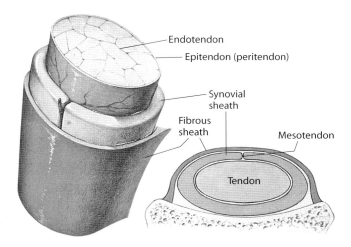

Figure 10.2. Left: A tendon within a tendon sheath. Right: Cross-section of a tendon within a tendon sheath.

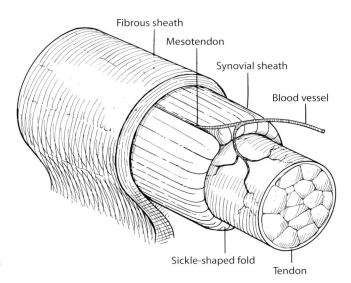

Figure 10.3. The sickle-shaped fold at the proximal limits of a tendon sheath.

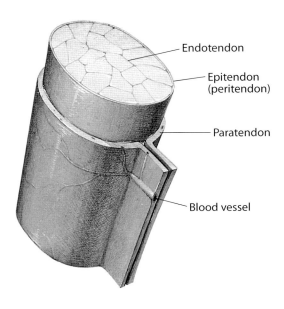

Figure 10.4. A tendon within a paratendon.

insertions only supply the proximal and distal ~25% of the tendon, while the paratendon and mesotendon are assumed to play an important role in other areas. There are also intratendinous vessels, interconnected by a diffuse capillary network, which travel more than 25% of the length in the portion of the tendon that is covered by paratendon.[3]

Healing

There are two generally accepted patterns of tendon healing, classified as intrinsic and extrinsic. The primary difference between the two patterns is the origin of the cellular components which migrate into the injured area, multiply, and eventually produce collagen, which is remodeled into a functional bridge between the severed tendon ends. The intrinsic pattern is characterized initially by an inflammatory phase and the in-growth of macrophage-like cells which stimulate fibroblast migration from the epitendon and the endotendon. The extrinsic pattern is characterized by the in-growth of cells from either the paratendon or, to a very limited extent, from the tendon sheath. Vascular elements follow cellular migration in both forms of healing.

Extrinsic healing is the most important and possibly the exclusive pattern of healing following severe disruption/transection of an equine tendon. Unfortunately, the end result of extrinsic healing is compromised by the formation of peritendinous adhesions, which decrease the gliding function of the tendon. While limited passive motion tends to promote intrinsic healing, immobilization promotes extrinsic healing. This situation constitutes a major dilemma in the management of equine tendon lacerations, since limb immobilization is required to prevent disruption of the repair site and healing process.

Although the biological sequence of events leading to tendon healing is the same as for other tissues, the time frame to progress from the inflammatory phase through the proliferative phase and finally the remodeling phase stretches over days, weeks, and months, respectively.[3,4] In general, the vascular and cellular reactions of the inflammatory phase may extend well into the second week of repair. The tendon repair is weakest between the fifth and seventh days post-wounding, presumably because of the lysis of the fibrocellular clot. The repair phase (14–45 days) results in a fibrovascular callus that forms around the tendon, coalescing all structures in the wound. During the maturation phase (45–120 days), the fibroblasts and collagen fibers begin to orient themselves longitudinally. At 45 days, collagen synthesis and lysis reach equilibrium. At 90 days early collagen bundle formation is seen, and at 120 days the bundles appear much like those of a normal tendon. However, in vivo tensile strength studies indicate that it takes approximately 240 days before the repair site reaches a strength equivalent to that of the adjacent normal tendon.[3,5,6]

Clinical Diagnosis

Severed Flexor Tendons

Flexor tendon lacerations are common injuries. In both the fore limb and hind limb they occur in the palmar/plantar metacarpal/metatarsal and pastern regions. These injuries almost always result from impact with sharp objects in the environment. Barbed wire is probably the single most common cause for these injuries.

The clinical signs associated with lacerated flexor tendons consist of alterations in limb conformation as well as gait deficits, and these will vary depending on the structures involved. The simplest and most effective way to assess loss of tendon function due to complete transection is to observe the animal during controlled ambulation. The distal interphalangeal (DIP) and metacarpophalangeal (MCP)/metatarsophalangeal (MTP) joints undergo a certain degree of characteristic hyperextension depending on which flexor support structure has been transected. Complete transection of the superficial digital flexor tendon (SDFT) results in mild hyperextension of the MCP/MTP joint (fetlock drop) during weight bearing (Figure 10.5). When the SDFT deep digital flexor tendons (DDFT) are severed, the MCP/MTP and the DIP joints simultaneously hyperextend during weight bearing—this is evidenced by a dropped fetlock and toe elevation (Figure 10.6). If both the flexor tendons and the suspensory ligament are cut, the fetlock will rest on the ground with the toe pointing up (Figure 10.7). Because of anatomic considerations, a laceration below the fetlock will usually involve only the deep digital flexor tendon and the digital sheath. In these cases the toe elevates when weight is placed on the foot (Figure 10.8).[4,7–9]

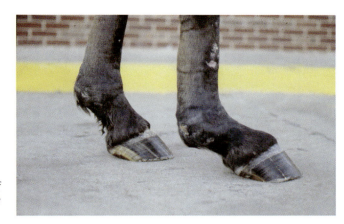

Figure 10.5. Example of mild hyperextension (fetlock drop) of the left fore metacarpophalangeal joint resulting from complete transection of the superficial digital flexor tendon.

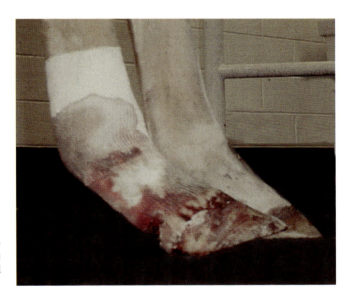

Figure 10.6. Mild hyperextension of the right rear metatarsophalangeal and distal interphalangeal joints associated with complete transection of both the superficial and deep digital flexor tendons.

Digital palpation is often useful in determining the extent of damage to tendons which are not completely transected. This can be done in the conscious horse but it is easier and more informative with the use of general anesthesia. A technique which can be useful is passively flexing and extending the distal joints while simultaneously palpating the tendons. This permits assessment of the overall integrity of the tendon and the extent of partial lacerations. Partial lacerations of the flexor tendons are very significant because a partial thickness injury can progress to full thickness without appropriate bandage splinting and/or casting.

Severed Extensor Tendons

Loss of extensor function in the distal limb occurs when a major extensor tendon is transected. The common digital extensor tendon (CDET) and the long digital extensor tendon (LDET) are the major extensor tendons of the thoracic and pelvic limbs, respectively. Transection of either of these will result in loss of extensor function in the distal limb. The clinically apparent gait deficit is a knuckling forward of the fetlock when the limb is advanced (Figure 10.9). There is no loss of ability to bear weight nor is there hyperextension of the MCP/MTP

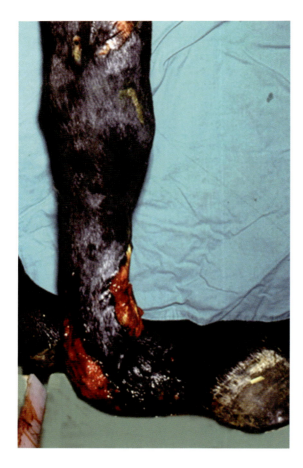

Figure 10.7. Both flexor tendons and the suspensory ligament of the right fore limb were completely transected. Note the fetlock is resting on a block of wood and there is only slight elevation of the toe. The toe is only being slightly elevated because the extensor tendons were also transected.

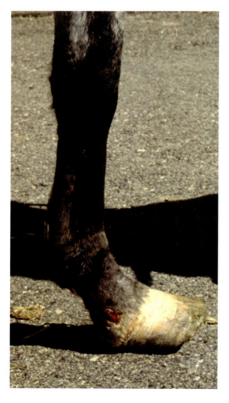

Figure 10.8. An example of transection of the deep digital flexor tendon only in the pastern region of the right fore limb. Generally, lacerations below the fetlock involve only the deep digital flexor tendon and the digital sheath. Note that the toe is elevated but the fetlock joint is in a correct anatomic position when weight is placed on the foot.

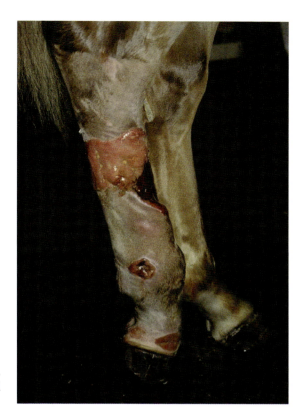

Figure 10.9. Knuckling of the right rear fetlock joint associated with compromised extensor function resulting from lacerated long and lateral digital extensor tendons.

or DIP joints with the limb in appropriate anatomic position.[10] Severance of the lateral digital extensor in the fore limb or hind limb will generally not cause any gait deficit in the horse.

Partial severance of an extensor tendon is often diagnosed by careful digital palpation. As with partial transection of a flexor tendon, these injuries are significant because a partial thickness laceration could become full thickness without appropriate bandage splinting and exercise restriction.

Lacerated Paratendon

Laceration of the paratendon, particularly those that are perpendicular to the limb's long axis, can be problematic. Standard approaches of suturing and bandaging, even with fresh, clean, sharp wounds, tend to fail via dehiscence, usually seen between the 7th and 10th days after suturing. The problem occurs when the tendon, paratendon, subcutaneous tissues, and skin attempt to heal together; this repair is disrupted due to the unrestricted and independent movement of the tendon relative to more superficial tissues. While infection is often implicated as the culprit, continued attempts to reconstruct the wound after healthy granulation tissue forms generally lead to failure.

Clinically, the problem is recognized after dehiscence of the sutured wound where a separate focus of granulation tissue emanates from the lacerated paratendon site at the wound center. A circular cleft in the granulation tissue surrounds this focus and a ring of granulation tissue surrounds the cleft (Figure 10.10). When the limb is flexed or extended, the central focus of granulation tissue moves independent of the surrounding granulation tissue. This same problem can be seen in wounds to the paratendon that have been left to heal by second intention. Generally, healing will not proceed in these wounds until the limb is immobilized.[3]

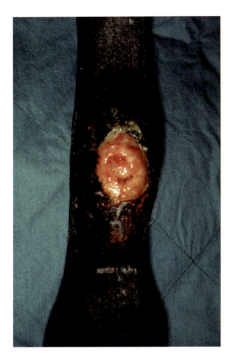

Figure 10.10. Typical appearance of a wound over the superficial digital flexor tendon which involved the skin and subcutaneous and paratendon tissues. Note the circle of granulation tissue surrounding the central focus of granulation tissue with a cleft between them. The circle of granulation tissue is formed from the subcutaneous tissue and the central focus of granulation tissue is formed from the paratendon. This wound had been treated surgically (sutured) on three separate occasions followed by bandaging. Wound dehiscence occurred at 7 to 10 days following each attempt at suturing.

Wound Location

The importance of wound location relates to the healing difficulties encountered when tendon lacerations are located in a sheathed region as opposed to those situated in a non-sheathed region.[11,12] The *sine qua non* of appropriate treatment of these injuries is a sound knowledge of the anatomic boundaries of the tendon sheaths. Basically, the palmar/plantar surface of the fetlock and both the dorsal and palmar/plantar surfaces of the carpus and tarsus are the regions in which synovial tendon sheaths are found. In the non-sheathed regions, tendons are enveloped by a highly vascular connective tissue called the paratendon. The non-sheathed regions are in the mid-metacarpal and metatarsal zones.[3,4]

Treatment

Flexor Tendon Severance

Non-sheathed Regions

The ultimate goal of any tendon repair is to restore limb function. Three basic principles of tendon surgery must be strictly adhered to in order to achieve this. Each of these principles should be considered an objective: (1) minimize the post-tenorrhaphy gap, (2) avoid compromising the tendon's intrinsic blood supply, and (3) prevent/reduce adhesion formation. These goals are harder to achieve in the sheathed regions than in the non-sheathed regions. The recommended treatment protocol has been divided into seven steps. Although these steps must be adapted to each case, close observance of them will maximize the functional outcome.[9]

Step 1: Immobilization of the injured limb. The neurovascular structures of the distal limb must be preserved. To achieve this, the distal limb should be supported with a well-padded splint. The commercially available Kimzey Leg Saver (Kimzey, Woodland, CA) is one of the most effective in immobilizing the distal limb (Figure 10.11). Alternatively, a splint can be constructed using polyvinyl chloride (PVC) material. The PVC pipe splint is applied to the dorsal surface of the fore limb or the plantar surface of the hind limb (Figures 10.12a,b).

To be most effective, in both cases the splint should extend down to the ground level. The fetlock is pulled dorsally into the splint in the case of a fore limb laceration, whereas the foot is pulled in a plantar direction into the splint in the case of a hind limb laceration. In both situations the fetlock is stabilized in slight flexion. Splinting also reduces the risk for further damage during transportation of the horse to a surgical facility. This initial

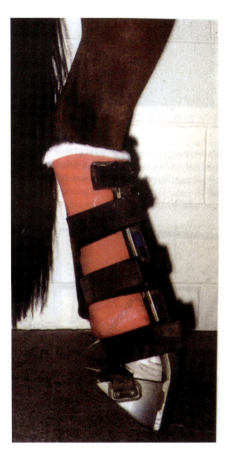

Figure 10.11. A Kimzey™ leg brace affixed to the right hind limb.

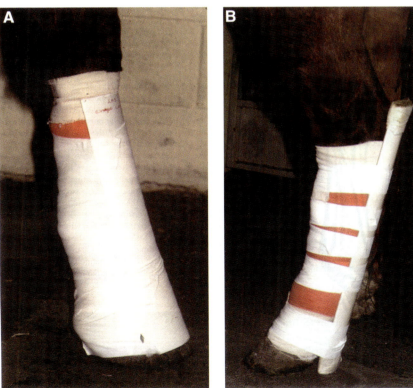

Figure 10.12. (A) A PVC splint affixed to the dorsal aspect of the forelimb. (B) A PVC splint affixed to the plantar aspect of the hind limb.

step is crucial to the overall success of the treatment. For more information regarding splinting and casting techniques, see Chapter 16.

Step 2: Treatment for shock and infection. With most flexor tendon lacerations there is a potential for significant hemorrhage from major arteries in the area, including the median artery in the fore limb and the dorsal metatarsal artery in the pelvic limb. In wounds which are distal to the fetlock, the digital arteries are often severed. Patients should be evaluated for hypovolemia prior to the use of chemical restraint and the induction of general anesthesia. Pale mucous membranes and a high pulse rate are indicative of significant blood loss, in which case treatment for shock with volume replacement is warranted. Active hemorrhage can be controlled in most cases with pressure bandaging or direct ligation.

Many tendon lacerations are either highly contaminated or infected at the time of presentation. Antibiotic treatment in the form of penicillin (22,000 IU/kg twice daily intramuscularly or four times daily intravenously) or cefazolin (10 mg/kg three times daily intravenously or intramuscularly) and gentamicin (6 mg–8 mg/kg once daily intravenously or intramuscularly) or amikacin (14 mg/kg once daily intravenously or intramuscularly) is recommended. The antibiotic regimen is maintained for 2 to 6 weeks, depending on the patient's response.[13]

Step 3: Debridement, hemostasis, and irrigation. Although initial blood vessel ligation and wound lavage can be achieved in the standing sedated horse, definitive layered debridement, hemostasis, lavage, and tenorrhaphy are best performed under general anesthesia. The objective is to upgrade the wound from a severely contaminated status to one which is suitable for tenorrhaphy or grafting. The *sine qua non* of this step is meticulous layered debridement. All contaminated (infected) and devitalized (avascular) tissues must be excised (Figures 10.13a,b). This usually includes frayed tendon ends, paratendon, subcutaneous tissues, and skin margins. Hemostasis is critical at this stage; this not only includes major vascular components which may have been damaged at the time of injury but also minor sources of hemorrhage encountered during the debridement process.

Irrigation of the wound is critical. Large volumes of 0.1%–0.2% povidone-iodine (PI) solution (10 ml–20 ml of 10% PI in 1 L lactated Ringer's solution) are required. This concentration of PI is bactericidal within 15 seconds and has minimal deleterious effects on tissues. The solution should be delivered at 10–15 PSI. Delayed wound closure is used for the most severely contaminated and infected wounds. In these cases the limb is best immobilized in a Kimzey Leg Saver splint. (A more complete discussion will follow.)

Step 4: Tenorrhaphy. Recent literature has clearly documented the importance of this procedure, which is performed because it minimizes the tendon gap, reduces adhesion formation, and maximizes post-operative healing strength.[12,14–25] Tenorrhaphy is recommended even if there is a tendon deficit.[14] The suture pattern favored by the authors is the three-loop pulley (Figure 10.14).[20] Compared to other suture patterns, the three-loop pulley is desirable for a number of reasons: (1) it is most resistant to gap formation, (2) it is easy to place, (3) it uses less suture material, (4) it does not cause distortion of tendon ends, and (5) it is minimally disruptive to the intrinsic vasculature.

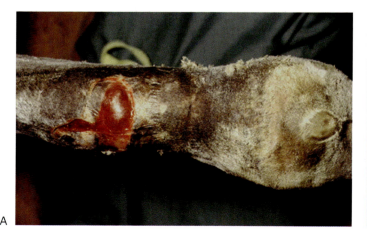
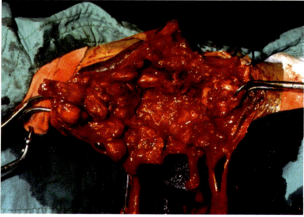

A   B

Figure 10.13. (A) A 4-day-old severely contaminated/infected wound. (B) The same wound as in (a) following extensive layered debridement. Both the superficial and deep digital flexor tendons were transected. A partial transection (<25%) of the suspensory ligament was also present. Delayed tenorrhaphy was used in this case.

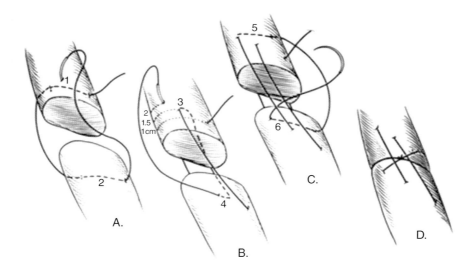

Figure 10.14. Illustrates placement of three-loop pulley suture pattern.

A slowly-absorbed synthetic monofilament suture material is preferred because it circumvents the potential formation of suture sinus while retaining sufficient post-operative tensile strength.[24-31] Either size 2 polydioxanone (PDS™, Ethicon, Sommerville, NJ) or size 1 polyglyconate (Maxon™, Sherwood-Davis and Geck, St. Louis, MO) is recommended. The suture pattern should extend for at least 1.5 cm into the proximal and distal segments of the lacerated tendon because the cut ends of the tendon undergo post-injury collagenolysis. This results in weakening, and consequently a reduced holding power of the suture. A potential means of overcoming tenorrhaphy gap involves bioabsorbale tendon plates. This technique has been shown to provide increased strength in the early post-operative phase of tendon healing, which could decrease the time required for external coaptation.[32]

In some situations it is impossible to eliminate gap via tenorrhaphy. In these cases special attention is paid to closing the paratendon, which provides the extrinsic vascular and cellular elements necessary for healing.

Partially transected flexor tendons (<75%) are generally not sutured, whereas those that are transected >75% should be. Debridement and other appropriate treatments to rid the wound of contamination and/or infection should be performed prior to suturing, and a cast should be applied to the limb subsequently.[3]

Step 5: Wound closure. At this juncture the wound has been upgraded from a contaminated or severely contaminated status to a clean one. Closure is performed in a stepwise fashion, paying particular attention to the highly vascular paratendon which provides a resistant barrier to infection between the tenorrhaphy and the superficial layers of the wound. Furthermore, the paratendon provides the extrinsic vascular and cellular elements responsible for tendon healing, so by apposing it over the tenorrhaphy, early scar formation is encouraged. This is of consequence since the early scar tissue eventually remodels into a new tendon tissue. The subcutaneous tissues and skin should be closed to further support healing and circumvent formation of exuberant granulation tissue.

In the case of a contaminated wound, tenorrhaphy and wound closure are generally performed 5 to 6 days after the initial debridement and wound cleansing. This delay allows the wound to be upgraded to a clean state. During this time the limb is maintained in a splint and the bandage is changed as needed, generally daily at first and then every other day. Once the decision is made to perform the tenorrhaphy, granulation tissue is debrided and the paratendon incised to expose the tendon ends. Hyper-flexion of the fetlock brings the tendon ends as close together as possible, which facilitates suturing.[3]

Step 6: Post-operative immobilization. The distal limb should be immobilized with the digit in slight flexion in an effort to negate flexor strain in the immediate post-operative period. Although a Kimzey splint can be used, immobilization is best achieved with a fiberglass cast. Four weeks of external coaptation is required following tenorraphy,[9] while a 6-week period is recommended in the absence of tenorrhaphy. The opposite limb should be kept in a support bandage and in some cases an Equine Digital Support System™ (EDSS) padded shoe is recommended in an effort to prevent the development of support limb laminitis.

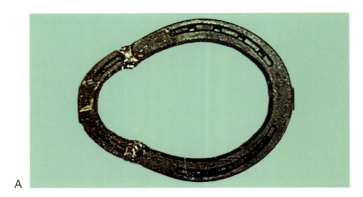

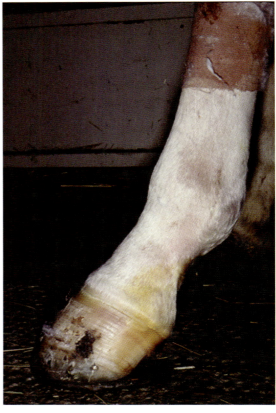

Figure 10.15. (A) Example of an extended heel shoe. (B) The extended heel shoe applied to the hind hoof.

The cast is removed while the horse is standing and sedated to circumvent another general anesthesia, and then a heel extension shoe is applied if the deep digital flexor tendon was involved. This shoe counteracts hyperextension of the DIP joint and is required for several months (Figures 10.15a,b).[9] Following cast removal, a support bandage is applied to the limb and maintained for 3 more weeks.

Step 7: Convalescent protocol. The time of convalescence is proportional to the severity of the injury. In general, following cast removal the horse is confined to a stall and small run for an additional 6 weeks. At 12 weeks, hand walking can begin and gradually can increase in frequency and duration during the next 3 to 6 weeks. Controlled exercise consisting of walking or ponying is preferred to pasture turnout. Once the horse is sound at a walk and trot and ultrasound examination shows extensive fibrosis and mature scar tissue, the patient can be turned out to pasture. The total convalescence period ranges from 6 to 12 months before a horse is returned to full work.[9]

Sheathed Regions

Tendon lacerations occurring within the sheathed regions are problematic for two reasons. First, these lacerations heal poorly within the confines of the tendon sheath. In fact, one study showed that transected DDFT healed in such a way that the SDFT and the DDFT became one flexor unit with reduced functionality.[12] The palmar aspect of the transected DDFT formed an adhesion to the dorsal aspect of the SDFT so that the two structures became one. Although somewhat functional, the healing was weaker than that which holds two ends of a lacerated tendon together in a non-sheathed zone. Additionally, horses were three out of five lame at the jog 6 months after tenorrhaphy of the DDFT within the digital sheath. Delayed healing was attributed to the lack of extrinsic vascular supply due to the physical barrier created by closing the tendon sheath. Thus, it is recommended that the tendon sheath be left partially open to allow in-growth of the vascular and cellular elements required for healing.

Second, the potential for septic tenosynovitis is a reality that must be dealt with.[3,33] These injuries should always be treated as if they are or will become infected. Preventing septic tenosynovitis is as important as the tenorrhaphy itself.

To prevent infection the sheath should be irrigated with several liters of lactated Ringer's solution delivered either through a needle or arthroscope sleeve placed within the sheath in a site remote to the wound. This effectively flushes the sheath from within outward. If the wound is very clean and of short duration (<3 hours), primary repair/closure may be effected after the wound and tendons are meticulously debrided. Following tenorrhaphy the sheath is either left open or a window is created laterally and medially to the repair site so that the surrounding extrinsic blood supply and cells can support the healing process. The subcutaneous tissues are closed over these openings in the sheath.[3] After closure of the wound, a broad-spectrum antibiotic such as amikacin (500–750 mg) can be injected into the tendon sheath. Amikacin has good activity against equine orthopedic pathogens and resistance to amikacin is less likely compared to gentamicin. A cast should be applied following intrathecal injection. A parenteral broad spectrum peri-operative antibiotic (e.g., penicillin, 22,000–44,000 IU/kg q6–12hours IV, and gentamicin, 6.6 mg/kg/ q24 hours IV [administered slowly]) beginning within 2 hours of surgery and continued for at least 24 hours is recommended.

If the wound is heavily contaminated, and of >3 hours duration, it is considered infected. Treatment for septic tenosynovitis consists of the same approach to flushing/lavage and layered debridement plus regional limb perfusion and the installation of a fenestrated polyethylene tube, which is used as the ingress portal of an intrasynovial lavage system (Figure 10.16). Regional limb perfusion administered either intravenously or intraosseously allows delivery of a high concentration of an antimicrobial to the affected site (Figures 12.1–4). For more information on the technique, see chapters 9 and 12.

To install the partially fenestrated tube, the non-fenestrated portion is placed in the wound and advanced in a retrograde manner so that it exits at the proximal extent of the digital sheath. The fenestrated portion of the tube remains within the sheath while the non-fenestrated portion is external and sutured to the skin to secure it in place. A Penrose drain can exit through an incision in the distal extent of the tendon sheath, thereby establishing an ingress/egress system to flush the entire sheath from proximal to distal (Figure 10.17).

Partially fenestrated drains usually require rinsing with heparinized saline to maintain patency. Following flushing, the limb is supported in a Kimzey splint for recovery and during stall confinement (Figure 10.11). The sheath is flushed several times daily. Following flushing, full-strength heparin is instilled for as long as the tube is functional. The actual time the drain is left in place varies according to patency and need. If the drain is patent and flushing the sheath is effective, the drain may be left in place for several days. If flushing becomes a problem

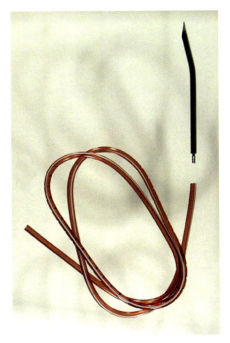

Figure 10.16. Example of a fenestrated drain that can be used to irrigate the digital sheath.

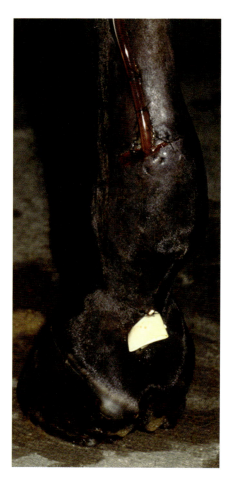

Figure 10.17. Example of an ingress-egress irrigation system. The non-fenestrated portion of the irrigation tube is exiting through the proximal extent of the digital sheath at the laceration site; it was sutured to the skin to secure it in place. The fenestrated portion of the tube remains within the sheath. A Penrose drain exits through an incision in the distal extent of the tendon sheath, thereby establishing an ingress/egress system to flush the entire sheath from proximal to distal.

because the drain is plugged with fibrin, it should be removed. Drains that are dysfunctional for whatever reason act as foreign bodies and are rapidly contaminated, serving as a source of infection.

The solution that is routinely used for flushing is lactated Ringer's or lactated Ringer's and 0.1% povidone-iodine. This can be followed by lavage with a 10% DMSO solution. Antibiotics can be instilled directly into the tendon sheath (through the ingress portion of the drain) after each flush. Systemic broad-spectrum antibiotics as used for wounds <3 hours old are continued for 10–14 days followed by the administration of Trimethoprim sulfa 15 mg/kg q12 PO for an additional 7 to 10 days. See Chapter 9 for more information regarding the treatment of wounds involving synovial structures.

Delayed tenorrhaphy is performed when the sheath is free of infection, generally after 4 to 6 days of flushing and antibiotic therapy. The technique is performed as previously described and the sheath is either left open or fenestrated to allow extrinsic support for healing. Delayed tenorrhaphy is recommended for wounds that have a high level of contamination and/or devitalized tissue. This allows the surgeon to minimize the deleterious effects of septic tenosynovitis and hopefully increase the chances for a successful tenorrhaphy.

Other important aspects of therapy include pre- and post-operative bacteriologic culture/sensitivity, synovial cytologic analysis, and sequential ultrasonographic exams.

Prognosis

The prognosis for flexor tendon lacerations has been reported as "guarded to good" depending on the series of cases being studied. The best prognosis is a 50% chance of return to athletic endeavors.[34,35] As for the outcome of cases with partial transection of the flexor tendons, there have not been enough reported cases to provide a reliable prognosis at the time of this writing.

Extensor Tendon Severance

Non-sheathed Regions

The vast majority of extensor tendon injuries occur in the mid-metacarpal or mid-metatarsal regions, which are non-sheathed. The wounds are often avulsive in nature, resulting in considerable soft tissue loss (Figure 10.18).

All of the surgical principles described previously for flexor tendon lacerations are applicable to extensor tendon lacerations. However, due to the large soft tissue defects which often accompany these wounds it is often difficult and not necessary in most cases to perform a tenorrhaphy. An exception is a transection of an extensor tendon close to or at the level of the fetlock. Tenorrhaphy, using size 0 or 1 monofilament synthetic absorbable suture, is recommended in these cases, because without suturing the tendon ends do not heal readily.

Following wound care, external splinting is required for approximately 4 to 5 weeks, after which a support bandage is applied until healing is complete. During this time the tendon will adhere to the dorsal periosteum of the cannon bone and extensor function will be restored. See Chapter 16 for more information regarding bandage splinting.

Sheathed Regions

All the aforementioned treatment approaches for lacerated flexor tendons in sheathed zones apply to extensor tendons, with prevention of septic tenosynovitis representing the primary treatment goal.

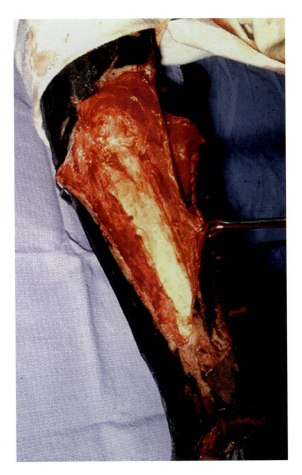

Figure 10.18. An extensive avulsive wound over the dorsal metatarsus resulted in complete transection of the extensor tendons.

Prognosis

The prognosis for extensor tendon lacerations is generally favorable. Even when a large gap is present between tendon ends, the horse usually learns to flip the digit forward to avoid knuckling. The severed tendon ends rapidly become adherent to the periosteum and extensor function is restored.[7,31] Return to athletic soundness was reported in 62% of cases in which the long and lateral digital extensor tendons were lacerated and in 80% of cases in which the long digital extensor tendon alone was lacerated.[34]

Paratendon Lacerations

Laceration of the paratendon can present a surgical challenge because of the propensity of these wounds to dehisce. This is especially true when the wound is perpendicular to the long axis of the tendon.[3] The reason for this remains undefined, but movement between the paratendon and subcutaneous tissues and skin has been incriminated. Prevention of this problem is relatively simple and depends on good surgical principles as well as immobilization in a cast or splint for 2 to 3 weeks after the wound is sutured. If the problem already exists, debulking the wound of granulation tissue (Figure 10.10) should precede suturing and cast application (Figure 10.19). If a tissue deficit dictates second intention wound healing, the application of a cast or a bandage splint is generally all that is needed (Figure 10.20).

Prognosis

In the authors' experience the prognosis for treatment of paratendon lacerations is very favorable as long as the affected region is immobilized, using a cast or bandage splint, for 2 to 3 weeks and if infection is not a problem.

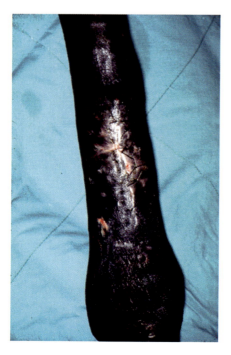

Figure 10.19. The wound in Figure 10.10 after removal (debulking) of granulation tissue, suturing, and cast application for a 2-week period.

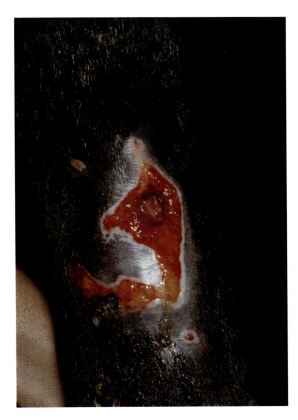

Figure 10.20. A non-healing wound, overlying an extensor tendon that involved the paratendon. Note the central focus of granulation tissue with a cleft between it and the surrounding granulation tissue. This wound healed following immobilization in a bandage splint for 2 weeks.

Conclusion

Over the last two decades the precision of equine tendon surgery has been honed to a point that return to function can be expected and often is achieved. This is largely the result of clinical research which has helped modify and refine repair techniques to the point of making surgical repair the accepted treatment modality. Tendon repair is a surgical discipline that has huge potential for the application of clinical studies. Topics currently under investigation include autologous tendon grafting,[36,37] growth factor application,[38–40] xenografting with porcine small intestinal submucosa (SIS),[41] and stem cell implantation.[42] At this juncture, the area in which therapeutic efficacy has been documented most extensively is autologous tendon grafting. Recent investigations have shown a 6-fold increase in tenorrhaphy strength between 4 and 6 weeks post-repair. The procedure is technically simple and applicable to almost any repair situation. More clinical trials must be performed and reported before a precise verdict on therapeutic efficacy can be reported (Figures 10.21 and 10.22).[37]

Incorporation of growth factors into suture material or another slow release modality is an area which will continue to be investigated. Epidermal growth factor and insulin-like growth factor (IGF-I) have been shown to stimulate tenoblast migration in vitro,[38] while PDGF-BB increased collagen type I gene expression of equine tendon in explant culture.[40] One in vivo study showed that intra-tendinous injections of IGF-I brought about positive effects on tendon healing.[39] Specifically, intralesional injection of 2 μg of recombinant human IGF-I every other day for 10 injections reduced the size while augmenting cell proliferation and collagen content and mechanical stiffness of the lesions. What is needed now is the appropriate delivery mechanism so that growth factors can be concentrated at the actual tenorrhaphy site.

Porcine small intestinal submucosa xenografts for tendon repair have not been investigated in equine tendons. Promising results were obtained when SIS was transplanted into rabbit tendon.[41] The grafts were accepted and remodeled into new tendon-like tissue. The remodeling process was positively influenced by subjecting the repaired tendons to partial or full range motion. Conversely, when SIS was used to augment

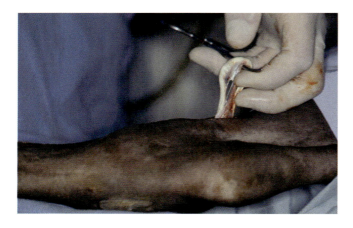

Figure 10.21. Harvest of the lateral digital extensor tendon for use as an autologous tendon graft.

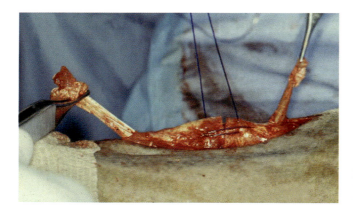

Figure 10.22. An autologous tendon graft (ends held with forceps) is being incorporated into a deep digital flexor tenorrhaphy.

surgical repair of large chronic rotary cuff tears, clinical efficacy could not be demonstrated.[43] For more information regarding the use of extracellular matrix scaffolds, see Chapter 3.

Stem cell implantation is another area which has some very real potential and applicability to tendon repair/healing situations. Although little data is available to document the actual ability of stem cells to accelerate tendon healing, anecdotal evidence makes this an area worthy of a future investigative effort. In fact, two recent reports have documented a positive effect of adipose-derived adult stem cells[42] and mesenchymal stem cell and bone marrow mononucleated cells[44] on tendon healing.

References

1. Evans JH, Barbenel JC: Structural and mechanical properties of tendon related to function. Equine Vet J 1975;7:1
2. Goodship AE, Birch HL, Wilson AM: The pathobiology and repair of tendon and ligament injury. Vet Clin North Am Eq Pract 1994;2:323
3. Stashak TS: Management of wounds associated with tendons, paratendons, and tendon sheaths. In TS Stashak, ed. *Equine wound management (1st edition)*. Philadelphia: Lea and Febiger, 1991, p.238
4. Jann HW, Pasquini C: Wounds of the distal limb complicated by involvement of deep structures. Vet Clin North Am Eq Pract 2005;21:145
5. Baxter GM: Retrospective study of lower limb wounds involving tendons, tendon sheaths or joints in horses. Proc Am Assoc Equine Pract 1987;33:715
6. Manske PR, Gelberman RH, Vande Berg JS, et al: Intrinsic flexor-tendon repair. A morphological study in vitro. J Bone Joint Surg Am 1984;66:385
7. McIlwraith CW: Diseases and problems of tendons, ligaments and tendon sheaths. In TS Stashak, ed, *Adam's Lameness in Horses (4th edition)*. Philadelphia: Lea and Febiger, 1987, p.472
8. Pasquini C, Jann HW, Pasquini S, et al: *Guide to clinics lameness* (vol. 2). Texas: SUDZ Publishing, 1995, p.160

9. Jann HW: Current concepts and techniques in the management of tendon lacerations. Clin Tech Equine Pract 2004;3:215

10. Belknap JK, Baxter GM, Nickels FA: Extensor tendon lacerations in horses: 50 cases (1982–1988). J Am Vet Med Assoc 1993;203:428

11. Honnas CM, Schumacher J, Watkins JP, et al: Diagnosis and treatment of septic tenosynovitis in horses. Comp Cont Ed Pract Vet 1991;13:301

12. Jann H, Blaik M, Emerson R, et al: Healing characteristics of deep digital flexor tenorrhaphy within the digital sheath of horses. Vet Surg 2003;32:421

13. Brumbaugh GW: Use of antimicrobials in wound management. Vet Clin North Am Equine Pract 2005;21:63

14. Jann HW, Alexander JW: Using a modified three-loop pulley tenorrhaphy to repair avulsion of the gastrocnemius tendon in dogs. Vet Med 1996;9:841

15. Pruitt DL, Manske PR, Fink B: Cyclic stress analysis of flexor tendon repair. J Hand Surg (Am) 1991;16:701

16. Krackow KA, Thomas SC, Jones LC: A new stitch for ligament-tendon fixation. J Bone Joint Surg Am 1986;68:764

17. Spurlock GH: Management of traumatic tendon lacerations. Vet Clin North Am Equine Pract 1989;5:575

18. DeKlerk AJ, Jonck LM: Tendon response to trauma lacerations. Vet Clin North Am Equine Pract 1989;5:575

19. Bertone AL, Stashak TS, Smith FW, et al: A comparison of repair methods for gap healing in equine flexor tendon. Vet Surg 1990;19:254

20. Jann HW, Good JK, Morgan SJ, et al: Healing of transected equine superficial digital flexor tendons with and without tenorrhaphy. Vet Surg 1992;21:40

21. Nixon AJ, Stashak TS, Smith FW, et al: Comparison of carbon fiber and nylon suture for repair of transected flexor tendons in the horse. Equine Vet J 1984;16:93

22. Bertone AL: Tendon lacerations. Vet Clin North Am Equine Pract 1995;11:293

23. Davis CS, Smith RKW: Diagnosis and management of tendon and ligament disorders. In JA Auer and JA Stick, eds. *Equine surgery (3rd edition)*. Philadelphia: Saunders/Elsevier, 2006, p.1086

24. Jann HW, Stein LE, Good JK: Strength characteristics and failure modes of locking-loop and three-loop pulley suture patterns in equine tendons. Vet Surg 1990;19:28

25. Easley KJ, Stashak TS, Smith FW, et al: Mechanical properties of four suture patterns for transected equine tendon repair. Vet Surg 1990;19:102

26. Jann HW, Stein LE, Good JK, et al: A comparison of nylon, polybutester, and polyglyconate suture materials for long digital flexor tenorrhaphy in chickens. Vet Surg 1992;21:234

27. Fackelman GE: Tendon surgery. Vet Clin North Am Large Anim Pract 1983;5:381

28. Bovane RB, Bitar H, Adreae PR, et al: In vivo comparison of four absorbable sutures: Vicryl, Dexon Plus, Maxon, and PDS. Can J Surg 1998;31:43

29. Sanz LE, Patterson JA, Kamath R, et al: Comparison of Maxon suture with Vicryl, chromic catgut, and PDS sutures in facial closure in rats. Obstet Gynecol 1988;71:418

30. Crowson CL, Jann HW, Stein LE, et al: Quantitative effect of tenorrhaphy on the intrinsic vasculature of the equine superficial digital flexor tendon. Am J Vet Res 2004;65:279

31. Jann HW: Equine tendon lacerations. Proc Am Coll Vet Surg Equine 2000;10:72

32. Jenson PW, Lillich JD, Roush, JK et al: Ex vivo strength comparison of bioabsorbale tendon plates and bioabsorbale suture in a 3-loop pulley pattern for repair of transected flexor tendons from horse cadavers. Vet Surg 2005;34:565

33. Honnas CM, Schumacher J, Watkins JP, et al: Diagnosis and treatment of septic tenosynovitis in horses. J Am Vet Med Assoc 1991;199:1616

34. Foland JW, Trotter GW, Stashak TS, et al: Traumatic injuries involving tendons of the distal limbs in horses: A retrospective study of 55 cases. Equine Vet J 1991;23:422

35. Taylor DS, Pascoe JR, Meagher DM, et al: Digital flexor tendon lacerations in horses: 50 cases (1975–1990). J Am Vet Med Assoc 1995;206(3):342

36. Valdes-Vasquez MA, McClure JR, Oliver JL, et al: Evaluation of an autologous tendon graft repair method for gap healing of the deep digital flexor tendon in horses. Vet Surg 1996;25:342

37. Reiners SR, Jann HW, Stein LE, et al: An evaluation of two autologous tendon grafting techniques in ponies. Vet Surg 2002;31:155

38. Jann HW, Stein LE, Slater DA: In vitro effects of epidermal growth factor or insulin-like growth factor on tenoblast migration of absorbable suture material. Vet Surg 1999;28:268

39. Dahlgren LA, van der Meulen MCH, Bertram JEA, et al: Insulin-like growth factor-I improves cellular and molecular aspects of healing in a collagenase-induced model of flexor tendonitis. J Orthop Res 2002;20:910

40. Haupt JL, Donnelly BP, Nixon AJ: Effects of platelet-derived growth factor-BB on the metabolic function and morphologic features of equine tendon in explant culture. Am J Vet Res 2006;67:1595

41. Hodde JP, Badylak SF, Shelbourne KD: The effect of range of motion on remodeling of small intestinal submucosa (SIS) when used as an Achilles tendon repair material in the rabbit. Tissue Eng 1997;3:27

42. Dahlgren LA, Haupt JL, Yeager AD, et al: Adipose-derived adult stem cells improve aspects of tendon regeneration. Proc Am Coll Vet Surg 2006;35:E5

43. Iannotti JP, Codsi MJ, Kwon WY, et al: Porcine small intestine submucosa augmentation of surgical repair of chronic two-tendon rotator cuff tears. J Bone Joint Surg Am 2006;88:1238

44. Crovace A, Lacitignola L, De Siena R, et al: Regeneration of extracellular matrix in collagenase induced tendonitis model in the horse using cultured bone marrow mesenchymal cells and bone marrow mononucleated cells, controlled with placebo: preliminary results. Proc Am Coll Vet Surg 2006;35:E5

11 Free Skin Grafting

Jim Schumacher, DVM, MS, Diplomate ACVS, MRCVS, and Jacintha M. Wilmink, DVM, PhD, Diplomate RNVA

Introduction

Skin grafting should be considered for a full-thickness skin defect that cannot heal by epithelialization and contraction or be closed using conventional suturing techniques or sliding flaps. Many large, full-thickness wounds at or below the carpus and hock are best treated with a skin graft because wounds in these regions are incapable of significant contraction, and if not grafted, heal unsatisfactorily with the formation of exuberant granulation tissue or a dense fibrogranuloma.[1] Although most wounds of the neck and trunk heal effectively by second intention, large wounds in these regions may also benefit from skin grafting, which markedly reduces the time required for healing. The purpose of this chapter is to describe the principles and various techniques of free skin grafting, the advantages and disadvantages of each technique, and the effects of grafts on the wound. Proper care of the wound, before and after grafting, is described so that failure of the graft can be avoided.

Classification of Grafts

The two basic types of skin grafts are the pedicle skin graft and the free skin graft. A pedicle skin graft is a full-thickness graft that remains joined to the donor site by a vascular pedicle so that the graft does not depend on the vascularity of the recipient site to survive. Wounds healed with a pedicle graft have a good cosmetic appearance because the graft is composed of all layers of skin. Pedicle grafts are not commonly applied to wounds of horses because mobilizing an adequate amount of skin to advance a pedicle graft can be difficult.[2]

A free skin graft is a section of skin that has been detached from its vascular supply and relocated to a wound at another site where it must create a new vascular connection to the wound bed to survive. A free graft can be classified according its source; the most common type is the autograft, or isograft, which is a graft that is relocated from one area to another on the same individual. An allograft, or homograft, is a graft that is transferred between two members of the same species, whereas a xenograft, or heterograft, is a graft that is transferred from a member of one species to a member of another. Although allografts and xenografts develop vascular connections to the recipient wound, the graft is eventually rejected because the host mounts an immune response against it.[3,4] An autograft is the most common and practical type of graft applied to wounds of horses due to the minimal immune response induced in the host. An allograft or xenograft is sometimes applied to a wound on a horse as a biological dressing.[5-7]

Free skin grafts can also be classified as full-thickness or split-thickness. A full-thickness graft is composed of epidermis and the entire dermis, whereas a split-thickness graft is composed of epidermis but only a portion of the dermis. The thickness of split-thickness grafts can vary and is determined by the relative amount, rather than the absolute amount, of dermis included in the graft, because thickness of the dermis varies between individuals and between regions on an individual.[8-10]

Full- or split-thickness skin grafts are applied to the surface of wounds as sheet grafts or are embedded within the wound as island grafts. Each technique of grafting has its advantages and disadvantages, and the choice of technique depends on circumstances such as the location and size of the wound, required cosmetic appearance, available instrumentation, and bias of the surgeon, as well as the financial resources of the owner.

Requirements for Graft Acceptance

Nearly any type of tissue is capable of supporting a free graft except bone that is devoid of periosteum, tendon devoid of paratendon, or cartilage devoid of perichondrium.[11-14] Tissues less likely to accept a free graft are adipose tissue, joint capsules, and ligaments. The presence of small areas of incompatible tissue within a wound, such as tendon, can still be covered with a graft owing to the phenomenon of vascular bridging. Vascular bridging is a process whereby a portion of a graft overlying a small, avascular portion of the wound is re-vascularized by capillaries from the vascularized portion of the graft.[13,15] Full-thickness grafts are more effective than split-thickness grafts at bridging avascular portions of the wound due to better collateral circulation within the dermis.[15]

To accept a free graft, the wound should be vascularized and free of infection and necrotic tissue. Fresh wounds, created surgically or by accident, are the most capable of accepting a free graft because they are highly vascular and have not had time to become infected.[10,16,17] Granulating wounds can also accept grafts, though not as readily as can fresh wounds. An advantage of postponing grafting of a large fresh wound until fibroplasia is well under way is that contraction rapidly decreases the size of the wound after granulation tissue forms, allowing it to be covered by a smaller graft.

Physiological Events Associated with Graft Acceptance

Re-vascularization

The graft is initially adhered to the wound by fibrin, which binds to exposed collagen within the graft.[11,18-20] Vessels and fibroblasts from the wound invade the fibrin clot within 48 to 72 hours, and by the tenth day, the graft is firmly attached to the wound. The graft is nourished initially by plasmatic imbibition, or plasmatic circulation, a process whereby plasma is imbibed passively by capillary action into the exposed lumen of the graft's vessels.[11,19,21] During the stage of plasmatic imbibition, which typically lasts about 48 hours, the graft has no blood supply of its own, and cells in the graft have depressed mitotic activity resulting from low oxygen tension. The graft becomes edematous and remains so until it re-vascularizes.

After the first 2 days, new capillaries from the wound cross the fibrin matrix to anastomose with capillaries in the graft, a process called inosculation.[11,19,21,22] Inosculation occurs mainly in the central region of the graft.[23] Following inosculation, new capillaries from the wound invade other vessels within the graft and cut new vascular channels into its dermis, a process referred to as neovascularization. The graft re-vascularizes between the fourth and fifth day after being applied to the wound, and lymphatic circulation is re-established by 7 days. Restoration of vascular and lymphatic circulation resolves edema.[22]

Graft Regeneration

The epidermis of the graft becomes hyperplastic after grafting and may die and slough in some areas, exposing pale dermis beneath it (Figure 11.1).[12,16] The exposed dermis may closely resemble granulation tissue

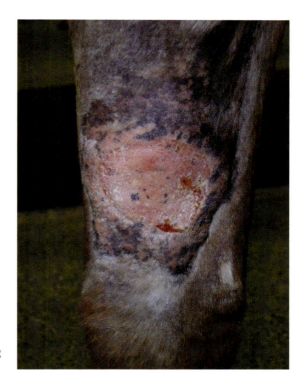

Figure 11.1. The entire epidermis of this graft has sloughed, exposing pale dermis beneath it. This dermis may resemble granulation tissue.

but can be differentiated from it by its paler color. Epithelial cells that migrate from the hair follicles and the eccrine glands within the dermis soon cover the dermis.

Split-thickness skin grafts remain covered with flaky debris for several months, until the eccrine glands regenerate.[16] They usually regain pigmentation starting at about 1 month (Figure 11.2). Hair begins to appear between 4 and 6 weeks,[16] though it often grows abnormally long, which may be due to the origin of the graft.[9,24,25] The origin is usually the trunk, where the local temperature is higher than that of the limbs. Transfer of the graft to a cooler area (e.g., the distal portion of a limb) may stimulate hair growth.

Nerves enter the base and margins of the graft and reconstruct its innervation pattern by following vacated neurolemmal sheaths.[26] Split-thickness grafts become re-innervated more rapidly but to a lesser extent than do full-thickness grafts.[11,26] Sensation to split-thickness grafts of humans usually returns between 7 and 9 weeks but is incomplete and patchy.[27] Humans sometimes develop hyperesthesia of the grafted wound,[12,26] and judging from incidents where horses have mutilated the healed, grafted wound, some horses likely also suffer from this condition.

Graft Contraction

Recoil of elastin fibers within the deep layers of the dermis causes a graft to contract immediately after harvest.[28] This contraction is referred to as primary graft contraction. Full-thickness grafts contract more than do split-thickness grafts, and as the proportion of dermis within split-thickness grafts increases, so does the amount of primary contraction. The significance of primary contraction is minor for sheet grafts because it is reversed when the graft is stretched and attached to the wound margins.

Contraction after the graft has been accepted is referred to as secondary graft contraction, which in reality represents contraction of the wound itself rather than the graft. Wound contraction is brought about by the action of myofibroblasts, and skin grafts have been shown to inhibit wound contraction in humans and other species, perhaps by accelerating the life cycle of myofibroblasts.[28] The relative thickness of the graft's dermis, the stage of healing of the recipient bed at the time of grafting, and the percentage of area grafted determine the extent to which a skin graft inhibits wound contraction.[28,29]

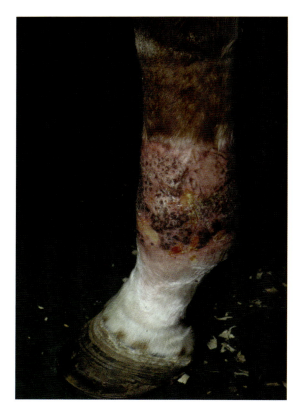

Figure 11.2. This split-thickness skin graft is beginning to pigment. Split-thickness grafts that have sloughed their epidermis are eventually epithelialized and usually begin to develop pigment by about 1 month.

The effect of the skin graft on wound contraction is influenced by physical or biochemical differences between the superficial and deep portions of the dermis.[28,29] Granulating or fresh wounds of humans and rats that receive a full-thickness graft tend to contract less than those receiving a split-thickness graft, even when the full-thickness graft is thinner than the split-thickness graft. This indicates that the deep portion of the dermis may suppress the formation of myofibroblasts in the granulation tissue, or their contraction.[30] On the other hand, the fractional rate of contraction between wounds in horses that received either a full-thickness or split-thickness graft did not differ significantly.[31]

Skin grafts applied to wounds of humans prevent wound contraction; they are applied for this purpose because wound contraction in humans, especially of large wounds over flexor surfaces, often results in contracture or distortion of one or more joints.[3,11] Conversely, skin grafts applied to granulating wounds of horses seem to stimulate, rather than inhibit, wound contraction, as demonstrated in an equine clinical trial. Granulating wounds that receive Meek micrografts (see Island Grafting) contract more than do those that are not grafted.[32] Moreover, wound contraction in horses before or after grafting is generally considered beneficial because it accelerates wound closure and rarely, if ever, causes joint contracture.

Stimulation of wound contraction in horses after grafting may result from the presence of certain cytokines in the dermis of the graft, although these have not yet been identified. Additionally and concomitantly, the reduction of chronic inflammation and thus the concentration of several contraction-inhibiting mediators (e.g., prostaglandin [PG]E$_1$, PGE$_2$, interferon [IFN]γ, tumor necrosis factor [TNF]α, interleukin [IL]-1, and IL-6) while the wound is being prepared for grafting could increase the rate of contraction.[32]

Reduction of inflammation is also affected by covering the wound with a graft and reducing the area of exposed granulation tissue. The exposed, superficial portion of granulation tissue in an open wound usually contains many leukocytes, indicating the presence of inflammation, whereas leukocytes are not normally found beneath the leading edge of advancing epithelium. As the latter advances to cover the wound, the concentration of leukocytes in the superficial portion of granulation tissue decreases, indicating resolution of inflammation. An immediate effect of grafting a wound is reduction of the area of exposed granulation tissue, which in turn reduces inflammation. Decreased inflammation then optimizes conditions for wound contraction and epithelialization.

The influence of skin grafts on wound contraction may also depend on mechanical factors. Fixing a (meshed) sheet graft to a wound under slight tension may influence the granulation tissue by partially relieving the mechanical stress exerted on it by the environment. This, in turn, favors myofibroblast apoptosis, as suggested by in vitro studies of fibroblasts in collagen lattices.[33] The disappearance of myofibroblasts reduces wound contraction, however, and although this is important in preventing contractures in humans, it is disadvantageous in horses, where wound contraction is beneficial. Whether fixation or certain characteristics of a (meshed) sheet graft result in disappearance of myofibroblasts and thus reduced contraction of equine wounds is not known, but one author (Wilmink) has the impression that wounds of horses contract less after receiving a meshed split-thickness sheet graft than after receiving split-thickness island grafts (e.g., Meek micrografts).

In general, the responsiveness of the wound to dermal factors of grafts is determined by the age of the granulation tissue, and hence the concentration and state of differentiation of the myofibroblasts.[31,34,35] Wound contraction is reduced when wounds are grafted soon after wounding, when myofibroblasts are not yet present, and when grafting mature, fibrotic granulation tissue from which myofibroblasts have disappeared.

Causes of Graft Failure

Failure of skin grafts to be accepted can be caused by infection, inflammation, fluid accumulation beneath the graft, and motion.[9,12,20,21,25,28] Infection is reported to be the most common cause of failure in both humans[36,37] and horses.[38]

Infection

Although the surface of granulation tissue has a resident bacterial population, abundant blood vessels and phagocytic cells within the tissue act as a barrier against bacterial invasion.[3,11,13,20,39,40] The wound becomes infected only when the tissue concentration of bacteria exceeds the ability of humoral and cellular defenses to destroy the microorganisms; this concentration is generally estimated to be 10^5 organisms per gram of tissue in a sutured wound or a wound covered with a graft. Skin graft survival is better correlated to the concentration of bacteria in the wound than to any other factor;[36,37] therefore, a wound should not be grafted if it is found, by quantitative bacterial analysis, to contain more than 10^5 bacteria per gram of tissue.

Although the bacterial concentration in the wound is an important consideration, the concentration necessary to infect a wound can be much less than 10^5 per gram of tissue for some bacteria, particularly β-hemolytic streptococci.[20,39] β-hemolytic streptococci, more so than other common types of bacteria, produce proteolytic enzymes destructive to both the graft and the wound. These enzymes degrade the graft's fibrinous attachment to the wound by catalyzing the conversion of plasminogen to plasmin, which digests fibrin.[20,41] Pseudomonads also weaken a graft's fibrinous attachment by producing elastase, which specifically damages elastin in the dermis of the graft, a protein to which fibrin attaches.[20]

Inflammation

Although infection is reported to be the most common cause of graft failure in horses,[38] chronic inflammation, inherently present during second intention healing of wounds on the distal limbs of horses, may be at least as important because it deteriorates the quality of the granulation bed and results in the production of moderate amounts of purulent exudate,[42,43] both of which negatively influence graft acceptance. Grafts applied to wounds of horses may, therefore, be at greater risk of failure than grafts applied to wounds of other species. Wounds of ponies are less prone to chronic inflammation, and therefore may better accept a graft, though this has not yet been specifically investigated.

Fluid Accumulation

Accumulation of fluid such as blood, serum, or exudate beneath a graft prevents fibrin from attaching the graft to the wound bed and obstructs graft vascularization.[13,21] Although a graft can survive for several days by imbibing nutrients from blood or serum, the graft perishes if capillaries from the wound are incapable of traversing the fluid within this time. To prevent a hematoma or seroma from forming beneath a graft, a hemorrhagic wound should be grafted only after hemorrhage has ceased. A slight amount of hemorrhage from a wound may cease, however, when a graft is applied, because production of fibrin beneath the graft may stimulate hemostasis. If hemostasis cannot be achieved at the time of surgery, the graft should be stored for later application (see Storing Split-thickness Sheet Grafts). Meshing the graft before applying it to a wound at risk of producing fluid, such as a hemorrhagic wound or one over an open synovial cavity, allows escape of fluid that would otherwise accumulate between the graft and the wound bed. To avoid severe hemorrhage at the time of grafting, exuberant granulation tissue should be excised well in advance of grafting. Excision of the wound at the time of grafting, usually performed with the aim of removing slightly protruding or poor quality granulation tissue and creating a fresh, slightly bleeding wound surface, should be limited to the superficial aspect of the granulation tissue. Thereafter, the graft should be firmly compressed against the wound with a bandage to enhance hemostasis.

Motion

To establish vascular connections, the graft must remain immobile. Shearing forces between the graft and the wound, caused by movement of the bandage, disrupt the fibrin seal, impairing plasmatic imbibition and vascularization. Shearing forces occur when the wound is located in a highly mobile region, such as over a joint, but can usually be prevented by application of a splint or cast. Open grafting (i.e., grafting without bandaging) is a technique sometimes used to avoid shear forces and is especially useful when grafting a wound located in a region hard to bandage, such as the trunk (see Aftercare of the Recipient Site). Shearing forces that occur during dressing changes can be prevented by using non-adherent dressings and by immobilizing the horse with sedation.

Fibrin glue has been used to encourage graft acceptance in humans by increasing the strength of the adhesive bond between the graft and the wound bed.[41] Fibrin glue enhances acceptance of skin grafts not only in this manner but also by providing hemostasis and enhancing phagocytosis. Regrettably, a trial using fibrin glue to attach autogenous, split-thickness skin grafts to experimentally created wounds on the dorsal aspect of the metacarpi and metatarsi of horses did not support its use to decrease the incidence of graft failure.[44]

Grafting Techniques

Preparation of the Wound

The wound must be properly prepared to optimize a graft's chances of survival. The most important factors to consider when evaluating a wound's readiness for grafting are its vascularity and whether it appears free of infection.[11] Grafting should be postponed if the vascularity of the wound seems inadequate to support a graft or if the wound appears to be infected or has an increased susceptibility to infection.

Fresh tissue accepts a graft more readily than does granulation tissue, and new granulation tissue accepts a graft more readily than does mature granulation tissue because vascularity diminishes upon maturation.[39] Consequently, fibrous, poorly vascularized granulation tissue should be excised to below the margin of the skin edge so that new, vascular granulation tissue can form prior to grafting.[9] Granulation tissue can usually be excised with the horse standing because it is poorly innervated.

When granulation tissue is allowed to proliferate for several days after wounding or after excision, the interval between graft application and the time at which it begins to vascularize (i.e., the phase of plasmatic imbibition) can be reduced from about 48 to 24 hours.[45] Postponing grafting in such cases provides time for sprouting capillaries, capable of rapidly re-vascularizing the graft, to proliferate in the wound. A wound that is allowed to develop sprouting capillaries for several days prior to grafting is referred to as a "prepared wound." In clinical practice, however, the term wound preparation implies more than postponing grafting until capillaries begin to sprout.

A wound should be examined thoroughly for infection or susceptibility to infection prior to grafting. A wound, particularly a slow healing one or one with a draining tract, should be assessed for the presence of a foreign body and for evidence of damage to bone, ligaments, tendons, or a synovial structure. Involved bone should be examined radiographically for evidence of an osseous sequestrum or septic osteitis. Granulation tissue of slowly healing or non-healing wounds, particularly those that appear pruritic, should be examined histologically for the presence of larvae of the equine stomach worm, *Habronema*, or for cutaneous neoplasms such as sarcoids or carcinomas because these may resemble granulation tissue (Figure 11.3).

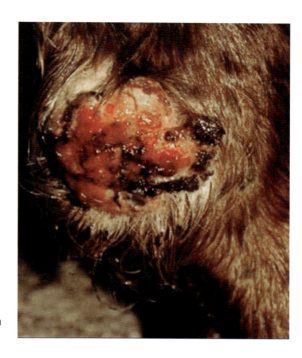

Figure 11.3. Some cutaneous neoplasms, such as this sarcoid on a fetlock, resemble granulation tissue.

The bacterial status of a wound to be grafted is usually assessed qualitatively, rather than quantitatively, because quantifying the concentration of bacteria in a wound is time-consuming and often impractical, and because the type of bacteria in the wound is sometimes more important than the concentration of bacteria.[20] A wound is assumed to be infected if it shows signs of inflammation such as redness, swelling of the wound and surrounding area, and/or formation of exudate. A wound should not be grafted if it shows signs of infection, but unfortunately, even a wound without signs of infection may contain an infective concentration of bacteria.[37] A wound that is suspected of being infected should be cultured for bacteria, and isolates should be tested for susceptibility to antimicrobial drugs.

Wound infection is most often caused by *Streptococcae* or *Pseudomonas* spp. Resolving a streptococcal wound infection is relatively easy because this organism is nearly always susceptible to penicillin or other β-lactam antibiotics.[39,46,47] Occasionally, however, other bacteria in the wound secrete β-lactamase, an enzyme that inactivates most β-lactam antibiotics.[46] The efficacy of the β-lactam antibiotic against streptococci is maintained if the β-lactam antibiotic administered is effective against β-lactamase producing bacteria also present in the wound. The efficacy of the β-lactam antibiotic can also be maintained by concomitant administration of potassium clavulanate, or clavulanic acid, an inhibitor of β-lactamase.[46] Potassium clavulanate has no therapeutic value when administered alone; most commonly, potassium clavulanate is combined with amoxicillin or ticarcillin.

Pseudomonas infection, which is also highly detrimental to grafts, can be recognized by the characteristic bluish-green exudate and odor of grape juice produced by the bacteria. Pseudomonads are usually sensitive to aminoglycoside antibiotics, polymyxin-B sulfate, silver sulfadiazine, or mafenide acetate (Sulfamylon, Bertek Pharmaceuticals, Sugarland, TX).[48]

Topical administration of an antimicrobial drug to an infected, granulating wound is often more successful in resolving infection than is systemic administration of the same antimicrobial drug. Systemically administered antimicrobial drugs often fail to reach a therapeutic concentration within granulation tissue and at its surface in spite of its good blood supply because fibrin at the base of the granulation tissue prevents adequate penetration of the drug[11,49] and may also serve to physically isolate bacteria within clefts at the surface of the granulation bed.

In general, the most effective method of decreasing infection and/or chronic inflammation in a wound that contains exuberant granulation tissue is to excise the granulation tissue to the level of or slightly below the margin of the surrounding skin. Most bacteria, inflammatory cells, and debris are simultaneously removed, improving local wound conditions. Exuberant granulation tissue should be excised several days before grafting, and a pressure bandage should be applied to control hemorrhage. When excision is performed at least 24 hours in advance of grafting, time is provided for the development of budding capillaries that subsequently vascularize the graft.[45] The bandage should be changed daily after excision, until the wound appears ready for grafting. The concentration of bacteria in the wound can be further reduced by topical application of a broad-spectrum antimicrobial drug (as described earlier), which at the same time decreases the inflammatory response.

The chronic inflammation often present in wounds on limbs of horses can be further reduced with a single topical application of a corticosteroid, such as triamcinolone acetonide, 2 days before surgery, which may improve graft acceptance.[32,42,43] The potentially negative influence of the corticosteroid on angiogenesis is offset by reduction of the detrimental effect of inflammation on graft acceptance.

A granulating wound capable of accepting a free graft is firm, flat, vascular, and red, and contains only a few clefts. It should not bleed easily, and discharge from the wound should be slight and sero-sanguinous or only slightly purulent (Figure 11.4).[3] Adherence of a dressing to the wound bed by fibrin as well as advancing epithelium at the wound's margin are both useful indicators that a wound is free of infection and receptive to grafting.

At the time of grafting, the recipient bed should be prepared by clipping or shaving the hair surrounding the wound, taking care to first cover the wound with moistened swabs. The skin surrounding the wound can be cleansed with surgical soap, but the wound itself should be cleansed only by rinsing it with physiological saline or a balanced electrolyte solution because detergent found in surgical soap is cytotoxic and increases the wound's susceptibility to infection.[50] The surface of the wound can then either be rubbed with a gauze sponge to remove fibrinous debris, or its most superficial layer can be excised (i.e., 2 mm to 3 mm). This excision is best done before the graft is harvested to allow time for the wound to cease hemorrhaging. Slight hemorrhage caused by superficial excision may enhance formation of fibrin, which enables the graft to adhere to the wound surface. Too much hemorrhage, however, may hinder graft re-vascularization. The wound should not be scraped because such an action damages the surface of the wound and makes it irregular.

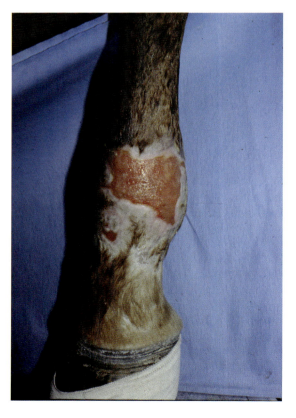

Figure 11.4. This granulating wound is firm, flat, vascular, and red and is likely capable of accepting a free skin graft.

Preparation of the Donor Site

Because harvesting a graft, especially one of split-thickness, creates a blemish at the donor site, the site should be inconspicuous. The area selected for harvest depends on the intended method of grafting and whether the graft is to be harvested with the horse standing or anesthetized.

Hair can be removed from the donor site by clipping with a #40 clipper blade, shaving using a guarded razor (i.e., one with a recessed blade), or chemical depilation. Shaving or depilating the hair at the donor site may improve the performance of a power dermatome. The direction of hair growth remains visible when the donor site is clipped, but when hair is removed completely by shaving or by depilation, the graft should be marked to indicate the direction of hair growth. After the donor site is prepared for surgery, it should be rinsed with water or physiological saline solution to remove residue detrimental to the graft such as surgical soap or isopropyl alcohol.

Grafting Techniques

Island Grafting

An island graft, sometimes referred to as an implantation or a seed graft, is a small piece of skin that is implanted either into or onto a wound.[51–53] Island grafts are usually implanted into granulation tissue of horses, rather than applied to the wound surface (with exception of the Meek micrografts), to prevent shearing forces between the dressing and the graft. The different types of island grafts applied to wounds of horses are punch grafts, pinch grafts, tunnel grafts, and modified Meek micrografts. Island grafts are applied to wounds to increase the area of epidermis from which epithelialization can proceed.

Punch Grafting

Punch grafts are full-thickness plugs of skin harvested and implanted into granulation tissue using skin biopsy punches. Punch grafts are harvested directly from the horse (Figure 11.5) or from a full-thickness piece of skin (Figure 11.6), usually excised from the cranial pectoral region.[54] Punch grafts harvested directly from the horse should be collected at a relatively inconspicuous site such as the ventrolateral aspect of the abdomen, the perineum, or the portion of the neck that lies beneath the mane, because wounds created at the donor site heal with small scars.

Technique. The donor site is clipped, scrubbed, and desensitized by subcutaneous administration of local anesthetic solution, or if the perineum is the donor site, by administering caudal epidural anesthesia. Grafts should be harvested about 1 cm apart and in a symmetrical pattern in an effort to improve the cosmetic appearance of the donor site (Figure 11.5).[38] The small wounds created by the biopsy punch can be left unsutured to heal by

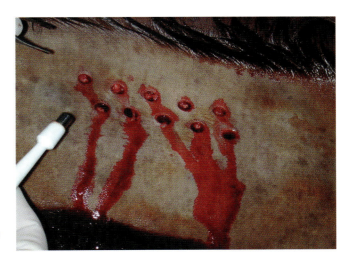

Figure 11.5. Punch grafts have been harvested directly from the neck of this horse.

second intention, but closing each wound with a staple or suture speeds healing and may decrease scarring. Prior to implantation, subcutaneous fascia should be sharply excised from each graft to expose dermal vasculature and encourage plasmatic imbibition and inosculation.[55] Subcutaneous tissue can be excised from the dermis while the graft is still attached to the wound bed. The biopsy punch is rotated until it penetrates only the full thickness of skin. One edge of the graft is elevated, using Brown-Adson thumb tissue forceps, to expose the attached subcutaneous tissue, which is incised from the dermis using a #15 scalpel blade.[56]

Because removing subcutaneous tissue from each small plug of skin is tedious, some clinicians prefer to harvest punch grafts from a full-thickness section of skin from which the subcutaneous tissue has been removed (Figure 11.6). This section of skin is usually harvested from the cranial pectoral region, where the skin is relatively mobile.[54] A 10 cm × 4 cm section of skin provides a sufficient number of grafts to cover most wounds, and the resulting wound on the chest can be sutured easily.[57] The chest wound is closed in one or two layers, and a tie-over (e.g., stent) bandage is sutured to the closed incision to decrease tension on the wound (Figure 11.7). The excised strip of skin is stretched and fixed, dermal side up, to a sterile piece of plastic, cardboard, or

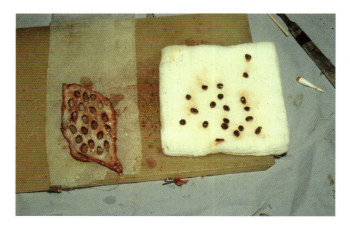

Figure 11.6. These punch grafts were harvested from a full-thickness section of skin excised from the cranial pectoral region. Subcutaneous tissue was sharply excised from the section of skin to expose the dermis prior to harvesting the grafts with a biopsy punch.

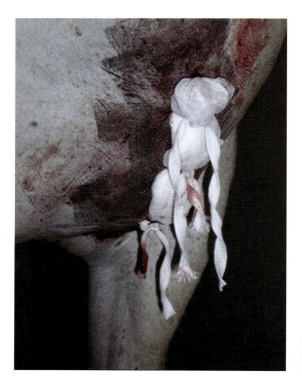

Figure 11.7. The wound created after excising a full-thickness section of skin from the chest is sutured in one or two layers, and a tie-over bandage is sutured to the closed incision to decrease tension on the wound.

Styrofoam or to a sterile polypropylene block, and subcutaneous tissue is sharply excised to expose the dermis (Figure 11.8). Plugs are cut from the skin with a 5 mm–8 mm diameter skin biopsy punch. The grafts are covered with a sterile gauze sponge moistened with physiological saline until implantation (Figure 11.6).

The recipient holes in the wound should be created before the grafts are harvested to ensure that hemorrhage has stopped before the grafts are implanted. The holes should be created in a symmetrical pattern, about 6 mm apart.[54] A common mistake is making the holes too deep. The depth of the recipient holes should correspond to the thickness of the grafts.[54] Creation of the holes should begin distally and proceed proximally so that the hemorrhage emanating from the holes does not obscure the portion of the wound that has not yet been perforated.[55] Inserting a cotton-tipped applicator into the holes prevents a blood clot from forming within and facilitates locating the holes for subsequent graft insertion.[57] A hemorrhage-free wound for grafting can be ensured by creating the recipient holes at least an hour in advance of implantation. In anticipation of primary graft contraction, the recipient holes should be created with a slightly smaller biopsy punch than that used to harvest the grafts. For example, if the grafts are harvested with a 6 mm diameter biopsy punch, the holes should be created with a 4 mm diameter biopsy punch. The holes should be lavaged to remove blood clots before inserting the grafts. Each graft is inserted into a recipient hole (Figure 11.9), using a hemostat or tissue forceps with the graft oriented according to the direction of its hair growth. The grafted wound is covered with a non-adherent dressing and then bandaged.

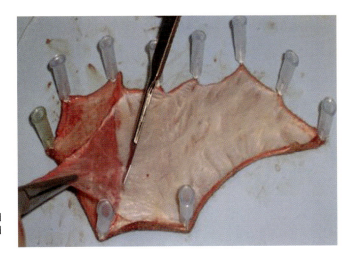

Figure 11.8. This section of skin has been stretched and fixed to a sterile piece of plastic. Subcutaneous tissue is being excised to expose the dermis.

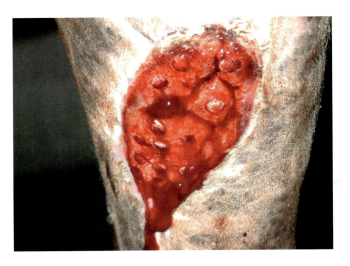

Figure 11.9. The recipient holes in this granulating wound have been filled with punch grafts.

Acceptance and Appearance. About 60% to 75% of the grafts can be expected to survive.[57] The superficial, pigmented portion of many of the grafts may slough between the first and second week, exposing the pale underlying dermis, which may be similar in appearance to surrounding granulation tissue. Difficulty in identifying many of the grafts and the presence of sloughed portions of graft on the primary dressing may convince the clinician that a number of grafts have been lost. But by 3 weeks, the pale grafts can easily be recognized by the pink rim of migrating epithelium that surrounds them.[54] The time required for epithelium to fully cover the remaining wound surface after migrating epithelium is first noted is inversely proportional to the wound area covered with viable plugs. Wounds to which punch grafts have been applied heal with an epithelial scar from which emerge sparse tufts of long hair that often grow in various directions. This cosmetic problem can be largely eliminated by orienting the grafts during implantation according to the direction of their hair growth.

Advantages and Disadvantages. Punch grafting requires little expertise and neither expensive nor sophisticated equipment, and it and can be performed with the horse standing. The grafts are often accepted into recipient wounds that are not suitable for sheet grafting, such as wounds in regions of high motion.[54] The grafts are independent of one another, and so rejection of one graft bears no effect on acceptance of other grafts. Punch grafting is usually reserved for small to moderate sized wounds and for circumstances in which cosmetic appearance of the healed wound is not important.

Pinch Grafting

Pinch grafts, sometime referred to as Reverdin grafts, are small disks of skin that are harvested by excising an elevated cone of skin and then implanted into pockets created in granulation tissue.[16,47,51–53,58] The perineum and the portion of the neck that lies beneath the mane are common donor sites for harvesting pinch grafts from horses because small scars created at these locations are relatively inconspicuous.

Technique. The donor site is prepared in the manner described for punch grafting. A cone of skin is tented with a tissue forceps, a hypodermic needle with a bent point, or a suture needle and excised with a scalpel blade.[47,51–53,58] A disk of optimal size is about 3 mm in diameter.[51] A disk of this diameter is thin toward its periphery but nearly full-thickness toward its center. The grafts are covered with a sterile gauze sponge moistened with physiological saline solution until they are implanted.

As for punch grafting, implantation of pinch grafts should begin distally and proceed proximally so that the hemorrhage emanating from sites of implantation does not obscure the portion of the wound that has not yet been implanted. To implant a pinch graft, a #15 scalpel blade is stabbed into the granulation tissue at an acute angle to the wound to create a shallow pocket into which the pinch graft is inserted (Figure 11.10). The pockets are created about 3 mm–5 mm apart.[51] The graft is placed on the wound, proximal to the pocket, with its epidermal side up. It is pushed into the pocket using a straight suture needle, hypodermic needle, mosquito hemostat, or the scalpel blade used to make the pocket. No consideration need be given to the direction of hair

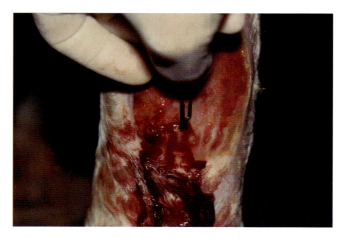

Figure 11.10. A shallow pocket, into which a pinch graft can be inserted, is created by stabbing a #15 scalpel blade into the granulation tissue at a severely acute angle.

growth on the graft upon insertion because in addition to being tedious, orienting the hair in its proper direction has little effect on the cosmetic outcome.

To speed implantation, three or more grafts can be placed on the wound, each several centimeters proximal to the proposed site of implantation. While the grafts remain adhered to the wound by hydrostatic pressure, the surgeon creates a pocket distal to a graft and pushes the graft into it using the same scalpel blade that was used to create the pockets. This technique enables the surgeon to create and implant the pockets in quick succession, without looking away from the wound. Alternatively, each graft can be inserted into the granulation tissue, without making a pocket, using a curved mosquito hemostat. The graft is grasped in the midepidermal region and inserted obliquely, from proximal to distal, into the granulation tissue, after which the hemostat is opened to create more space for the graft. This technique is much quicker than making separate pockets using a scalpel blade (T Stashak, personal communication).

The small, partial-thickness wounds created at the donor site can be left unsutured to heal by second intention, but closing each wound with a staple or suture speeds healing and may decrease scarring. The grafted wound is covered with a non-adherent dressing and then bandaged.

Acceptance and Appearance. The grafts initially appear as dark spots on the wound. The thin layer of granulation tissue overlying each graft sloughs, usually between the first and second week,[51] and frequently, so does the superficial, pigmented portion of the graft. The exposed, pale dermis may be difficult to distinguish from surrounding granulation tissue, giving the impression that the entire graft has sloughed. By 3 weeks, however, grafts are surrounded by a pink rim of advancing epithelium, making them easy to identify. Epithelium migrating from the wound margin and from the periphery of each graft rapidly coalesces to cover the entire wound. Even when conditions for grafting are unfavorable, at least 50%–75% of the grafts are usually accepted.[51] The healed wound is covered by epithelium containing scattered islands of hair.

Advantages and Disadvantages. Pinch grafting, like punch grafting, requires little expertise and is economical because only basic instruments are required and the procedure can be performed with the standing horse.[54] Pinch grafts, like punch grafts, can survive in a granulation bed that is not suitable for sheet grafting, such as a wound in an area of high motion.[52,59] Like punch grafts, pinch grafts are independent of one another; therefore, rejection of one graft has no effect on acceptance of other grafts. Pinch grafting is tedious, however, and therefore is usually reserved for small wounds. The cosmetic appearance of a wound healed with pinch grafts is poor (Figure 11.11).

Tunnel Grafting

Tunnel grafts are thin strips of skin implanted into tunnels created in granulation tissue.[2,60,61] Granulation tissue covering the grafts is removed days later, by which time the grafts have re-vascularized. Grafts can be split-thickness or full-thickness and can be harvested from a number of sites on the horse using a variety of techniques. They can be implanted with the horse standing or anesthetized.

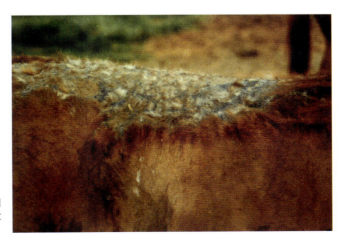

Figure 11.11. The wound on the back of this horse was healed with pinch grafts. The back is covered by an epithelial scar that contains scattered islands of hair.

Technique. Split-thickness or full-thickness tunnel grafts can be harvested from the ventral region of the flank or from the portion of the neck that lies beneath the mane or the cranial pectoral region.[2,60,61] After clipping and scrubbing the donor site, linear wheals, 2 cm–3 cm wide and slightly longer than the width of the wound to be grafted, are created along the longitudinal axis of the donor site by subcutaneously injecting physiological saline when the graft is to be harvested with the horse anesthetized, or local anesthetic solution when the graft is to be harvested with the horse standing.

A long, straight Doyen intestinal forceps is applied to the base of each wheal, causing skin to protrude slightly above the jaws of the forceps.[2,60,61] The amount of skin that bulges above the jaws determines the width and thickness of the graft. If a graft longer than the jaws of the forceps is required, two intestinal forceps are applied end to end. Skin that protrudes above the jaws is excised with a scalpel blade. If the graft is split-thickness, the partial-thickness wound at the donor site can be closed or left open to heal by epithelialization. If the graft is full-thickness, its dermis should be exposed by excising subcutaneous tissue and the wound at the donor site should be closed with sutures or stainless steel skin staples. Another option is to harvest an elliptical, 2 cm–3 cm wide, full-thickness section of skin that is slightly longer than the width of the wound.[56] After exposing its dermis, the section of skin is divided into 2 mm–3 mm wide strips (Figure 11.12).

To implant a graft into the wound, the jaws of a long, thin, rat-tooth, alligator forceps are inserted into granulation tissue at the edge of the wound and pushed through it at a depth of about 5 mm–6 mm until they emerge at the opposite wound margin.[2,61] One end of the graft is grasped by the jaws of the forceps and pulled through the newly-created tunnel, taking care to orient its epidermis toward the overlying surface of the wound (Figure 11.13). The grafts should be implanted about 2 cm apart.[61]

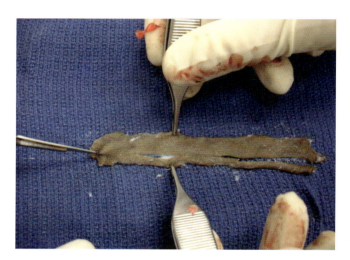

Figure 11.12. A full-thickness section of skin, harvested from the neck of a horse, is being divided into 2 mm wide strips for implantation in a granulating wound. Courtesy of Dr. P. Rakestraw.

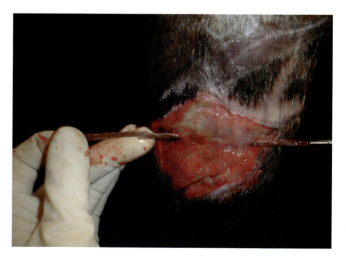

Figure 11.13. To implant a tunnel graft, one end of the graft is grasped by the jaws of an alligator forceps, which has been pushed through the granulation tissue at a depth of 5 mm or 6 mm, then dragged through the tunnel created by the forceps, with the epidermis facing the surface of the wound. Courtesy of Dr. P. Rakestraw.

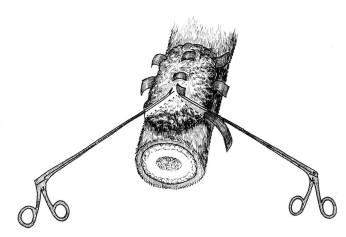

Figure 11.14. To implant a tunnel graft in a wound too convex to be spanned by alligator forceps, the forceps is inserted at the wound's margin and exited in the center of the wound. The graft is grasped by the jaws of the forceps and dragged back through the wound. The end of the forceps is re-inserted at the wound's opposite margin and exited close to the site of entry of the graft in the center of the wound. The end of the graft is grasped by the jaws of the forceps and pulled back through the wound. Courtesy of K. Abney.

To permit easy entry and exit of the forceps, the graft should be implanted perpendicular to the long axis of the limb in granulation tissue that protrudes slightly above the margin of the skin.[61] The graft is implanted in two steps if the wound is too convex to be spanned by the alligator forceps, or if the forceps is too short to completely span the wound.[2,60,61] In either situation, the end of the forceps is inserted at the margin of the wound, pushed through the granulation tissue, and exited in the center of the wound. The graft is grasped by the jaws of the forceps and dragged back through the newly-created tunnel. The end of the forceps is re-inserted into the granulation bed at the opposite wound margin, pushed through the granulation tissue, and exited at or close to the site of entry of the graft in the center of the wound. The free end of the graft is grasped by the jaws of the forceps and pulled back through the second tunnel (Figure 11.14).

The protruding ends of the implanted grafts are fixed to the margin of the wound with a suture, staple, or cyanoacrylate glue. The wound is covered with a non-adherent dressing and then bandaged. Six to 10 days after being implanted, the grafts are exposed, with the horse sedated or anesthetized, by excising overlying granulation tissue.[2,60,61] This is done by running a scalpel blade over a small, malleable probe inserted into the tunnel superficial to the graft. Overlying granulation tissue can also be excised with a twisted, doubled piece of 0.30 mm wire threaded through the tunnel.[60] The edges of the tunnel are trimmed with a bistoury.

Acceptance and Appearance. Complications of tunnel grafting include failure to locate buried grafts and inadvertent dislodging of a graft while attempting to expose it.[61] These difficulties can best be avoided by exposing the grafts with the horse anesthetized or by applying a tourniquet proximal to the wound to enhance visibility by eliminating hemorrhage. About 60%–80% acceptance of the grafts can be expected.[60,61] The healed wound is covered by pigmented epithelium that migrates from the margin of the wound and from the margin of each graft. Within this epithelium are linear, divergent tufts of hair.

Advantages and Disadvantages. Tunnel grafting is useful in wounds located in regions of high motion, such as the dorsal aspect of the hock, because the grafts are immobilized by granulation tissue, which protects them from shear forces that develop between the bandage and the wound.[60,61] Like pinch and punch grafts, tunnel grafts are independent of one another, and so rejection of one graft has no effect on acceptance of other grafts. Like other techniques of island grafting, tunnel grafting is economical because only basic instruments are required and the procedure can often be performed with the horse standing. On the downside, tunnel grafting is limited to granulating wounds, and removing granulation tissue overlying the grafts is tedious. Furthermore, locating the grafts within the granulation tissue can be difficult.

Modified Meek Technique

The modified Meek technique of skin grafting, a combination of split-thickness sheet and island grafting, has recently been evaluated in horses.[25] This technique, introduced in the 1990s as a method of grafting burn wounds of humans, uses split-thickness, 3 mm² islands of skin, referred to as micrografts. The technique has proved particularly suitable for grafting wounds of severely burned patients who lack large donor sites because greater expansion ratios can be achieved with these split-thickness micrografts than with meshed sheet grafts, and because all harvested skin can be applied.[62] Moreover, micrografts are less susceptible to infection and inflammation than a meshed sheet graft, which improves the acceptance of Meek micrografts in wounds of poor quality.[62,63] These same advantages also apply to wounds of horses.[25]

Technique. The Meek micrografting equipment consists of a cutting block, a frame, and a pneumatic or hand-driven motor. The micrografts are obtained from a split-thickness section of skin, harvested with the horse anesthetized, usually from the abdomen or ventrolateral aspect of the thorax (See Split-Thickness Sheet Grafting, below). The split-thickness graft is placed, dermal side down, on a cork template measuring 4.2 cm² then trimmed exactly to the size of the template. The cork template, with graft, is placed on a cork holder, which is placed in a cutting block (Figure 11.15) and the composite is passed through the motor-driven or hand-driven Meek micrograft machine where 13 circular knives cut the skin into 14 strips, each 3 mm wide (Figure 11.16). The machine cuts the skin, but not the cork. The cork holder is then rotated 90 degrees, replaced onto the cutting block, and again passed through the Meek micrograft machine. The second passage produces 196 (i.e., 14 × 14), 3 mm², split-thickness grafts. Adhesive spray is applied to the epidermal layer of the grafts, which are glued to a pre-folded, pleated, polyamide gauze (e.g., plissé) (Figure 11.17) with a predetermined expansion factor of 1:3, 1:4, 1:6, or 1:9. An expansion of 1:3 is preferred for horses because availability of skin is usually not a problem. The cork template is carefully removed and the plissé is expanded in two directions, separating the 196 micrografts to a fixed distance. The supporting aluminum backing is peeled off the gauze, which is then

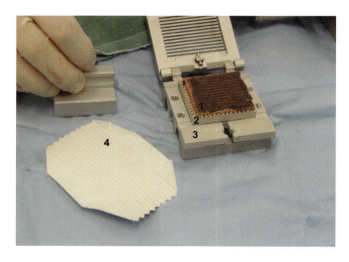

Figure 11.15. To create Meek micrografts, a split-thickness graft is placed on a 4.2 cm² cork template and trimmed exactly to the size of the template (1), placed on a square cork holder (2), and then placed in a cutting block (3). More to the left is a plissé 1:3 (4). Reprinted with permission.[25]

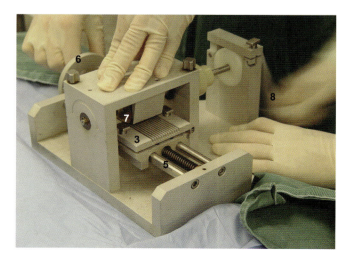

Figure 11.16. The cutting block (3) is placed on the guiding axes (5) of a Meek micrograft machine and moved by a hand wheel (6) under a bridge, where 13 circular knives (7) cut the skin into 14 strips, each 3 mm wide. A Meek micrograft machine is shown with a hand drive (8) instead of a pneumatic motor for turning the knives. Reprinted with permission.[25]

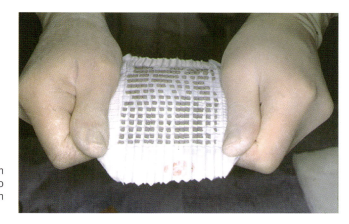

Figure 11.17. The epidermal side of the cut graft sprayed with an adhesive and glued to the plissé is being unfolded in two directions to separate the micrografts. Reprinted with permission.[25]

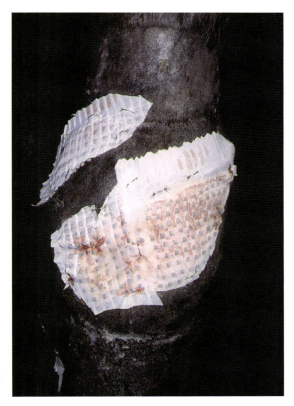

Figure 11.18. The expanded plissé is cut to the appropriate size and sutured or stapled to the wound. Reprinted with permission.[25]

trimmed to the appropriate size and sutured or stapled to the wound (Figure 11.18). The wound is protected with a bandage or a cast.

Acceptance and Appearance. Noticeable effects produced by the grafts on the granulation tissue are seen when the bandage is changed or the cast is removed after 10 days.[25] When the cast is removed, most wounds that were suffering from exuberant granulation tissue and/or chronic inflammation before grafting appear flat, smooth, and less inflamed, and the rates of contraction and epithelialization appear to have increased substantially.[25] These effects may result from the action of cytokines present in the dermis of the grafts. Although any type of graft that includes the dermis may have such an effect, dermal contact with the wound after Meek micrografting is greater than after the other types of island grafting because of the high number of islands and

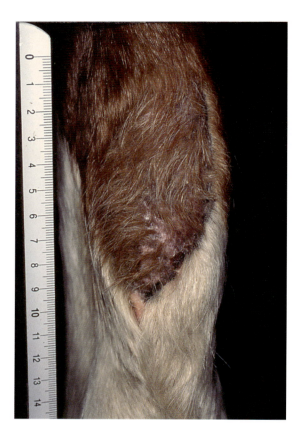

Figure 11.19. Wounds healed with Meek micrografts have regular though somewhat thinner than normal hair growth. Hairs usually grow longer than at the donor site or the area surrounding the wound.

because the grafts are split-thickness. The micrografts can be applied closely together and uniformly in the same direction. The distance between the grafts diminishes as the wound contracts, which allows for fast wound coverage and a good functional and cosmetic result. Most wounds that receive Meek micrografts are healed within a month, regardless of the wound's size and location.[25] Hair growth occurs from most of the grafts and is regular, though somewhat thinner and longer than normal, and hair color is the same as that at the donor site (Figure 11.19).

Advantages and Disadvantages. As with other techniques of island grafting, the Meek micrografting technique creates small islands of skin independent of one another, so that rejection of one or more grafts has no effect on acceptance of other grafts. In contrast, partial detachment of a sheet graft due to infection or movement may propagate into other areas of the graft, resulting in complete loss of the graft. Meek micrografts are, therefore, better accepted by poor quality wounds than are sheet grafts and can be applied in higher numbers than can other types of island grafts. Because granulation tissue is not damaged by this technique, obviating bleeding, clot formation, and additional inflammation, Meek micrografts are more readily accepted than are other types of island grafts. Grafts up to 1.2 mm in thickness can be applied, with good acceptance, and these thick grafts provide more hair follicles than do thin sheet grafts. The micrografts can be applied closely and uniformly, which results in faster epithelialization, and with the hair properly oriented in the wound, which improves the cosmetic outcome. Acceptance of micrografts is nearly 95% and is reported to be better than that achieved with any other type of skin grafting performed in horses.[25] Functional and cosmetic results are consistently good.

A disadvantage of the micrografting technique is that the horse must be anesthetized to harvest the split-thickness skin required. Equipment to harvest the split-thickness skin and the micrografting machine are relatively expensive but comparable to that required for harvesting and meshing sheet grafts (See Instrumentation.)

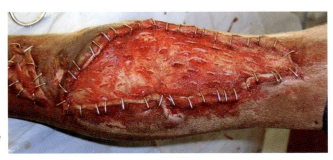

Figure 11.20. This graft has been attached to a wound on the dorsal surface of the fetlock using staples.

Sheet Grafting

Full-Thickness Sheet Grafting

Technique. A full-thickness graft is usually harvested from the cranial pectoral region, where the skin is relatively mobile.[57,64] The graft is usually harvested and the donor site sutured with the horse sedated, after desensitizing the donor site with a local anesthetic solution. The excised skin is stretched and fixed, dermal side up, to a sterile piece of cardboard or Styrofoam or to a sterile polypropylene block. Subcutaneous tissue on the undersurface of the graft obstructs plasmatic imbibition and inosculation and so must be sharply excised to expose the dermis and its vasculature (Figure 11.8).[21,59,64] Hair follicles in the dermis are visible when the subcutaneous tissue has been removed. Grafts are attached to the recipient site with staples or sutures (Figure 11.20). Attaching the graft to the recipient site with slight tension keeps the small dermal vessels open for plasmatic imbibition and inosculation.[58]

Acceptance and Appearance. Full-thickness grafts are not as readily accepted as split-thickness grafts because of their greater requirement for nourishment and fewer exposed blood vessels.[3,21,35,65] Circumstances at the recipient site must be ideal for a full-thickness graft to be accepted because it has few blood vessels available for imbibition of plasma or for inosculation. Although a full-thickness skin graft can successfully be applied to healthy, new granulation tissue,[31] this type of grafting is usually reserved for fresh, uncontaminated wounds.[3,10,11,16,39]

Advantages and Disadvantages. Wounds healed with a full-thickness skin graft have a superior cosmetic appearance and resist trauma better than do those healed with a split-thickness sheet graft or with island grafts.[3,10,35,38,59] Furthermore, full-thickness sheet grafts can be harvested and applied with the horse standing and in the absence of sophisticated equipment.

The horse's lack of redundant donor skin limits the practicality of full-thickness grafting to relatively small wounds, provided that the surgeon intends to suture the donor site after harvesting the graft. The amount of graft that can be harvested from the cranial pectoral area is governed by the capacity of the donor site to be sutured; therefore, the largest graft that can usually be safely harvested is an ellipse not exceeding 8 cm at its widest point. The owner should be forewarned that the donor site might dehisce but reassured that a wound in the cranial pectoral region heals rapidly by contraction, leaving little scarring.

A full-thickness graft can be meshed and expanded to cover a wound larger than the graft itself (see Meshing Sheet Grafts), but full-thickness skin of horses is too thick to be easily meshed using most commercial meshgraft dermatomes.

Split-Thickness Sheet Grafting

Instrumentation. A split-thickness graft is composed of epidermis and a portion of dermis. To harvest a split-thickness graft, the dermis must be split using a power-driven dermatome, drum dermatome, or free-hand knife.

Power-driven Dermatomes. A power-driven dermatome harvests a split-thickness skin graft with predictable depth and width using a rapidly oscillating blade, which is set in a housing and driven by an electric motor or gas turbine. Examples of commonly used power-driven dermatomes are the Stryker electric dermatome (Electric Dermatome, Stryker Electro-Surgical Unit, Orthopedic Frame Co., Kalamazoo, MI), Brown pneumatic or electric dermatome (Brown Dermatome, Zimmer, Warsaw, IN), Padgett electric dermatome (Padgett Model B Dermatome, Padgett Instruments, Kansas City, MO), and Humeca electric dermatome (Humeca Models D42 and D80, Humeca Instruments, Enschede, The Netherlands). A pneumatic dermatome generally provides a smoother harvest than does an electric dermatome of the same type because the cutting head of the pneumatic dermatome oscillates more rapidly.[21] Different types of power-driven dermatomes may vary in their ability to smoothly harvest, and some of the newer types of electric dermatomes may harvest skin as smoothly as do pneumatic dermatomes.

The Davol-Simon skin graft dermatome (Davol-Simon Dermatome, Davol Inc., Cranston, RI) is a relatively inexpensive dermatome powered by a rechargeable battery.[13,14] It uses a disposable, nonadjustable cutting head that harvests a graft with a fixed width of 3 cm and a fixed thickness of 0.38 mm. A graft of these dimensions is too thin to impart a good cosmetic appearance to wounds of horses, but a graft harvested with this dermatome may be useful for covering relatively small wounds when cosmetic appearance is not important. Pinch or punch grafts could also be considered for such wounds, however.

The Humeca dermatome is small and maneuverable and is powered by a rechargeable battery. It has a fixed width of either 42 mm or 80 mm, which can be reduced, if necessary, with clamps. The D42 model has the exact width necessary for harvesting skin to be used in the Meek micrograft machine. Thickness of cut can be adjusted from 0 mm–1.2 mm; therefore, the dermatome is capable of harvesting thick split-thickness grafts that contain a large concentration of hair follicles. Unlike some power dermatomes, the Humeca dermatome is usually capable of easily harvesting skin from the ventral surface of the abdomen of horses. In rare situations in which the Humeca dermatome is unable to grip the skin in this region, a firm area, such as the ventrolateral aspect of the thorax, can be used as an alternative donor site. The ability of a power dermatome to split skin in compliant areas, such as the ventral aspect of the abdomen, also depends on the skin's elasticity. Harvesting skin with a power dermatome presents similar problems in humans, where harvesting the elastic skin of children is more difficult than harvesting the relatively inelastic skin of adults.

A power-driven dermatome allows harvesting of grafts of precise width and thickness, but the widest graft that can be harvested with many power dermatomes is only 76 mm to 80 mm. Although a power-driven dermatome can be operated with only a minimal amount experience, the dermatome requires skilled maintenance and may fail to operate properly at critical moments. Because power-driven dermatomes are expensive, they are generally found only at equine referral centers.

Drum Dermatomes. The drum dermatome consists of a portion of a drum, which is coated with an adhesive, and a knife. A section of skin adheres to the drum as the drum is rolled across the skin, and the knife oscillates back and forth on a piston to precisely split the dermis at a predetermined thickness.

Using a drum dermatome, the surgeon can harvest a graft with the exact dimensions of the wound to be grafted by applying glue to an area on the drum that is identical to the dimensions of the wound, so that as the drum is rotated, only the adhered portion of skin is cut.[11] The drum dermatome requires no external power source and allows anyone to harvest a uniform section of skin with only minimal training.[10,11,21] The drum dermatome is not as expensive as a power-driven dermatome, although it is considerably more expensive than a free-hand dermatome. A major disadvantage of the drum dermatome for harvesting grafts from horses is that the length of the graft is limited by the circumference of the drum. An example of a drum dermatome is the Padgett Manual Dermatome (Z-PD-100R, Padgett Instruments, Inc., Kansas City, MO), of which the drum has a diameter of 10.2 cm and a circumference of 31.9 cm.

Free-hand Dermatomes. Large grafts to cover wounds of horses can be harvested with any one of a variety of free-hand dermatomes designed specifically for harvesting skin of humans. The Watson skin grafting knife (Watson Skin Grafting Knife, Padgett Instruments, Inc., Kansas City, MO), a modification of the Braithwaite knife, has an adjustable roller in front of a disposable blade and can harvest a graft 100 mm wide. Because the depth of cut is primarily controlled by the adjustable roller, only a moderate amount of practice is required to develop proficiency in harvesting uniform, split-thickness grafts with this knife. The position of the adjustable roller is controlled by a knob marked with calibrations at one end of the roller (Figure 11.21) and a lock at the other end (Figure 11.22). The thickness of graft corresponding to each calibration is learned by experience. The depth of cut depends not only on the distance of the roller from the blade, but also on the angle of incidence at which the knife is held, as well as the pressure applied to the knife while cutting.[39] By applying greater pressure to the knife or by increasing the knife's angle of incidence, the thickness of the graft can be increased without changing the position of the roller.

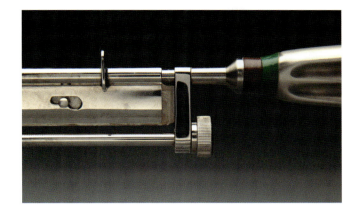

Figure 11.21. The position of the adjustable roller on the Watson skin graft dermatome is controlled by a knob marked with calibrations at one end of the roller.

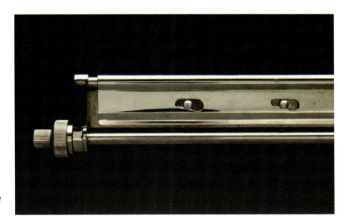

Figure 11.22. A knob located on one end of the knife locks the position of the roller.

A free-hand knife is far less expensive than a power-driven dermatome, requires significantly less maintenance, has fewer parts to malfunction, is easy to clean and sterilize, and can be easily transported. Arguably, the greatest advantage of a free-hand knife over a power-driven dermatome is that with the former, skin can be harvested consistently from the ventral surface of the abdomen, which is a difficult feat using some power-driven dermatomes. Additionally, wider grafts can be harvested with the free-hand knife than with most power-drive dermatomes.

Harvesting a Split-Thickness Sheet Graft. Harvesting a split-thickness graft leaves a large epithelial scar; therefore, cosmetic appearance should be considered when selecting a donor site. A split-thickness graft is usually harvested from a horse at the ventral surface of the abdomen or the ventrolateral surface of the thorax, caudal to the elbow.[1,24,25,64,66] The ventral surface of the abdomen is the least conspicuous site from which to harvest a split-thickness graft on a horse. To successfully harvest with a power-driven dermatome other than the Humeca dermatome, however, a surface firmer than the ventral surface of the abdomen, such as the ventrolateral surface of the thorax, is often required. Split-thickness skin is most easily harvested from the ventral aspect of the abdomen with a free-hand knife.

To harvest from the ventrolateral surface of the thorax or abdomen using a power dermatome, the horse can be positioned in either lateral or dorsal recumbency (Figure 11.23). The donor site is prepared for aseptic surgery, but draping is optional. The mobile skin at the ventrolateral surface of the thorax is stabilized by assistants who stretch the skin with towel clamps. Lubricating the blade and donor site with physiological saline reduces friction. The blade can also be lubricated with a light coating of mineral oil, which does not seem to adversely affect graft acceptance.[3,14] Mineral oil should not be used when harvesting a sheet using the Meek micrografting technique because the oil adversely affects adhesion of the grafts to the plissé. Slight tension is applied by the surgeon or an assistant to the cut end of the graft as it is harvested. When the desired length of graft has been harvested, the graft is transected by tilting the dermatome outward.

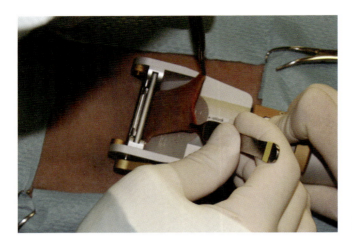

Figure 11.23. A graft is being harvested from the ventral abdomen using a Humeca power dermatome, with the horse in lateral recumbency.

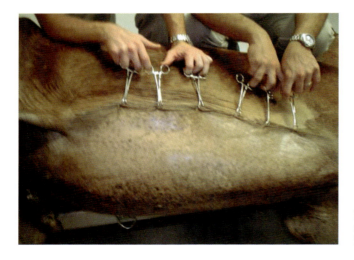

Figure 11.24. Stabilizing the skin with towel clamps is not usually necessary but may be somewhat helpful when harvesting skin from the ventral abdomen.

To harvest skin from the most ventral surface of the abdomen using a free-hand knife, the horse is positioned on a table in lateral recumbency. The ventral portion of the abdomen must protrude over the edge of the table so that the surface of the table does not impair manipulation of the knife. The donor site is prepared for aseptic surgery, but draping is not necessary and may interfere with manipulation of the knife.

Harvesting usually begins at the umbilicus and proceeds cranially. Stabilizing the skin of the ventral abdomen by stretching it with towel clamps is not usually necessary but may be helpful (Figure 11.24). Depressing the abdomen inward with the non-dominant hand while harvesting with the dominant hand flattens the abdomen slightly, enabling a wider graft to be harvested. The knife is applied to the abdomen with moderate pressure at an acute angle of about 5°–10°, and the dermis is cut using a sawing motion, while concentrating on moving the blade up and down rather than forward (Figure 11.25). This sawing motion causes the margin of the graft to assume a saw-toothed appearance. An assistant should apply slight, uniform tension to the cut end of the graft during harvesting. The knife and donor site should be lubricated with physiological saline solution or mineral oil to reduce friction between the knife and the abdomen.

After several centimeters of graft have been harvested, the surgeon should cease cutting and examine the graft and donor site to determine whether the graft is being harvested at the proper thickness before continuing. Thickness can be judged by examining the graft for translucency and the donor site for the pattern of bleeding.[13,14] A shallow cut through the dermis severs many small vessels and creates a semi-transparent graft, whereas a deep cut severs fewer but larger vessels and creates a more opaque graft. The depth of cut can be changed by repositioning the adjustable roller, changing the pressure applied to the knife, or changing the

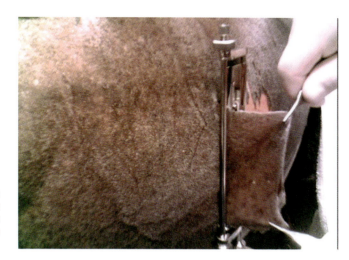

Figure 11.25. To harvest skin from the ventral abdomen, the free-hand knife is pressed against the abdomen at an acute angle of about 5°–10° using moderate pressure, and the dermis is cut using a sawing motion. An assistant should apply tension to the cut end of the graft.

knife's angle of incidence. Harvesting a thin, split-thickness skin graft is much more difficult than harvesting a thick one. The graft is transected by tilting the knife outward. If the graft is to be meshed and fully expanded, it should be considerably longer than the wound to which it is to be applied because expansion shortens the graft.

Judging the depth at which a graft should be harvested is difficult because the dermis varies in thickness between horses and between donor sites.[9] Split-thickness grafts between 0.63 mm and 0.76 mm thick, harvested from the hip, lateral gaskin, or ventral abdomen or thorax, have good durability and moderate to good hair coverage,[9,17] whereas split-thickness grafts that are 0.5 mm or less thick and harvested from these same areas lack durability and have sparse or no hair coverage.[17] An aim of split-thickness grafting is to provide satisfactory hair coverage at both the donor and recipient sites, although this is rarely achieved.[35] Grafts with good hair coverage may leave the donor site devoid of hair.

By purposely harvesting a thin split-thickness graft, a second split-thickness graft, composed only of dermis, can be harvested from the same site. The recipient site is covered partly with one graft composed of both epidermis and a portion of the dermis and partly with another graft composed solely of a portion of the dermis. This second graft contains no epidermis, but epithelialization proceeding from adnexa within the transplanted skin eventually resurfaces the dermis.[67] This "two-layer" technique of harvesting split-thickness grafts may be useful for grafting exceptionally large wounds, such as burn wounds that cover much of the back. Another option for covering such large wounds is to use the Meek technique with an expansion of 1:9.

Meshing Sheet Grafts. A split- or full-thickness sheet graft can be applied to a wound as a solid or meshed (i.e., fenestrated) sheet. The principal reason for meshing a sheet graft is to enable it to uniformly cover a wound larger than the graft itself.[1,9,11,13,21,64,66,68,69] Meshing a sheet graft also prevents blood, serum, or exudate from becoming interposed between the newly applied graft and the wound, thus improving the likelihood of graft adherence. A meshed sheet graft conforms to an irregular surface better than does a solid sheet graft and because it can expand, it has a greater tolerance to motion. Fibrin fills the fenestrations, increasing the graft's stability on the wound.[38] Meshing also enables a topically applied antimicrobial agent to uniformly contact a large portion of the wound.

A graft can be meshed manually with a scalpel blade or mechanically with a meshgraft dermatome. An example of a relatively inexpensive, commonly used, meshgraft dermatome is the Padgett mechanical skin mesher (Mesh Skin Graft Expander, No. Z-PD-170, Padgett Instruments, Kansas City, MO), which consists of staggered parallel rows of blades housed in an aluminum block and a Teflon-covered rolling pin. The graft is positioned on the block, dermal side down, and pressed into the cutting blades with the rolling pin. The cutting blades fenestrate the graft in a staggered pattern that allows the graft to be expanded to 3 times its original area.

The Zimmer mechanical skin mesher (Zimmer Meshgraft Dermatome, Zimmer, Warsaw, IN) is more sophisticated and expensive but can create different patterns of fenestrations that allow the graft to be expanded to 1.5, 3, 6, or 9 times its original area (Figure 11.26). The graft is placed dermal side down on a grooved plastic carrier selected according to the amount of expansion desired, and the graft and carrier are advanced through the mesher by turning a hand crank. The pattern of grooves stamped onto the plastic carrier determines the distance between cuts. The graft must be placed on the grooved surface of the carrier because if placed on its smooth side, the graft is shredded into thin, spaghetti-like strips.

The width of grafts routinely harvested with the skin graft dermatome should be considered prior to purchasing a meshgraft dermatome. Grafts close to 100 mm wide can be harvested with a free-hand skin graft knife, but a graft wider than 76 mm cannot be fitted into a Zimmer mechanical skin mesher. Grafts up to about 110 mm wide, however, can be fitted onto the cutting surface of the Padgett mechanical meshgraft dermatome described previously. Although the Padgett mechanical skin mesher accommodates a graft only up to 135 mm long, a longer graft can be meshed in sections.

Full-thickness sheet grafts of horses, except those of foals, are difficult to mesh on commercial mechanical skin meshers and so must usually be meshed manually. To manually mesh a sheet graft, the graft is fixed to a cutting board, such as a sterile piece of cardboard or Styrofoam, and staggered, parallel rows of incisions are created in the graft. The more numerous and the longer the incisions, the greater is the expansion. Meshing a graft manually is tedious, especially if the graft is large or if it must be greatly expanded.

Expanding a meshed graft uniformly exposes portions of the wound within the fenestrations, and so the amount of wound exposed by the fenestrations depends on the extent to which the graft is expanded. Expanding a meshed graft to cover a wound delays healing because each portion of the wound exposed within a fenestration must heal by contraction and epithelialization. Portions of the wound covered by the meshed graft heal primarily, whereas the exposed portions of the wound rapidly epithelialize because meshing the graft provides an extensive border from which epithelial cells can migrate and proliferate.[1,24] The healed wound is eventually covered with a uniform pattern of diamond-shaped scars beneath which dermis is absent. The more a graft is expanded at application, the more apparent are the epithelial scars within the grafted wound. These scars diminish in size, however, as the grafted wound contracts.[1,10,24,39] The size of epithelial scars can be minimized by applying the graft to the wound in such a way that the fenestrations are parallel to the long axis of the limb.[64]

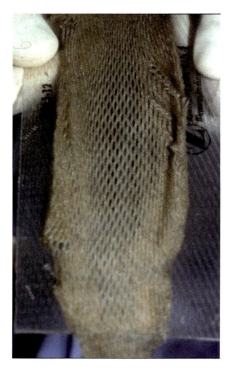

Figure 11.26. This split-thickness graft was meshed with a Zimmer meshgraft dermatome using a carrier that provided a 1–1.5 expansion ratio.

Applying Sheet Grafts. The graft should be applied so that the direction of hair growth conforms to that of the surrounding skin. A graft harvested from the anesthetized horse can be sutured or stapled to the wound's margin. In the standing horse, the margin of the wound must be desensitized using local or regional anesthesia prior to graft fixation. An alternative method is to overlap and glue the margin of the graft to the wound margin using cyanoacrylate glue (Super Glue, Loctite Co., Cleveland, OH), which obviates the necessity of desensitizing the wound margin. This is only possible, however, when ample skin has been harvested to permit overlap of the graft onto the surrounding skin (Figure 11.27). The overlapped and glued portion of the graft eventually desiccates and sloughs. This portion separates without harming the rest of the graft as the underlying epidermis desquamates. Applying the graft after the horse recovers from general anesthesia shortens the time of anesthesia and eliminates the possibility of damage to the graft that might occur during recovery.

A graft applied to a small wound in a non-mobile region need only be fixed to the wound's margin because within minutes of graft application, fibrin firmly fixes the graft to the wound's surface.[10,16] A graft applied to a wound that is large or is in a region that is difficult to immobilize, such as the dorsum of a fetlock or hock, can be further secured to the wound with simple interrupted sutures placed through the fenestrations of the graft to reduce shearing forces. In the standing horse, this can be done without anesthetizing the granulation tissue because granulation tissue is not innervated. A fresh wound, however, must first be desensitized using local or regional anesthesia prior to suturing a graft to its base. Sutures can be removed after 1 week, when graft acceptance is certain. Simple interrupted catgut sutures tied with a square knot are easily removed after several days by applying gentle traction to one end of the suture with a hemostat because swelling of the suture causes the knot to unravel when tension is applied to it.

Acceptance and Appearance. The thickness of the dermis of a split-thickness graft greatly influences both the graft's acceptance and the wound's healed appearance.[3,17,21,28,39,65,70] A graft that contains a large portion of dermis is more durable and imparts a better cosmetic appearance than a graft that contains a small portion of dermis. Conversely, a graft that contains a small portion of dermis is more likely to be accepted than one containing a large portion of dermis because a thin graft has reduced metabolic demands compared to a thick one. Further-

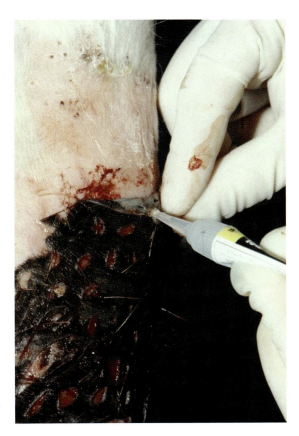

Figure 11.27. This graft is being attached in a standing horse by overlapping and gluing the margin of the graft to the margin of the wound.

more, a thin graft has more exposed cut vessels than does a thick one because blood vessels branch as they ascend the dermis. The more cut vessels are exposed, the better the absorption of nutrients from the wound during the phase of plasmatic imbibition, and the more rapidly the graft re-vascularizes.

Clinical studies of the effects of hyperbaric oxygen therapy (HBOT) on split-thickness grafts applied to wounds of people as well as an experimental study of the effects of HBOT on pedicle grafts and free grafts on rats showed that HBOT improves graft survival.[71-73] An experimental study of the effects on HBOT on grafted wounds of pigs, however, showed that HBOT is detrimental to grafts,[74] and a study of the effects of HBOT on survivability of skin grafts applied to wounds of horses showed that daily, 1-hour administration of HBOT for 1 week decreased viability of full-thickness grafts applied to either fresh or granulating wounds.[75] Although HBOT reduced graft edema, it negatively affected neovascularization, probably because it reduced the oxygen gradient between the wound and the graft. Tissue hypoxia is an important stimulus for neovascularization, which is essential for graft acceptance. Reducing the oxygen gradient between the wound and the graft with HBOT results in elimination of mediators of angiogenesis, subsequently reducing neovascularization, which decreases graft viability.

Advantages and Disadvantages. The split-thickness sheet graft is more versatile than the full-thickness graft because it can be harvested in sheets large enough to cover wounds too large to be covered by a full-thickness graft and because it is more readily accepted than the full-thickness graft.[3,39,65] The appearance and durability of a wound healed with a split-thickness skin graft is poorer than that of a wound healed with a full-thickness skin graft; it is comparable to that of a wound healed with Meek micrografts, but is better than that of a wound healed with the other island grafts. Unlike island grafts, which are independent of one another, failure of a portion of a sheet graft, either split- or full-thickness, may result in loss of the entire graft. Harvesting a split-thickness graft is far less convenient and more expensive than harvesting a full-thickness graft or island grafts, because the horse must be anesthetized.

Aftercare

Aftercare of the Recipient Site

The grafted wound is covered with a sterile, non-adherent dressing such as rayon polyethylene dressing (Release, Johnson and Johnson Products Inc., New Brunswick, NJ), cotton non-adherent film dressing (Telfa Sterile Pads, Covidien Animal Health/Kendall, Dublin, OH), or petrolatum-impregnated gauze dressing (Adaptic, Johnson and Johnson, Inc., New Brunswick, NJ), which is secured to the wound with conforming rolled gauze. If the grafted wound is located in a region that is hard to immobilize, such as the dorsal or palmar/plantar aspect of the fetlock or hock, shearing forces between the dressing and the graft can be decreased by securing the primary dressing to the wound with staples or with elastic adhesive tape instead of rolled gauze.[38]

The secondary layer of the bandage should be absorbent to wick bacteria and destructive enzymes away from the wound and bulky to limit motion of the limb. If the grafted wound is located in a highly mobile region, a cast can be applied to completely immobilize the distal portion of the limb and thus eliminate shear forces acting between the bandage and the graft. If casting the limb is impractical, a splint or Robert Jones bandage may suffice. Grafted wounds over the dorsal aspect of the hock can be effectively immobilized by applying a bandage cast splint. (See Chapter 15 for information on how to make the cast splint.)[56] A grafted wound in a less mobile region, such as the dorsal surface of the metacarpus or metatarsus, is usually sufficiently immobilized with a simple bandage.

The bandage should not be changed for 4 to 5 days after grafting to avoid disturbing the fragile vascular and fibrinous attachments of the graft to the wound. A cast can be left in place for approximately 10 days. When infection with virulent bacteria such as *Streptococcus* and *Pseudomonas* spp. is a common problem in the hospital, the bandage should be changed sooner and frequently following grafting. Changing the bandage allows application of an appropriate antimicrobial drug to the wound and removes bacteria and destructive enzymes.

Streptococci or pseudomonads can rapidly destroy a graft, and so prompt recognition of infection, coupled with topical application of an antimicrobial drug likely to be effective in resolving the infection, is necessary. Exudate from a grafted wound that appears infected should be cultured for bacterial growth and antimicrobial susceptibility of isolates should be determined. While awaiting results, a broad-spectrum antimicrobial agent such as ticarcillin with potassium clavulanate (Timentin, GlaxcoSmithKline, Research Triangle Park, NC), effective against both β-hemolytic *Streptococcus* and *Pseudomonas* spp., should be applied topically to the wound.[48] If the affected limb has been immobilized in a cast, and if the wound is at high risk of developing a streptococcal or pseudomonas infection, a broad-spectrum antimicrobial drug should be applied to the wound at regular intervals through an infusion tube placed on the surface of the grafted wound and exited through the top of the cast. By 5 days after grafting, fibrous and vascular attachments between the graft and the wound are secure enough that loss of graft from infection or motion becomes unlikely.

Great care should be taken during initial bandage changes to avoid disturbing the delicate fibrinous and vascular connections between the wound and the graft. Removing the primary dressing may be difficult if it adheres to the wound via fibrin. Tight adherence of the dressing to the wound indicates that the graft is also tightly adhered and that graft acceptance is proceeding unhindered by infection or motion. Saturating the primary dressing with physiological saline solution may ease removal of the dressing, but if this proves difficult, the dressing should be left in place until the next scheduled bandage change. The dressing can most easily be removed by grasping one end and pulling it parallel to the wound. Pulling the dressing perpendicular to the wound tends to place excessive traction on the graft.

Exuberant granulation tissue sometimes proliferates through the fenestrations of an expanded meshed graft or in between island grafts, obscuring the grafts and retarding migration of epithelium. A corticosteroid applied to the grafted wound causes the exuberant granulation tissue to regress, allowing epithelialization to proceed unhindered. Although a corticosteroid may reduce the rate of epithelialization, exuberant granulation tissue exerts even more detrimental effects on this process.[9,76–78]

Ideally, a grafted wound should be protected by a bandage until it is completely epithelialized because bandaging produces conditions conducive to epithelialization. If bandaging becomes impractical prior to complete epithelial coverage, however, small, non-epithelialized areas within the grafted wound can be allowed to heal beneath a scab, which soon develops when the wound is left exposed.

A grafted wound in a region difficult to bandage, such as the trunk, can be protected with a tie-over, or stent, bandage.[2,9,55] Movement of the wound does not create shear forces between the wound and the tie-over bandage because the latter is attached to the wound. To apply a tie-over bandage, a pile of gauze, placed over a non-adherent dressing, is positioned next to the wound and secured with the long ends of interrupted sutures inserted at regular intervals around the wound margin. A bandage applied to the grafted wound provides pressure, which prevents fluid from accumulating beneath the graft and also protects the graft from the environment, but pressure on a graft is not indispensable for graft acceptance. A grafted wound located in a region that is difficult to bandage, such as the back, or a grafted wound at risk of developing infection can be left unbandaged, a practice referred to as "open grafting."[10,21] Leaving the wound uncovered eliminates shear forces that occur between a bandage and the graft and prevents accumulation of exudate, which can cause the graft to macerate. If a grafted wound is left uncovered, precautions such as applying a neck cradle or tying the horse must be taken to prevent the horse from disturbing the exposed graft.

Because some horses suffer from hyperesthesia at the grafted wound, tying a horse or applying a neck cradle may be prudent when bandaging is discontinued, to prevent the horse from damaging its grafted wound. Applying an ointment such as lanolin or petroleum jelly to the healed donor and recipient sites of a split-thickness graft may reduce scaling, which results from dysfunction of eccrine glands at these sites, and prevents the occurrence of small splits in epithelium.[3]

Aftercare of the Donor Site

The donor site of a split-thickness graft is similar to a deep abrasion and contains many exposed nerve fibers. To relieve pain, an analgesic drug such as phenylbutazone should be administered before the graft is harvested and for several days following surgery.

A scab of blood and fibrin, often containing bedding material, rapidly forms over the donor site of a split-thickness graft. Beneath this scab, proliferating epithelial cells from the margin of the wound and the remaining adnexa migrate to cover the surface of the site. A horse whose donor site is at the ventrolateral surface of the thorax may show signs of discomfort, such as a stilted gait, until the wound is covered with a scab. The scab that develops at the donor site of a split-thickness graft should not be removed, despite its contaminated appearance (Figure 11.28), because this interferes with epithelialization and is painful to the horse.

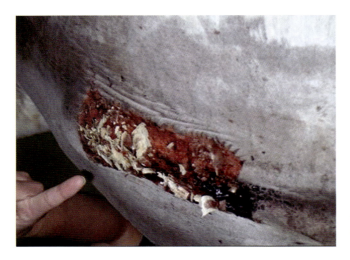

Figure 11.28. A scab at the donor site of a split-thickness graft is contaminated with bedding material. Removing the scab interferes with epithelialization and is painful.

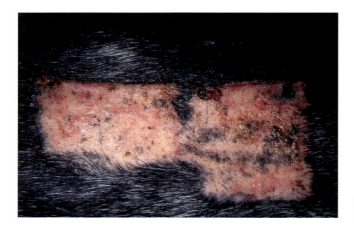

Figure 11.29. Harvesting a split-thickness graft leaves an unsightly scar at the donor site.

Gauze applied to the donor site immediately after harvesting adheres to the wound by fibrin and may provide some relief from discomfort. The dressing, which soon becomes dry and hard, spontaneously separates from the wound 1 to 2 weeks later. A stored skin graft from another horse can also be used to cover the donor site and, if temporarily accepted, might provide better analgesia.

The donor site is covered by pink epithelium, usually within 1 to 3 weeks, but the time required for complete epithelialization depends on the depth at which the graft was harvested. Epithelium covers the donor site more quickly when a thin skin graft is harvested because the most superficial layers of the dermis contain the greatest quantity of adnexa.[11,17] Pigment soon appears in the new, pink epithelium, blackening the epithelial scar. The donor site heals with prominent epithelial scarring when split-thickness grafts between 0.63 mm and 0.76 mm thick are harvested (Figure 11.29).[1,17]

To speed healing of the donor site and to decrease scarring, one author (Schumacher) has sutured the partial-thickness donor site of 76 mm wide, split-thickness grafts harvested from the ventrolateral surface of the thorax. Although the sutured, partial-thickness donor site heals rapidly, narrow epithelial scars associated with the suture tracts develop in response to the tremendous tension required to close the wound and result in a blemish no less unsightly than the large epithelial scar of an unsutured donor site (Figure 11.30).

One author (Wilmink) always excises the 42 mm wide partial-thickness wound created by harvesting with a Humeca dermatome (Figure 11.31). To close the resulting full-thickness wound, the adjacent skin must be undermined (Figure 11.32). Relief incisions, or occasionally an H plasty, may be required to close wider wounds.

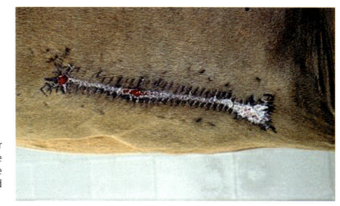

Figure 11.30. Suturing the partial-thickness wound at the donor site on the ventrolateral surface of the thorax decreases the width of the scar. The epithelial scars that develop along the suture tracts compromise the appearance of the healed wound.

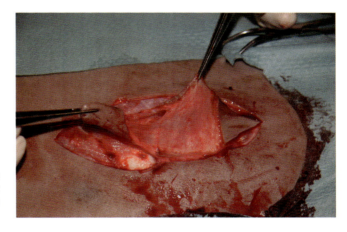

Figure 11.31. Excising the remaining part of the dermis creates a full-thickness wound at the donor site. The wound created at the donor site with a 42 mm wide Humeca dermatome can usually be closed primarily.

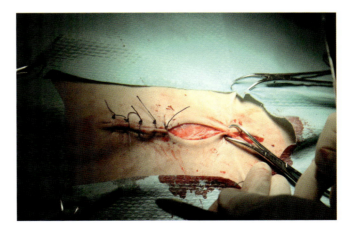

Figure 11.32. After undermining the wound margins, the donor site is sutured.

The full-thickness wound usually heals by primary intention when sutured (Figure 11.33), but even if it is left open or dehisces, the resulting scar is smaller than that which would develop were the partial thickness wound (abrasion) not excised. This is because the full-thickness wound heals primarily by contraction, thus minimizing the area that heals by epithelialization. Moreover, removing the abrasion relieves pain at the donor site. Therefore, excising the deep abrasion at the donor site to create a full-thickness wound after harvesting a split-thickness graft is an effective method to reduce scarring at the donor site and to relieve pain.

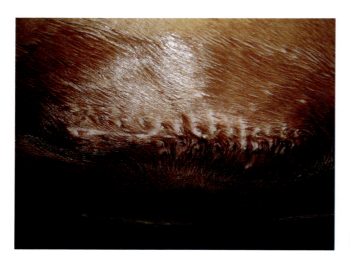

Figure 11.33. Appearance of the healed donor site after excising the abrasion and suturing the full-thickness wound.

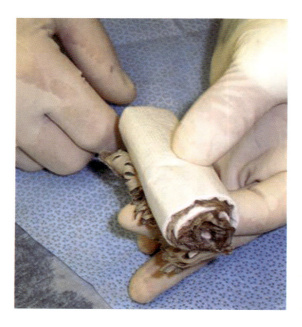

Figure 11.34. To prepare a skin graft for storage, the graft is placed on a sterile dressing with the epidermis next to the dressing, and the dressing-graft composite is rolled up.

Storing Split-Thickness Sheet Grafts

Autografts and allografts can be used successfully after being stored in a refrigerator in gauze swabs that have been soaked in either physiological saline or lactated Ringer's solution.[3,13,21] Skin can be stored in a refrigerator for even longer when placed in a tissue culture medium, such as McCoy's 5A medium, to which a small volume of serum has been added.[79–82] McCoy's 5A medium is a balanced electrolyte solution containing amino acids, vitamins, dextrose, and a pH indicator (phenol red). The concentration of serum in the storage medium should be between 10% and 33%.[83] A concentration of serum greater than 33% decreases the storage life of the graft by stimulating its metabolic activity. Antigenic reaction of the serum to the graft is prevented by using pooled, homologous serum, the horse's own serum, or a commercially available, antibody-free, equine serum.[81] When using pooled, homologous serum or the horse's own serum, however, the medium must be agitated periodically to prevent it from coagulating.

To prepare a skin graft for storage, it is placed epidermis side down on a sterile gauze dressing. The gauze-graft composite is rolled up, with the gauze facing out (Figure 11.34), and placed in a sterile container with approximately 1 mL to 2.5 mL of the McCoy's 5A medium for each square centimeter of stored graft.[81,83] The stored graft should have access to air.[82] The nutrient medium should be examined every few days for a color shift produced by a change in pH. A change in color from cherry-red to orange-yellow indicates that metabolites have accumulated to a dangerous concentration, necessitating immediate use of the graft or replacement of the medium. Only half of the storage medium should be replaced because complete replacement may be detrimental to the graft.[81]

Skin from humans has been stored successfully in a nutrient medium at refrigeration temperature for 6 to 8 weeks.[81,82] Wounds of horses have been grafted successfully using autografts stored for 3 weeks at 4°C, in a solution composed of McCoy's 5A medium and horse serum, with consistently good results.[79] One author (Schumacher) has successfully applied allografts stored in this manner for 8 to 12 weeks to wounds of horses. Skin has been preserved in raw honey, at 4°C or room temperature, for up to 12 weeks.[84] An equine skin graft stored in honey by Schumacher appeared histologically healthier at 3 weeks than a graft obtained from the same horse at the same time and stored in McCoy's 5A medium and serum.

Harvesting more skin than is necessary to cover a wound is sometimes beneficial because the surplus can be stored to cover defects created by a slough in the primary graft. A skin graft obtained at the same time a wound is created, such as when a cutaneous neoplasm is excised, can be stored for delayed grafting of that wound if excision is accompanied by excessive hemorrhage. Delayed graft application decreases the likelihood of hematoma or seroma formation beneath the graft. A graft harvested when a horse is anesthetized for treatment of a wound, such as removal of an osseous sequestrum or lavage of an open joint, can be stored until the wound's condition has improved enough to permit grafting.

A stored graft is more readily accepted than a fresh one because those stored for 24 hours or more undergo anaerobic metabolism, which causes release of metabolites that encourage rapid vascularization of the graft.[85] A graft that has been stored for 24 hours or more is referred to as a "prepared graft," and by placing it on a "prepared wound" (see Preparation of the Wound), the phase of plasmatic imbibition is decreased to less than 8 hours. A graft stored for autografting, if not used on the donor, can be used as a biological dressing for a wound on another horse (see Use of Allografts and Xenografts).

Use of Allografts and Xenografts

A cutaneous allograft (i.e., a skin graft harvested from one animal and transferred to a wound of another of the same species) or a cutaneous xenograft (i.e., a skin graft harvested from one animal and transferred to a wound of another of a different species) can be used to dress wounds of horses. Cutaneous allografts obtained from cadavers and xenografts obtained from pigs have been used extensively since the middle of the last century to temporarily dress large wounds on humans but have been used infrequently to dress wounds of horses.[5,6,86,87] The use of cutaneous allografts to dress wounds of horses has only recently been reported.[7] Viable, cutaneous allografts can be harvested from refrigerated cadavers within 24 hours after death.[82] An allograft seems to survive for at least 2 weeks after being applied to a wound on a horse. The duration of survival is often difficult to determine, however, because even when the superficial layers of the graft seem desiccated, the deeper layers may still remain viable and firmly attached to the wound by fibrous and vascular connections.[7]

A wound can be temporarily dressed with a cutaneous allograft or xenograft when autografting is economically or physically impractical. A cutaneous allograft or xenograft applied to a wound on a human or horse stimulates angiogenesis and allows epithelialization to proceed rapidly beneath it, unimpeded by complications such as infection and the formation of exuberant granulation tissue.[5-7,10,82,86,88] A cutaneous allograft or xenograft vascularizes before it is rejected, which further enhances its ability to defend the wound against infection.[4] Even a graft that is rejected before it can vascularize may protect the wound from bacterial infection, possibly by trapping bacteria in the fibrin that attaches the graft to the underlying wound.[5,6,11,20,40,89] An allograft or xenograft can be used to test the preparedness of a wound for grafting. A wound capable of accepting an allograft or xenograft is healthy enough to accept an autograft.

The use of cutaneous porcine xenografts as substitutes for allografts to dress wounds of humans arose because of the short supply of cadaveric allografts. Clinical comparisons between allografting and xenografting of wounds in humans have shown that cutaneous porcine xenografts adhere poorly, allow higher bacterial counts in the wound, and cause a more intense immunological rejection than do allografts.[4] A study examining the use of allografts to dress small experimental limb wounds of horses showed no apparent advantages over non-biological dressings in promoting healing.[7] When used clinically to cover large wounds of horses, however, the allograft appears to prevent formation of excessive granulation tissue and infection. Additionally, allografted wounds require far fewer bandage changes than do wounds covered with a non-biological dressing.

Conclusion

Skin grafting should not be regarded as an option of last resort. It should be considered for any open wound that cannot be closed primarily, especially if the wound is in an area where healing by second intention is likely to be prolonged or result in a large epithelial scar, such as a wound on the distal limb. Although skin grafting may seem like an expensive method of therapy, a horse with a large wound can often be treated more economically by grafting than by a lengthy period of bandaging, and the horse can be returned more quickly to function. Sophisticated grafting instruments manufactured for use in humans, such as power and meshgraft dermatomes, are relatively expensive, but frequent use of these instruments may warrant their purchase. Moreover, only a moderate amount of expertise is required to use these instruments. Full-thickness grafting and most types of island grafting require only common, basic surgical equipment.

Small limb wounds can be easily grafted with pinch, punch, or tunnel grafts to speed healing when the cosmetic result is not important. The use of full-thickness grafts can be considered for small wounds when the cosmetic result is important. Large limb wounds can be best grafted with split-thickness, meshed sheet grafts or Meek micrografts. Meek micrografts are well accepted, reduce healing time, and improve the cosmetic appearance of the healed wound compared to the other types of island grafts. Full-thickness grafts are less suitable for large limb wounds because they have a greater chance of being rejected and because large, full-thickness grafts are less available. Grafting a wound on the trunk is necessary only when the wound is so large that wound contraction alone is insufficient for healing, resulting in a large area that must heal by epithelialization, or when the wound is in an area such as the back where the durability of healed tissue is important. Grafting these large wounds with pinch or punch grafts is often too tedious; therefore, application of a split-thickness meshed sheet graft or Meek micrograft may be a better option. Fixation is usually a problem for wounds on the trunk, and thus micrografts may be more suitable because they are less vulnerable to movement.

A split-thickness graft cannot easily be harvested when the horse is not anesthetized. Therefore, when a horse cannot be anesthetized, pinch, punch, tunnel, or full-thickness grafts are the only options. The selection of the type of graft also depends on the availability of equipment and the expertise of the surgeon.

References

1. Booth LC: Split-thickness autogenous skin transplantation in the horse. J Am Vet Med Assoc 1982;180:754
2. Wilson DG: Applications of skin grafting in large animals. Probl Vet Med 1990;2:442
3. Bell R: *The use of skin grafts*. New York: Oxford University Press, 1973, p. 6
4. May S: The effects of biological wound dressings on the healing process. Clin Materials 1991;8:243
5. Diehl M, Ersek RA: Porcine xenografts for treatment of skin defects in horses. J Am Vet Med Assoc 1980;177:625
6. Diehl M, Jeanmonod CA, Muller M, et al: Porcine skin as temporary covering of extensive skin defects in the horse. Schweizer Archiv fur Tierheilkunde 1979;121:23
7. Gomez JH, Schumacher J, Swaim S, et al: Effects of three biological dressings on healing of cutaneous wounds on the limbs of horses. Can J Vet Res 2004;68:49
8. Boyd CL: Equine skin autotransplants for wound healing. J Am Vet Med Assoc 1967;151:1618
9. Meagher DM, Adams OR: Split-thickness autologous skin transplantation in horses. J Am Vet Med Assoc 1971;159:55
10. Peacock E: *Wound repair (3rd edition)*. Philadelphia: WB Saunders, 1984, p. 187
11. Argenta LC, Dingman RO: Skin grafting. In E. Epstein, ed. *Skin surgery*. Philadelphia: WB Saunders, 1987, p. 129
12. Flowers RS: Unexpected postoperative problems in skin grafting. Surg Clin North Am 1970;50:439
13. Rothstein AS: Skin grafting techniques. J Am Podiatry Assoc 1983;73:79
14. Rudolph R, Fisher JC, Ninnemann JL: *Skin grafting*. Boston: Little, Brown and Co, 1979, p. 137
15. Gringrass PJ, Grabb WC, Gringrass RP: Skin graft survival on avascular defects. Plast Reconstr Surg 1975;55:65
16. Hogle RB, Kingrey W, Jensen EC: Skin grafting in the horse. J Am Vet Med Assoc 1959;135:165
17. Frankland AL: Autologous, split skin transplantation on the lower limbs of horses. Vet Rec 1979;104:590
18. Tavis MJ, Thornton JW, Harney JH, et al: Mechanism of skin graft adherence: collagen, elastin, and fibrin interactions. Surg Forum 1977;28:522
19. Mir Y, Mir L: Biology of the skin graft. Plast Reconstr Surg 1951;8:378
20. Teh B: Why do skin grafts fail? Plast Reconstr Surg 1979;63:323

21. Vistnes LM: Grafting of skin. Surg Clin North Am 1977;57:939
22. Converse JM, Smahel J, Ballantyne DL Jr, et al: Inosculation of vessels of skin graft and host bed: a fortuitous encounter. Br J Plast Surg 1975;28:274
23. O'Ceallaigh S, Herrick SE, Bluff JE, et al: Quantification of total and perfused blood vessels in murine skin autografts using a fluorescent double-labeling technique. Plast Reconstr Surg 2006;117:140
24. Hanselka DV: Use of autogenous meshgrafts in equine wound management. J Am Vet Med Assoc 1974;164:35
25. Wilmink JM, Van Den Boom R, Van Weeren PR, et al: The modified Meek technique as a novel method for skin grafting in horses: evaluation of acceptance, wound contraction and closure in chronic wounds. Equine Vet J 2006;38:324
26. Fitzgerald MJ, Martin F, Paletta FX: Innervation of skin grafts. Surg Gynecol Obstet 1967;124:808
27. Kernwein G: Recovery of sensation in split-thickness skin grafts. Arch Surg 1948;56:459
28. Rudolph R: Inhibition of myofibroblasts by skin grafts. Plast Reconstr Surg 1979;63:473
29. Corps BVM: The effect of graft thickness, donor site and graft bed on graft shrinkage in the hooded rat. Br J Plast Surg 1969;22:125
30. Hanson RR: Management of avulsion wounds with exposed bone. Clin Tech Eq Pract 2004;3:188
31. Ford TS, Schumacher J, Brumbaugh GW, et al: Effects of split-thickness and full-thickness skin grafts on secondary graft contraction in horses. Am J Vet Res 1992;53:1572
32. Wilmink JM, van Weeren PR: Treatment of exuberant granulation tissue. Clin Tech Eq Pract 2004;3:141
33. Grinnell F: Fibroblast biology in three-dimensional collagen matrices. Trends Cell Biol 2003;13:264
34. Bristol DG: Skin grafts and skin flaps in the horse. Vet Clin North Am Equine Pract 2005;21:125
35. French DA, Fretz PB: Treatment of equine leg wounds using skin grafts: thirty-five cases, 1975–1988. Can Vet J 1990;31:761
36. Krizek TJ, Robeson MC, Kho E: Bacterial growth and skin graft survival. Surg Forum 1967;18:518
37. Robson M, Krizek TJ: Predicting skin graft survival. J Trauma 1973;13:213
38. Booth L: Equine wound reconstruction using free skin grafting. Calif Vet 1991;45:13
39. Cason J: Skin grafting and diagnosis of depth of burn. In J. Cason, ed. *Treatment of burns*. London: Chapman and Hall, 1981, p. 135.
40. Eade GG: The relationship between granulation tissue, bacteria, and skin grafts in burned patients. Plast Reconstr Surg 1958;22:42
41. Currie LJ, Sharpe JR, Martin R: The use of fibrin glue in skin grafts and tissue-engineered skin replacements: a review. Plast Reconstr Surg 2001;108:1713
42. Wilmink JM, Stolk PWT, van Weeren PR, et al: Differences in second-intention wound healing between horses and ponies: macroscopic aspects. Equine Vet J 1999;31:53
43. Wilmink JM, van Weeren PR, Stolk PWT, et al: Differences in second-intention wound healing between horses and ponies: histological aspects. Equine Vet J 1999;31:61
44. Schumacher J, Ford TS, Brumbaugh GW, et al: Viability of split-thickness skin grafts attached with fibrin glue. Can J Vet Res 1996;60:158
45. Smahel J: Free skin transplantation on a prepared bed. Br J Plast Surg 1971;24:129
46. Boon RJ, Beale AS: Response of Streptococcus pyogenes to therapy with amoxicillin or amoxicillin-clavulanic acid in a mouse model of mixed infection caused by Staphylococcus aureus and Streptococcus pyogenes. Antimicrob Agents Chemother 1987;31:1204
47. James J: Skin grafting in difficult situations. Trop Doct 1999;29:41
48. Moore R: Antimicrobial therapy in horses. In P Colahan, AM Merritt, JN Moore, IG Mayhew, eds. *Equine medicine and surgery*. St. Louis: Mosby, 1999, p. 165
49. Robson MC, Edstom LE, Krizek TJ: The efficacy of systemic antibiotics in the treatment of granulating wounds. J Surg Res 1974;16:299
50. Edlich RF, Schmolka IR, Prusak MP, et al: The molecular basis for toxicity of surfactants in surgical wounds. J Surg Res 1973;14:277
51. Mackay-Smith MP, Marks D: A skin grafting technique for horses. J Am Vet Med Assoc 1968;152:1633
52. Davis JS: The use of small deep skin grafts. J Am Med Assoc 1914;63:985
53. Oien RF, Hansen BU, Hakansson A: Pinch graft skin transplantation for leg ulcers in primary care. J Wound Care 2000;9:217
54. Boyd CL, Hanselka DV: A skin punch technique for equine skin grafting. J Am Vet Med Assoc 1971;158:82
55. Lindsay WA: Step-by-step instructions for equine skin grafting techniques. Vet Med 1988;83:598
56. Stashak TS: *Equine wound management*. Philadelphia: Lea and Febiger, 1991, p. 271
57. Stashak TS: Skin grafting in horses. Vet Clin North Am Large Anim Pract 1984;6:215
58. Davis JS, Trout HF: Origin and development of the blood supply of whole thickness skin grafts: an experimental study. Ann Surg 1925;82:871
59. Ross GE, Jr: Clinical canine skin grafting. J Am Vet Med Assoc 1968;153:1759
60. Bjorck GTK, Twisselman K: Tunnel skin grafting in the equine species. Proc Am Assoc Equine Pract 1971;17:313

61. Lees MJ, Andrews GC, Bailey JV, et al: Tunnel grafting of equine wounds. Comp Cont Educ Pract Vet 1989;11:962
62. Kreis RW, Mackie DP, Vloemans AWFP, et al: Expansion technique for skin grafts: comparison between mesh and Meek island (Sandwich) grafts. Burns 1994;20:539
63. Zermani RGC, Zarabini A, Trivisonno A: Micrografting in the treatment of severely burned patients. Burns 1997;23:604
64. Hanselka DV, Boyd CL: Use of mesh grafts in dogs and horses. J Am Anim Hosp Assoc 1976;12:650
65. Valencia IC, Falabella AF, Eaglstein WH: Skin grafting. Dermatol Clin 2000;18:521
66. Hanselka DV, Milne FJ: Inexpensive mesh grafting technique in the horse. Proc Am Assoc Equine Pract 1975;21:191
67. Kogan L, Govrin-Yehudain J: Vertical (two-layer) skin grafting: new reserves for autologic skin. Ann Plast Surg 2003;50:514
68. MacMillan BG: The use of mesh grafting in treating burns. Surg Clin North Am 1970;50:1347
69. Tobin GR: The compromised bed technique. An improved method for skin grafting problem wounds. Surg Clin North Am 1984;64:653
70. Frankland AL, Morris PGD, Spreull JSA: Free, autologous, skin transplantation in the horse. Vet Rec 1976;98:105
71. Bowersox JC, Strauss MB, Hart GB: Clinical experience with hyperbaric oxygen therapy in the salvage of ischemic skin flaps and grafts. J Hyperbaric Med 1986;1:141
72. McFarland RM, Wermuth RE: The use of hyperbaric oxygen to prevent necrosis in experimental pedicle flaps and composite skin grafts. Plast Reconstr Surg 1966;37:422
73. Perrins DJD: Influence of hyperbaric oxygen on the survival of split skin grafts. Lancet 1967;1:868
74. Kalns JE, Dick EJ, Jr, Scruggs JP, et al: Hyperbaric oxygen treatment prevents up-regulation of angiogenesis following partial-thickness skin grafts in the pig. Wound Repair Regen 2003;11:139
75. Holder TE, Schumacher J, Donnell RL, et al: Effects of hyperbaric oxygen on full-thickness meshed sheet skin grafts applied to fresh and granulating wounds in horses. Am J Vet Res 2008;69:144
76. Baker BL, Whitaker WL: Interference with wound healing by the local action of adrenocorticoid steroids. Endocrinol 1950;46:544
77. Ehrlich HP, Hunt TK: The effects of cortisone and anabolic steroids on the tensile strength of healing wounds. Ann Surg 1969;170:203
78. Howes EL, Plotz CM, Blunt JW, et al: Retardation of wound healing by cortisone. Surg 1950;28:177
79. Schumacher J, Chambers M, Hanselka DV, et al: Preservation of skin by refrigeration for autogenous grafting in the horse. Vet Surg 1987;16:358
80. Hurst LN, Brown DH, Murray KA: Prolonged life and improved quality for stored skin grafts. Plast Reconstr Surg 1984;73:105
81. Gresham RB, Perry VP, Thompson VK: Practical methods of short-term storage of homografts. Arch Surg 1963;87:417
82. Brown JB, Fryer MP, Zaydon TJ: A skin bank for postmortem homografts. Surg Gynecol Obstet 1955;101:401
83. Allgower M, Blocker TGJ: Viability of skin in relation to various methods of storage. Texas Rep Bio Med J 1952;10:3
84. Gupta M: Preservation of split-skin grafts in honey: A preliminary report. Indian J Surg 1977;39:591
85. Smahel J: Preparation-phenomenon in a free skin graft. Br J Plast Surg 1971;24:133
86. Ambler J: Porcine xenografts to facilitate integumental wound healing. Vet Rec 1980;106:37
87. Marden DT: Use of pigskin to repair leg wounds in the horse. Vet Med Small Anim Clin 1974;69:771
88. O'Donoghue MN, Zarem HA: Stimulation of neovascularization—comparative efficacy of fresh and preserved skin grafts. Plast Reconstr Surg 1971;48:474
89. Burleson MD, Eiseman B: Mechanism of antibacterial effect of biological dressings. Ann Surg 1973;177:181

12 Management of Severely Infected Wounds

James A. Orsini, DVM, Diplomate ACVS; **Yvonne A. Elce**, DVM, Diplomate ACVS; **Beth Kraus**, DVM, Diplomate ACVS

Introduction

Wound management in equine patients can be very challenging. Bacterial infection of traumatic wounds or surgical incisions compromises healing and further complicates wound management. This chapter focuses on recent advances in the management of severely infected wounds, with particular attention paid to selection of antibiotic agents and methods for optimizing the delivery and efficacy of antibiotic drugs at the site of infection.

Bacterial infection of a wound generally is obvious clinically, because it comprises two readily identifiable elements:

- Swelling, heat, redness, and/or pain that is excessive for the type, size, or age of the wound
- Purulent exudate from or within the wound (other than exudate that may be found on the surface of the granulation bed)

Note: Purulent exudate may not be evident initially in patients with abscessation or deep infection of a surgical wound that was closed primarily.

Empiric antibiotic therapy is sufficient to resolve the infection in many cases. However, it may be inadequate in wounds infected with organisms that are not susceptible to the chosen antibiotic(s); patients with a compromised immune system; and tissues in which delivery and/or efficacy of the antibiotic at the site of infection is compromised by poor blood supply, local conditions (e.g., low pH, inflammatory debris), or the presence of sequestered bacteria associated with devitalized tissue, surgical implants, or a foreign body.

For our purposes, a wound infection is considered to be severe when it meets one or more of the following criteria:

- Any infection involving bone, a synovial structure (joint, tendon sheath, bursa), or a body cavity
- Any infection involving a surgical implant (metal plates, screws, pins, wires; surgical mesh; embedded suture material; etc.)
- Evidence of a systemic inflammatory response (e.g., malaise, fever, neutrophilia or neutropenia, hyperfibrinogenemia)
- Presence of Gram-negative bacteria on cytology or bacterial culture of the wound

Delayed wound healing and dehiscence of sutured wounds are other common features of severely infected wounds. By the same token, wounds that are slow to heal because of a compromised blood supply or defective immune function carry an increased risk for severe bacterial infection.

Initial Assessment

Initial assessment should include a review of the patient's medical history and a complete physical examination. The cause of the wound (e.g., traumatic or surgical) and the presence of surgical implants or the possibility of a non-surgical foreign body in the wound are important considerations that may influence wound management. Tetanus vaccination history should also be reviewed if the horse is being examined by a veterinarian for the first time.

The systemic status of the patient must be determined, both to direct immediate medical care and to identify any conditions that may compromise immune function or affect wound healing (e.g., severe hypoproteinemia, malnutrition, advanced pregnancy, concurrent systemic disease). A complete blood count and serum biochemistry profile are warranted during initial assessment and are used to monitor the response to treatment if abnormalities are found.

Involvement of musculoskeletal structures (especially a synovial structure, tendon, ligament, or bone) and other body systems should also be considered during initial assessment. For example, penetrating injuries to the body wall can lead to septic peritonitis or pleuritis and may even involve internal organs (bowel, lung, etc.). Similarly, traumatic wounds to the head may involve the paranasal sinuses, nasal cavity, orbit, and even the central nervous system. Traumatic neck wounds must be carefully evaluated to determine whether penetration of the pharynx, larynx, trachea, or esophagus has occurred.

Wound Evaluation

The severity and extent of the wound infection are determined by physical examination and, when necessary, radiography, contrast fistulography, and/or ultrasonography. Sterile gloves should be worn if the wound is digitally examined to avoid further wound contamination and to protect the clinician from exposure to potential human pathogens. (Note: Rinse the talc from the outer surface of the gloves before examining the wound digitally.)

Bacterial Culture and Cytology

In all cases of severe wound infection, assessment must include aseptic collection of tissue, synovial fluid, and/or exudate from the depths of the wound (i.e., from the primary site of infection) for bacterial culture and antibiotic sensitivity testing and for cytologic examination. This step should be performed before antibiotic therapy is initiated or, if the horse is already receiving antibiotics, before the regimen is changed. In the latter instance, it is best to discontinue antibiotic administration for 24–36 hours before sample collection, depending on the dosing interval being used (e.g. discontinue for 36 hours for antibiotics administered every 24 hours); otherwise the culture results may not reflect the true nature of the infection. When indicated, surgical implants (e.g., loose metal fixation devices, suture material) and other foreign objects at the site of infection should also be submitted.

These samples are sent to the laboratory in appropriate shipping containers and media for aerobic and anaerobic bacterial culture and antibiotic sensitivity testing and for cytologic examination. Synovial fluid samples should be placed into blood culture media (e.g., BBL Septi-Chek, Becton-Dickinson Co., Cockeysville,

MD). This step increases the probability of isolating the causal bacteria in cases of septic arthritis;[1] however, it delays results by another 24 hours. Anaerobes should be considered a distinct possibility when culture results are negative and in patients with osteomyelitis, abscess formation, or draining tracts.[2] Because time usually is of the essence, cytologic examination should also be performed in-house whenever possible.

It must be emphasized that samples for cytology and culture be collected from the primary site of infection. Exudate at the wound surface or from a draining tract frequently is contaminated with normal skin flora or environmental contaminants, and may not reflect the pathogen(s) primarily responsible for the wound infection. One should avoid contact with the skin and wound edges (if possible) when collecting specimens for bacterial culture and cytology. In some cases it may even be advisable to collect microbiologic samples via aseptic percutaneous aspiration from a site well away from the wound margins or by surgical biopsy.[2]

General Treatment Approach

The optimal treatment approach for a particular patient depends on the physical examination findings, wound type and location, and any treatment undertaken thus far. For patients with severely infected wounds, the general approach is as follows:

1. Stabilize the patient, if necessary, and address any factors that might affect resolution of the infection or delay wound healing; ensure adequate nutrition and fluid balance.
2. Administer tetanus prophylaxis (tetanus toxoid or antitoxin, depending on vaccination history) if the horse's tetanus vaccination status is questionable or unknown.
3. Start or continue systemic parenteral antibiotic therapy; while awaiting culture and sensitivity results, use broad-spectrum coverage that targets the most likely pathogens (see Antibiotic Selection).
4. Thoroughly debride the wound to improve the blood supply and reduce bacterial load; use local, regional, or general anesthesia as necessary; remove any devitalized tissue, foreign material, and nonessential surgical implants. (Note: If tissue samples or surgical implants are to be submitted for bacterial culture, they should be aseptically collected before beginning or changing antibiotic therapy.)
5. Copiously lavage the wound with sterile isotonic crystalloid fluids (e.g., physiologic saline, lactated Ringer's solution), using moderate delivery pressure (ideally, 13–15 PSI). Using a mildly alkaline solution as a buffer may enhance treatment efficacy, because the acidic environment of an infected wound can impede host defense mechanisms, inhibit the activity of certain antibiotics, and delay wound healing by interfering with cell proliferation and migration. Lavage with dilute antiseptic solution (e.g., 0.1%–0.2% povidone-iodine or 0.05% chlorhexidine) reduces the numbers of surface bacteria and can be performed following wound debridement. Antiseptics should not be used to lavage synovial structures, however. Antibiotics can be added to the final flush for synovial structures, body cavities, or wounds with extensive dead space. Chelating agents such as Tricide®, developed as antibiotic potentiators, can also be used at this point. (Tricide® is discussed later in this chapter).
6. Establish or allow continued dependent (ventral or distal) drainage from the wound as appropriate (e.g., leave part or all of the wound open or place a surgical drain that exits through the skin); consider use of vacuum-assisted closure (discussed later).
7. Start or continue basic wound care (e.g., wound dressing with a bandage or stent, frequent wound cleansing, repeated lavage and debridement as necessary, fly control, limitation on the patient's activity); evaluate any human health risks and instruct caregivers accordingly.
8. Start or continue nonsteroidal anti-inflammatory therapy as needed.
9. Consider local or regional antibiotic therapy to enhance delivery or concentration of antibiotics at the site of infection (see Modes of Delivery).
10. Reassess the patient daily.

Optimizing Antibiotic Therapy

Antibiotic therapy is not necessarily indicated for every wound in the horse, but it certainly is a critical component of management for patients with severely infected wounds. In these cases, either bacterial invasion has already overwhelmed the body's defenses or the mere presence of an infectious process is likely to have severely debilitating or even life-threatening consequences.

Table 12.1. Factors that may be involved in the development and persistence or progression of wound infection.

Bacterial	Number of contaminating bacteria ($>10^5$/g of tissue); virulence of contaminating bacteria; resistance to antibiotics.
Host—local	Type of tissue(s) involved (i.e., tissue's inherent vascularity and metabolic rate); local perfusion; severity of inflammatory response (e.g., ischemia exacerbated by edema or thrombosis, accumulation of cellular debris); presence of devitalized tissue; presence of hematoma, seroma, blood, or fibrin clots; presence of fibrosis (scarring or abscessation).
Host—regional	Location of the wound (e.g., environmental contamination with wounds on the distal limb, edema in dependent areas, poor drainage from wounds on the dorsum); gravitational effect on lymphatic drainage from the limb.
Host—systemic	Immune status; hydration status; cardiovascular function; nutritional status; presence of concurrent disorders (e.g., endotoxemia, anemia, hypoproteinemia, metabolic disorders).
Wound	Size and character of the tissue defect (e.g., width, depth, amount of tissue destruction or loss, dead space); cause (e.g., sterile surgery, blunt-force trauma, third-degree burn); presence of debris or foreign material (including sutures, drains, and other surgical implants) in the wound.
Human	Improper wound care (e.g., delayed care, inadequate lavage and debridement, insufficient stabilization or wound protection); further contamination through improper handling or hygiene; inappropriate use of antibiotics, corticosteroids, other medications that may impede recovery.

It must be remembered, however, that the presence of bacteria in a wound is only one factor involved in the development and the persistence or progression of wound sepsis. Local, regional, and systemic host factors as well as bacterial, drug, and human factors all play important roles (Table 12.1). In an otherwise healthy horse, the immune system is well equipped to prevent or resolve bacterial colonization of its tissues and repair tissue damage. Thus, at the same time one is pondering which antibiotic(s) to choose for a particular patient, equal time should be given to considering why this patient has been unable to resolve the infection and heal the wound.

In many cases, antibiotics have already been given, either by the primary-care veterinarian or the horse's caretaker (owner, trainer, farm/barn manager). The success of antibiotic therapy in these patients generally hinges on the following:

- Selecting the most appropriate antibiotic(s) for the patient, based on culture and sensitivity results
- Delivering and maintaining therapeutic concentrations of the appropriate antibiotic(s) at the site of infection for as long as needed (dictated by the patient's response)
- Minimizing adverse local, systemic, and environmental effects of the antibiotic(s) through selection of appropriate drug(s), dosage, delivery, and duration, based on the individual patient's needs

Antibiotic Selection

It bears repeating that bacterial culture and antibiotic sensitivity testing are essential in the successful management of severely infected wounds. No more time must be wasted on "trial" therapy with empiric antibiotic selections, particularly if antibiotics have already been used in the initial treatment of the wound. It is appropriate, however, to start empiric broad-spectrum antibiotic therapy while awaiting culture and sensitivity results (i.e., interim therapy), provided that all samples for culture and cytology are collected first. As mentioned earlier, cytologic evaluation of a Gram-stained smear of wound exudate or tissue is valuable in guiding antibiotic selection. It can be performed on site for immediate results.

Another important reason for performing culture and sensitivity testing is that pathogens resistant to multiple commonly used antibiotics are increasingly being cultured from hospitalized horses. These pathogens include methicillin-resistant *Staphylococcus aureus* (MRSA),[3–5] methicillin-resistant *S. epidermidis* (MRSE),[6] penicillin-resistant *Actinobacillus* sp.,[7] and aminoglycoside-resistant *Escherichia coli*.[8–10] In addition to confounding wound management, these pathogens can have important zoonotic implications, because they also are human pathogens. Therefore, when it comes to selection of antibiotics for the management of severely infected wounds, it is best to adopt the tenet, "Never assume."

Empiric Choices for Interim Therapy

In most cases, broad-spectrum antibiotic therapy is the best approach for initial treatment while awaiting culture and sensitivity results. The combination of penicillin G and gentamicin has been the mainstay of broad-spectrum systemic antibiotic therapy in adult horses for many years. However, penicillin G may not be the most appropriate choice in some circumstances.

Several common equine pathogens produce enzymes (β-lactamases, including penicillinase) which inactivate penicillin G; they include many *Staphylococcus* sp., most Gram-negative enteric organisms, and many *Bacteroides* sp. (including *B. fragilis*).[11] In wounds in which these organisms are likely to be present, a penicillinase-resistant penicillin (e.g., oxacillin) or a cephalosporin (e.g., ceftiofur, cefazolin, cephalothin) should be used in place of penicillin G. Alternatively, a combination of a synthetic penicillin (e.g., ampicillin, amoxicillin) and a β-lactamase inhibitor (e.g., clavulanate, sulbactam) can be added.

Table 12.2 summarizes antibiotic sensitivity data for various Gram-positive and Gram-negative pathogens isolated from horses at one large veterinary hospital in the United States. This information must serve as *a guide only* and should not be relied upon to replace sensitivity data from your clinical microbiology laboratory. Sensitivity patterns vary among geographic areas, and are influenced by the extent of antibiotic use in a particular population. Specifically, pathogens isolated from hospitalized horses or those on farms where antibiotics are frequently used are more likely to show antibiotic resistance than are pathogens isolated from horses on premises on which antibiotic use is less common.[10,11] This variability in sensitivity patterns is another good reason for performing culture and sensitivity testing on all severely infected wounds. One must also bear in mind that in vitro sensitivity does not guarantee satisfactory in vivo results. Numerous patient, pathogen, and drug factors interplay to determine the clinical outcome.

The bacteria that predominate on normal equine skin are *Bacillus* sp., non-hemolytic *Staphylococcus* sp., and *Micrococcus* sp.[12,13] Organisms isolated less frequently or in lower numbers include *Corynebacterium* sp. (varies by geographic region), *Streptomyces* sp., non-hemolytic *Streptococcus* sp., and other non-enteric genera.[13] Environmental contamination, particularly with fecal matter, and human contact can alter the normal skin flora. These contaminants often play an important role in wound infection, both with wounds of traumatic origin and in postoperative wound infections. Knowing which pathogens are likely to be found in particular types of wounds is helpful in guiding the initial selection of antibiotics.

The following is a brief discussion of empiric antibiotic therapy for specific types of wounds, based on the tissue(s) involved (Tables 12.3 and 12.4). Included are some general guidelines on duration of treatment. However, these broad recommendations need to be balanced against the clinical response observed by the clinician and supportive laboratory data (e.g., white blood cell count, fibrinogen).

Cellulitis/Lymphangitis

The organisms most often implicated in cases of cellulitis or lymphangitis in horses are coagulase-positive *Staphylococcus* sp. Less often, β-hemolytic *Streptococcus* sp., coagulase-negative *Staphylococcus* sp., Gram-negative aerobic bacteria, and/or anaerobes are involved.[11] Because the more commonly implicated organisms often are resistant to penicillin, initial therapy should comprise a cephalosporin plus an aminoglycoside (amikacin or gentamicin); enrofloxacin alone is a reasonable alternative in adult horses. Oxacillin may also be appropriate for penicillin-resistant staphylococcal infections.[11]

Treatment duration is based on the organism(s) isolated. As a rule, staphylococcal infections are more insidious in onset and incite a more chronic inflammatory response, requiring treatment for weeks or even months in some cases. The decision to discontinue treatment should be based on the health of the soft tissues and a negative culture (where possible). In marked contrast, streptococcal infections are more susceptible to antibiotics, so treatment duration generally is shorter than for staphylococcal infections, averaging 10–14 days.

In a series of 44 cases of primary and secondary limb cellulitis the authors concluded that the soft tissue infection is a life-threatening condition and affects the hind limbs 75% of the time.[14] Patients that were febrile on admission and developed laminitis while hospitalized were statistically less likely to survive to discharge.

Synovial Structures

In infected wounds of traumatic origin that involve synovial structures (joint, tendon sheath, bursa), the most common pathogens are Gram-negative enteric organisms, anaerobes, *Staphylococcus* sp., and *Streptococcus*

Table 12.2. In vitro sensitivity of equine pathogens to various antibiotics.*

Organism	Antibiotic sensitivity Drug tested (percentage of susceptible isolates)
Gram-positive bacteria	
Enterococcus faecalis	Ampicillin (100%), amoxicillin/clavulanic acid (100%), chloramphenicol (90%), tetracycline (90%), erythromycin (40%).
Enterococcus faecium	Ampicillin (90%), amoxicillin/clavulanic acid (90%), chloramphenicol (80%), tetracycline (70%), erythromycin (10%).
Rhodococcus equi	Ceftiofur (100%), ceftizoxime (100%), gentamicin (100%), trimethoprim-sulfonamide (100%), rifampin (88%), amikacin (87%), chloramphenicol (63%), erythromycin (63%), cephalothin (39%), tetracycline (25%).
Staphylococcus aureus	Chloramphenicol (97%), amikacin (94%), enrofloxacin (94%), rifampin (94%), cephalothin (91%), amoxicillin/clavulanic acid (88%), erythromycin (76%), ceftiofur (69%), oxacillin (67%), trimethoprim-sulfonamide (55%), gentamicin (45%), ceftizoxime (36%), tetracycline (36%), penicillin G (30%).
Coagulase-negative *Staphylococcus* sp.	Amikacin (100%), amoxicillin/clavulanic acid (100%), cephalothin (97%), rifampin (97%), enrofloxacin (96%), chloramphenicol (94%), tetracycline (81%), ceftiofur (77%), oxacillin (77%), ceftizoxime (74%), gentamicin (74%), trimethoprim-sulfonamide (74%), erythromycin (61%), penicillin G (13%).
Streptococcus zooepidemicus	Amoxicillin/clavulanic acid (100%), ampicillin (100%), ceftiofur (100%), ceftizoxime (100%), cephalothin (100%), chloramphenicol (100%), erythromycin (100%), penicillin G (100%), trimethoprim-sulfonamide (100%), rifampin (71%), gentamicin (7%), amikacin (0%).
Gram-negative bacteria	
Actinobacillus sp. (*A. suis*-like, *A. equuli, A. ligniersii*)	Amikacin (100%), amoxicillin/clavulanic acid (100%), ceftiofur (100%), ceftizoxime (100%), cephalothin (100%), chloramphenicol (100%), gentamicin (100%), penicillin G (100%), ampicillin (89%–100%), trimethoprim-sulfonamide (86%–100%), tetracycline (86%–100%), trimethoprim-sulfonamide (86%–100%), erythromycin (0%–30%).
Escherichia coli	Amikacin (100%), enrofloxacin (100%), ceftizoxime (97%), ceftiofur (94%), ticarcillin (94%), amoxicillin/clavulanic acid (93%), chloramphenicol (91%), gentamicin (86%), cephalothin (73%), tetracycline (71%), ampicillin (68%), trimethoprim-sulfonamide (60%).
Klebsiella pneumoniae	Amikacin (100%), ceftiofur (100%), ceftizoxime (100%), enrofloxacin (100%), ticarcillin (87%), chloramphenicol (80%), amoxicillin/clavulanic acid (79%), gentamicin (67%), trimethoprim-sulfonamide (67%), cephalothin (66%), tetracycline (54%), ampicillin (14%).
Pasteurella sp.	Amikacin (100%), amoxicillin/clavulanic acid (100%), ampicillin (100%), cephalothin (100%), chloramphenicol (100%), gentamicin (100%), penicillin G (100%), tetracycline (100%), trimethoprim-sulfonamide (100%), ceftiofur (83%), ceftizoxime (83%), enrofloxacin (83%), erythromycin (33%).
Salmonella sp. (*S. agona, S. typhimurium, S.* sp.)	Amikacin (100%), amoxicillin/clavulanic acid (100%), ceftiofur (100%), ceftizoxime (100%), cephalothin (100%), enrofloxacin (100%), tetracycline (73%–92%), ticarcillin (54%–91%), gentamicin (49%–82%), trimethoprim-sulfonamide (15%–82%), ampicillin (0%–82%), chloramphenicol (0%–82%).
Serratia marcescens	Ceftizoxime (100%), enrofloxacin (100%), ceftiofur (75%), tetracycline (50%), amikacin (0%), amoxicillin/clavulanic acid (0%), cephalothin (0%), chloramphenicol (0%), gentamicin (0%), ticarcillin (0%), trimethoprim-sulfonamide (0%).

*Organisms isolated from horses presented for treatment at the University of California–Davis during 1998[22]

sp.[11,15] Infection with more than one organism (polymicrobial infection) is common in these wounds. In infected surgical wounds involving synovial structures, the most common pathogens are *Staphylococcus* sp., *Enterobacter* sp., and *Pseudomonas* sp.[11,15] Therefore, an appropriate choice for interim antibiotic therapy with either type of wound is a cephalosporin plus amikacin (or gentamicin). Enrofloxacin is again a reasonable alternative in adult horses.[11]

Table 12.3. Empiric antibiotic choices for interim treatment* of infected wounds, based on the tissue(s) involved. Recommended dosages are given in Table 12.4.

Tissue(s) involved	Empiric antibiotic options
Cellulitis/lymphangitis	Ceftiofur + gentamicin/amikacin; OR enrofloxacin (adult horses only).
Synovial structures (joint, tendon sheath, bursa)	Ceftiofur + gentamicin/amikacin; OR enrofloxacin (adult horses only).
Distal limb, foot	Penicillin/ceftiofur + gentamicin/amikacin + metronidazole.
Bone or physeal cartilage	As for synovial structures.
Respiratory tract (e.g., penetrating neck or chest wound)	Penicillin (penicillin G or ampicillin) + gentamicin + metronidazole; ceftiofur and amikacin can be substituted for penicillin and gentamicin, respectively.
Bowel (e.g., penetrating belly wounds, open drainage for septic peritonitis)	Penicillin (penicillin G or ampicillin) + gentamicin; ceftiofur and amikacin can be substituted for penicillin and gentamicin, respectively.
Internal abscess	Penicillin (penicillin G or ampicillin) ± rifampin.
Muscle	Penicillin (penicillin G or ampicillin) ± metronidazole (for *Clostridium* sp.).

*Interim treatment: antibiotic therapy instituted while awaiting bacterial culture and antibiotic sensitivity results
Note: Enrofloxacin and other fluoroquinolones are not recommended for use in foals.

Table 12.4. Recommended systemic dosages for antibiotics commonly used to treat severe wound infections in horses.[2,11]

Drug	Dosage	Comments
Penicillins		
Penicillin G:		Penicillins are time-dependent antibiotics, so maintenance of blood and tissue levels with recommended dosing intervals is important.
Crystalline (sodium or potassium) penicillin	10,000–40,000 IU/kg IV or IM, q 4–6 h	Activity is reduced with low tissue pH and purulent exudate (e.g., abscesses, tissue necrosis). Na- and K-penicillin are unstable in solution, so each dose must be reconstituted immediately before use.
Procaine penicillin	22,000 IU/kg IM, q 12–24 h	K-penicillin should be given slowly (over 30 minutes) when administered IV. Potential for CNS excitation with procaine penicillin.
Ampicillin sodium	10–40 mg/kg IV, q 6–8 h	Little therapeutic advantage over penicillin G for most equine pathogens.
Oxacillin	20–40 mg/kg IV, q 6–8 h	Narrower spectrum than penicillin G, but resistant to penicillinases, so may be effective against penicillin-resistant *Staphylococcus* sp.
Ceftiofur	2.2–4.4 mg/kg IM, q 24 h (label dose) 5–10 mg/kg IV or IM, q 12 h (Gram-negative infections)	Label dose is based on studies using highly susceptible β-hemolytic *Streptococcus* sp. A higher dose is recommended for other susceptible pathogens (e.g., *E. coli*). Kinetic profile is slightly better for IM than for IV administration. Diarrhea and colitis have been reported in horses treated with higher than label doses. Unstable in solution, so unused portion must be used within 12 hours or refrigerated (and used within 7 days).

Table 12.4. *Continued*

Drug	Dosage	Comments
Aminoglycosides		
Gentamicin	7 mg/kg IV or IM, q 24 h	IV route is preferred.
		Efficacy is greatly decreased by low tissue pH and purulent material.
Amikacin	21 mg/kg IV or IM, q 24 h	Aminoglycosides are concentration-dependent antibiotics with a significant post-antibiotic effect, so once-daily dosing is effective and minimizes the risk for toxicity.
		Maintaining hydration also is important in minimizing toxicity.
		Avoid in patients with renal compromise.
		Monitor BUN and creatinine in systemically compromised patients.
Metronidazole	20–25 mg/kg PO, q 8–12 h or 15 mg/kg PO, q 6 h	Narrow spectrum of activity.
		Major indication is the treatment of infections caused by anaerobes, especially *Bacteroides fragilis*.
Enrofloxacin	IV: 5–5.5 mg/kg q 24 h PO: 7.5 mg/kg q 24 h OR 4 mg/kg q 12 h	Reserve for treatment of Gram-negative or staphylococcal infections resistant to other antibiotics.
		Avoid in foals (causes arthropathy in immature animals).
Rifampin	5–7.5 mg/kg PO, q 12 h	Excellent tissue and cell membrane penetration, active even at low pH and in presence of purulent material, but spectrum is limited and resistance develops easily.
		Always use in combination with high-potency antibiotics.
		Not practical to use nor well accepted by horses (may even cause inappetance).

IV: intravenous; IM: intramuscular; PO: oral (per os); BUN: blood urea nitrogen

Penetrating wounds to the distal limb frequently involve a synovial structure (e.g., digital tendon sheath, navicular bursa, and/or distal interphalangeal joint). Given the location of these wounds, a polymicrobial infection can be expected and typically includes Gram-negative enteric bacteria and, with penetrating wounds of the foot, anaerobes such as *Bacteroides* sp. Many species of *Bacteroides* are resistant to penicillin and also to ceftiofur, so metronidazole should be added to the broad-spectrum coverage provided by a cephalosporin (or penicillin) and an aminoglycoside.

As discussed previously for soft tissue infections, the health of the affected tissues and the type(s) of organism(s) isolated are important factors in determining duration of treatment. Generally, antibiotic treatment for several weeks is recommended, using a combination approach:

- Systemic antibiotic therapy (parenteral initially)
- Regional antibiotic perfusion
- Intrathecal lavage and antibiotic deposition
- Antibiotic-impregnated polymethylmethacrylate (PMMA) beads and/or collagen impregnated sponges

See Regional Perfusion of Antibiotics and Intrathecal Administration of Antibiotics.

Bone and Physeal Cartilage

Severely infected wounds involving bone commonly involve *Enterobacter* sp., *Streptococcus* sp., and *Staphylococcus* sp.[11] Following orthopedic surgery, the most common bacterial isolates from infected surgical wounds in horses include *S. zooepidemicus*, *S. aureus*, and α-*Streptococcus* sp.[16] In young foals, Gram-negative organisms may be more common, particularly in established infections involving physeal cartilage. Initial antibiotic selection is the same as for infected wounds involving a synovial structure: a cephalosporin plus an aminoglycoside, or enrofloxacin alone (in adult horses). Metronidazole may be added for penetrating wounds of the foot which involve the distal phalanx or navicular bone.

Infections involving internal fixation devices can be particularly problematic, and not just because the resulting osteolysis may lead to failure of the fixation device before the bone has adequately healed. While metallic surgical implants are designed to be inert insofar as they incite little or no host response, they can encourage some types of bacteria to proliferate. Bacteria which secrete a protective mucopolysaccharide glycocalyx (commonly referred to as a bio-film) when affixed to a metallic implant are more protected from host defense mechanisms and antibiotics. *S. epidermidis* is one such pathogen. Antibiotics alone cannot adequately eliminate these slime-producing bacteria once they colonize a metallic implant.[17]

Bone infections require a combination of surgical debridement and long-term antibiotic treatment, possibly for months if adequate debridement is not possible because of the location or extent of the infection or when surgical implants must remain in place to stabilize a fracture. A combined treatment protocol is recommended:

- Systemic antibiotic therapy (parenteral initially)
- Regional antibiotic perfusion
- Antibiotic-impregnated implants (see later in this chapter)

Repeated surgical debridement often is required to improve the local blood supply.

Respiratory Tract

Infected wounds that involve the respiratory tract, such as a neck wound which penetrates the trachea or pharynx or an open chest wound, frequently comprise combinations of Gram-positive aerobes (especially *S. zooepidemicus*), Gram-negative aerobes (e.g., *Actinobacillus* sp., *Pasteurella* sp., *E. coli, Klebsiella pneumoniae*), and anaerobes (e.g., *Bacteroides* sp., *Fusobacterium* sp., *Peptostreptococcus* sp.).[11]

In these cases a combination of penicillin (penicillin G or ampicillin) and gentamicin is a good choice for interim therapy, with metronidazole added to expand the anaerobic spectrum. Ceftiofur can be substituted for penicillin, and amikacin for gentamicin. This combination would also be an appropriate initial choice for neck wounds that penetrate the esophagus, because organisms which comprise the normal pharyngeal flora can be expected to predominate in these wounds.

Infections involving the respiratory tract may respond quickly, necessitating only a short course (5 to 10 days) of antibiotic therapy. In cases of severe pleuropneumonia, treatment may be required for several months and must include pleural lavage and drainage. The organism(s) isolated, specific anatomic location and tissue(s) involved, clinical response, and laboratory monitoring influence both treatment duration and outcome.

Gastrointestinal Tract

Infected wounds that involve the intestine, such as penetrating wounds to the abdomen or perineum, and open drainage of the peritoneal cavity in cases of septic peritonitis most often comprise Gram-negative enteric organisms, especially *E. coli* and *K. pneumoniae.* Anaerobes also are commonly isolated from the peritoneal cavity. The combination of penicillin (penicillin G or ampicillin) and gentamicin is an appropriate empiric choice in these cases; ceftiofur and amikacin are suitable substitutes.[11]

If an intra-abdominal abscess is suspected as the cause of peritonitis, *S. zooepidemicus* and, in the western parts of the U.S., *Corynebacterium pseudotuberculosis* should be considered as the primary pathogen. In such cases, a combination of penicillin (penicillin G or ampicillin) plus rifampin is an appropriate initial choice.[11]

Wound infections involving the gastrointestinal tract are particularly challenging, due to the potential for abscess formation with anaerobic organisms, the many recesses for bacterial sequestration within the peritoneal cavity, and the frequency with which multi-antibiotic-resistant Gram-negative aerobes are found in the equine large intestine. In addition, effective concentrations of the appropriate antibiotic(s) at the site of infection generally must be achieved primarily using the parenteral route. These factors all influence duration of treatment, which in most cases must be weeks long.

Peritoneal lavage is beneficial in some cases, as much for the removal of inflammatory cytokines and fibrin as for the removal of bacteria. However, thorough lavage of the entire peritoneal cavity and its contents is impossible in the horse. With this limitation understood, peritoneal lavage can be performed via laparotomy or laparoscopy. A technique for active (closed-suction) abdominal lavage and drainage in the standing horse has been described.[18]

Muscle

Clostridium sp. are likely in infected wounds that involve extensive muscle necrosis, particularly if gas pockets have formed within or between tissues. While clostridial myonecrosis is most often associated with intramuscular injections, it can also occur with deep wounds to the muscle. In these cases, immediate and aggressive therapy with penicillin (penicillin G or ampicillin), with or without metronidazole, may be critical for survival. *C. pseudotuberculosis* is another important pathogen to consider with deep muscle infection, particularly in the western U.S. It too is susceptible to penicillin G, although the addition of rifampin may be advantageous.

Infection involving muscle (septic myositis) is one of the more rewarding infections to manage because of the good blood supply to the tissue and the ease with which the area can be opened and drained if abscessation occurs. A combination of surgical debridement and both local and systemic antibiotic therapy generally yields a good outcome with these infections. Treatment duration ranges from days to several weeks.

The mainstays of antibiotic therapy in equine practice remain the penicillins (crystalline or procaine penicillin G, ampicillin), ceftiofur, aminoglycosides (gentamicin and amikacin), trimethoprim-sulfonamide combinations, enrofloxacin, and to a lesser extent tetracyclines, erythromycin, and chloramphenicol. When used appropriately, these antibiotics are effective in the vast majority of equine infections. Other antibiotics are required in very few instances, and in these cases there are factors to be considered which extend beyond the individual patient being treated.

Vancomycin

As mentioned earlier, reports of infections caused by multi-drug–resistant bacteria (e.g., methicillin-resistant *S. aureus* and *S. epidermidis* [MRSA and MRSE, respectively]) are on the rise in both human and veterinary medicine. Vancomycin, either alone or in combination with an aminoglycoside, is an option for serious staphylococcal and enterococcal infections that resist other antibiotic agents. A dosage used with good effect in horses with such infections is 7.5 mg/kg q 8 h, administered in saline by slow IV infusion over 30 minutes.[19]

However, vancomycin resistance in MRSA and enterococci is an increasing concern in human medicine. Vancomycin-intermediate *S. aureus* (VISA) strains have been reported in humans, and vancomycin-resistant enterococci (VRE) are widely reported in humans and farm animals, including horses. Of even more concern, vancomycin-resistant strains of *S. aureus* (VRSA) have begun to emerge in human hospitals.[19]

So far, no clinical cases involving confirmed isolates of VISA, VRSA, or VRE in horses have been reported. Nevertheless, veterinarians should be mindful of the existence of these organisms and their increasing prevalence in the human population. It is therefore recommended that vancomycin use in horses be limited to only those situations in which culture and sensitivity results clearly indicate that vancomycin is likely to be effective and for which there are no other reasonable alternatives.

Regional perfusion with vancomycin, either by IV or intraosseous (IO) administration, may help ameliorate this concern, at least for infections confined to the distal limb. Recent studies in horses showed that vancomycin (300 mg as a 0.5% solution in sterile isotonic saline) administered by IV or IO regional perfusion was well tolerated and achieved therapeutic concentrations in the synovial fluid and medullary sinusoidal plasma of the distal limb.[20,21] These modes of delivery, both described in detail later in this chapter, may serve to optimize the efficacy of vancomycin for susceptible distal limb infections and thereby minimize the risk for the development of bacterial resistance.

Imipenem-cilastatin

Imipenem (with cilastatin) is a carbapenem antibiotic that is used in human medicine, particularly in critically ill patients with infections caused by unidentified bacteria or multi-drug–resistant bacteria. Its spectrum of activity includes a wide range of Gram-positive and Gram-negative organisms, including multi-drug–resistant enteric pathogens (*E. coli*, *Klebsiella* sp., *Salmonella* sp.), *Pseudomonas aeruginosa*, and *Bacteroides fragilis*. Imipenem reportedly is safe for use in horses at a dosage of 10 mg–20 mg/kg by slow IV infusion q 6 h.[22] However, as with vancomycin, the development of resistance in currently imipenem-susceptible pathogens is a concern with overuse of this antibiotic. Empirical use of imipenem in horses should thus be avoided.

Azithromycin and Related Macrolides

Azithromycin and clarithromycin have gained popularity in equine practice in recent years, primarily because of their efficacy against *Rhodococcus equi*. However, their empirical use in horses with severely infected wounds is questionable, at best. While these antibiotics are highly effective in vitro against various Gram-positive equine pathogens, they offer little advantage over penicillin G and ceftiofur, and sensitivity of the most clinically important Gram-negative pathogens, including *E. coli, Klebsiella* sp., and *Salmonella* sp., is intermediate to poor.[9] These antibiotics should be used only when bacterial culture and sensitivity results clearly indicate that they are the most appropriate choice for the particular patient.

Modes of Delivery

In the majority of patients with severely infected wounds, systemic parenteral antibiotic therapy is indicated, at least initially. Local or regional modes of delivery may also be advantageous in individual cases, based on the characteristics of the wound, the antibiotic(s) chosen, and even the pathogen(s) involved. These modes of delivery include intrathecal injection (for wounds involving a synovial structure), regional intravenous or intraosseous perfusion (primarily for infections of the distal limb), and antibiotic-impregnated implants.

Intrathecal Injection of Antibiotics

For infected wounds involving a joint, tendon sheath, or bursa, injection of an appropriate antibiotic into the synovial space following lavage can be a very effective adjunct to systemic antibiotic therapy. At the dosages given below, supratherapeutic concentrations of each drug are delivered directly into the synovial space. In addition, if the synovial membrane is largely intact, the structure acts as a temporary depot or reservoir for the drug, thereby maximizing antibiotic efficacy at that site.

The following dosages are recommended for intrathecal injection of commonly used antibiotics: amikacin, 0.5 g–1 g; gentamicin, 150 mg–500 mg; ceftiofur, 150 mg; cefazolin, 250 mg–500 mg; crystalline (Na and K) penicillin, 2 million–5 million units.[23] These dosages appear to be effective and well tolerated, causing minimal damage to the synovial membrane or articular cartilage. Systemic antibiotic therapy is used concurrently at generally recommended dosages (Table 12.4).

It is important to practice proper sterile technique when performing intrathecal lavage and injection of antibiotics, even though the wound is already contaminated. The clinician must take care not to introduce other bacteria into the synovial space, and must be equally conscious of the zoonotic potential of infected wounds in horses.

Regional Perfusion of Antibiotics

Regional perfusion is another means of maximizing delivery of an antibiotic to the site of infection. This technique uses lower doses of antibiotic than systemic therapy with the same drug, so it maximizes drug efficacy while minimizing the risk of toxicity. Compared with systemic administration of an equal or higher dose of the drug, regional perfusion achieves much higher tissue and synovial fluid concentrations of antibiotic at the site.[24,25] Consequently, therapeutic concentrations of antibiotic can be achieved in severely or chronically infected wounds, even those containing poorly vascularized or necrotic tissue, as the antibiotic diffuses down a concentration gradient from the vasculature to the interstitial space.[23]

The technique is primarily used for wounds at or below the level of the carpus (Figure 12.1) or tarsus (Figure 12.2), because venous outflow proximal to the infected area must be occluded during the procedure—something that is easy to accomplish on the lower limb, but difficult to achieve on the proximal portion of the limb (at least in adult horses) and in most other parts of the body. Two basic options are available: intravenous (IV) perfusion and intramedullary or intraosseous (IO) perfusion. Each has its advantages and drawbacks (Table 12.5).

Preparation

IV Catheterization. For IV regional perfusion, any accessible vein of suitable size in the general vicinity of the wound can be used, provided that venous outflow proximal to the wound and the infusion site can be effectively

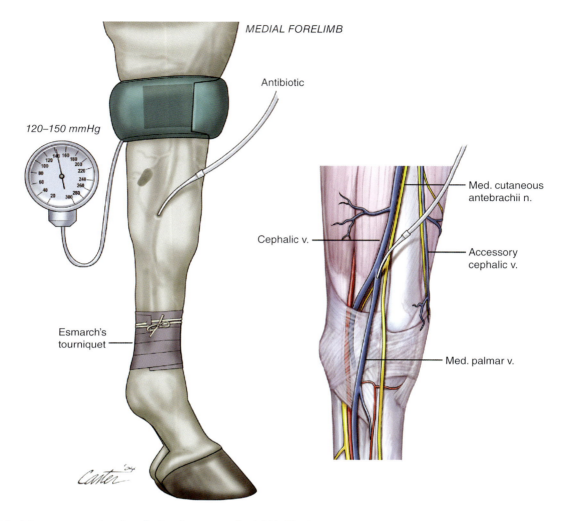

MEDIAL FORELIMB

120–150 mmHg

Antibiotic

Esmarch's tourniquet

Med. cutaneous antebrachii n.

Cephalic v.

Accessory cephalic v.

Med. palmar v.

Figure 12.1. Intravenous regional perfusion for carpus. Orsini JA, Elce Y, Kraus B: Management of severely infected wounds in the equine patient. *Clinical Techniques in Equine Practice, Vol 3*, 225–326, WB Saunders, 2004. Reprinted with permission from Elsevier.

occluded (see below). Preparation is essentially the same as for routine IV catheterization. In the conscious patient, sedation and local or regional anesthesia are used as needed. The skin over the vein is clipped and aseptically prepared. An IV catheter of appropriate size (either an over-the-needle or butterfly catheter) is inserted through the skin and into the vein, and a heparinized extension line with a stopcock or catheter cap is attached. The catheter is fixed in place for the procedure with glue, suture, or adhesive tape.

IO Catheterization. For IO perfusion (Figure 12.3), the largest and most accessible medullary cavity nearest the wound generally is used (e.g., distal tibia or proximal third metatarsus for perfusion of the tarsus), with the same caveat for occlusion of venous outflow discussed above for IV perfusion. Preparation is more involved than for IV perfusion, because a hole must first be drilled through the cortex of the bone and aseptic surgical technique must be used throughout the procedure. Sedation and regional anesthesia (perineural blocks or ring block) are necessary if the procedure is being performed in the conscious horse.

Following aseptic skin preparation, a 1 cm long incision is made through the skin, subcutis, and periosteum overlying the infusion site. A pilot hole is then drilled through the bone cortex and into the medullary cavity using a power drill and sterile drill bit of appropriate size for the cannula to be used (bone marrow needle, hollow bone screw, or simply the male adapter of an IV extension set). The cannula is inserted firmly into the hole such that it provides direct access to the medullary cavity. (Note: While the plastic tip of a sterile extension

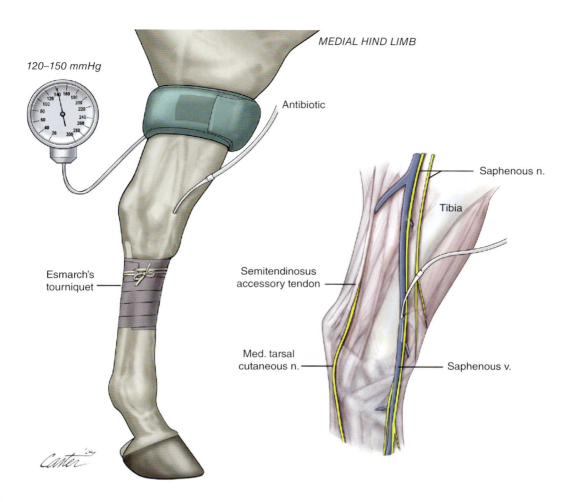

Figure 12.2. Intravenous regional perfusion for tarsus. Orsini JA, Elce Y, Kraus B: Management of severely infected wounds in the equine patient. *Clinical Techniques in Equine Practice, Vol 3*, 225–326, W.B. Saunders, 2004. Reprinted with permission from Elsevier.

Table 12.5. Comparison of intravenous (IV) and intramedullary (intraosseous; IO) perfusion for regional delivery of antibiotics in horses.

Procedure	Advantages	Disadvantages/limitations
IV perfusion	Quick and simple to perform. May be performed under sedation and local/regional anesthesia. Requires no special equipment. Achieves higher antibiotic levels in tissues and synovial fluid than IO perfusion.	Difficult or impossible if soft tissue swelling obscures the vein. Can cause phlebitis or local cellulitis, making repeated IV perfusion at that site difficult. In-dwelling IV catheters for repeat perfusion are difficult to maintain.
IO perfusion	Easier than IV perfusion if there is soft tissue swelling at the site. Can be repeated daily if necessary, with minimal adverse effects.	More involved procedure than IV perfusion. May need to be performed under general anesthesia initially. A hole must be drilled through the cortex. Perfusion is best performed using a bone marrow needle or hollow bone screw (leakage can occur with nonmetal inserts).

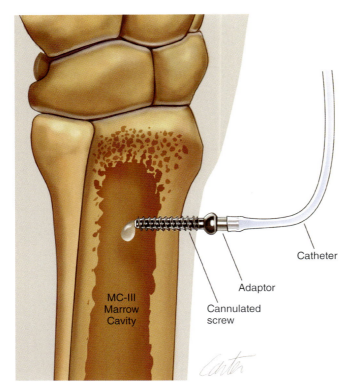

Catheter

Adaptor

MC-III
Marrow
Cavity

Cannulated
screw

Figure 12.3. Intraosseous perfusion—metatarsus. Orsini JA, Elce Y, Kraus B: Management of severely infected wounds in the equine patient. *Clinical Techniques in Equine Practice, Vol 3*, 225–326, W.B. Saunders, 2004. Reprinted with permission from Elsevier.

set can be used as the cannula, leakage around the cannula is more likely than when a bone marrow needle or bone screw is used.) When a metal cannula is used, a short extension line can be attached to facilitate delivery of the antibiotic solution.

Application of the Tourniquet(s)

With either procedure, the site to be perfused is isolated using tourniquets placed proximal and distal to the wound. (Note: For wounds distal to the fetlock, only the proximal tourniquet is used.) The proximal tourniquet prevents escape of the antibiotic into the systemic circulation during perfusion, and the distal wrap limits the volume of tissue being perfused, and thus dilution of the antibiotic in the extracellular fluid. An Esmarch bandage can be used as the distal tourniquet, applied from the hoof to just distal to the infected area. For wounds at or below the level of the fetlock, the Esmarch bandage can be used as the sole occlusive wrap; it is applied from hoof to distal metacarpus/metatarsus, unwrapped from distal to proximal, and secured just proximal to the catheter (Figure 12.4).

Use of an Esmarch bandage may be contingent upon the type of wound being treated, however. It may not be advisable when extensive cellulitis is present, because it may force bacteria-laden interstitial fluid into the lymphatic system. Instead of using an Esmarch bandage when performing IV regional perfusion, venous filling at the site to be perfused can be reduced by allowing blood to flow freely from the IV catheter for 30–60 seconds after the tourniquets are applied but before the antibiotic solution is perfused.[23]

Provided the tourniquet effectively occludes the venous outflow proximal to the wound, IV or IO perfusion can be performed either proximal or distal to the site of infection, depending on the nature and location of the wound. For example, in a heavily muscled horse, perfusion of the tarsus may most easily be achieved by IV or IO perfusion in the proximal metatarsal region. In these horses, the muscle mass in the gaskin may necessitate application of the tourniquet just a few inches proximal to the hock for effective occlusion, which leaves little room to insert the catheter proximal to the joint.

In one study, synovial fluid concentrations of amikacin in the tibiotarsal joint were higher after IO infusion of 1 g amikacin in 56 ml of fluid into the distal tibia than with infusion of 1 g amikacin in 26 ml of fluid into the

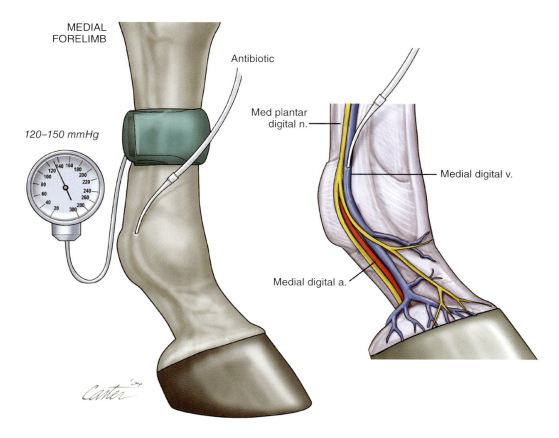

MEDIAL
FORELIMB

Antibiotic

120–150 mmHg

Med plantar
digital n.

Medial digital v.

Medial digital a.

Figure 12.4. Intravenous regional perfusion for the metacarpo/metatarso-phalangeal, proximal, and distal interphalangeal joints. Orsini JA, Elce Y, Kraus B: Management of severely infected wounds in the equine patient. *Clinical Techniques in Equine Practice*, *Vol 3*, 225–236, W.B. Saunders, 2004. Reprinted with permission from Elsevier.

proximal third metatarsus.[25] Nonetheless, perfusion distal to the joint resulted in antibiotic concentrations in the synovial fluid that were well above the minimum inhibitory concentration (MIC) for common equine pathogens, so when it is difficult or impossible to use the proximal site, perfusion distal to the wound is a reasonable alternative.

Dosage and Infusion Volume. Drug dosages recommended for regional limb perfusion in adult horses are as follows: amikacin >250 mg, up to 1 g; gentamicin 100 mg–300 mg; crystalline penicillin or ampicillin, 10 million–20 million units; and enrofloxacin 1.5 mg/kg.[25–27] Various studies in adult horses have reported regional limb perfusion with amikacin or gentamicin at a dosage of 1 g per site.[25,29] While adverse effects are minimal or clinically undetectable at this dosage, peak tissue and synovial fluid concentrations typically are 5 to >55 times greater than the MIC for common equine pathogens,[25] which suggests that lower dosages can be used effectively.

The efficacy of lower dosages has been demonstrated in horses with various septic conditions involving the digit.[26] However, a recent study indicated that an amikacin dosage of 250 mg was insufficient to maintain tissue and synovial fluid concentrations above the MIC for common equine pathogens once the tourniquet was removed.[28] Higher than recommended dosages are unnecessary and increase the potential for vasculitis and local tissue necrosis.[23,26] Enrofloxacin can cause vasculitis, even at the dosage required to achieve effective concentrations in target tissues and fluids (1.5 mg/kg).[28] A further risk with enrofloxacin and other fluoroquinolones is cartilage damage in immature animals, so these drugs should be used in immature horses only if no other alternative is available.

The total dose of drug to be delivered is diluted in sterile physiologic saline solution to the desired infusion volume. Total infusion volumes of 20 ml–60 ml are used in adult horses, depending on the size of the region being perfused. Volumes as small as 20 ml may be adequate for IV perfusion of the digit,[30] whereas up to 60 ml is used for IV perfusion of larger regions such as the carpus or tarsus and for IO perfusion.[23,25,27,29]

With either procedure (IV or IO perfusion), the tourniquet is left in place for a total of 30 minutes. When performing IV perfusion, the total volume is infused over 1–2 minutes, and the tourniquet is left on for the remainder of the 30-minute period. When performing IO perfusion, some clinicians advocate using a maximum infusion rate of 2 ml/minute to avoid excessive intramedullary pressure,[23] in which case the tourniquet is removed immediately after completing the infusion when using an infusion volume of 60 ml. Other clinicians routinely infuse the total volume over a 10-minute period, in both standing and anesthetized patients, without incident. When performing IO perfusion in the conscious horse, instilling a small amount of local anesthetic into the medullary cavity before perfusion avoids the restlessness exhibited by some patients during IO infusion under pressure.[31]

Aftercare. Once IV infusion is completed and the tourniquet(s) is released, the catheter is removed and digital pressure is applied over the vein for a few minutes to prevent bleeding. The site can then be covered with a sterile dressing. A small amount of perivascular swelling may be present for 24–48 hours afterward, but no other adverse effects are noted in most cases.

Following IO infusion and removal of the tourniquet(s) and cannula, the skin incision can be closed primarily or left open to heal by second intention; either way, the site is covered with a sterile dressing. Localized soft tissue swelling can be expected for a few days afterward, as can a small amount of serosanguineous discharge with incisions that are left open, but no treatment other than basic wound care is necessary. The cannula can also be left in place for several days if repeated IO perfusion is anticipated. In the interim, the port is capped and the site covered with a sterile dressing and protective bandage.[31]

With either technique, tissue and synovial fluid concentrations of the antibiotic remain well above the MIC of common equine pathogens for several hours.[25,29] Whether concentration-dependent antibiotics (e.g., aminoglycosides) or time-dependent antibiotics (e.g., penicillins) are used, this technique maximizes bactericidal activity in the perfused tissues. In many cases, only one treatment with regional perfusion is necessary,[24,26] provided that the pathogen involved is susceptible to the chosen drug. It is important to note, however, that systemic antibiotic therapy is used concurrently and for as long as clinically indicated.

Antibiotic-impregnated Implants

Antibiotic-impregnated implants, whether polymethylmethacrylate (PMMA) beads or biodegradable materials (e.g., cancellous bone, collagen sponges, plaster of paris, various polymers), are another means of effectively delivering therapeutic concentrations of antibiotic to the site of infection while minimizing systemic concentrations and thus toxicity of the drug.[23,32] Much higher local tissue concentrations of antibiotic can be achieved with this method than with systemic administration of the drug at recommended dosages.[23] In fact, use of antibiotic-impregnated implants may obviate the need for systemic antibiotic therapy, although in most cases both forms of therapy are used concurrently, for at least the first few days of wound management.

Antibiotic-impregnated implants are of particular value in the treatment of infected wounds that have a poor blood supply and in those containing surgical implants that must remain in place to preserve structural integrity until healing is advanced. By implanting the antibiotic-impregnated material in the wound, therapeutic concentrations of antibiotic are delivered directly to the target tissues, and continuous release of antibiotic from the implant sustains therapeutic concentrations in surrounding tissues for several days (and in some cases for weeks or months), depending on the elution characteristics of the antibiotic-implant combination.[23,32] Two other practical advantages of this form of antibiotic therapy are that it may be used alone for the treatment of infected wounds in intractable patients in which systemic therapy is difficult, and it allows the use of antibiotics that would be cost-prohibitive for systemic administration in a horse.[31]

Suitable Antibiotics

Antibiotics suitable for this use include aminoglycosides (e.g., gentamicin, amikacin, tobramycin, streptomycin), cephalosporins (e.g., cefazolin, ceftiofur), and penicillins.[23,32,33] For orthopedic infections, gentamicin-impregnated PMMA beads are used most often (Figure 12.5); if indicated, cephalosporin-impregnated PMMA beads can also be used.[23,33,34] Clinically, metronidazole mixed with hoof acrylic (Equilox, Equilox International,

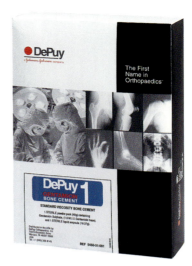

Figure 12.5. Bone cement with gentamicin. Courtesy of DePuy Orthopaedics, Inc. Orsini JA, Elce Y, Kraus B: Management of severely infected wounds in the equine patient. *Clinical Techniques in Equine Practice*, Vol 3, 225–236, W.B. Saunders, 2004. Reprinted with permission from Elsevier.

Pine Island, MN) has been useful for treatment of infections involving the foot.[23] Elution characteristics are poor for polymyxin B, tetracycline, and chloramphenicol, possibly because these drugs are inactivated during the exothermic hardening process or because they bind to the polymer in PMMA.[33]

Making Antibiotic-impregnated PMMA Beads

Currently, antibiotic-impregnated PMMA (AIPMMA) beads are not commercially available in the U.S. However, they are easily made by hand in clinical practice.[23,32,33,35] As a general guide, 1 g–4 g of the chosen antibiotic is added to 20 g of the dry PMMA polymer before the liquid monomer is added and mixed. When the decision is made to use more than one antibiotic for wound treatment (e.g., a cephalosporin plus an aminoglycoside), a separate batch of beads should be made for each antibiotic to avoid drug interactions or interference with elution of one or both drugs if the two antibiotics are combined in the same batch.[23,32]

One procedure for fabricating strings of AIPMMA beads uses three strands of #0 braided polyester suture material and a 6 mm diameter bead mold (Midwest Orthopedic Research Foundation, Orthopedic Biomechanics Laboratory, Minneapolis, MN) (Figures 12.6a–e). The antibiotic of choice (preferably in lyophilized form) is thoroughly mixed with the PMMA powder, then the liquid monomer is added in a powder-to-liquid ratio of 2:1. After mixing the powder and monomer together for 1 minute, the strands of suture material are overlaid onto one-half of the mold (Figure 12.6b), both halves of the mold are filled with the AIPMMA mixture, and the mold is closed, clamped tightly, and the AIPMMA allowed to harden in the mold for at least 10 minutes (Figure 12.6c). Upon unmolding (Figure 12.6d), any excess material is scraped from the surface of the beads to yield a string of smooth, spherical beads (Figure 12.6e).[36] These beads can be used immediately or stored in a sterile, airtight container for future use.

Clinical Use

The size and number of AIPMMA beads implanted in the wound are determined by the dimensions of the wound. The beads may be held in place by partially suturing the wound closed or by maintaining a sterile dressing (bandage, cast, or stent) over the wound.[33] Small beads can be implanted within a synovial space, although their presence can cause discomfort; limit the range of motion in diarthrodial joints; and result in synovitis, capsular fibrosis, and superficial cartilage erosion.[37]

Removal of the beads can be difficult after 10–14 days because they become encapsulated by granulation or fibrous tissue in the healing wound. Whether or not the beads are removed depends on the type of wound, ease of bead removal, and the likelihood of them causing functional impairment if left in place.[23,33] Beads implanted in a synovial space should be removed as soon as the infection is resolved (usually in fewer than 10

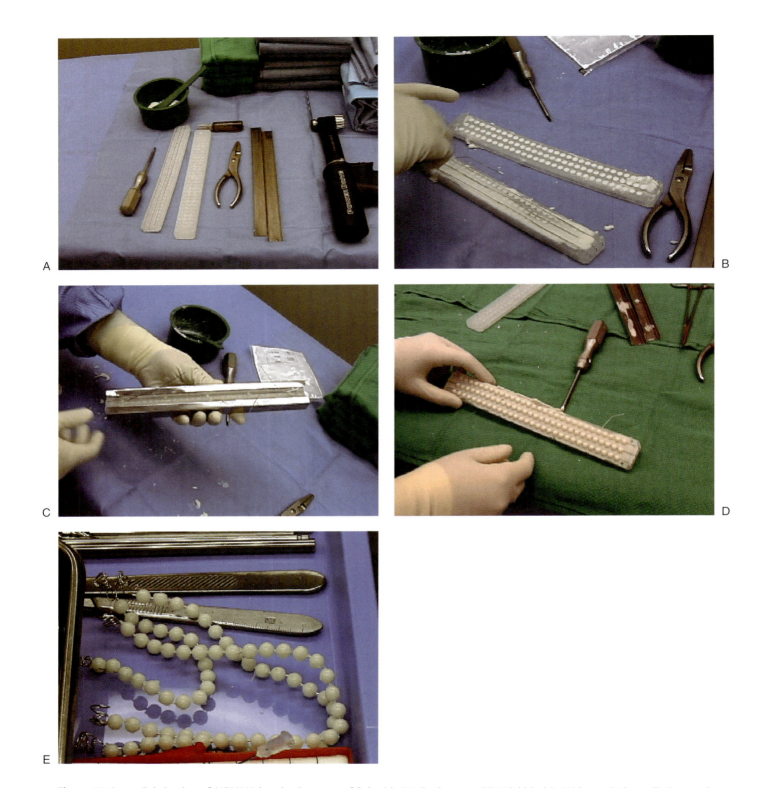

Figure 12.6a–e. Fabrication of AIPMMA beads. Courtesy of Schmidt AH, Tsukayama DT, Wickhind B, Midwest Orthopedic Research Foundation, Minneapolis. Orsini JA, Elce Y, Kraus B: Management of severely infected wounds in the equine patient. *Clinical Techniques in Equine Practice, Vol 3*, 225–236, W.B. Saunders, 2004. Reprinted with permission from Elsevier.

days).[37] In other locations, the beads may be left in place unless they are causing persistent drainage (i.e., foreign body reaction) or they are likely to interfere with athletic function in the future, or the elution characteristics of the antibiotic dictate replacement of the original beads with new implants.

Gentamicin-impregnated Collagen Sponges

Gentamicin-impregnated collagen sponges are biodegradable implants that may be superior to AIPMMA beads in certain types of wounds or clinical situations. Concentrations of gentamicin in wound exudate reportedly are higher for the first few days of treatment with collagen sponges than with AIPMMA beads. In addition, the collagen sponge is absorbed within 12–49 days of implantation, depending on the vascular supply to the region, so removal may be unnecessary.

Although clinical experience in horses is limited, in one report seven of eight horses with traumatic septic arthritis and/or tenosynovitis responded favorably to intrathecal treatment with gentamicin-impregnated collagen sponges. The sponges, which contained 130 mg of gentamicin (Collatamp G, Schering Corporation, UK), were implanted in the synovial cavity via an arthroscopic cannula.[38] These and other biodegradable implants may offer the clinician a means of maximizing therapeutic efficacy while minimizing further damage to structures with limited regenerative capacity, such as articular cartilage.

New Strategies for Enhancing Treatment Efficacy

Supplemental Immunoglobulins

Intravenous administration of pooled human immunoglobulins (Ig) is increasingly being used in human medicine to treat bacterial infections. Clinical studies have shown that combining the IV administration of Ig with IV antibiotics has a synergistic effect.[39] Immunoglobulins promote opsonization and phagocytosis of bacteria, neutralize toxins produced by bacteria, inhibit bacterial attachment and motility, and induce bacterial lysis by activating complement. Several mechanisms have been proposed to explain the synergism of supplemental Ig and antibiotics, including the delivery of antibodies specific to toxins released by antibiotic-lysed bacteria, antibodies specific to bacterial enzymes that destroy antibiotics (e.g., β-lactamases), or antibodies specific to epitopes that were unmasked by the action of the antibiotic.[39]

As good as it sounds, with the volume of Ig required, this approach is costly. In fact, it would be cost-prohibitive in most equine patients. But a study in mice offers a more economical alternative: local administration of Ig along with IV administration of an appropriate antibiotic. In that study, survival in mice with burn wounds infected with a virulent strain of *P. aeruginosa* was at least double that found with either treatment alone when local (sub-eschar) injection of pooled polyclonal human Ig (Gammagard S/D, 98% pure IgG protein fraction, Baxter Healthcare Corp., Glendale, CA) was combined with IV ceftazidime. Furthermore, this combination approach substantially decreased the effective dose of each component (Ig and antibiotic).[39]

Although not yet studied in horses, this treatment approach has important implications for the management of severe wound infections in horses. Commercial equine Ig products are widely available for parenteral use in adult horses and foals. Provided that the wound is amenable to either local injection or regional perfusion with an Ig product, the addition of Ig to the treatment regimen could enhance the efficacy of antibiotic therapy, and thus wound management, in a cost-effective manner.

Antibiotic Potentiation by Chelating Agents

Based on evidence that the chelating agent ethylenediaminetetra-acetic acid (EDTA) causes fatal structural damage to the cell walls of Gram-negative bacteria, a group of researchers at the University of Georgia explored the use of chelating agents as antibiotic potentiators. Tricide® (Molecular Therapeutics, Inc., Riverbend Laboratories, Athens, GA), a third-generation chelator which contains buffered disodium EDTA dehydrate, is the product of that research. Originally formulated for use in human burn patients with multi-drug–resistant bacteria, Tricide® is now used for a variety of human and veterinary applications, including bacterial and fungal skin infections in fish and otitis externa, dermatitis, keratitis, rhinitis, fistulous tracts associated with bone plates, endometritis, sinusitis, and cystitis in multiple animal species and humans.[40]

Many bacterial proteases are calcium dependent; therefore, treating infected wounds with a chelating agent may reduce the additional damage caused by bacterial infection and thereby accelerate wound healing.

Furthermore, by damaging the bacterial cell wall, third-generation chelating agents such as Tricide® potentiate the antibacterial effect of antibiotics, reducing the MIC and minimal bactericidal concentration (MBC) of antibiotics and thus rendering bacteriostatic drugs bactericidal and multi-drug–resistant bacteria susceptible to even "low class" antibiotics.[39]

Tricide® is used primarily as a wound flush and in wound dressings. It can be used alone or combined with appropriate antibiotic(s) in the lavage solution or dressing. At the concentration recommended by the manufacturer, it is non-toxic to tissues. However, absorption through full-thickness skin defects is minimal, so this agent appears to be of value only in killing bacteria on the wound surface or lining a draining tract. Even so, it may aid in the management of severely infected wounds in horses by decreasing the total number of bacteria in the wound. The patient's immune system and antibiotics delivered to the infected tissues by systemic or regional perfusion may then be able to do the rest.

Other Topical Antibiotic Substances

Topical products containing ionic silver, such as silver sulfadiazine or a silver chloride-impregnated wound dressing, can also substantially decrease the numbers of pathogenic bacteria with which they come in contact.[41] In fact, ionic silver is bactericidal against a wide range of clinically important Gram-positive and Gram-negative equine pathogens, including *E. coli, K. pneumoniae, P. aeruginosa, S. equi* subsp. *zooepidemicus,* and *S. aureus.*[41] However, as with chelating agents, these products exert their antibiotic effect just at the wound surface.

Even so, these and other topical antibiotic products may still play an important role in the management of severely infected wounds. Simply lowering the numbers of bacteria in a wound to below 10^5 bacteria/gram of tissue by using an antibacterial lavage solution can be sufficient in an immunocompetent patient to allow wound healing to proceed normally.[42] Topical antibiotic and antiseptic products also suppress bacterial growth in the dressing materials, a potential source of recontamination of the wound.[43] Topical wound medications used in horses have recently been reviewed[43] and are covered in Chapter 3.

Vacuum-assisted Closure

Vacuum-assisted closure (VAC) is a method of wound therapy that has been used in human medicine for several years. Its primary use is to manage wound infections, accelerate wound closure, and facilitate skin grafting. Experimentally, application of controlled subatmospheric pressure to a wound results in an increase in local tissue blood flow, reduction in edema at the wound margins, acceleration of granulation tissue formation, and reduction in bacterial numbers in the wound.[45] Clinical use in human medicine has demonstrated VAC to be of great benefit in managing a wide variety of acute and chronic wounds, including contaminated open chest and abdominal wounds as well as infected wounds involving exposed tendon, bone, or surgical implants.[46–50]

The procedure involves application of subatmospheric pressure (typically 125 mm Hg) to the wound either continuously or intermittently (e.g., cycles of 5 minutes on/2 minutes off) until healing is advanced.[45] Sterile, open-cell polyurethane foam, cut to fit the dimensions of the wound, is packed into the wound; the entire wound is then covered by a waterproof adhesive barrier drape which forms an airtight seal with the skin at the wound margins. Before completing the seal, an evacuation tube is seated between the foam dressing and the barrier drape; the proximal end of the tube exits under the barrier drape and is connected to a small vacuum pump which applies negative pressure to the dressing, and thus to the wound bed (Figure 12.7). A combination of foam dressing and evacuation tube as a single piece is now available in various sizes.

In ambulatory large animal patients, the vacuum pump is suspended from the ceiling above the stall and the coiled tubing from a large animal IV extension set is inserted between the evacuation tube and pump to allow the animal to move about the stall and lie down without disconnecting the pump. Battery powered VAC units have now been developed for use in human medicine. Compact and lightweight, these portable units are ideal for use in horses because they can be attached to the horse's body, blanket, or harness. Depending on the nature of the wound, they may even permit the horse to be exercised (e.g., hand walked) while the pump continues to maintain suction.

A recent report describes the use of VAC in the management of two extensive neck wounds in a horse.[51] This technique has since been used successfully on a variety of other wounds (clean and contaminated) in large animal patients. Use of the VAC on contaminated or severely infected wounds requires only minor modifications to the basic technique. Prior to use on an infected wound, the wound is debrided, if possible, and then

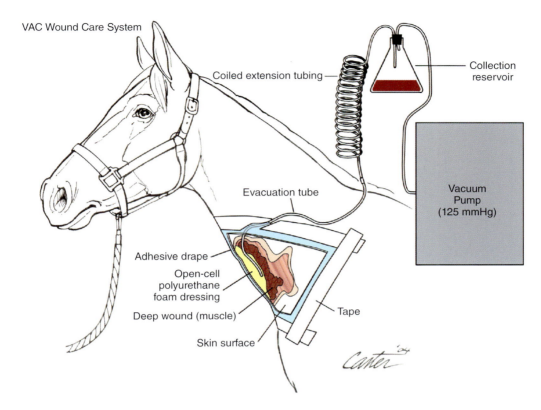

Figure 12.7. Vacuum assisted closure. Orsini JA, Elce Y, Kraus B: Management of severely infected wounds in the equine patient. *Clinical Techniques in Equine Practice, Vol 3*, 225–236, W.B. Saunders, 2004. Reprinted with permission from Elsevier.

copiously lavaged. Antibiotics can be added to the lavage solution or to the final flush in an effort to further reduce bacterial numbers. Initially, the foam dressing is changed every 24 hours (whereas for noninfected wounds it is changed every 48–72 hours). As the infection is brought under control and the wound begins to close, the dressing changes can be extended to every 48 hours (KD Gemeinhardt, DVM, personal communication).

Hyperbaric Oxygen Therapy

Hyperbaric oxygen (HBO) therapy involves the inhalation of 100% oxygen within a specialized chamber that is pressurized to 2 to 3 times normal atmospheric pressure. During treatment, the increased alveolar oxygen tension results in increased blood oxygen tension, and thus increased tissue oxygen tensions. Even poorly perfused tissues can benefit (provided there is at least some blood supply to the area), as the oxygen is driven from the hyperoxygenated plasma into the tissues.[52,53]

This therapy aids in tissue repair through a number of specific cellular mechanisms, beyond merely correcting tissue hypoxia.[52,53] This is particularly relevant because it enhances epithelialization, collagen deposition, fibroplasia, angiogenesis, and bacterial killing—processes which are impaired in the presence of tissue hypoxia.[52,53] Increasing the oxygen tension in ischemic tissue may also improve the efficacy of antimicrobial therapy as the activity of certain antimicrobial drugs (e.g., aminoglycosides, sulfonamides, fluoroquinolones) is reduced under hypoxic or anoxic conditions. It is even suggested that HBO may enhance the activity of certain antimicrobial drugs by inhibiting biosynthetic reactions in bacteria.[52]

Hyperbaric oxygen therapy is a relatively recent addition to equine medicine, owing to the logistical challenges of adapting this human tool to the horse, because the patient must spend at least 60 minutes within the pressurized chamber during an HBO treatment (Figure 12.8). Numerous centers now offer HBO therapy for horses. Controlled studies of HBO therapy in horses are still lacking,[54] but clinical experience indicates that it

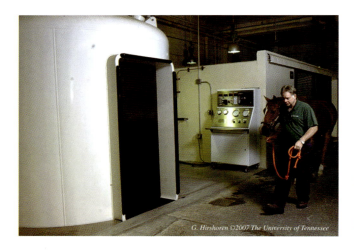

Figure 12.8. Hyperbaric oxygen chamber for horses. The hyperbaric chamber is used for wound healing therapy at the University of Tennessee College of Veterinary Medicine in Knoxville, Tennessee. Greg Hirshoren © 2007. The University of Tennessee.

is a useful adjunct to standard medical and surgical care for a variety of conditions, including burns, ischemic injuries, and infected wounds.[52]

Hyperbaric oxygen therapy is well tolerated in most horses. Contraindications remain to be fully explored, but logically they include untreated pneumothorax, high fever (which may predispose the patient to oxygen toxicity), emphysema, upper airway obstruction, and thoracic surgery.[52]

Biotherapy

Maggots may be used medically to assist with wound debridement, a procedure referred to as biosurgery. These larval insects preferentially feed on necrotic tissue, leaving a relatively clean wound bed.[55] (See Chapter 1 for further details.) The use of medical leeches (hirudotherapy) is also worthy of consideration for wounds in areas suffering extensive venous congestion. While hardly new, hirudotherapy has recently been rediscovered and embraced by human plastic and reconstructive surgeons. In addition to ingesting blood and consequently relieving congestion in the area of application, the secretions of the leech have anticoagulant, vasodilatory, bacteriostatic, and anesthetic properties.[56]

Monitoring Response to Therapy

Horses with severely infected wounds must be monitored frequently (at least once a day initially) until the infection is resolved. Provided that an appropriate treatment plan is implemented, a positive response to therapy (e.g., reduction in inflammation, purulent exudate, and lameness; improvement in attitude and appetite; resolution of fever; improvement in white blood cell count and fibrinogen concentration) should be seen within a few days. Antibiotic therapy should continue until signs of infection have resolved completely and wound healing is proceeding as expected.

The case should be reviewed if there is no improvement within 3 to 4 days of starting or changing treatment. Depending on the circumstances, physical examination and routine blood work are repeated, the wound is further explored and debrided, and bacterial culture and antibiotic sensitivity testing is repeated. The treatment plan is then adjusted accordingly. For example, if systemic antibiotic therapy alone was chosen initially, local or regional antibiotic therapy can be added.

Culture and sensitivity testing is repeated as often as necessary until wound healing is advanced; a single culture may not be enough in severely infected wounds. The procedure has few drawbacks and offers the potential for important gains. The clinician should not hesitate to repeat culture and sensitivity testing if there is a poor response to treatment or if signs of infection recur during or after discontinuing therapy. It may also be wise to repeat culture and sensitivity testing during prolonged antibiotic therapy and within a week of discontinuing antibiotic therapy for wounds with polymicrobial infections or infections involving multi-resistant organisms.

Once the infection is resolved, methods for enhancing wound healing can be considered. Depending on availability and on the nature and location of the wound, these methods include delayed closure with suture material, vacuum-assisted closure (discussed above), topical application of growth factors or extracellular matrix material,[44,57] and skin grafting.

Conclusion

Severely infected wounds can be challenging to manage. Most will require a combination of surgical debridement and adjunctive therapy to include one or several of the following: (1) systemic, regional, and/or local antimicrobials; (2) nutritional support; (3) copious lavage; (4) ventral or continuous drainage; (5) anti-inflammatory medications; (6) supplemental immunoglobulins; (7) vacuum-assisted closure; (8) hyperbaric oxygen therapy; and (9) biotherapy. Once a treatment plan has been established and implemented, monitoring the response of the wound guides the clinician until the desired outcome has been achieved.

References

1. Montgomery RD, Long IR, Milton JL, et al: Comparison of aerobic culturette, synovial membrane biopsy, and blood culture medium in the detection of canine bacterial arthritis. Vet Surg 1989;18:300
2. Spurlock SL, Hanie EA: Antibiotics in the treatment of wounds. Vet Clin North Am: Eq Pract 1989;5:465
3. Hartmann FA, Trostle SS, Klohnen AAO: Isolation of methicillin-resistant *Staphylococcus aureus* from a postoperative wound infection in a horse. J Am Vet Med Assoc 1997;211:590
4. Seguin JC, Walker RD, Caron JP, et al: Methicillin-resistant *Staphylococcus aureus* outbreak in a veterinary teaching hospital: potential human-to-animal transmission. J Clin Microbiol 1999;37:1459
5. Walther B, Friedrich AW, Brunnberg L, et al: Methicillin-resistant *staphylococcus aureus* (MRSA) in veterinary medicine: a "new emerging pathogen"? [Article in German] Berl Munch Tierarztl Wochenschr 2006;119:222
6. Trostle SS, Peavey CL, King DS, et al: Treatment of methicillin-resistant *Staphylococcus epidermidis* infection following repair of an ulnar fracture and humeroradial joint luxation in a horse. J Am Vet Med Assoc 2001;218:554
7. Smith MA, Ross MW: Postoperative infection with *Actinobacillus* spp in horses: 10 cases (1995–2000). J Am Vet Med Assoc 2002;221:1306
8. Bentley AP, Barton MH, Lee MD, et al: Antimicrobial-induced endotoxin and cytokine activity in an in vitro model of septicemia in foals. Am J Vet Res 2002;63:660
9. Jacks SS, Giguere S, Nguyen A: In vitro susceptibilities of *Rhodococcus equi* and other common equine pathogens to azithromycin, clarithromycin, and 20 other antimicrobials. Antimicrob Agents Chemotherap 2003;47:1742
10. Dunowska M, Morley PS, Traub-Dargatz JL, et al: Impact of hospitalization and antimicrobial drug administration on antimicrobial sensitivity patterns of commensal *Escherichia coli* isolated from the feces of horses. J Am Vet Med Assoc 2006;228:1909
11. Wilson WD: Rational selection of antimicrobials for use in horses. In Proceedings, 47th Annual Convention of the American Association of Equine Practitioners. San Diego, CA, American Association of Equine Practitioners, 2001;47:75
12. Hague BA, Honnas CM, Simpson BR, et al: Evaluation of skin bacterial flora before and after aseptic arthrocentesis in horses. Vet Surg 1997;26:121
13. Galuppo LD, Pascoe JR, Jang SS, et al: Evaluation of iodophor skin preparation techniques and factors influencing drainage from ventral midline incisions in horses. J Am Vet Med Assoc 1999;215:963
14. Adam EN, Southwood LL: Primary and secondary limb cellulitis in horses: 44 cases (2000–2006). J Am Vet Med Assoc 2007;231:1696
15. Schneider RK, Bramlage LR, Moore RM, et al: A retrospective study of 192 horses affected with septic arthritis/tenosynovitis. Equine Vet J 1992;24:436
16. MacDonald DG, Morley PS, Bailey JV, et al: An examination of the occurrence of surgical wound infection following equine orthopaedic surgery (1981–1990). Equine Vet J 1994;6:323
17. Rimoldi RL, Haye W: The use of antibiotics for wound prophylaxis in spinal surgery. Orthop Clin North Am 1996;27:47
18. Nieto JE, Snyder JR, Vatistas NJ, et al: Use of an active intra-abdominal drain in 67 horses. Vet Surg 2003;32:1
19. Orsini JA, Snooks-Parsons, C, Stine L, et al: Vancomycin for the treatment of methicillin-resistant staphylococcal and enterococcal infections in 15 horses. Can J Vet Res 2005;69:278
20. Rubio-Martinez LM, Lopez-Sanroman J, Cruz AM, et al: Evaluation of safety and pharmacokinetics of vancomycin after intravenous regional limb perfusion in horses. Am J Vet Res 2005;66:2107
21. Rubio-Martinez LM, Lopez-Sanroman J, Cruz AM, et al: Medullary plasma pharmacokinetics of vancomycin after intravenous and intraosseous perfusion of the proximal phalanx in horses. Vet Surg 2005;34:618
22. Orsini JA, Moate PJ, Boston RC, et al: Pharmacokinetics of imipenem-cilastatin following intravenous administration in healthy adult horses. J Vet Pharmacol Ther 2005;28:355

23. Anderson BH, Ethell MT: Modes of local drug delivery to the musculoskeletal system. Vet Clin North Am (Equine Pract) 1999;15:603

24. Whitehair KJ, Bowersock TL, Blevins WE, et al: Regional limb perfusion for antibiotic treatment of experimentally induced septic arthritis. Vet Surg 1992;21:367

25. Scheuch BC, Van Hoogmoed LM, Wilson WD, et al: Comparison of intraosseous or intravenous infusion for delivery of amikacin sulfate to the tibiotarsal joint of horses. Am J Vet Res 2002;63:374

26. Santschi EM, Adams SB, Murphey ED: How to perform equine intravenous digital perfusion. In Proceedings, 44th Annual Convention of the Am Assoc Equine Pract. Baltimore, MD, American Association of Equine Practitioners 1998;44:198

27. Butt TD, Bailey JV, Dowling PM, et al: Comparison of 2 techniques for regional antibiotic delivery to the equine forelimb: intraosseous perfusion vs. intravenous perfusion. Can Vet J 2001;42:617

28. Parra-Sanchez A, Lugo J, Boothe DM, et al: Pharmacokinetics and pharmacodynamics of enrofloxacin and a low dose of amikacin administered via regional intravenous limb perfusion in standing horses. Am J Vet Res 2006;67:1687

29. Whitehair KJ, Blevins WE, Fessler JF, et al: Regional perfusion of the equine carpus for antibiotic delivery. Vet Surg 1992;21:279

30. Redden RF: A technique for performing digital venography in the standing horse. Equine Vet Educ (American Edition) 2001;3:172

31. Tate LP, Berry CR, King C: Comparison of peripheral-to-central circulation delivery times between intravenous and intraosseous infusion in foals. Equine Vet Educ (American Edition) 2003;5:254

32. Swalec Tobias KM, Schneider RK, Besser TE: Use of antimicrobial-impregnated polymethyl methacrylate. J Am Vet Med Assoc 1996;208:841

33. Holcombe SJ, Schneider RK, Bramlage LR, et al: Use of antibiotic-impregnated polymethylmethacrylate in horses with open or infected fractures or joints: 19 cases (1987–1995). J Am Vet Med Assoc 1997;211:889

34. Booth TM, Butson RJ, Clegg PD, et al: Treatment of sepsis in the small tarsal joints of 11 horses with gentamicin-impregnated polymethylmethacrylate beads. Vet Record 2001;148:376

35. Blackford JT, Latimer FG, Valk N: How to make and use antibiotic-impregnated poly(methylmethacrylate) beads to treat infected wounds in horses. In Proceedings, 43rd Annual Convention of the Am Assoc Equine Pract. Phoenix, AZ, American Association of Equine Practitioners 1997;43:145

36. Ramos JR, Howard RD, Pleasant RS, et al: Elution of metronidazole and gentamicin from polymethylmethacrylate beads. Vet Surg 2003;32:251

37. Farnsworth KD, White NA II, Robertson J: The effect of implanting gentamicin-impregnated polymethylmethacrylate beads in the tarsocrural joint of the horse. Vet Surg 2001;30:126

38. Summerhays GE: Treatment of traumatically induced synovial sepsis in horses with gentamicin-impregnated collagen sponges. Vet Rec 2000;147:184

39. Felts AG, Grainger DW, Slunt JB: Locally delivered antibodies combined with systemic antibiotics confer synergistic protection against antibiotic-resistant burn wound infection. J Trauma 2000;49:873

40. Ritchie BW, Wooley RE, Kemp DT: Use of potentiated antibiotics in wound management. Vet Clin Exot Anim 2004;7:169

41. Adams AP, Santschi EM, Mellencamp MA: Antibiotic properties of a silver chloride-coated nylon wound dressing. Vet Surg 1999;28:219

42. Peyton LC, Connelly MB: Evaluation of quantitative bacterial counts as an aid in the treatment of wounds in the horse. Equine Vet J 1983;15:251

43. Stashak TS: Wound Infection: Contributing factors and selected techniques for prevention. In Proceedings, 52nd Annual Convention of the Am Assoc Equine Pract, San Antonio, TX, American Association of Equine Practitioners 2006;52:270

44. Farstvedt E, Stashak TS, Othic A: Update on topical wound medications. Clin Tech Equine Pract 2004;3:164

45. Morykwas MJ, Argenta LC, Shelton-Brown EI, et al: Vacuum-assisted closure: a new method for wound control and treatment: animal studies and basic foundation. Ann Plast Surg 1997;38:553

46. Argenta LC, Morykwas MJ: Vacuum-assisted closure: a new method for wound control and treatment: clinical experience. Ann Plast Surg 1997;38:563

47. de Lange MY, Schasfoort RA, Obdeijn MC, et al: Vacuum-assisted closure: indications and clinical experience. Eur J Plast Surg 2000;23:178

48. Scheufler O, Peek A, Kania NM, et al: Problem-adapted application of vacuum occlusion dressings: case report and clinical experience. Eur J Plast Surg 2000;23:386

49. Wu SH, Zecha PJ, Feitz R, et al: Vacuum therapy as an intermediate phase in wound closure: a clinical experience. Eur J Plast Surg 2000;23:174

50. DeFranzo AJ, Argenta LC, Marks MW, et al: The use of vacuum-assisted closure therapy for the treatment of lower-extremity wounds with exposed bone. Plast Reconstr Surg 2001;108:1184

51. Gemeinhardt KD, Molnar JA. Vacuum-assisted closure for the management of a traumatic neck wound in a horse. Equine Vet Educ (American Edition) 2005;7:35

52. Slovis NM. Review of Hyperbaric Medicine. In Proceedings, 51st Annual Convention of the Am Assoc Equine Pract, Seattle, WA, American Association of Equine Practitioners 2005;51:153

53. Hopf HW, Rollins MD. Wounds: An overview of the role of oxygen. Antioxidants and Redox Signaling 2007;9:1183

54. Holder TE, Schumacher J, Donnell RL, et al: Effects of hyperbaric oxygen on full-thickness meshed sheet skin grafts applied to fresh and granulating wounds in horses. Am J Vet Res 2008;69:144

55. Dart AJ, Dowling BA, Smith CL: Topical treatments in equine wound management. Vet Clin North Am: Equine Practice 2005;21:77

56. Ben-Yakir, S: Veterinary hirudotherapy, or the therapy that sucks. In 2006 Proceedings, Annual Conference of the Am Holistic Vet Med Assoc. Louisville, KY, 2006:359

57. Badylak SF: Extracellular matrix as a scaffold for tissue engineering in veterinary medicine. Clin Tech Equine Pract 3:2004:164

13 | Burn Injuries

R. Reid Hanson, DVM, Diplomate ACVS and ACVECC

Introduction

Burns are uncommon in horses, with the majority resulting from barn fires. Thermal injuries may also result from contact with hot solutions; electrocution or lightning strike; friction as in rope burns, abrasions, and radiation therapy; and chemicals such as improperly employed topical drugs or maliciously applied caustic agents.[1,2]

Most burns are superficial, easily managed, inexpensive to treat, and heal in a short time. Serious burns, however, can result in rapid, severe burn shock or hypovolemia with associated cardiovascular changes. Smoke inhalation and corneal ulceration are also of great concern.[1,2] Management of severe and extensive burns is difficult, expensive, and time consuming. The large surface area of the burn dramatically increases the potential for loss of fluids, electrolytes, and calories. Burns covering up to 50% or more of the body are usually fatal, although the depth of the burn also influences mortality. Massive wound infection is almost impossible to prevent because of the difficulty of maintaining a sterile wound environment. Long-term care is required to prevent continued trauma, because burn wounds are often pruritic and self-mutilation is common. Burned horses are frequently disfigured, preventing them from returning to full function. Therefore, it is imperative that prior to treatment the patient be carefully examined, with particular attention paid to cardiovascular function, pulmonary status, ocular lesions, and the extent and severity of the burns. Cost of treatment and prognosis should be thoroughly discussed with the owner.[1-4]

This chapter will review the classification and mechanism of burn injury. The pathophysiology of burn injury and pulmonary injury will be discussed as they relate to the physical exam findings and appropriate treatment for immediate disorders as well as long-term wound care. Complications and nutritional needs will also be addressed.

Classification of Burns

Burns are classified according to the depth of the injury.[1-3] First degree burns involve only the most superficial layers of the epidermis. These burns are painful and characterized by erythema, edema, and desquamation of the superficial layers of the skin. The germinal layer of the epidermis is spared and the burns heal without complication (Figure 13.1).[4]

Second degree burns involve the epidermis and can be superficial or deep. Superficial second degree burns involve the stratum corneum, stratum granulosum, and a few cells of the basal layer. Tactile and pain receptors remain intact. Because the basal layers of the epidermis remain relatively uninjured, superficial second degree burns heal rapidly, within 14–17 days with minimal scarring (Figure 13.2).[5] Deep second degree burns involve all layers of the epidermis, including the basal layers. These burns are characterized by erythema and edema at the epidermal-dermal junction, necrosis of the epidermis, accumulation of white blood cells at the base of the burn zone, and eschar (slough produced by a thermal burn) formation, and they cause minimal pain (Figure

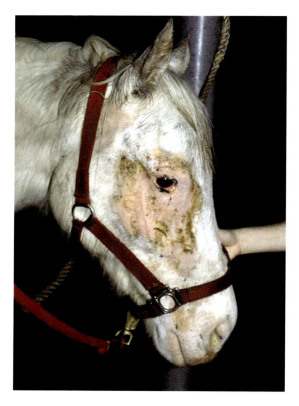

Figure 13.1. First degree burn of the right facial and periocular regions. This type of burn involves only the most superficial layers of the epidermis. These burns are painful and characterized by erythema, edema, and desquamation of the superficial layers of the skin. The germinal layer of the epidermis is spared and the burns heal without complication. Reprinted from Veterinary clinics of north america, Vol 21, R. Reid Hanson, Management of burn injuries, p. 106, (2005), with permission from Elsevier.

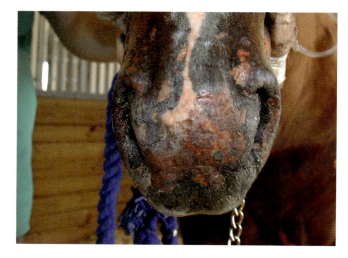

Figure 13.2. Superficial second degree burn of the nose. Tactile and pain receptors remain intact. Because the basal layers of the epidermis remain relatively uninjured, superficial second-degree burns heal rapidly, within 14–17 days with minimal scarring.

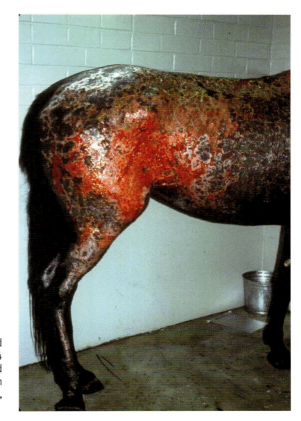

Figure 13.3. Deep second degree burn of the right dorsum and right hind limb. Deep second degree wounds may heal spontaneously in 3 to 4 weeks if care is taken to prevent further dermal ischemia that may lead to full-thickness necrosis. Reprinted from Veterinary Clinics of North America, Vol 21, R. Reid Hanson, Management of burn injuries, p. 107, (2005), with permission from Elsevier.

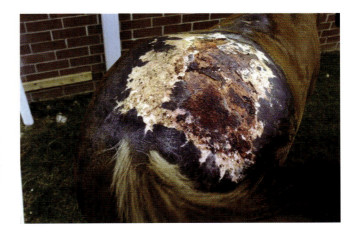

Figure 13.4. Third degree burn of the dorsal gluteal region incurred during a barn fire due to hot asphalt roof shingles falling on the horse. The central burn area is surrounded by deep and superficial second degree burns. Reprinted from Veterinary Clinics of North America, Vol 21, R. Reid Hanson, Management of burn injuries, p. 108, (2005), with permission from Elsevier.

13.3).[1,3] The only germinal cells spared are those within the ducts of sweat glands and hair follicles. Deep second degree burn wounds may heal spontaneously in 3 to 4 weeks if care is taken to prevent further dermal ischemia that may lead to full-thickness necrosis. In general, deep second degree burn wounds, unless grafted, heal with extensive scarring.[5]

Third degree burns are characterized by loss of the epidermal and dermal components, including the adnexa. The wounds range in color from white to black (Figure 13.4). There is fluid loss and a marked cellular response at the margins and deeper tissue, eschar formation, lack of pain, shock, wound infection, and possible bacteremia and septicemia. Healing occurs by contraction and epithelialization from the wound margins or acceptance of an autograft. These burns are frequently complicated by infection. Fourth degree burns involve all of the skin and underlying muscle, bone, ligaments, fat, and fascia (Figure 13.5).[6]

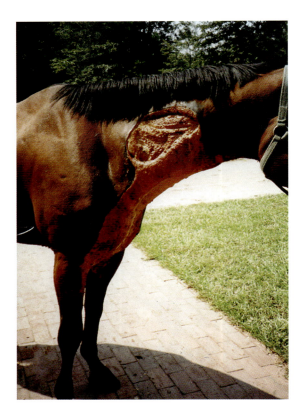

Figure 13.5. Fourth degree burn of the right cervical region and pectoral area due to acid. Fourth degree burns involve all of the skin and underlying muscle, bone, ligaments, fat, and fascia. Reprinted from Veterinary Clinics of North America, Vol 21, R. Reid Hanson, Management of burn injuries, p. 108, (2005), with permission from Elsevier.

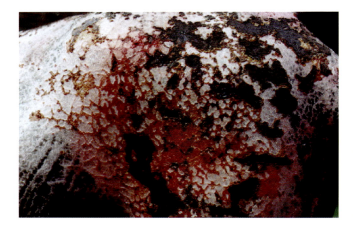

Figure 13.6. Deep second degree burn of the left hind limb. The central burn area is surrounded by less severe skin burns, illustrating the dissipating radiating effects of the heat and damage to the skin. Reprinted from Veterinary Clinics of North America, Vol 21, R. Reid Hanson, Management of burn injuries, p. 109, (2005), with permission from Elsevier.

Mechanism of Burn Injury

The extent of tissue destruction depends upon the temperature of the heat source, duration of exposure, blood supply, and local environment of the wound.[6] At onset there are three levels of injury: the central zone of coagulation, the intermediate zone of vascular stasis, and the outer zone of hyperemia. The central zone of coagulation corresponds to the area that was closest to the heat source. At temperatures >45°C, protein denaturation exceeds the capacity for cellular repair and cell death ensues. The severity of injury decreases radially from this center as heat is dissipated (Figure 13.6).

Adjacent to the coagulation core is an intermediate zone of vascular stasis caused as dermal vessels thrombose during the initial 24 hours following injury. The damaged cells in this zone will survive only under ideal circumstances. The use of heparin and thromboxane inhibitors may moderate the amount of tissue damage in this zone by limiting the number of thromboses developing in the affected area.[7] The outer region is the zone of hyperemia where epidermis is lost but the dermis remains intact and cellular recovery is rapid.

In humans, the total body surface area affected and the depth of the injury correlate highly with the degree of morbidity and mortality associated with thermal injury. New blood markers, such as serum cholinesterase and inflammatory cytokines, have been introduced to assist in the prognosis of morbidity and mortality, beyond the traditional vital signs. At this time, however, these are available only for research purposes.[8]

Pathophysiology

Burn Injury

Following severe burns there is a dramatic cardiovascular effect termed burn shock, which resembles hypovolemic shock. A dramatic increase in local and systemic capillary permeability occurs in response to heat and the release of cytokines, prostaglandins, nitric oxide, vasoactive leukotrienes, serotonin, histamine, and oxygen radicals.[9] Local tissue damage results from massive protein coagulation and cellular death. In the immediate area of the burn, arteries and venules constrict and capillary beds dilate. Capillary wall permeability is increased in response to vasoactive amines released as a result of tissue damage and inflammation. These vascular responses result in fluid, protein, and inflammatory cells accumulating in the wound; ensuing vascular sludging, thrombosis, and dermal ischemia lead to further tissue damage. Tissue ischemia continues for 24–48 hours after injury and is caused by the local release of thromboxane A_2.

Before any change in blood or plasma volume, there is a dramatic drop in cardiac output due to circulating levels of myocardial depressant factors. Fluid loss into the extravascular space leads to an acute reduction in blood volume. With reductions in blood volume and cardiac output, peripheral and pulmonary vascular resistance increase, peripheral tissue perfusion decreases, and organ failure ensues.[9]

The extent of fluid loss parallels the severity of the burn. Fluid losses result in increased heat loss from evaporation and an increased metabolic rate. The heat loss is in part responsible for increased oxygen consumption and metabolic rate as the horse tries to generate heat. Depletion of fat stores and some endogenous protein supplies are two means whereby metabolic compensation is achieved. In turn, this hyper-metabolic rate leads to weight loss, a negative nitrogen balance, and delayed wound healing. Thus, the nutritional condition of the patient prior to injury is a prime prognostic consideration.

In burn injury the vascular compartment remains permeable to proteins up to 15 nm in size, including albumin.[10] With moderate thermal injury, up to 2 times the total plasma albumin pool can be lost from the vascular compartment. Loss occurs both through the open wound and into the extravascular space. Protein concentration can reach 3 g/dl in the extracellular fluid, which is sufficient to cause large fluid shifts because of differences in osmotic pressure.[11] The resultant burn edema is clinically recognized within 60 minutes of injury.[12]

Electrolyte disturbances accompany the fluid and protein shifts. Immediately after a burn, hyperkalemia may occur because of cellular disruption and potassium leakage. When counterbalanced by increased mineralocorticoid secretion, the urinary sodium-potassium ratio is reversed and a subsequent potassium deficit may develop 3 to 5 days after injury.[13] Simultaneously, hypernatremia may result as sodium is reabsorbed after restoration of vascular membranes. Protein concentrations, circulatory volume, and electrolyte concentrations should be measured frequently during replacement therapy.[13]

Anemia is not usually a significant concern immediately following a burn. Anemia can, however, become a problem in patients with burns exceeding 30% of the total body surface area. Early anemia resulting from red cell hemolysis and splenic sequestration may be present but is often masked by hemoconcentration. Initial anemia is caused by the immediate destruction of red blood cells by heat and wound hemorrhage. Subsequently, erythrocyte loss occurs from both intravascular and extravascular removal of damaged cells, as well as during eschar removal. Thrombocytopenia may result from platelet aggregation on damaged capillary endothelium. If damage is extensive, a hemorrhagic diathesis may result from exhaustion of clotting factors.

Immunoglobulin levels in the serum drop; the lowest values are reached 2 days following a burn. Serious defects in neutrophil function such as inefficient chemotaxis, impaired phagocytic rate, and bactericidal capacity have also been observed in severely burned horses. Their combined effect leads to a compromised host that is prone to infection.[14] This translates clinically to the fact that most deaths in severely burned human patients are due to burn wound sepsis; burn patients are also at risk for developing sepsis secondary to pneumonia, catheter-related infections, and suppurative thrombophlebitis.[15]

Host metabolic rate increases in a curvilinear fashion in proportion to the size of the thermal injury exceeding 10% of the total body surface area. This causes a 1°–2°C increase in core body temperature and increases in oxygen consumption, fat degradation, and protein and glucose utilization.[16] Caloric expenditure and protein catabolism are greater in burn injury than in any other physiologic stress state. In patients with burns exceeding 30% of the total body surface area, energy expenditure doubles and fuel substrates are metabolized at 2 to 3 times the normal rate.[16] Caloric and protein intakes must be rapidly adjusted to avoid the rapid depletion of skeletal muscle, delayed wound healing, and impaired cellular defense mechanisms.[16,17] Environmental temperatures should be kept between 28° and 33°C to minimize the metabolic expenditure required to maintain the elevated core temperatures.[16,17]

Inhalation Injury

Inhalation injury is a common sequella of closed-space fires. It develops through three mechanisms: direct thermal injury, carbon monoxide poisoning, and chemical insult. Direct thermal injury causes edema and obstruction of the upper airway, but because of the efficient heat exchange capacity of the nasopharynx and oropharynx, superheated air is cooled prior to entering the lower respiratory tract.

Carbon monoxide interferes with oxygen delivery in several ways.[18] It has a 230–270 times greater affinity for oxygen, thus shifting the oxygen-hemoglobin curve to the left. The resultant carboxyhemoglobin is incapable of oxygen transport. Carbon monoxide also binds to myoglobin, thereby impairing oxygen transport to muscles.[18] Carbon monoxide is excreted by the lungs at a rate related to ambient oxygen tensions. In room air, carbon monoxide has a half-life of 3 to 4 hours. An increase in oxygen tensions promotes the dissociation of carbon monoxide and hemoglobin; thus 100% oxygen therapy reduces the half-life to 30–40 minutes. Hyperbaric oxygen therapy at 2.5 atmospheres further decreases the half-life to 22 minutes.[19]

Chemical insult depends on the material that was burned.[20] Combustion products such as hydrogen cyanide, hydrochloric acid, phosgene, sulfuric acid, and aldehydes may induce severe tracheobronchitis when combined with the moisture in the airways. Initially, only erythema may be present, but chemical injury continues as long as chemical-covered carbon particles remain attached to the airway mucosa; particle size determines where damage will occur within the respiratory tree (Figure 13.7). Combustion products cause increased pressure within the pulmonary artery, peribronchial edema, mucosal sloughing, bronchoconstriction, decreased mucociliary transport, and bacterial clearance, as well as altered surfactant activity.[20] Significant pulmonary ventilation/perfusion mismatches may subsequently develop.[21]

Pulmonary infection is a potential complication of smoke inhalation. Alveolar macrophages, the primary cellular defenders in the lung, are increased in number after injury but display decreased phagocytic and bactericidal functions. Susceptibility to pulmonary infection, pulmonary edema, and lung dysfunction increases greatly in patients that also suffer cutaneous thermal injury. The relationship between inhalation and surface

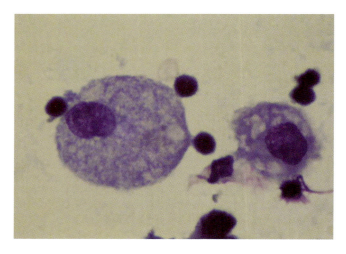

Figure 13.7. Carbon particles associated with alveolar macrophages in the bronchoalveolar lavage due to smoke inhalation injury. Chemical injury continues as long as chemical-covered carbon particles remain attached to the airway mucosa; the size of the particles determines where damage will occur within the respiratory tree. Reprinted from *Veterinary Clinics of North America*, Vol 21, R. Reid Hanson, Management of burn injuries, p. 112, (2005), with permission from Elsevier.

burns is unclear but appears to be additive. Major cutaneous burns alone have been reported to cause pulmonary dysfunction in as many as 25% of patients, whereas inhalation injury increases the morbidity and mortality rates for a given cutaneous thermal injury.[22]

Exam Findings

Physical Exam Findings

Because heat is slow to dissipate from burn wounds, it is often difficult to accurately evaluate the amount of tissue damage in the early period following injury. The extent of the burn depends on the size of the area exposed, while the severity relates to the maximum temperature the tissue attains and the duration of overheating. This explains why skin injury often extends beyond the boundaries of the original burn.[23] A complete physical examination should be performed on any burned animal before the wound is evaluated. Only after the patient's condition is stable should the burn wound be assessed.

Physical criteria used to evaluate burns include erythema, edema, and pain; blister formation; eschar formation; presence of infection; body temperature; and cardiovascular status.[23] In general, erythema, edema, and pain are favorable signs because they indicate that some tissue is viable, although pain is not a reliable indicator of wound depth.[23] Often, time must elapse to allow progression of tissue changes in order for an accurate evaluation of burn severity to be made (Figures 13.8 and 13.9).

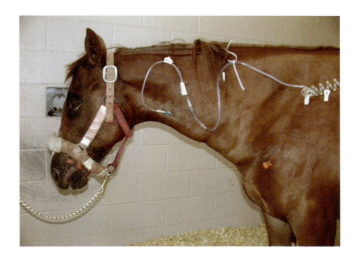

Figure 13.8. Severe burn edema along the ventral neck region 24 hours after injury due to a barn fire. Reprinted from Veterinary Clinics of North America, Vol 21, R. Reid Hanson, Management of burn injuries, p. 114, (2005), with permission from Elsevier.

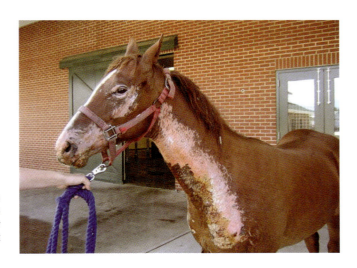

Figure 13.9. Same horse as in Figure 13.8. The extent of the burn is more evident after the skin has sloughed in response to latent thermal injury to the skin. Reprinted from Veterinary Clinics of North America, Vol 21, R. Reid Hanson, Management of burn injuries, p. 114, (2005), with permission from Elsevier.

Burns are most commonly seen on the back and face. Erythema, pain, vesicles, and singed hair are present, depending on the extent of the injury (Figure 13.10). Increases in heart and respiratory rates accompany abnormal discoloration of mucous membranes. The burned horse may exhibit blepharospasm, epiphora, or both, which signify corneal damage (Figure 13.11). Coughing may indicate smoke inhalation while a fever signals or confirms a systemic response to injury.

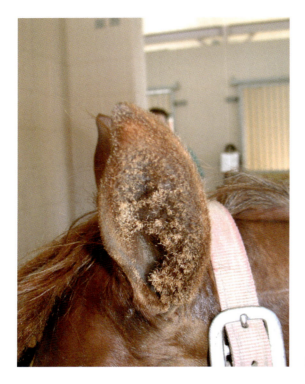

Figure 13.10. Singed hair due to heat generated from a barn fire.

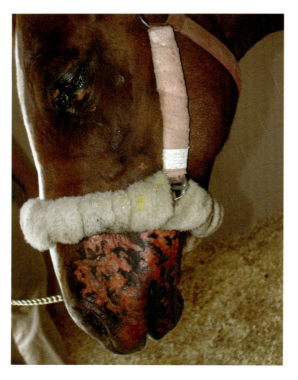

Figure 13.11. Blepharospasm, epiphora, and severe erythema with loss of epithelium of the muzzle due to a barn fire.

Laboratory Findings

Initial laboratory data including complete blood count, clotting profile, serum chemistry, urinalysis, arterial blood gas, and carbon monoxide concentration as well as chest radiographs and bronchoalveolar lavage are helpful in the preliminary evaluation.[6]

Laboratory findings may reveal a low total protein concentration with anemia that may be severe and steadily progressive. Hemoglobinuria may be detected. Hyperkalemia may be present initially but hypokalemia is more likely later in the course of the condition and is often associated with fluid therapy. Evidence of hemolysis or hemoglobinuria in a horse that has suffered cutaneous burns is indicative of severe burn trauma and potential complications such as pigment nephropathy and renal failure.[24]

Percentage Body Surface Area Burn Related to Prognosis

The percentage of total body surface area involved usually correlates with mortality, whereas the depth of the burn determines morbidity.[11] The rule of 9 is used in humans to estimate the total body surface area involved. This method allows an estimation of prognosis according to the extent of the burn. Each arm represents 9%, each leg 18%, the head with neck 9%, and the thorax and abdomen each 18% of body surface area.[4] Special care should be taken to identify injury to major vessels of the lower limbs and presence of eye, perineal, tendon sheath, and/or joint involvement.

Although specific guidelines do not exist for burned large animals, euthanasia should be recommended for those with deep partial-thickness to full-thickness burns involving 30%–50% of the total body surface area.[13,25] The availability of adequate treatment facilities, cost of treatment, and pain experienced by the horse during long-term care should be considered when deciding whether or not to treat. Because convalescence may take up to 2 years, euthanasia is often an acceptable alternative.[26]

Treatment

Burn Shock

With burn shock, large volumes of balanced electrolyte solution are generally chosen unless serum electrolyte analysis dictates otherwise. In patients with burns exceeding 15% of the total body surface area, intravenous fluid therapy is required to avoid circulatory collapse.[27,28] Inadequate fluid resuscitation results in decreased renal and gastrointestinal perfusion that could lead to gastrointestinal bacterial translocation and sepsis.[27,28] Administration of isotonic fluids at a rate of 2 ml–4 ml/kg for each percentage of surface area burned is recommended, but fluid resuscitation is best titrated to maintain stable and adequate blood pressure.[16] An alternative is to use hypertonic saline solution (4 ml/kg) with plasma, hetastarch, or both, followed by administration of additional isotonic fluids.

If there has been smoke or heat inhalation injury, crystalloid administration should be limited to the amount that normalizes circulatory volume and blood pressure. Continuation of the same rate of administration of electrolyte solutions following the resolution of burn shock leads to edema in excess of any improvement in cardiovascular dynamics.[28] Two to 10 liters of plasma is an effective albumin source as well as an exogenous source of antithrombin III against coagulopathies. Hydration, lung sounds, and cardiovascular status should be monitored carefully during fluid administration by clinical assessment and PCV/TP measurement.

Flunixin meglumine (0.25 mg–1 mg/kg IV q 12–24 h) is an effective analgesic. Cyclooxygenase (COX)-2 inhibitors are a new class of nonsteroidal anti-inflammatory drugs that selectively block the COX-2 enzyme, which impedes the production of prostaglandins that cause pain and swelling. Because the COX-2 enzyme does not play a role in the normal function of the stomach or intestinal tract, medications which selectively block COX-2 do not present the same risk of injuring the stomach or intestines. Firocoxib (0.1 mg/kg PO SID) is a newly developed COX-2 inhibitor for the horse. Although COX-2 inhibitors would seem beneficial in the management of burn patients, Firocoxib is currently approved only for use in musculoskeletal pain. Pentoxyfylline (8 mg/kg IV q 12 h) is used to improve the flow properties of blood by decreasing its viscosity. Administration of dimethylsulfoxide (DMSO) (1 g/kg IV) for the first 24 hours may decrease inflammation and pulmonary edema. If pulmonary edema is present and is unresponsive to DMSO and furosemide treatment, dexamethasone can be administered once at 0.5 mg/kg IV.

Pulmonary Injury

Maintenance of airway patency, adequate oxygenation and ventilation, as well as stabilization of hemodynamic status are the cornerstone of therapy for smoke inhalation injury. Intervention and respiratory support are essential, even before the diagnosis of respiratory injury is confirmed. Nasal or tracheal insufflation with humidified 100% oxygen counteracts the damaging effects of carbon monoxide and facilitates clearance by decreasing its half-life in the blood. Oxygen insufflation rates of 15–20 l/minute can be achieved through a tracheostomy and should be continued until the patient is able to autonomously maintain normal oxygenation. Humidification can relieve excessive airway drying or mucous plugging.

Nebulizing with N-acetyl cysteine and heparin and using humidified air will reduce the formation of pseudomembranous casts and aid in the clearance of airway secretions.[21,22] If there is respiratory distress with low arterial oxygen tensions, a tracheostomy is indicated to attempt to remove large obstructive pseudomembranous tracheobronchial casts that have formed.[29] Nebulized DMSO will help decrease lung fluid formation.[21,22] The beta adrenergic agonist albuterol can be aerosolized to reduce bronchospasm. DMSO and heparin may protect against airway damage caused by smoke.[30–33] Maintenance of optimal fluid status is essential. Patients with concurrent surface burns and inhalation injury require 2 ml per percentage burn per kg more fluid than those with cutaneous burns alone to support adequate cardiac and urine output.[34]

Antibiotics and corticosteroids do not influence survival rates and should not be routinely administered to smoke inhalation patients. Systemic antimicrobials are indicated only for proven infections, the incidence of which increases 2 to 3 days after smoke inhalation. Intramuscular penicillin is effective against oral contaminants colonizing the airway. Gentamicin was shown to improve hemodynamics in ovine septic shock after smoke inhalation injury.[35] If signs of respiratory disease worsen, a transtracheal aspirate should be submitted for culture and sensitivity testing, and the antibiotic regimen adapted accordingly.[30,34]

Patients with suspected significant smoke inhalation should be observed closely for several hours and hospitalized in the presence of extensive burns. Therapy must be adjusted according to the clinical response and the results of serial blood gas analyses, complete blood counts, chest radiographs, airway endoscopy, and cultures. Successful treatment depends on continuous patient reassessment as well as early and aggressive patient care.

Wound Care

First degree burns are generally not life-threatening and thus are simply managed. Topical therapy in the form of cool compresses, cold-water baths, and wound coverings may provide relief from pain. Additional pain control can be achieved with nonsteroidal anti-inflammatory drugs or narcotics.

Second degree burns are associated with vesicles and blisters. These vesicles should be left intact for the first 24–36 hours following formation, because blister fluid provides protection from infection and the presence of a blister is less painful than the denuded exposed surface. After this interval the blister is partially excised and an antibacterial dressing such as silver sulfadiazine (Silvadene, Par Pharmaceutical, Inc., Spring Valley, NY) is applied to the wounds while an eschar is allowed to form.[1,2,11]

Third degree burns can be difficult to manage. The patient's condition should be stabilized as rapidly as possible prior to undertaking wound management. Destruction of the dermis leaves a primary collagenous structure called an eschar. Dry exposure is a treatment method that respects the principle that bacteria do not thrive on a dry surface. The goals of therapy are to keep the wound dry and protected from mechanical trauma. Heat and water loss from the uncovered wound, however, are a disadvantage of this approach.

There are several methods to treat burn wounds in the horse, and the choice depends on the extent and location of the injury. Full-thickness burns can be managed by occlusive dressings (closed technique), continuous wet dressings (semi-open technique), eschar formation (exposed technique), or excision and grafting.[23]

The closed method relies on the use of occlusive artificial dressings. Wound cleansing and debridement are performed at each of the frequent dressing changes. Temporary dressings can, by adhering to the underlying wound bed, decrease the bacterial population, reduce heat and water loss, protect the bed of granulation tissue, and hasten wound healing. However, with large burns, frequent bandage changes and debridement can be painful, and extensive bandaging may not be feasible or affordable in some patients.[23]

With the semi-open method, the eschar is left in place but kept covered with an antimicrobial-soaked dressing such as silver sulfadiazine (Silvadene, Par Pharmaceutical, Inc., Spring Valley, NY). The dressing provides protection against trauma, bacterial contamination, and evaporative losses. The wet dressings enhance eschar removal.[23]

With the open technique the wound is left exposed to the air to form its own biologic barrier composed of exudate, collagen, and layers of dead skin, known as the burn eschar. The eschar does not prevent bacterial contamination nor heat nor water evaporation, and the depth of tissue destruction may be marginally increased during the drying process. The eschar is covered with an antibacterial agent twice daily. Wound contraction does not occur while the eschar is intact. The eschar is sloughed by bacterial collagenase activity within 4 weeks.[36] The exposed bed can then be grafted or allowed to contract.

Eschar excision and grafting are useful for smaller burns but cannot be used for large burns because of lack of donor skin. Commercially available xenografts (porcine skin) can be used to cover large defects following excision; however, the cost can be prohibitive.[1,11] Amnion, however, functions as a protective barrier for the wound, prevents fluid and protein loss, controls the growth of bacteria, and reduces pain at the wound site. The physical structure of amnion is similar to that of skin and it contains growth factors that enhance fibroplasia; therefore, it is a viable alternative for burn wounds that are treated with the closed method. Thus, while early excision of the eschar has substantially decreased the incidence of invasive burn wound infection and secondary sepsis in humans, eschar excision and open treatment are not practical for extensive burns in horses because of the likelihood of environmental contamination and massive losses of fluid and heat.[23] The most effective and practical therapy for large burns in horses is the open method, leaving the eschar intact, combined with continuous application of antibacterial agents.[1,2,23]

Initially, the surrounding hair should be clipped and the wound debrided of all devitalized tissue.[11] Attempts should be made to cool the affected skin using an ice- or cold-water bath. Copious lavage with a sterile 0.05% chlorhexidine solution should be performed.[11] A water-based antibiotic ointment such as silver sulfadiazine should be applied liberally to the affected areas to prevent heat and moisture loss, protect the eschar, prevent bacterial invasion, and loosen necrotic tissue and debris. This slow method of debridement allows removal of necrotic tissue as it is identified, thereby preventing erroneous removal of healthy germinal layers. The eschar is allowed to remain intact with gradual removal, permitting it to act as a natural bandage until it is ready to slough.

A calcium alginate wound dressing with acemannan hydrogel (CarraGinate, Carrington, Irving, TX) absorbs 30 times its weight in exudate, prevents further eschar formation by keeping tissues moist, and will not interfere with the activity of topical antibiotics, which can be applied before the gel or mixed with it.

Although bacterial colonization of large burns in horses is not preventable, the wound should be cleansed 2 or 3 times daily and a topical antibiotic reapplied to reduce the bacterial load to the wound. Occlusive dressings should be avoided because of their ability to produce a closed wound environment, which may encourage bacterial proliferation and delay healing.

Systemic antibiotics do not favorably influence wound healing, fever, or mortality, and can encourage the emergence of resistant microorganisms. Additionally, circulation to the burned areas is often compromised, making it highly unlikely that parenteral administration of antibiotics can achieve therapeutic levels at the wound. Short-term prophylactic intravenous antibiotic therapy may be indicated in the immediate post-burn period if quantitative biopsy cultures or a more rapid slide dilution method yield more than 100,000 cells/g of tissue.

The most commonly used topical antibacterial for the treatment of burns is silver sulfadiazine in a 1% water miscible cream. It is a broad-spectrum antibacterial agent that can penetrate the eschar. Silver sulfadiazine is active against Gram-negative bacteria, especially *Pseudomonas*, with additional effectiveness against *S. aureus*, *E. coli*, *Proteus*, *Enterobacteriaceae*, and *C. albicans*.[11,23,28] It causes minimal pain upon application but must be used twice a day because it is inactivated by tissue secretions.

One *in vitro* study found that a 1% silver sulfadiazine/0.2% chlorhexidine digluconate product (Silvazene, Sigma Pharmaceuticals, Melbourne, Australia) was more cytotoxic to the tissue when compared to a 1% silver sulfadiazine (Flamazine, Smith & Nephew Healthcare, Hull, UK) and a silver-based dressing (Acticoat, Smith & Nephew Healthcare, Hull, UK).[37]

Recent evidence suggests that the compound delays the wound healing process and that silver may have variable but serious cytotoxic activity in a range of host cells. It is recommended in human burn patients that silver levels in plasma and/or urine be monitored.[38] A review of 410 papers comparing the effectiveness of silver sulfadiazine cream to normal dressings in promoting healing in burn patients without infection found no direct evidence of improved healing or reduced infection with silver sulfadiazine.[39] Although pseudo-eschar formation that may preclude wound evaluation as well as transient leukopenia, skin hypersensitivity, and the development of bacterial resistance have all been reported in humans, silver sulfadiazine has few systemic effects and provides good results in the horse.[23,28,40]

Aloe vera is a gel derived from a yucca-like plant that has antithromboxane and antiprostaglandin properties.[41] It is reported to relieve pain, decrease inflammation, stimulate cell growth, and kill bacteria and fungi.

Although used successfully in the acute treatment of burns, it may actually delay healing once the initial inflammatory response has resolved.[41] Aloe vera and silver sulfadiazine are good first choices in antibiotic therapy for burns and are used extensively in human medicine.

Other effective topical antimicrobials include mafenide acetate, chlorhexidine, povidone iodine, and gentamicin sulfate ointment. Nitrofurazone (Furacin, Phoenix Pharmaceuticals, Inc, St. Joseph, MO) has a fairly narrow range of antibacterial activity, it may induce resistance, and it does not penetrate the eschar very well. Chlorhexidine (Nolvasan, Fort Dodge Animal Health, Fort Dodge, IA) is active in vitro against a broad spectrum of Gram-positive and Gram-negative vegetative bacteria. A potential drawback is that *Proteus* and *Pseudomonas* have developed or possess an inherent resistance to this product and it has no effect against fungi or Candida.[42] Because of its cationic nature, chlorhexidine binds strongly to skin, mucosa, and other tissues; therefore, it is very poorly absorbed, thus minimizing excessive systemic absorption and toxicity. Chlorhexidine can be applied as a cream or solution.

Povidone-iodine (Betadine, Purdue Frederick Co., Norwalk, CT) causes some patient discomfort but is effective against bacteria, yeast, and fungi. Its hyperosmolality causes severe hypernatremia and acidosis due to water loss such that it should not be used on extensive burns where systemic absorption is likely.[34] Depression of the immune system has also been reported in humans.[34] Gentamicin (Gentamicin sulfate ointment USP, Clay-Parks Labs, Inc., Bronx, NY) is excellent for serious Gram-negative infections but should be used only in selected cases because resistance can develop and it may be nephrotoxic in patients with renal problems.

Topical aqueous antibacterial preparations have also been used to treat burns. The solution (mixture of nitrofurazone, glycerin, and distilled water) can be applied to the wound as a mist from a spray bottle several times a day.[1] The nitrofurazone kills bacteria while the moisture loosens the eschar and promotes debridement. Other agents that are occasionally used topically include neomycin, bacitracin, and polymixin B. Their use is generally associated with the rapid development of bacterial resistance and systemic toxicity. For this reason they are not recommended for routine use in long-term wound care.[40]

It is appropriate to change antibacterial creams according to clinical results. In large burns, quantitative wound biopsy analysis is advantageous. Wound flora densities of more than 10^5 organisms/g tissue predispose the patient to bacterial invasion of healthy tissue.[36] Conversion of superficial wound sepsis to full-thickness infection with the risk of systemic sepsis is prevented by administering local antibiotics. The use of systemic antibiotics is not recommended because they are ineffective in penetrating the avascular eschar, where the risk of contamination is greatest.[40]

Many burn patients suffer pruritis such that measures must be taken to prevent self-mutilation of the wound. Reserpine, normally used in the horse as a long-acting tranquilizer, can be effective in decreasing the urge to scratch by successfully breaking the itch-scratch cycle.

Hyperbaric Oxygen

Hyperbaric oxygen (HBO) is designed to increase oxygen delivery to local ischemic tissue and, by a variety of primary and secondary mechanisms, to facilitate wound healing (Figure 12.8). At normal atmospheric pressure (atm), most of the oxygen in blood is carried by hemoglobin, with minimal additional oxygen dissolved in the plasma. By administering high concentrations of oxygen under increased pressure (2 atm–2.4 atm), the dissolved oxygen in the blood can be significantly increased, resulting in a ~30% increase in oxygen-carrying capacity. At a standard treatment pressure of 2.4 atm, an arterial PO_2 of 1,500 mmHg can be achieved, which increases the driving pressure for diffusion of oxygen into the tissue and increases the diffusion distance by 3- to 4-fold. Even though treatment sessions are relatively brief, oxygen tensions may remain elevated in subcutaneous tissue for several hours after exposure.[43,44]

The postulated mechanisms of a beneficial effect of HBO on burn wounds are decreased edema due to hyperoxic vasoconstriction, increased collagen formation, and improved phagocytic killing of bacteria.[45] In a trial comparing burn treatment with and without HBO in 16 human patients, the mean healing time was significantly shorter in the group receiving HBO.[44] On the other hand, among 266 patients with burns who were treated with HBO and 609 who were not, there were no significant differences in mortality and length of hospital stay.[46] Preliminary results of a randomized, controlled trial using HBO at a burn center were reported recently; among 125 patients randomly assigned to usual burn care or usual burn care plus HBO, the outcomes were virtually identical.[47]

Nutritional Needs/Requirements

Assessment of nutritional intake is performed with a reliable weight record. Weight loss of 10%–15% during the course of illness indicates inadequate nutritional intake. Nutritional support can include both parenteral and enteral routes; the latter is superior.[22] Early enteral feeding not only decreases weight loss but also maintains intestinal barrier function by minimizing mucosal atrophy. This reduces bacterial and toxin translocation and the potential for subsequent sepsis.[22]

Gradually increasing the grain, adding fat in the form of 4 oz–8 oz of vegetable oil, and offering free-choice alfalfa hay increases caloric intake. Stanozolol (Winstrol-V, Pfizer, New York, NY; 0.55 mg/kg IM) is an anabolic steroid that may be used to help restore a positive nitrogen balance by improving appetite and promoting weight gain. It can be given on a weekly basis for up to 4 weeks. If smoke inhalation is a concern or there is evidence of burns around the face, the hay should be water-soaked and fed on the ground in a well-ventilated environment to facilitate mastication and minimize aspiration.[23]

Complications

Burn wounds are very pruritic.[2,23] Significant self-mutilation through rubbing, biting, and pawing can occur if the horse is not adequately restrained or medicated. Usually the most intense pruritic episodes occur in the first weeks following injury, during the inflammatory phase of repair and eschar sloughing. To prevent extreme self-mutilation the animal must be cross-tied and/or sedated during this time. Other complications include habronemiasis, keloid-like fibroblastic proliferations, sarcoids, and other burn-induced neoplasia.[2,26] Hypertrophic scars, which commonly develop following deep second degree burns, generally remodel in a cosmetic manner without surgery, within 1 to 2 years. Because scarred skin is hairless and often depigmented, solar exposure should be limited. Chronic non-healing areas should be excised and autografted to prevent neoplastic transformation. Delayed healing, poor epithelialization, and complications of second intention healing may limit the return of the animal to its previous uses.

Skin Grafts

Burns heal slowly and many weeks may be required for the wound to close by granulation, contraction, and epithelialization (Figures 13.12, 13.13, 13.14). Closure of the burn wound either by suturing or skin grafting

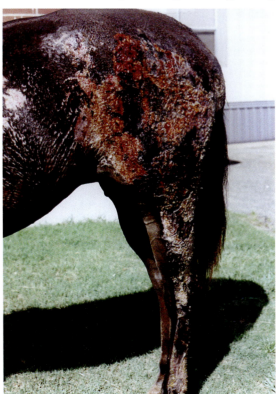

Figure 13.12. Deep second degree and third degree burns of the dorsum and left hind limb 8 days post injury. Marked erythema and early eschar formation are present.

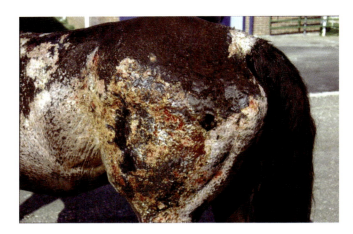

Figure 13.13. Same horse as in Figure 13.12, 5 weeks after injury. The eschar is still present centrally. The wounds are cared for with twice-daily application of silver sulfadiazine and removal of the loose eschar. Note the peripheral epithelialization of the wound.

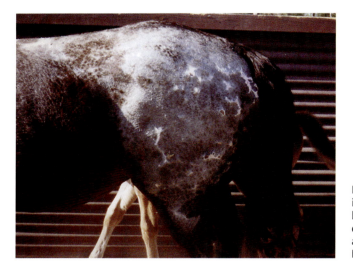

Figure 13.14. Same horse as in Figure 13.13, 7 months post injury. The entire wound has epithelialized. The skin is thin and brittle due to sparse subcutaneous tissue. Reprinted from Veterinary Clinics of North America, Vol 21, R. Reid Hanson, Management of burn injuries, p. 121, (2005), with permission from Elsevier.

following eschar removal allows for more rapid healing and superior pain relief, and prevents loss of heat, water, and protein-rich exudate from the wound surface. Burns involving only the superficial dermis heal well within 3 weeks and do not need grafting. Conversely, deep partial-thickness wounds require several months to heal, during which time bacterial contamination of the wound develops. Second-intention healing generates a thin and hairless epithelium which is vulnerable to trauma. Excision followed by grafting of the wound is recommended in these cases. Full-thickness grafts from a cadaver donor can be used as a dressing early in the clinical course of the burn to encourage healing, while split-thickness autogenous mesh grafts can be applied once healthy granulation tissue has formed. Early excision and grafting may also benefit horses that do not tolerate daily wound debridement and cleansing.

Conclusion

Extensive thermal injuries in horses can be difficult to manage. The large surface of the burn dramatically increases the potential for loss of fluids, electrolytes, and calories. Burns are classified according to the depth of injury: first degree burns involve only the most superficial layers of the epidermis; second degree burns involve the entire epidermis and can be superficial or deep; third degree burns are characterized by loss of the epidermal and dermal components; and fourth degree burns involve all of the skin and variable amounts of underlying muscle, bone, and ligaments.

Burns cause local and systemic effects. Routine use of systemic antibiotics is not recommended in burn patients. Topical medications should be water-based to facilitate cleaning and minimize toxicity. They are easily applied and removed, do not interfere with wound healing, and can be readily excreted or metabolized.

Weight loss of 10%–15% during the course of illness is indicative of inadequate nutritional intake. Gradually increasing the grain, adding fat in the form of vegetable oil, and offering free-choice alfalfa hay increase caloric intake.

During the past 2 decades, there have been many advances in burn therapy, including improved respiratory care, better use of topical and parenteral antibiotics, early debridement, and parenteral nutrition. HBO therapy is a promising treatment modality that has the potential to be an ideal supplemental therapy for burn injury and its associated complications in the horse.

References

1. Fubini SL: Burns. In N. Edward Robinson ed. *Current therapy in equine medicine (2nd edition)*. Philadelphia: WB Saunders, 1987, p.639
2. Fox SM: Management of a large thermal burn in a horse. Comp Cont Educ Pract Vet 1988;10:88
3. Baxter GM: Management of burns. In Pat Colahan, Ian Mayhew, Alferd Merritt, Jim Moore, eds. *Equine medicine and surgery (4th edition)*. Goleta: American Veterinary Publication Inc, 1991, p.1843
4. Warden GD: Outpatient care of thermal injuries. Surg Clin North Am 1987;67:147
5. Robson MC, Heggars JP: Pathophysiology of the burn wound. In Hugo Carvajal, Donald Parks, eds. *Burns in children—pediatric burn management (1st edition)*. St Louis, MO: Year Book Medical Publishers, 1988, p.27
6. Provost PJ: Thermal Injuries. In: Jorge Auer, John Stick, eds. *Equine surgery (2nd edition)*, Philadelphia: WB Saunders, 1999, p.179
7. Bietner R, Chem-Zion M, Sofer-Bassukevitz Y: Therapeutic and prophylactic treatment of skin burns with several calmodulin antagonists. Gen Pharm 1989;20:165
8. Marko P, Layon AJ, Caruso L, et al: Resuscitation and trauma anaesthesia. Curr Opin Anaesthesiol 2003;16:183
9. Carleton SC: Cardiac problems associated with burns. Cardiology Clin 1995;13:257
10. Dernling RH: Fluid replacement in burned patients. Surg Clin North Am 1987;67:15
11. Fox SM: Management of thermal burns, Part 1. Comp Cont Educ Pract Vet 1985;7:631
12. Till GO, Guilds LS, Mahroughi M: Role of xanthine oxidase in thermal injury of skin. Am J Pathol 1989;135:195
13. Johnston DE. Burns: Electrical, chemical and cold injuries. In Doug Slatter, ed. *Textbook of small animal surgery (1st edition)*. Philadelphia: WB Saunders, 1985, p.516
14. Hansbrough JF, Zapata O, Sirvent RI, et al: Immunomodulation following burn injury. Surg Clin North Am 1987;67:69
15. Church D, Elsayed S, Winston B, et al: Burn wound infections. Clin Microbiol Rev 2006;19:403
16. Herndon DN, Curreri PW, Abston S: Treatment of burns. Cur Probl Surg 1987;24:341
17. Gamelli RL: Nutritional problems of the acute and chronic burn patient. Arch Dermatol 1988;124:756
18. Young CJ, Moss J: Smoke inhalation: diagnosis and treatment. J Clin Anesth 1989;1:377
19. Mayes RW: ACP Broadsheet No. 142: Measurement of carbon monoxide and cyanide in blood. J Clin Pathol 1993;46:982
20. Walker HL, McLeod CG, McManus WF: Experimental inhalation injury in the goat. J Trauma 1981;21:962
21. LaLonde C, Demling R, Brain J: Smoke inhalation injury in sheep caused the particulate phase, not the gas phase. J Appl Physiol 1994;77:15
22. Nguyen TT, Gilpin DA, Meyer DA: Current treatment of severely burned patients. Ann Surg 1996;223:14
23. Geiser D, Walker RD: Management of large animal thermal injuries. Compend Cont Educ Pract Vet 1985;7:S69
24. Norman TE, Chaffin KM, Johnson MC: Intravascular hemolysis associated with severe cutaneous burn in five horses. J Am Vet Med Assoc 2005;226:2039
25. Fox SM, Goring RI, Probst CW: Management of thermal burn injuries, part II. Compend Cont Educ Pract Vet 1986;8:439
26. Schumacher J, Watkins JP, Wilson JP, et al: Burn-induced neoplasia in two horses. Equine Vet J 1986;18:410
27. Deitch EA: Nutritional support of the burn patient. Crit Care Clin 1995;11:735
28. Orsini, JA, Divers TJ: Burns and acute swelling. In Jim Orsini, Tom Divers, eds. *Manual of equine emergencies (2nd edition)*. Philadelphia: WB Saunders, 2003, p.300
29. Kemper T, Spier S, Barratt-Boyes SM, et al: Treatment of smoke inhalation in five horses. J Am Vet Med Assoc 1993;202:91
30. Muller MJ, Herndon DN: The challenge of burns. Lancet 1994;343:216
31. Brown M, Desai M, Traber LD: Dimethylsulfoxide with heparin in the treatment of smoke inhalation injury. J Burn Care Rehabil 1988;9:22

32. Cox CS Jr, Zwischenberger JB, Traber DL, et al: Heparin improves oxygenation and minimizes barotrauma after severe smoke inhalation in an ovine model. Surg Gynecol Obstet 1993;176:339

33. Kimura R, Traber L, Herndon D, et al: Ibuprofen reduces the lung lymph flow changes associated with inhalation injury. Circ Shock 1988;24:183

34. Herndon DN, Barrow RE, Traber DL, et al: Extravascular lung water changes following smoke inhalation and massive burn injury. Surg 1987;102:341

35. Maybauer MO, Maybauer DM, Traber LD, et al: Gentamicin improves hemodynamics in ovine septic shock after smoke inhalation injury. Shock 2005;24:226

36. Heimbach DM: Early burn excision and grafting. Surg Clinic North Am 1987;67:93

37. Fraser JF, Cuttle L, Kempf, et al: Cytotoxicity of topical antimicrobial agents used in burn wounds in Australasia. ANZ J Surg 2004;74:139

38. Atiyeh BS, Costagliola M, Shady N: Effect of silver on burn wound infection control and healing: Review of the literature. J Burn 2006;33:139

39. Hussain S, Ferguson C: Silver sulfadiazine creams in burns. Emerg Med J 2006;23:929

40. Monafo WW, Freedman B: Topical therapy for burns. Surg Clin North Am 1987;67:133

41. Swaim SF: Topical wound medications: A review. J Am Vet Med Assoc 1988;190:1588

42. Prince HN, Nonemaker WS, Norgard RC: Drug resistance studies with topical antiseptics. J Pharm Sci 1978;67:1629

43. Davidson JD, Siddiqui A, Mustoe TA: Ischemic tissue oxygen capacitance after oxygen therapy—new physiologic concept. Undersea Hyperbar Med 1996;23(suppl):57

44. Thom SR: Hyperbaric oxygen therapy. J Int Care Med 1989;4:58

45. Cianci P, Lueders H, Lee H, et al: Adjunctive hyperbaric oxygen reduces the need for surgery in 40–80% burns. J Hyperb Med 1988;3:97

46. Niu AKC, Yang C, Lee HC, et al: Burns treated with adjunctive hyperbaric oxygen therapy: a comparative study in humans. J Hyperb Med 1987;2:75

47. Brannen AL, Still J, Haynes MS, et al: A randomized prospective trial of hyperbaric oxygen in a referral burn center population. Undersea Hyperb Med 1995;22:(Suppl):11

14 Sarcoid Transformation at Wound Sites

Derek C. Knottenbelt, OBE, BVM&S, DVMS, Diplomate ECEIM, MRCVS

Introduction

Horses have been affected by sarcoids for centuries,[1] but the condition was first described by Jackson in 1936.[2] Sarcoids occur in all equine populations with a prevalence varying between 2% and 8%. This unique, benign fibroblastic tumor is by far the most prevalent skin neoplasm of horses. Other equidae, including donkeys, mules, and zebras, are also affected. Conversely, the role of sarcoid in wound healing failure has only recently come to light.[3]

The equine sarcoid has six different clinical manifestations that can be effectively correlated with the underlying pathology.[4]

Occult sarcoid: The mildest and most superficial form is called the occult form. It is characterized by a vague (often circular) change in the hair coat color or density. The epidermis is thickened and there is invariably at least one small nodule within the affected area.

Nodular sarcoid: The nodular form is solid and often spherical. Lesions of this type can vary widely in size and number; some involve the dermis while others are entirely subcutaneous.

Verrucose sarcoid: The verrucose form is "warty" in appearance and usually ill-defined. The size can vary widely from limited zones to extensive plaques.

Fibroblastic sarcoid: The fibroblastic form is fleshy and exophytic in appearance and is usually exudative and infected. Lesions can be pedunculated or sessile with a broad base. The latter type is that most commonly involved in wound healing problems.

Mixed sarcoid: Mixed sarcoids showing characteristics of several of the other types are relatively common, occurring both spontaneously and in association with certain types of wounds.

Malignant sarcoid: The malignant form is a rare and very dangerous expanding invasive tumor. It can arise spontaneously at some body sites and may also develop when a milder form (most often the fibroblastic type) is subjected to repeated inappropriate interference. While this form is rare, it can develop in sarcoid-contaminated wounds, especially if repeated surgeries are performed (usually in response to suspected exuberant granulation tissue).

Occult and nodular forms seldom have any relationship to wound healing, except where they are subjected to incomplete surgical removal or are directly traumatized by wounding episodes.

A high proportion of the sarcoid fibroblasts have papilloma viral genomic inclusions.[5,6,7] Attempts to replicate sarcoid occurrence by injection of various papilloma virus particles have resulted in the development of a transient sarcoid-like tumor with spontaneous resolution and seroconversion to the virus used.[8] This does not impart immunity to sarcoid development later in life. Although there have been numerous attempts to transplant sarcoid tissue and cells into different sites on the affected horse or to other genetically unrelated horses, transfer of sarcoid cells across the horse results, as might be expected, in a new sarcoid.

Transmission of cells between horses can result in development of classic sarcoid lesions with a typical natural history, but in others the cells are unable to survive. This is probably related to major histocompatibility (MHC)/equine leukocyte antigen (ELA) status of the individual.

The findings from the transmissibility and induction studies suggest that the virus implicated in the pathogenesis of sarcoid (bovine papilloma virus [BPV-1]) is not necessarily the major player in the epidemiology of the disease. Transfer of a cell from one site to another suitably receptive one on the same animal would likely result in cell survival and clonal replication. Also, it would seem likely that individual sarcoid cells would be transmissible between horses. However, a cell transferred from one animal to another (allograft) may or may not be viable, depending on the characteristics of the cells themselves and the extent of tissue compatibility between the donor and recipient. The precise placement of the grafted donor cell into subcutis, dermis, or epidermis will also have a significant influence on its survivability; unless the cell is placed in a suitably supportive "growth medium," it will not survive. However, it is certainly true that de novo sarcoids occur from time to time, and these are likely the result of virally induced genomic inclusion.

Horses have a reputation for non-healing wounds, particularly those involving the distal limb (carpus/tarsus and below). While the prevalence of non-healing (chronic or refractory) wounds is possibly higher than in other species, the reputation for non-healing may be exaggerated. Most equine wounds will heal if the clinical inhibitory factors such as infection, movement, necrotic tissue, foreign body, etc. are removed. However, when a wound is affected by a sarcoid, the healing process will inevitably be suspended, often indefinitely. Sarcoid transformation of wounds is therefore one of the most serious complications associated with skin wounds in horses.[3]

Both types of fibroblastic sarcoids and verrucous sarcoids are especially encountered as a complication of traumatic or surgical wound healing, but not exclusively, if sarcoids are present at other sites on the animal.[3,9,10,11] There are significant differences in the type of sarcoid that develops in wounds at different anatomical sites. Sarcoids developing in wounds on the trunk tend to be verrucous and tend to remain superficial, while those on the limbs tend toward the invasive, fibroblastic type.

Wounds affected by sarcoid transformation are often overlooked, mainly because of the visual similarity of the sarcoid tissue with granulation tissue or keloid/hypertrophic scar. The main clinical challenges are therefore centered on the recognition of sarcoid transformation in a wound and the lack of consistently effective treatment options for such circumstances.

This chapter will focus mainly on the clinical features of sarcoid transformation and the challenges of treating those wounds in which sarcoid is identified.

Etiopathogenesis

In naturally occurring and experimental wounds, the healing processes are instigated immediately (see Chapter 1, Physiology of Wound Healing). These healing processes are well defined and the mechanisms for graft-take are also known (Chapters 1, Physiology of Wound Healing, and 11, Free Skin Grafting). Both of these have important implications for sarcoid transformation and the processes required to manage the problem and heal the wound.

The size and type of wound that is susceptible to sarcoid transformation is not the major issue. Even small wounds such as injection sites and single insect bites can be transformed into non-healing, sarcoid-contaminated, chronic wounds. Surgical wounds can easily be affected either naturally or by accidental or inadvertent iatrogenic transfer of sarcoid tissue into the wound during surgery (e.g., castration sites).

The time scale for the development of sarcoid at a wound site is a major variable. In some cases, the transformation is obvious early in wound healing, while in others it may occur much later—even long after the wound has appeared to heal (months or years).

Sarcoid transformation within a wound can arise in several ways.

- Injury (traumatic or surgical) to sarcoid-affected skin. In this case the wound involves sarcoid tissue, and if the wound extends into normal skin adjacent to the sarcoid, the entire wound is susceptible to sarcoid development (Figure 14.1).
- Sarcoid development at a wound site in normal skin when there are sarcoids at other sites (Figure 14.2). In this case there is either transmission of sarcoid cells or (less convincingly) virus from the sarcoid site into the wound bed. Cell transfer from a sarcoid to a wound bed at another site could easily take place and the "autograft" of cells would result in a high probability of cell survival in the wound site. Vector transmission provides the only plausible explanation for this transfer, whether a virus or a transformed (tumorous) fibroblast is the accepted mechanism. There is no evidence to support a hematogenous dissemination of either sarcoid-transformed cells or virus or genomic particles of the virus.[12]
- Sarcoid transformation occurring at a wound site when there are no sarcoids at other sites but there is contact with horses having sarcoids (Figure 14.3). Here it is suggested that the sarcoid cells, or less convincingly, virus particles are transferred from a sarcoid site on another horse into the wound bed, probably by a vector. It is reasonable to suppose that this transmission would be less likely to permit development of a sarcoid by virtue of the reduced chance of tissue compatibility between the donor and the recipient. If the transfer involved a virus, then a predictable tumor resulting in clonal expansion would seem far less plausible. The rate of development of many sarcoids in wound beds is at odds with the possibility of transfer of virus particles.

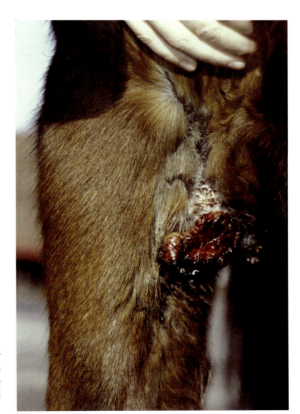

Figure 14.1. This horse sustained an accidental wire cut to its axilla over a site that was already affected by occult and verrucose sarcoid. The sarcoid had been quiescent for at least 4 years, but within weeks of the relatively trivial injury the region had deteriorated badly into a deep and invasive fibroblastic lesion.

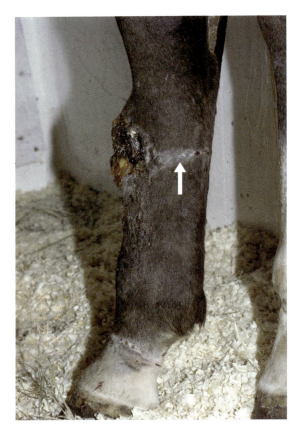

Figure 14.2. This circumferential laceration around the mid-cannon region healed remarkably well except for the area dorsally. The horse had several other occult and verrucose sarcoids on the medial thigh and axillary regions. Several attempts were made to excise the "granulation tissue" and graft the early "granulating" wound bed after each procedure. Histological examination of the granulation tissue obtained from each debridement later confirmed that the tissue was in fact almost pure fibroblastic sarcoid. Note the remarkably good healing that had taken place away from the sarcoid region (white arrow).

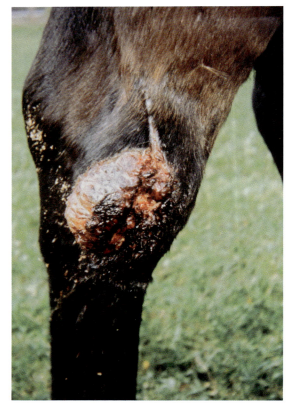

Figure 14.3. This horse sustained a deep laceration to the lateral aspect of the hock. The wound healed along most of its length but was slow to close at the distal extent. The proximal scar can be appreciated. Two attempts were made to excise the "granulation tissue." Fortunately, the tissues from each excision had been retained in formalin solution and when these were submitted, a mixture of sarcoid and infected granulation tissue was identified histologically. The horse had no other sarcoids and there were no cattle in the vicinity. However, two other horses in the same field had several small ulcerated fibroblastic/nodular sarcoids and several verrucose lesions each.

- A wounded horse is in contact with a source of bovine papilloma virus (BPV) (usually infected cattle). It seems highly improbable that the virus allegedly responsible for sarcoids is transmitted from a bovine papilloma into the wound bed to induce a predictable clonal tumor transformation. The virus is possibly ubiquitous and there is no material difference between horses with sarcoids and those without sarcoids in the detection of virus on the skin.[13]

  Iatrogenic transfer of sarcoid into a surgical site can occur when surgical instruments (or even hypodermic needles) are used at a sarcoid site and then for a surgical procedure at another site (Figure 14.4).

- Failure to remove all sarcoid cells during surgical treatment of sarcoids. In this case both residual sarcoids and cells released into the wound bed are responsible for recurrence. Exacerbation is common under these circumstances and this may explain why it occurs following biopsy (Figures 14.5a, 14.5b).

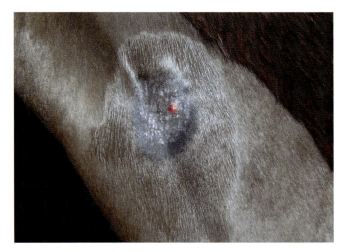

Figure 14.4. This verrucose sarcoid with occult skin changes in a roughly circular shape developed at the site of an intravenous injection. The same needle had been used to infiltrate this site with local anesthetic solution immediately after infiltration of a sarcoid site prior to biopsy. The lesion developed over a period of 5 weeks; there was no evidence at all of a pre-existing sarcoid at this site.

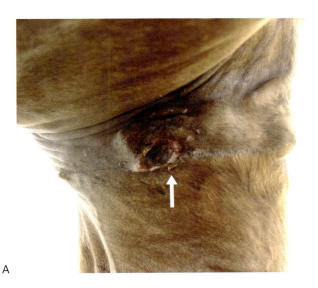

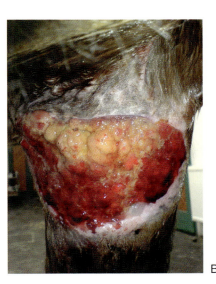

A

B

Figure 14.5. (A) This horse had been subjected to surgical excision of an axillary sarcoid some 8 months prior to photo. A second attempt was made to remove the lesion in the center of the scar (arrow). (B) Wound dehiscence and massive exacerbation developed over the ensuing months.

The time required for this to occur is very unpredictable. Wound dehiscence, failure of the wound to epithelialize, a lack of wound contraction, or any combination of these may be indicators of recurrence of the disease.

Larger wounds may be more susceptible to the development of sarcoids than smaller wounds in the following situations: (a) in normal skin when there are sarcoids at other sites, (b) in a wound site when there are no other wounds but there is contact with horses having sarcoids, or (c) a wounded horse is in contact with a source of BPV (usually infected cattle). Although needle puncture sites can develop sarcoid complications (Figure 14.4), small wounds heal more quickly and so it would seem that the risk of a prolonged exposure to vector transmissions is less likely overall than in a large open wound that is left exposed for a longer time. The anatomic proximity of a sarcoid to a wound can have an influence on the likelihood of sarcoid transformation (Figures 14.6a, 14.6b), but this may depend more on the feeding behavior of possible vectors.

A high fly population in warm, still weather results in far more fly activity on the horse. Flies prefer to feed on sarcoids, especially if they are ulcerated. A wound occurring nearer an open sarcoid lesion clearly provides a better chance of cell survival if transfer takes place via the fly (Figures 14.7a, 14.7b). Biting flies appear to have a reduced tendency to transfer sarcoid cells to wounds because they do not prefer to feed on ulcerated tissue.

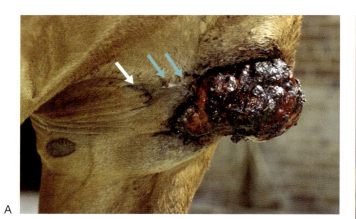

A

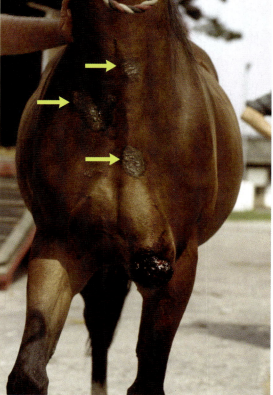

B

Figure 14.6. (A) This pony sustained a wire laceration across the front of the left shoulder. The white arrow points to the scar. The wound appeared to heal well at first, but around 4 weeks post injury an "exuberant granulation tissue mass" developed at the most lateral extent of the wound. Several smaller fibroblastic growths developed along the wound site shortly afterwards (blue arrows). (B) Clinical examination showed the main bulk to be very extensive subcutaneously and identified several occult and verrucose sarcoids in the adjacent regions (yellow arrows). Biopsy confirmed the main mass and the smaller ones to be pure sarcoid.

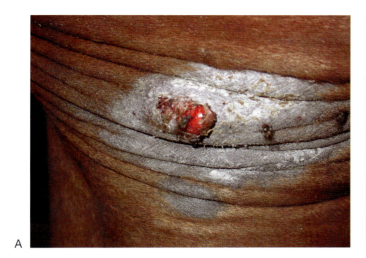
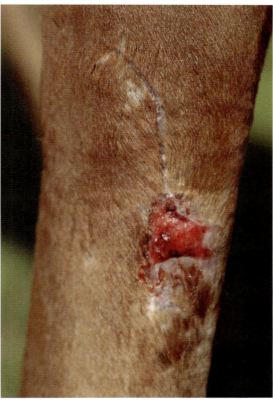

Figure 14.7. (A) The sarcoid illustrates the preferential feeding pattern of certain species of fly for sarcoid tissue (note the flies present in the photo). (B) This horse sustained a minor injury to the medial metatarsal region that failed to heal in a localized area. Biopsy of the site was undertaken because of the presence of sarcoid at other sites, and it revealed almost pure sarcoid features. Flies were noted by the owner to move between the fresh wound site and the sarcoid.

When sarcoids are diagnosed on the limbs of horses there is a high probability that a wound (e.g., ranging from a minor abrasion to a full-thickness laceration) was present first; spontaneous sarcoid development does not commonly occur in the limb regions below the femoro-tibial joint (stifle) and the humero-radial joint (elbow) in the absence of skin trauma.

Flies have been implicated in the epidemiology of sarcoids; it is possible that they act as vectors for the BPV particles. Transferring the virus to the wound bed, however, would be most unlikely to result in the predictable development of a fibroblastic tumor within a relatively short time period. Simple infection of a fibroblast with the virus should result in random integration of the genome and therefore a random set of cell clones with different properties. In reality, the pattern of integration is clonal; this can only occur if the cells are identically affected (i.e., they were a clonal expansion of a single transformed cell). It seems far more likely that the sarcoid-transformed cell is transferred physically from a sarcoid site to a wound site. In this event, the anatomic location of the wound has an important bearing on the type of sarcoid induced. Transfer of tumor cells to limb wounds (e.g., elbow/stifle and below) tends to induce fibroblastic sarcoids (Figure 14.8), while body and neck wounds more commonly develop verrucous sarcoid (Figure 14.9).[3,11]

This may relate to local factors rather than any particular feature of the cell itself. It is well known that wounds on the trunk heal by contraction, while those on the limb tend to heal more by epithelialization. However, this is not a matter of any obvious cellular differences in the fibroblasts responsible for contraction. Rather, it is suggested that this is due to local effects (see Chapter 1).

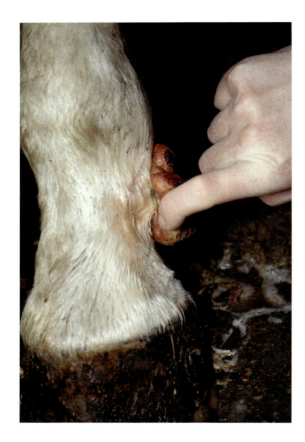

Figure 14.8. A pedunculated sarcoid developed at one of a number of small wire wound sites that had occurred several months previously. The horse had several other superficial sarcoids in the head and axilla. Diagnosis was confirmed upon biopsy.

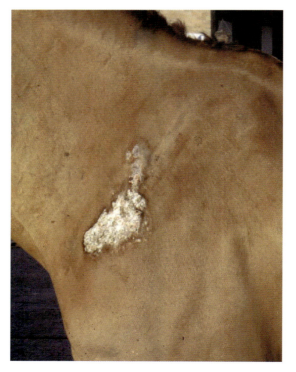

Figure 14.9. This horse sustained a large degloving wound on its shoulder from a fall. The horse had several types of sarcoids at other sites. The wound appeared to heal reasonably well but was left with this verrucose area that was confirmed histologically as sarcoid.

Clinical Aspects

A detailed general history of the horse and a specific history of the wound should be obtained at the outset. It is important to establish concurrent or previous sarcoid involvement. Even if treatment has appeared to be effective, the horse will remain genetically prone to the disease. Moreover, it is easy to overlook in-contact animals, yet a brief but focused summary of these can help, especially if any has sarcoids. Given the familial tendencies to sarcoids, related horses may be particularly important epidemiologically. Horses with sarcoids at other sites are far more likely to have this complication than those without, but close contact with an affected horse may be a significant factor.

Wounds occurring during summer (fly season) are far more predisposed to sarcoid involvement, and the longer the wound remains uncovered the greater the opportunity for transformation to take place (Figure 14.10). In the author's experience, contact with cattle is not a common feature of sarcoid-contaminated wounds; it is extremely unlikely that direct viral infection can or will result in sarcoid development at a wound site.

A physical examination should always be carried out because concurrent factors such as infection, movement, impaired local blood supply, necrotic tissue, or foreign bodies can inhibit wound healing, and small sarcoids can be detected at other sites that may have been overlooked.

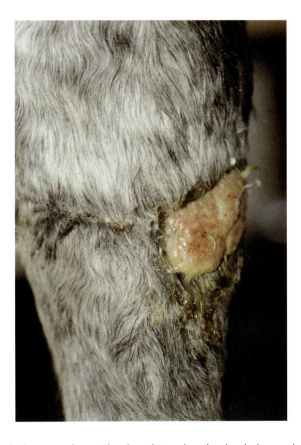

Figure 14.10. Most of this horizontal wire wound over the dorsal tarsal region healed remarkably well following excellent wound care, despite a 3-day delay in seeking veterinary attention. However, the medial limit failed to heal over many months, and perhaps justifiably, suspecting the problem to be exuberant granulation tissue, several vain attempts at surgical debridement and even an attempt at pinch grafting were performed. It was diagnosed with sarcoid upon biopsy. The lesion had a broad flat (sessile) base. The horse had no other sarcoids but several in-contact horses were affected.

Sarcoid transformation at wound sites is recognized in several forms.

- A common feature of sarcoid-contaminated wounds is early wound dehiscence for no apparent reason. Often the suture line breaks down in spite of careful closure and excellent wound management. This can occur within days of wounding if the wound is left uncovered and is attacked by flies. The problem seems to be more likely if the horse has ulcerated sarcoids at other sites. Use of a delayed primary closure technique may increase the opportunity for deposition of transformed cells in the wound bed. Any unexpected wound breakdown should alert the clinician to the possibility of sarcoid transformation.
- Following surgical excision of sarcoid tumors, any healing delay or wound dehiscence usually indicates that sarcoid tissue remains in the wound bed, even if the wound eventually appears to heal. More commonly, the wound left to heal by second intention does not show the normal healing tendency; static or indolent wound beds or even expanding surgical sites can occur when sarcoid cells are still present (Figure 14.10). Recurrence at such sites can occur at any time in the future, from days to many years.[9] Laser surgery may reduce the risks of recurrence,[14] but these recurrences remain a significant factor in all surgical sites involving known sarcoid tissue, whether left to heal by second intention or closed surgically.

  Although the earliest signs of sarcoid transformation/involvement in wound sites are subtle (wound breakdown, unhealthy granulation tissue, or lack of wound contraction), later evidence is far more obvious. Delays in the management of granulation tissue beyond the period when the wound bed reaches the epithelial level or repeated attempts to excise exuberant granulation tissue that fails to resolve the problem will result in much more obvious sarcoid development. The value of diagnostic pathology in cases in which granulation tissue is excised cannot be overstated; if a sarcoid is detected it will require a significant change in the management plan and the prognosis of the case.
- There are some anatomic differences in the clinical manifestations of sarcoids; limb wounds appear to have a greater tendency to develop fibroblastic sarcoids, either the type 1 (pedunculated) fibroblastic form or the type 2 (sessile) fibroblastic sarcoid (Figure 14.10). In contrast, the trunk and neck have a greater tendency to develop verrucose, or less commonly, occult sarcoid forms (Figures 14.4 and 14.9). On the head, either fibroblastic or verrucose sarcoids can develop in the wound sites. The anatomic differences coincide with the known facts that wound contraction is less obvious on the limb than on the body wounds and exuberant granulation tissue is more common in wounds of the distal limb (carpus/tarsus and below) than it is in wounds of the trunk. These regional differences in normal healing are attributed to local factors rather than any particular differences in fibroblast behavior[15] and it seems likely that the same local factors influence the behavior of the sarcoid-transformed fibroblasts. However, the specific factors responsible for these anatomic differences with respect to sarcoids are far from clear.

Identification

In the earliest stages it is often impossible to recognize sarcoid transformation at a wound site. Granulation tissue and bacterial pyogranuloma can appear remarkably similar to a wound that is either exclusively sarcoid or one that contains sarcoid tissue in addition to micro-abscessation and granulation tissue (Figures 14.11a–c). Similarly, a keloid or hypertrophic scar can easily be mistaken for a verrucose sarcoid and vice versa (Figures 14.11d, 14.11e).

The management of exuberant granulation tissue and sarcoids are very different and it is therefore important to establish whether a sarcoid is involved in a non-healing wound. The development of nodular sarcoids within wound beds is rare, although the fibroblastic form may have a generally nodular appearance.

Martens, et al.[16] described a polymerase chain reaction (PCR) method for the identification of sarcoid cells taken by swabbing the suspected sarcoid lesions. It is reasonable to expect that this method would be very helpful in the detection of sarcoid cells in wound beds, no matter how few of them there were, but it is not widely available as a commercial procedure.

Identification of sarcoid lesions (of any of the recognized six types)[4] at other sites on the body should immediately alert the clinician to the possibility of sarcoid transformation in a wound.

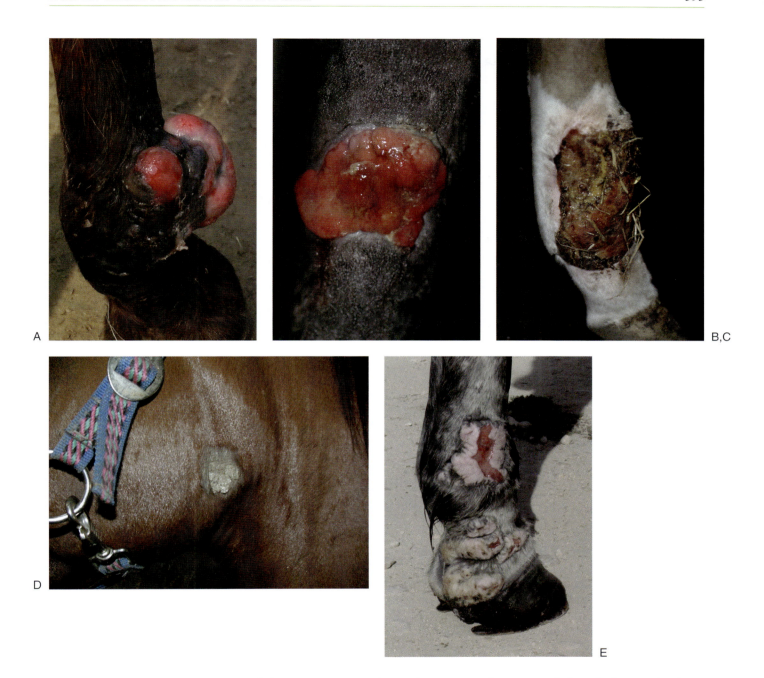

Figure 14.11. The clinical appearance of the more common primary changes occurring at wound sites. Each example shown developed in a wound. (A) Fibroblastic sarcoid. (B) Exuberant granulation tissue. (C) Pseudomycetoma/pyogranuloma. (D) Verrucose sarcoid. (E) Keloid/hypertrophic scar.

Differential Diagnosis of Sarcoid-Contaminated Wounds

The differential diagnosis of sarcoid transformation is complicated by the fact that there may be admixtures of granulation tissue, scar tissue, and infection within the wound. In some cases sarcoids can be suspected, and in a few, sarcoid transformation is quite obvious to an experienced clinician. However, the majority of cases are difficult to diagnose, at best. The differential diagnoses for equine sarcoids in wound sites include:

- (Exuberant) granulation tissue (Figure 14.11b)
- Staphylococcal pyogranuloma (Pseudomycetoma) (Figure 14.11c)

Table 14.1. Main differentiating clinical features for sarcoid-affected wounds.

	Fibroblastic sarcoid	Granulation tissue	Pyogranuloma/ pseudomycetoma	Verrucose sarcoid	Keloid/hypertrophic scar
Appearance	Figure 14.11a	Figure 14.11b	Figure 14.11c	Figure 14.11d	Figure 14.11e
Keratinization	No	No	No	Yes	Yes
Proliferation	Yes	Yes	Yes	Possible	Yes
Ulceration	Yes	Yes	Yes	No	No
Vascularization	High	High	Moderate	Low	Low
Exudation	Yes	Yes	Yes/Low	No	No
Bacterial culture	Mixed commensals	Mixed pathogens/ commensals	Staphylococci	Commensals only	Commensals only

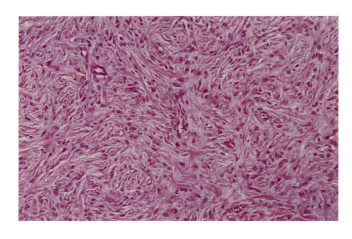

Figure 14.12. The histological appearance of the equine sarcoid, demonstrating the characteristic whorling patterns of the fibroblasts and the random/chaotic arrangements of the capillaries. There is little extracellular matrix and the mitotic index is very low, despite a clinically rapid growth rate.

- Fungal granuloma (e.g., Pythium spp., Conidiobolus coronata, etc.)
- Foreign body granuloma
- Keloid scars, which can closely resemble verrucose sarcoids (Figure 14.11e)

Various features enable differentiation of these clinical conditions (Table 14.1).

Pathology

Histologic examination of the tissues excised from a normally healing wound characteristically reveals organizing granulation tissue with a well recognized parallel arrangement of new blood vessels (Figure 1.6). The process where by this tissue is formed has been outlined in Chapter 1, and certainly it is well recognized by pathologists. Although granulation tissue from a chronic, granulating, non-healing wound may exhibit some possible causative factors (e.g., bacterial or fungal infection, foreign matter, necrotic tissue, etc.), the normal underlying structure of the granulating wound bed is invariably recognizable.

The histologic appearance of sarcoids, both within a wound site and in other sites, is well documented.[17] There is little difference in the histologic features between sarcoids at wound sites and those occurring without the history of a wound at the site, except where admixtures of sarcoid and granulation tissue occur. Histologic characteristics include fibroblastic proliferation with cells arranged in a whorling pattern (Figure 14.12). Random or chaotic fibroblast arrangements are common. The fibroblasts themselves can show anisocytosis (abnormal variations in cell size) and anisokaryosis (abnormal variation in nuclear size in the cells). Mitoses can be variable in number but usually they are low or rare. The extent and features of the extracellular matrix also vary.

The absence of overlying epithelium in tissues taken from ulcerated fungating sarcoid lesions can cause a diagnostic challenge in some cases. The first descriptions of the equine sarcoid were made by Jackson, who in 1936 identified a variable epithelial component to the typical sarcoid.[2] Skilled pathologists usually have little difficulty in recognizing the full range of sarcoid types, even in the absence of epidermis. The diagnosis is, however, heavily dependent on the collection of a truly representative sample of tissue and this is a major problem in many cases in which sarcoid and granulation tissue are admixed.

Biopsies taken by shaving off the surface of a granulating wound bed can be misleading and may show infected, ulcerated granulation tissue only. A far better representation of the true nature of the non-healing tissues is obtained by a core biopsy taken into the depth of the tissue. Deep core biopsies may reveal sequential "layers" of sarcoid and granulation tissue or nests of sarcoid tumor cells. Sampling of only one tissue type or inappropriate histologic preparation of the sections may therefore be deceptive; a single small biopsy may show only sarcoid, only pyogranuloma, or only granulation tissue. Treatment based on the biopsy alone may therefore be wrong. It is thus very important to examine the lesion closely and if necessary obtain several deep biopsies using a wide biopsy punch (6 mm–8 mm) if at all possible; this will maximize the chances of a correct diagnosis.

Biopsy technique is important. The site should not be scrubbed or otherwise molested. It is not usually necessary to use local anesthesia (both sarcoid and granulation tissue are usually free of nerve endings). If a remote nerve block can be performed, then that is preferred to local infiltration that commonly causes severe inflammation within minutes. A suspicious area of granulation tissue, such as denser nodular region, should be sampled. More commonly, it is not possible to identify a site, so several 6 mm–8 mm biopsy punch samples should be taken from the central portion of the tissue, with each one placed in an individual pot of formalin solution. It is useful to photograph the sites so that the pathologist can see what was sampled at each site. Samples taken from the skin margin are not usually very helpful; moreover, they are ill-advised because the tumor will be encouraged to extend further into the normal skin. Small lesions can be subjected to excisional biopsy with the precautions outlined below in Treatment/Management. Verrucous changes in wound sites are biopsied in the same way, although in many of these the skin edge could be included.

The value of biopsy cannot be overstated. The findings will influence the therapeutic approach and the prognosis. In all cases in which "granulation tissue" is removed during wound management, all excised tissue should be submitted. Sometimes a morphological diagnosis of fibroma, fibropapilloma, neurofibroma, neurofibrosarcoma, Schwannoma, low-grade fibrosarcoma, or spindle cell tumors of various types is made because of the variations in matrix type and staining characteristics. This should not divert the clinician from a diagnosis of sarcoid transformation because the behavior of the cells within the wound bed is variable and affected by many other concurrent problems including infection, foreign body, necrotic tissue, movement, etc.

Co-involvement of sarcoid and granulation tissue occurs with some frequency. Regardless of the amount of sarcoid tissue found in the wound, it is clear that it will inhibit healing. Although the physiological processes involved are not yet known, preliminary findings suggest that angiogenesis and fibroplasia are supported, whereas epithelial cell replication is specifically inhibited. The selective support and inhibition is likely mediated either by alterations in the cytokines expressed by the transformed fibroblasts or a secondary effect that alters the natural cytokine profile in the wound, biasing it toward the same situation as a chronic non-healing wound.[10] This may explain the truly fibroblastic and hemorrhagic nature of many cases showing sarcoid-contaminated granulation tissue.

Treatment/Management

Clinical management of "normal" sarcoids is a considerable challenge, and this is significantly increased when the condition afflicts a wound site. The fact that there are many suggested treatments for a sarcoid probably indicates that none is ideal in every circumstance. The options for treatment of wounds affected by sarcoid transformation are even less promising. At the present time it is hard to envision a treatment that would preferentially destroy sarcoid fibroblasts while leaving the normal cells intact. The implications of this are that whatever method is employed must destroy or remove all affected sarcoid cells because residual cells replicate and a new sarcoid will develop. It is widely recognized that recurrences tend to be more aggressive than the first population of sarcoid cells.

The conflict between treatment in which normal cell behavior needs to be encouraged and nurtured and the requirement for destruction of tumor cells in sarcoids underlines the critical need for an appropriate diagnosis. The difficulty of managing a complex mixture of sarcoid and granulation tissue in a wound is therefore a major clinical problem. Indeed, the current best practice for management of unhealthy or exuberant granulation tissue (surgical debridement, topical antibiotics and steroids, wound dressings, and grafting) is specifically contra-indicated in the management of most sarcoid lesions.

Unless a sarcoid tumor can be totally removed, its growth will recur. Attempts to skin graft a sarcoid-affected wound site will always fail. Similarly, repeated excision of sarcoid or sarcoid-containing granulation tissue will simply result in recurrence and more usually exacerbation. *Surgical excision of sarcoid must be complete.*

Management of injuries involving skin affected by a sarcoid is invariably difficult. Not only does the skin lack its normal elasticity and healing properties, but the wound site may well have been seeded with sarcoid cells—each of which results in a clonal expansion and further sarcoid tumors.

The anatomic site involved has a major bearing on the choice of treatment as well as the prognosis. Management of normal wounds is problematic, and this is more so in limb wounds. It is not surprising, then, that sarcoid-contaminated limb wounds are one of the most demanding therapeutic challenges in wound management. Currently available treatment options include:

- Surgery: surgical excision, cryosurgery, laser surgery, and combinations of surgical treatments
- Immunomodulatory therapy (using foreign/exogenous proteins such as Bacillus Calmette-Guerin, Regressin®, Equimune®, etc.)
- Topical or intralesional cytotoxic/antimitotic/caustic chemicals
- Photodynamic therapy
- Radiation
- Homeopathy/natural medicines

Surgery

Surgical methods, including skin grafting of various forms, are commonly used to manage granulating wounds. Before embarking on any such procedure the surgeon is strongly advised to consider whether a sarcoid involves the wound bed. If it does, skin grafting and surgical debridement will invariably fail (Figure 14.13).

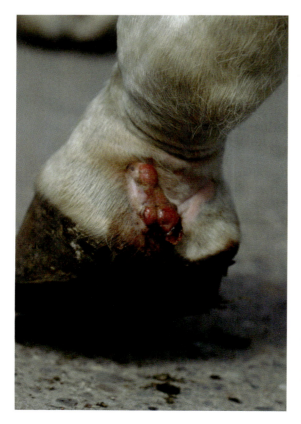

Figure 14.13. Multiple fibroblastic sarcoids developed at the site of a wire wound over the palmar pastern/heel bulb region. The injury had occurred some months previously; although part of the wound healed rapidly, this area had failed to heal. Pinch grafts were used after surgical debridement of the granulation tissue on three occasions, but failed to help. The horse had no other sarcoids and no contact with cattle.

Sharp Surgery

Surgical excision alone of a sarcoid-transformed wound site is usually unsuccessful and recurrence of the tumor is very common for a number of reasons. Probably the most significant are:

- Anatomic limitations: Very often, insufficient skin is available, after excision, to close the wound. Additionally, distal limb wounds affected by sarcoid tissue are commonly over joints or tendons/ligaments, which limits the opportunities for complete excision with suitable margins. There is little that the surgeon can do to overcome these anatomic limitations, although skin grafting of the operative site may be considered if a large area of tissue is exposed.
- Sarcoid tissue is frequently invasive in wounds, making it impossible to define a safe excisional margin that will ensure removal of all sarcoid tissue (even when anatomical limitations are not restrictive). This problem can be minimized by careful selection of cases and by ensuring that the sarcoid has not had any previous clinical or other ill-advised interference that might have encouraged a wider dissemination of the sarcoid tissues. Owners (and regrettably, some veterinarians) frequently attempt to manage the wound without any consideration of the implications of such interference, which may simply exacerbate the risks associated with any treatment, especially surgical removal.
- The operative site can be seeded with sarcoid cells from the incised lesion or directly from "rub-off" from the surface of an ulcerated lesion during surgical handling. Covering the exposed ulcerated sarcoid-contaminated tissue with a gauze swab or a plastic aerosol dressing is a wise precaution, as is the use of the "one cut, one blade" principle of "clean surgery." In this technique, each instrument is used only once and then discarded. This applies to surgical blades, scissors, forceps, and suture material/needles. This will at least limit the risks of direct cell transfer across the wound site. Laser surgery reduces the risks of this problem. An alternative to covering the exposed contaminated ulcerated sarcoid is to remove it to just below the skin level using electrosurgery, after which the site is prepared for surgical excision. Using separate gloves and instruments and the previously described principle of "clean surgery" prior to excision remains fundamental to success.

Sharp surgical excision of a sarcoid is not discriminatory unless the precise margin of the tumor can be defined and a safe excision margin, one that will ensure removal of all sarcoid-contaminated tissues without compromising the natural anatomy of the involved region, is identified. Failure to remove every cell of the tumor will result in recurrence along the wound scar (Figure 14.14).

In a few circumstances the surgeon may, however, differentiate larger or smaller masses of sarcoid tissue and may be fortunate enough to visualize the true margins of the tumor. It is clearly impossible to discriminate between normal tissue and sarcoid during routine surgery without the benefit of intraoperative frozen section pathology, so a high chance of failure remains. To overcome this problem to some extent, a wider margin of excision can sometimes be achieved but the excessive removal of healthy tissues has the potential to delay or complicate healing.

Adjunctive measures to surgery are used in some countries where the combined sarcoid-granulation tissue bed is surgically excised and the resulting wound bed cauterized by direct thermal cautery or cryosurgical necrosis. Although this may seem harsh and crude, the results are anecdotally reported to be

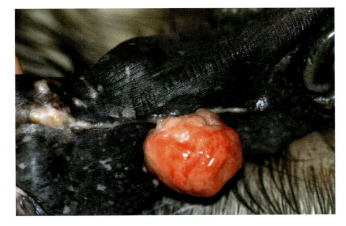

Figure 14.14. A nodular type sarcoid was removed from the penile skin some 10 weeks previously with laser surgery. Most of the wound healed well but this fibroblastic lesion developed in the wound scar. The possibilities of "cell seeding" or residual "root" were considered. The laser surgery was repeated with good results.

acceptable and better than surgical excision alone; this probably reflects the importance of preventing deposition of viable sarcoid cells in the wound bed. Other adjunctive measures to surgery will be described in the subsequent sections.

Cryosurgery

Cryonecrosis achieved by rapid freezing to temperatures below −35°C followed by slow thawing after each freeze (freeze-thaw cycle) has been used widely for many years in the management of both sarcoid tumors[18] and, regrettably, exuberant granulation tissue. The procedure is described in standard surgical texts and it should, by rights, work well. However, defining the margin of the affected tissue and ensuring that the freeze extends to this point is always difficult, even when a defined sarcoid is present, let alone when sarcoid and granulation tissue are mixed. The method is not discriminatory—both normal and neoplastic tissues are destroyed and extensive tissue necrosis necessarily follows treatment. Given that necrosis is an undesirable feature of wound healing, poor overall results are typically achieved. The requirement for repeated procedures adds to the shortcomings of this method.

Cryosurgery has also been used in an adjunctive fashion to cauterize the wound bed subsequent to surgical debulking of the sarcoid or sarcoid-granulation complex on the premise that cryonecrosis is easier to achieve when the bulk of the abnormal tissue has been removed. Hemorrhage at the site is a significant complication, however, and the method, either as an adjunctive treatment or a sole treatment, has little to commend it in the management of fibroblastic-sarcoid–contaminated wounds.

Cryoantigen-induced regression of sarcoids at remote sites has been described,[19] but this report makes no specific comment on the effects of performing the procedure on a remote lesion to influence the behavior of sarcoid tissue in a transformed wound. The author has not observed this effect and it is unreasonable to expect a benefit/cure in a sarcoid-contaminated wound following treatment of another remote sarcoid with cryosurgery.

Laser Surgery

Laser surgical excision/ablation has been described[20,21] and is a relatively acceptable technique because the wound margins are not seeded with sarcoid cells during the procedure. Either CO_2-YAG laser or diode laser can be used. Apart from the described advantages, the method has the same constraints as other surgical therapies in that it is impossible to ascertain that all of the sarcoid has been removed. Laser excision of granulation tissue alone boasts some advantages over sharp surgery from the reduced blood loss and from the extra "die back" at the margin of the excision site as damaged cells along the margin are sloughed. Although this may delay healing, it is unlikely to be significant compared to the effects of residual sarcoid tissue within the wound bed. Laser surgery in non-wound–related sarcoids is reported to carry a high chance of success[21] but its use in sarcoid-affected wounds is not reported.

Destruction of residual sarcoid cells in the wound bed with wide/extensive superficial laser exposure may reduce the recurrence rate but will also damage normal cells. There is merit in this process, however, because sarcoid cells are very damaging to the healing process and commonly result in recurrence and exacerbation.

Immunomodulatory Therapy

Immunotherapy

Exogenous proteins derived largely from *Bacillus* spp. bacteria ([BCG]/Regressin®/Equimune®) have been used for many years in the treatment of neoplastic conditions including equine sarcoid.[22,23,24] It has been suggested that the mechanism of action is related to altered immune cell function.[25] There are no specific reports of its use in the management of sarcoid-contaminated wound beds. However, there have been suggestions that it is more effective in treating periocular sarcoids and much less effective on the distal limb. Indeed, there is a possibility that the method is contraindicated on sarcoid-containing wound beds on the limbs below the elbow and stifle.[26] For as yet unexplained reasons, there is a possibility of active bacterial replication if the live bacillus is injected into wound sites contaminated with sarcoid, on the distal limb in particular. This is a very serious complication and may reflect localized or general immunological compromise. In the author's experience this method is an unwise choice in any case.

Combinations of treatment are probably more likely to bring success than any single one. Recent reports have suggested that the use of intralesional injections of Interleukin-2 (IL-2) in conjunction with intralesional cisplatin for naturally occurring sarcoids carries better prognosis than when either is used alone. However, this report makes no mention of sarcoid-contaminated wounds.[26]

Autogenous Vaccines

There is a full range of irrational immunologically-based approaches, including autogenous vaccines manufactured from macerated cells taken from the wound bed/sarcoid and "magic" treatments using blood extracted from the horse and "treated" in some undefined manner before being injected back into the horse. None of these treatments has any clinical rationale or therapeutic benefit. Indeed, it is possible that many cases are in fact exacerbated by these therapies.[26-29] However, there are some reports of regression in a limited number of lesions treated in this way.[30] The possible use of vaccines in sarcoid-contaminated wounds, as opposed to naturally occurring sarcoids, has not been reported. The sudden and complete spontaneous disappearance of "naturally occurring" sarcoids in 1%–5% of cases is a recognized phenomenon;[9] this implies that an immunological approach could be exploited. However, this is not, in the author's experience, a feature of sarcoid-contaminated wounds of any variety in any location.

Topical or Intralesional Cytotoxic/Antimitotic/Caustic Chemicals

Topical Chemotherapy

Many topical agents such as inorganic (heavy) metal salts (arsenic, antimony and zinc salts, silver nitrate), plant extracts (such as *Sanguineus canadensis*) often mixed with metal salts such as zinc chloride, and modern antimitotic compounds such as 5-fluorouracil and retinoids such as tazarotene, have been used to treat sarcoids for many years. Some of these, such as the material being tested at Liverpool University (named AW4-LUDES) may be applicable to some sarcoid-transformed wounds (Figures 14.15a–d).

Nevertheless, most are unsuitable for sarcoid-contaminated wounds because of their non-discriminatory and caustic necrotizing nature. Conventional surgical, laser surgical, or cryosurgical debulking of a large sarcoid-contaminated mass from a wound will clearly help by reducing the amount of topical material used and the depth it has to penetrate to be effective.

The best approach using the topical compounds is therefore to debulk the lesion by any suitable surgical means and then (usually after 24–36 hours to stem hemorrhage) to apply a gentle but effective topical therapy such as 5% 5-fluorouracil to the wound bed (twice daily for 7 days, then once daily for 7 days is a recommended course in the author's experience). This relatively gentle approach allows the 5-fluorouracil cream to penetrate the wound bed and hopefully reduce the number of residual active sarcoid cells. Unfortunately, in common with steroid-based creams (which can also be used in some circumstances), there is an obvious deleterious effect on the natural inflammatory processes upon which wound healing relies.

The use of stronger, caustic materials such as copper sulfate, silver nitrate, and herbal extracts such as *XXTERRA*® (Indian mud [*Sanguineus canadensis*/blood root extract] with zinc chloride) can be tried, but this author does not recommend these for either sarcoids or sarcoid-contaminated wounds. The efficacy is low and some have a highly destructive nature. Others simply exacerbate the condition. Topical application of AW4-LUDES, based on a combination of heavy metals (in low concentrations) with a high concentration of 5-fluorouracil and natural oils, is currently under trial at Liverpool University. This author has used this approach for many years with good results (Figure 14.15). Although there have also been enough failures to encourage further development, it is relatively easy and economical and carries a reasonable success rate (around 58%). The inadequacy of all available topical treatments underscores the need to develop more effective topical and systemic methods of eliminating sarcoid cells from wound beds.

Intralesional Chemotherapy

Intralesional administration of an antimitotic or cytotoxic material minimizes adverse systemic effects associated with chemotherapeutic agents normally delivered intravenously in large doses, while providing for exposure of tumor cells to high concentrations of the chemotherapeutic agent. Treatment of naturally occurring

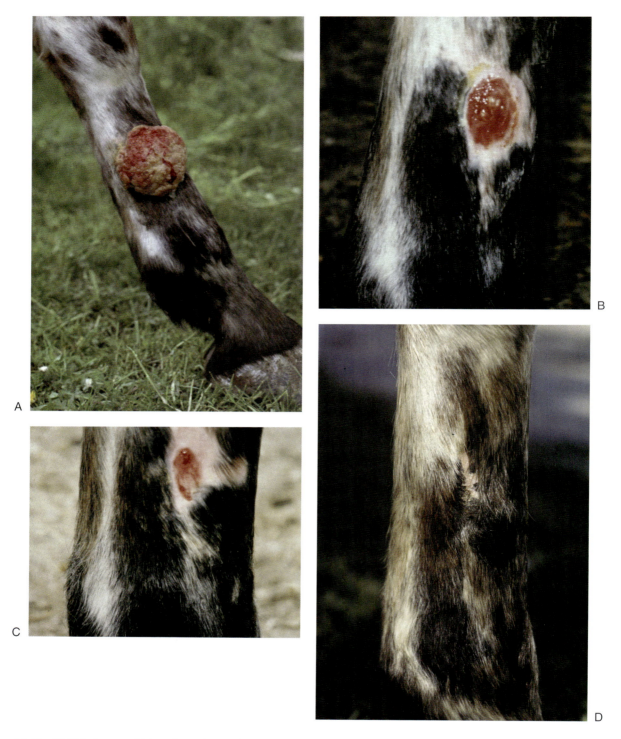

Figure 14.15. (A) This 8-year-old Appaloosa horse developed a fibroblastic sarcoid in a wound site on the dorsolateral metacarpal region. The lesion had a palpable and visible subcutaneous component. It was treated with the material known as AW4-LUDES. (B) The same horse, 6 weeks after treatment and (C) 8 weeks after treatment. (D) The outcome was highly satisfactory. No recurrence was reported at 4 years post-treatment, with only a small pink scar visible.

sarcoids (as opposed to wound-related sarcoids) using intralesional injection of stable emulsions of cisplatin in sesame oil[30] or implantation of slow-release cisplatin beads has been reported.[31] These have all been used to reasonable effect in some sarcoid cases. They all tend to be highly destructive to tissues and so may not be appropriate for sarcoid-contaminated wounds on the limbs and the face in particular. Furthermore, there are no clinical reports of any trials carried out with these materials on sarcoid-transformed/-contaminated wounds. As with other methods, all sarcoid cells must be destroyed, preferably without damaging normal cells—a combination that is virtually impossible to achieve with any known method. Still, with care and close clinical supervision, some very difficult sarcoids can be managed economically in this way (Figures 14.15a–d).

It is important owners be advised of the possible untoward effects that can occur when these methods are used. Complete destruction of the sarcoid tissue will necessarily involve some collateral damage, which makes sarcoid-affected wounds over vital structures such as joints, synovial sheaths, nerves, blood vessels, tendons, and ligaments particularly risky to treat. Furthermore, sarcoid involvement of these specific locations can be a critical and limiting factor for both the efficacy of treatment and the prognosis for the patient. That said, these treatment approaches may be the only methods that are practical. The reality is that failure to treat the affected wound correctly or completely will result in a progressively more problematic wound with an increasing risk of recurrence and exacerbation.

Photodynamic Therapy

Photodynamic therapy with hypericin has been evaluated in naturally occurring sarcoids.[17] Although there was a reduction in the tumor size, total resolution was not achieved. Several other agents, for example, 5-aminolevulinic acid, can also be used topically and possibly systemically prior to exposure of the site to an appropriate wavelength of light (usually ultraviolet). Chromophore materials such as melanin, methylene blue, riboflavin, etc. also can be applied prior to laser exposure or surgery to improve the rate of tumor cell destruction.

This is theoretically an attractive option given the rich blood supply in many sarcoid-contaminated wounds. There is no standardized approach available yet, and it is difficult to calculate the correct amount of photodynamic agent and the amount of light required to resolve any particular lesion/type. The main problem seems to be one of achieving sufficient penetration into deep lesions, and in spite of quite severe necrosis following the treatment, the sarcoid commonly regrows sooner or later, often in higher proportion than granulation tissue. There are no reports of extensive clinical trials of this method as a means to treat sarcoid treatment.

Radiation

Radiation (interstitial or topical brachytherapy or teletherapy) is the gold standard against which other treatment methods can be compared. It is highly effective but is limited by availability and the high costs of all forms of radiation treatment. Correctly applied, it is the best approach to treat sarcoid-contaminated fibroblastic lesions on the distal limb and other sensitive areas such as the eyelid. Ionization of tumor cells destroys cellular proteins and thus forces cell death, which normally occurs at the end of the natural life span of the cell. Therefore, the effects of all forms of radiation are likely to be slow, and it can take more than 12 months for treatment to be effective. Unwanted radiation of tendon and bone may become apparent long after the sarcoid has resolved because the turnover rate of tenocytes and osteocytes is low and their life span is much longer.

Healing is characterized by repeated episodes of acute inflammation, discharge, and secondary infection. However, radiation is not discriminatory and so healthy healing processes (fibroplasia, angiogenesis, and epithelialization) can also be adversely affected and there may be anatomical restrictions and secondary complications. These include synovial, articular, periosteal, and vascular damage in the immediate vicinity of the targeted tissue. Focused teletherapy will of course minimize these problems, but defining the entire affected area is a major challenge.

Although there are problems associated with the use of radiation in the management of sarcoid and sarcoid-contaminated wounds, the overall results are far better provided that a suitable calculated dose of radiation can be delivered. The expectation is that although normal cells are also affected (possibly equally or even more severely than sarcoid cells), repair is ensured by the normal cells derived from the unaffected surrounding tissues. Thus, the reparative process is normalized even though the time scale may be much prolonged.

The cosmesis is usually excellent. While there are no reports of comparative therapeutic studies involving wound-related sarcoids, in the author's experience the outcome of sarcoid treatment with radiation is excellent and better than that achieved with all other treatment options. However, owners should be aware that the treatment is slow to deliver its maximum effect. Regrettably, there are few veterinary facilities with suitable radiotherapy equipment for horses.

Teletherapy

Radiation can be applied directly via teletherapy using gamma (electromagnetic) or beta (high-energy electrons) radiation delivered from a linear accelerator either in a single beam or in a focused system of multiple low-level beams. Repeated general anesthesia is required in most circumstances but it may be possible to radiate a distal limb lesion effectively in a standing horse under strictly controlled conditions. Accurate dosimetry and fractionation are essential and there is little information on the sensitivity of transformed fibroblasts to either form of radiation. There are insufficient cases reported to provide a definitive prognosis, but where teletherapy can be applied it is likely to be highly effective.

Brachytherapy

Various forms of interstitial brachytherapy, including gold[198] in pellet form and platinum-sheathed linear iridium[192] sources, have been used routinely to treat sarcoids[32–36] and the methods are equally applicable to sarcoid-contaminated wounds. Accurate dosimetry is essential to achieve a good result without causing secondary/unwanted radiation damage in normal tissues. Probably the biggest hindrances are the logistics of the procedure and cost, which is prohibitive in most circumstances. The limited size of lesion that can be radiated in this way is usually a major obstacle; this can be partially overcome through surgical debulking immediately prior to irradiation. Set against the difficulties, the method carries an exceptionally good prognosis when compared to other methods. Properly executed, the author has found that more than 85% of sarcoids, including those at wound sites, will be resolved. Typical to all forms of radiation, the effects are slow to develop and there may be episodes of secondary infection and waves of tissue necrosis. The surrounding area will usually lose any pigmentation, so a pink scar and surrounding white hairs are a common feature.

Topical brachytherapy involving strontium[90] plaques or ruthenium patches are not applicable to wounds contaminated with sarcoid because beta emissions have poor penetration and consequently a correspondingly low efficacy. Furthermore, this particular technology is only suitable for extremely small areas and so is impractical.

Homeopathy/Natural Medicines

In the author's experience these are consistently useless and in many instances there is a considerable deleterious effect through neglect of a deteriorating tumor. Exacerbations and extensions are far more common than any resolutions. Many such attempts are borne out of a combination of client dissatisfaction (usually a result of poor efficacy of the chosen method of treatment and poor communication by the veterinarian with the owner) or some owners looking for an inexpensive treatment! Pure chemical applications (including inorganic arsenic salts and zinc chloride) and plant extracts with known biological effects such as blood root and aloe vera can have an effect but are unlikely to resolve the problem and their use should be very carefully considered at the outset.

Summary of Treatment

In conclusion, the treatment of sarcoid-transformed wounds is always likely to be problematic; the lack of any significant controlled study makes the selection of treatment difficult. Availability of particular treatments, cost, logistics, and client/owner compliance are just a few of the several factors to consider when designing a treatment regimen.

Where verrucous lesions occur on the body, topical cytotoxic or antimitotic applications and wide surgical excision followed by focused antimitotic treatment of any limited areas of regrowths would seem to be the best option. Fibroblastic lesions on the limbs produce a serious therapeutic challenge. The objective must be to remove all abnormal sarcoid tissue and this must usually be done in stages. Surgical debulking (including laser surgery, cryosurgery, or hyperthermia) or photodynamic therapy followed by topical application of cytotoxic medications is usually the preferred option. The difficulties are compounded by the invasive nature of many of these lesions and the need to destroy the last sarcoid cell. In many cases this will have implications for underlying vital structures including joints, tendons, nerves, blood vessels, and bone/periosteum. Radiation delivered by interstitial brachytherapy or preferably teletherapy is likely to be the best treatment with the least complications.

Prognosis

The pathological behavior of the equine sarcoid makes it virtually impossible for a sarcoid-affected wound to heal. There is, however, a significant and important difference in the prognosis for wounds affected by sarcoid on the trunk and those on the limbs (Figure 14.16).

Normal traumatic wounds on the limbs of horses have a somewhat unfair and largely unjustified reputation for non-healing; non-healing is principally due to the presence of complicating factors that tend to inhibit healing. Sarcoid transformation of the wound bed is possibly the most important of these factors simply because there are few, if any, reliably effective treatments that have any chance of resolving the problem. Because sarcoid-contaminated wounds on the trunk and neck tend to contract and tend to develop into verrucous lesions, and because the trunk is far more tolerant of skin loss, sarcoid-contaminated wounds in these anatomical regions have a reasonable prognosis.

On the limbs, early wound dehiscence is a common feature of sarcoid transformation. Inhibition of epithelialization and wound contraction are also cardinal features of the sarcoid-transformed wound bed. The prognosis for a transformed limb wound is poor without treatment because the normal reparative processes are suspended. The prognosis for limb wounds contaminated with sarcoid tissue is also adversely affected by the extreme difficulty with any of the currently available treatments. Either the treatment is effective in removing

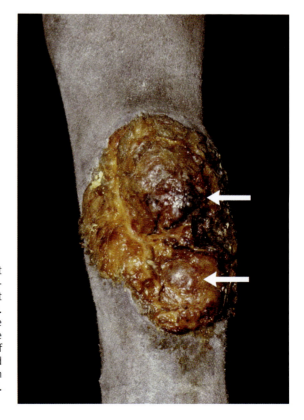

Figure 14.16. A small area of skin necrosis was caused by an overly tight bandage. The early stages of wound management included regular dressing changes; following sloughing of the eschar, the small wound was left open to heal. Within 4 weeks the wound had deteriorated to this position. Because the horse had sarcoids elsewhere, biopsies were taken from the two major nodular areas (arrows). Shave biopsies taken from the surface layers showed infected granulation tissue with small areas suspicious of sarcoid. A deep central biopsy showed irregular areas of sarcoid and granulation tissue. Treatment proved impossible. Repeated attempts with both topical and surgical management simply resulted in exacerbation. The horse was euthanized.

all sarcoid tissues, but causes unacceptable consequences, or the treatment is ineffective and the sarcoid returns, usually more aggressively.

The prognosis of sarcoid-transformed body wound sites is far better because the sarcoid remains relatively quiescent and localized. Topical treatments such as AW4-LUDES or 5-fluorouracil or even blood root and zinc chloride ointments (XXTERRA) can be singularly effective in treating these, even though this may be a prolonged process requiring several courses of therapy. Often the sites are in any case amenable to repeated topical applications and so persistence can result in a cure while scarring is nonetheless inevitable.

Prevention

Prevention is far better than any current treatments for the sarcoid-transformed wound. Pre-emptive measures taken at the time of wounding will have a profound limiting effect on the tendency toward sarcoid transformation within the wound bed. Immediate covering of a wound and in particular, prevention of fly contact, are vital measures. Following veterinary treatment of a wound on a horse with a sarcoid, or where the wounded horse is in contact with other sarcoid-infected subjects, the wound should remain protected until it has clearly healed and flies will not be attracted to the site. Fly repellants and petroleum jelly can be used to restrict fly contact. Clearly, there is a much reduced chance of a sarcoid developing at the site when these measures are taken immediately after wounding. However, the longer wounds are left open and the higher the fly population, the greater the risk of sarcoid transformation.

Owners of horses with sarcoids should be given specific instructions concerning the immediate measures that should be applied in the event that the horse sustains an injury. The wound must be covered as soon as possible and remain so until healing is complete. Prevention of fly contact seems to be a major issue and so these measures apply more to seasons when flies are a problem. The presence of other horses with sarcoids in the vicinity may also be an important issue and so it is generally wise to educate owners in immediate wound care so that healing is rapid and uncomplicated.

Conclusion

The equine sarcoid is a problematic skin disease with a disturbingly high number of suggested treatments,[36,37] thus implying that none is universally applicable. There are significant and possibly critical differences between sarcoid-transformed wounds and sarcoids occurring without apparent wounding (i.e., naturally occurring sarcoids) and this is reflected in the difficulties with treatment.

Although sarcoid transformation in wound sites has probably been present for many years, there has been little recognition of its significance as an important cause of wound healing failure. In spite of the variable proportion of sarcoid-to-granulation tissue that occurs in affected wounds, the clinical appearance remains constant: On the limbs the wound tends to develop a granulation tissue/fibrous tissue mixture which is often very difficult to differentiate clinically from pure granulation tissue. Most sarcoids that occur on the limb regions below the stifle/elbow are at sites of skin injury and develop into aggressive fibroblastic lesions; therefore, these are always likely to create difficulty with treatment. The combination of an aggressive tumor-transformed wound bed and anatomical restrictions makes predictions on cures ill-advised. Transformation occurring in body wounds tends to develop into a more obvious sarcoid-like verrucose lesion and may therefore be more readily recognized. These are also far more amenable to treatment.

While the clinical appearance of exuberant granulation tissue and pyogranuloma can be very similar to the sarcoid (whether partial or complete), treatments for these conditions are very different. Treatment that is suitable for proud flesh (cutting back and grafting) usually serves only to exacerbate sarcoid tissue. It is imperative, therefore, that all wounded horses be subjected to proper professional physical examination and care.

Among the large number of publications on sarcoid treatment, little or no mention is made about the specific problems of sarcoid-transformed wounds. This may reflect the lack of appreciation of the problem or the lack of efficacy of most treatments available today. Individual veterinarians will have their own preferred methods for treating excess granulation tissue but lack of response to therapy is a strong indicator of an "unrecognized" problem—the wound wants to heal if it can. The possibility of sarcoid involvement in non-healing wounds should never be overlooked. It follows that any tissues removed from a granulating wound should be submitted for histological examination and where sarcoids are noted on the horse, or where the wound involves sarcoid-affected skin, the site should be biopsied before embarking on any therapy that may be contra-indicated.

There is an urgent need to explore novel ways of managing sarcoid-contaminated wounds; immunological methods are possibly the ultimate goal.

References

1. Erk N: A study of Kitab al-Hail wal-Baitar, written in the second half of the ninth century by Muhammed Ibn ahi Hizam. Hist Vet 1976;1:101
2. Jackson C: The incidence and pathology of tumours of domestic animals in South Africa. Ondes J Vet Sci Anim Ind 1936;6:241
3. Knottenbelt DC: Sarcoid transformation at wound sites. *Equine wound management* London, WB Saunders, 2003, p.31
4. Knottenbelt DC: A suggested clinical classification for the equine sarcoid. Diag Tech Eq Med 2005;3:278
5. Reid SWJ, Smith KT, Jarrett WFH: Detection, cloning and characterisation of papillomaviral DNA present in sarcoid tumours of *Equus asinus*. Vet Rec 1994;135:430
6. Bloch N, Breen M, Spradbrow PB: Genomic sequences of bovine papillomaviruses in formalin fixed sarcoids from Australian horses revealed by polymerase chain reaction. Vet Microbiol 1994;4:163
7. Nasir L, Reid SW: Bovine papillomaviral gene expression equine sarcoids. Virus Res 1999;61:171
8. Voss JL: Transmission of the equine sarcoid. Am J Vet Res 1969;30:183
9. Broström H: Equine Sarcoids: A clinical, epidemiological and immunological study. PhD Thesis, University of Uppsala, Stockholm, Sweden 1995, p.9
10. Cochrane CM: An investigation into equine wound healing and sarcoid formation. PhD Thesis. University of Liverpool, Liverpool, UK 1996, p.67
11. Knottenbelt DC: Equine wound management: Are there significant differences in healing at different sites on the body? Vet Derm 1997;8:273
12. Nasir L, McFarlane ST, Torrntegui BO, et al: Screening for bovine papillomavirus in peripheral blood cells of donkeys with and without sarcoids. Res Vet Sci 1997;63:289
13. Bogaert L, Martens A, De Baere C, et al: Detection of bovine papillomavirus DNA on the normal skin and in the habitual surroundings of horses with and without equine sarcoids. Res Vet Sci 2005;79:253
14. Marti E, Lazary S, Antczak DF, et al: Report of the first international workshop on equine sarcoid. Equine Vet J 1993;25:397
15. Wilmink JM, Nederbragt H, van Weeren PR, et al: Differences in wound contraction between horses and ponies are not caused by inherent contraction capacity of fibroblasts. Equine Vet J 2001;33:499
16. Martens A, De Moor A, Ducatelle R: PCR detection of bovine papilloma virus DNA in superficial swabs and scrapings from equine sarcoids. Vet J 2001;161:280
17. Laursen BA: Behandling af equine sarcoider med krokirurgi. Dansk Vet Tidskr 1987;70:97
18. Lane GJ: The treatment of equine sarcoids by cryosurgery. Equine Vet J 1977;9:127
19. Vingerhoets M, Diehl M, Gerber H, et al: Traitement de la sarcoide equine au laser a gaz carbonique. Schweiz Arch Tierheilk 1988;130:113
20. Carstangen B, Jordan P, Lepage OM: Carbon dioxide laser as a surgical instrument for sarcoid therapy—a retrospective study on 60 cases. Can Vet J 1997;38:773
21. Flemming DD: BCG therapy for equine sarcoid. In: NE Robinson, ed. *Current therapy in equine medicine* Philadelphia, WB Saunders, 1983, p.539
22. Misdorp W, Klein WR, Ruitenberg EJ, et al: Clinicopathological aspects of immunotherapy by intralesional injections of BCG cell walls or live BCG in bovine ocular squamous cell carcinoma. Canc Immun Immunoth 1985;20:223
23. Owen RR, Jagger DW: Clinical observation on the use of BCG cell-wall–fraction in the treatment of periocular and other equine sarcoids. Vet Rec 1987;120:548
24. Davies M: Bacillus Calmette-Guérin as an antitumour agent. The interaction with cells of the mammalian immune system. Biochem Biophys Acta 1982;651:143
25. Pascoe RR, Knottenbelt DC: *Manual of equine dermatology* London, WB Saunders, 1999 p.244
26. Spoormakers TJ, Klein WR, Jacobs JJ, et al: Comparison of the efficacy of local treatment of equine sarcoids with IL-2 or cisplatin/IL-2. Can Immunol Immunother 2003;52:179
27. Knottenbelt DC, Walker JA: Topical treatment of the equine sarcoid. Equine Vet Educ 1994;6:72
28. Knottenbelt DC, Edwards SER, Daniel EA: The diagnosis and treatment of the equine sarcoid. In Practice 1995;17:123
29. Kinnunen RE, Tallberg T, Stenback H, et al: Equine sarcoid tumour treated by autogenous tumour vaccine. Anticancer Res 1999;19:3367
30. Theon AP: Cisplatin treatment for cutaneous tumours. In: NE Robinson, ed. *Current therapy in equine medicine* (4th edition), Philadelphia, WB Saunders, 1997, p.372
31. Hewes CA, Sullins K: Use of cisplatin-containing biodegradable beads for treatment of cutaneous neoplasia in equidae: 59 cases (2000–2004), J Am Vet Med Assoc 2006;229:1617

32. Wyn-Jones G: Treatment of periocular tumours of horses using radioactive gold[198] grains. Equine Vet J 1979;11:3
33. Wyn-Jones G: Treatment of equine cutaneous neoplasia by radiotherapy using iridium[192] linear sources, Equine Vet J 1983;15:361
34. Turrel JM, Stover SM: Iridium 192 interstitial brachytherapy of equine sarcoid. Vet Radiol 1985;26:20
35. Theon A, Pascoe JR: Iridium 192 interstitial brachytherapy for equine periocular tumours: Treatment results and prognostic factors in 115 horses. Equine Vet J 1994;27:117
36. Knottenbelt DC, Kelly DF: The diagnosis and treatment of periorbital sarcoid in the horse: 445 cases from 1974–1999. Vet Ophthal 2000;3:169
37. Genetzky RM, Biwer RD, Myers RK: Equine sarcoid: Causes, diagnosis and treatment. Comp Cont Educ Pract Vet 1983;5:416

15 Lasers: Effects on Healing and Clinical Applications

Kenneth E. Sullins, DVM, MS, Diplomate ACVS

Introduction

Veterinary laser surgery had its beginnings in the 1980s, which was a period of basic research and trial of the effects of laser energy on tissue and its comparison to conventional and other evolving modalities. The preferred wavelengths became the carbon dioxide (CO_2) and Nd:YAG lasers, which were also commonly used by physicians who were likewise involved in the developmental stages of laser surgery.

Progress and dissemination of the technology in veterinary medicine were somewhat hampered by cost of the equipment. However, in the 1990s, a more affordable waveguide-delivered CO_2 laser came to the market. Although limited somewhat by power and available accessories, this very workable technology was responsible for an explosion in the number of lasers used in private practices (particularly small animal) in the U.S., and, it increased the awareness of laser surgery in general.

Lasers are used in general surgery to reduce intraoperative hemorrhage and postoperative swelling, and the directly applied heat is bactericidal at the point of contact. Tissue can be debulked or debrided by vaporization, and specific tissue can be targeted by wavelength selection. The laser is well suited for reconstructive procedures where tissue is to be excised for primary closure. There is good evidence that subsurgical laser (low-level laser therapy [LLLT]) energies can stimulate or inhibit cellular activity.

The aim of this chapter is to briefly describe laser energy and to point out its purported advantages, including its effects on tissue healing. Prerequisites to safe and effective clinical application and essentials of laser physics and laser-tissue interaction are provided. The healing effects of LLLT will be reviewed.

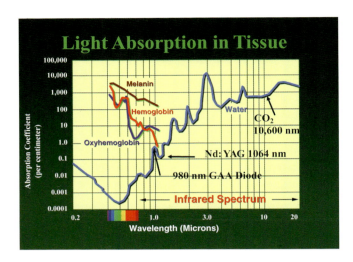

Figure 15.1. Tissue absorption of laser light of wavelengths (in nanometers) common in veterinary surgery. The visible spectrum is indicated by the rainbow along the lower axis. The absorption of light for various tissue types and water is shown on the vertical axis. Modified unpublished Lumenis, Inc. illustration.

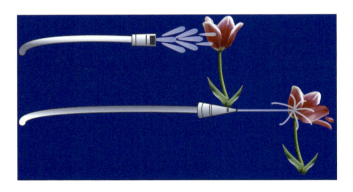

Figure 15.2. The principle of power density is illustrated by two water hoses transmitting identical flows of water. The upper hose delivers a sprinkle of water through a larger aperture, whereas the lower hose delivers a more forceful jet of water through a smaller diameter aperture.

Laser Energy

LASER is an acronym for "light amplification by stimulated emission of radiation." Monochromatic coherent light emits from a medium that has been excited by application of energy and it travels with little divergence over distance and exerts an effect on target tissue. In contrast, multichromatic radiant light from an incandescent light bulb does not concentrate sufficient energy to affect tissue. The source of the light is the laser medium and is usually reflected in the name of the laser. A CO_2 laser uses that gas to generate the energy; Nd:YAG lasers use a combination of neodymium, yttrium, aluminum, and garnet as the source. Each material generates light with a specific wavelength. The wavelengths of these lasers lie in the infrared spectrum, which begins after the visible spectrum of light (Figure 15.1).

Although laser light may not be visible, wavelength is analogous to "color" and determines the specific tissue interaction of that laser. Wavelengths used most commonly in veterinary medicine today include the far-infrared (farther away from visible light on the electromagnetic spectrum) CO_2 (10,600 nm) and two near-infrared lasers: the Nd:YAG (1,064 nm) and the gallium aluminum arsenide (GAA) diode (980 nm) with similar tissue interactions (Figure 15.1).

The rate at which energy is delivered to the tissue is measured in watts (W = 1 joule/second), which is a setting on the laser console. Much more important is power density (energy per unit of area of tissue in watts/cm^2) (Figure 15.2), which is determined by the power setting of the machine and the diameter of the laser beam at the tissue. The total energy delivered to tissue (J/cm^2) is the fluence. Power density decreases as the square of the increase in spot size, as the handpiece is moved away from the tissue (defocused) (Figure 15.3).

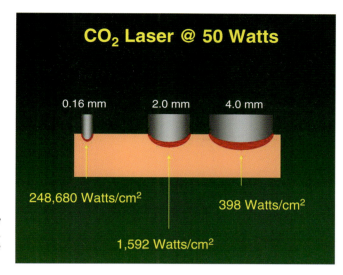

Figure 15.3. This illustration depicts the change in power density when a fixed energy beam is delivered in varying spot sizes. Power density changes as does the square of the diameter of the spot size. Modified unpublished Lumenis, Inc. illustration.

Laser Surgery

Advantages and Selection

The purported advantages of surgical lasers over conventional surgery are reduction of hemorrhage[1-3] and postoperative pain.[4-7] Swelling of the surgical site may also be reduced due to sealing of capillaries and lymphatics, which reduces postoperative swelling in the affected tissues.[5,6]

For incision or dissection, CO_2 lasers deliver the most physiologic results, and pulsed delivery produces noticeably better results than continuous delivery (see below).[3] While contact delivery of Nd:YAG or GAA lasers can be similarly applied, collateral heating of tissue is significantly greater than with CO_2 lasers. This difference is attributed to the difference in laser-tissue interactions. Carbon dioxide lasers vaporize very narrow bands of tissue when the light contacts the tissue water. The near-infrared wavelengths delivered by the Nd:YAG or GAA lasers are not absorbed by water, so a direct laser effect is exerted only on darkly pigmented tissue (Figure 15.1). Near-infrared laser energy can be converted to heat at the tip of a contact delivery device for an incision, but a greater amount of surrounding tissue heating occurs, similar to that generated by electrosurgery. Tension sufficient to separate tissues as the incision progresses is essential for incision/excision of tissue; without it tissue simply boils.

Hemostasis

Laser incisions provide readily apparent hemostasis of vessels ≤2 mm; vessels with visible lumens should be ligated. Active blood flow dissipates the laser energy and prevents coagulation, so blood flow must be stemmed to coagulate the vessel. If the walls are compressed to stem flow, the contacting vessel walls can then be "welded" together with a low power density; more energy will simply transect the vessel. A sufficiently rigid contact tip used to deliver the laser energy can be used to compress the vessel and deliver the energy simultaneously. A contact tip on an Nd:YAG or GAA laser can be inserted into a visible lumen approximating the same diameter as the fiber for temporary coagulation. The CO_2 laser produces noticeable reduction in hemorrhage along incisions, but will be less effective on larger vessels.

Penetration of Laser Energy into Tissue

Penetration of laser energy into tissue depends primarily upon the absorption length of the wavelength of the laser light and secondarily upon power density. A (noncontact) laser is simply light of various wavelengths which is absorbed differently by specific tissues (Figure 15.4). When applied to tissue that doesn't absorb that particular wavelength, the laser energy will pass through without effect. For example, CO_2 laser energy, which

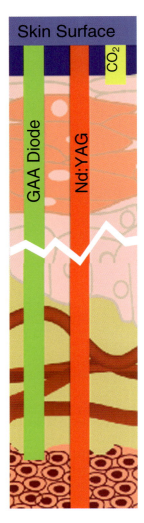

Figure 15.4. Relative depths of penetration of common laser wavelengths into skin (not to scale). The CO_2 laser (yellow) penetrates very little due to its profound absorption by water in skin, whereas the two near-infrared wavelengths, which are unaffected by tissue water, may travel full thickness through skin depending upon pigment. Modified unpublished Lumenis, Inc. illustration.

is completely absorbed by tissue water, will exert a profound effect on the cornea, while an Nd:YAG laser, whose energy is absorbed almost exclusively by dark pigment, will pass through the cornea with no effect but will exert a profound effect upon the dark iris or retina.

Superficial vaporization or coagulation of tissue can be safely accomplished using a CO_2 laser because it penetrates significantly less than a millimeter into the tissue, and the surgeon can observe its effect. An Nd:YAG or GAA diode laser can affect deeper tissues that can't be seen, such as the darkly pigmented skin on the opposite side of the cartilage of an ear where a wound is being debrided.

Note that coagulation of tissue protein is not the same as hemostasis. In this common usage of the term, coagulation refers to denaturing of protein grossly evident by blanching and contraction of tissue. Ideally, such tissue will be imperceptibly replaced as the wound heals. Carried to excess, a slough will follow.

CO_2 Laser Incision/Collateral Heating and Necrosis

For the most physiologic laser skin incision, the CO_2 laser is the best choice because collateral heating of tissue can be minimized so the wound margins resemble incisions created by a steel blade. However, insufficient power density will result in inefficient laser surgery with excessive collateral heating of tissue, often followed by marginal tissue slough.

With a small spot size, a single pass with efficient movement across the tissue, and adequate tension on the tissue, 5,000 W/cm^2 is a minimally sufficient power density to avoid collateral thermal necrosis.[6] However, most

Table 15.1. Author's preferences for laser equipment and technique.

Laser	Description	Capacity	Accessories	Preference for skin incision	Comments
CO$_2$ laser	Articulated arm with 125 mm focusing handpiece. Minimum spot size 0.16 mm.	Minimum 30 W.	Computerized pattern scanner.	30–50 W pulsed mode. Power density 149,283–248,806 W/cm^2 in continuous mode. Much higher in pulsed mode.	Sterilize handpiece for aseptic procedures. Better hemostasis in continuous mode if wound is to be left open.
GAA diode laser	Quartz fiber delivery.	25–50 W.	600 and 1,000 micron quartz fibers. Handpiece to hold fibers.	1,000 micron fiber sculpted down to approximately 600 micron at the tip.	25 W is insufficient for noncontact vaporization. 600 micron fiber too fragile for general surgery. Sterilize fibers for aseptic procedures.
Nd:YAG laser		100 W.	Gas cooled.	Conical sapphire tip.	Impractical to own both diode and Nd:YAG lasers.
Smoke evacuator	Manufactured for laser smoke evacuation. Many brands available.		Spare filters.		Performance drops off quickly when filter fills. Change promptly. Sterilize hose for aseptic procedures.

experienced surgeons apply a significantly higher power density (Table 15.1). The novice tends to reduce the power and move tentatively or by "sketching," which causes the laser to remain on the tissue longer while increasing the width of the wound and collateral heating. It should be no surprise that seemingly uncomplicated elective incisions dehisce. The wound margins slough from the initial thermal injury and the sutures just fall away.

Continuous Laser Energy

There is more than one way to achieve an adequate power density. A CO$_2$ laser in continuous mode at 50 W delivered through a 125 mm focusing handpiece with a 0.16 mm focused spot size yields a power density of 248,880 W/cm^2, or a waveguide-delivered CO$_2$ laser at 8 W through a 0.4 mm ceramic tip delivers approximately 6,300 W/cm^2. The former will produce an incision more efficiently but should be moved quickly across the tissue to confine the effect to the skin. The latter will produce an acceptable incision if tension is adequate to separate tissue and the waveguide is passed once and quickly across the skin. The skin defect will be 0.24 mm wider than the former with a perfect incision, which isn't clinically significant. The author prefers the first technique in a pulsed mode. This concept must be borne in mind when evaluating the literature. Incisions created with the CO$_2$ laser were reported to have reduced tensile strength upon healing and more necrosis and inflammation compared to steel (scalpel) incisions, but the laser incisions were created using a power density of 1,990 W/cm^2.[2] This is like comparing a razor blade incision to one made with electrosurgery.

Pulsed Laser Energy

Pulsed laser energy is a mode whereby very high power densities are produced repeatedly for very short intervals. The net effect is that an incision is made with essentially no collateral heating using the same total energy as continuous laser energy at a much lower setting (Figure 15.5). This is the preferred technique for making incisions that will be sutured primarily. Collateral heating is further reduced by using shorter pulse durations. One study demonstrated pulse durations >100 ms increased collateral tissue damage,[8] and another found 7.5 ms pulses to be similar to scalpel incisions.[3]

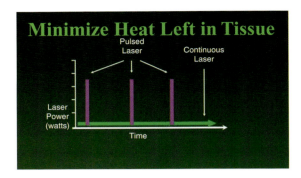

Figure 15.5. Pulsing higher power densities for short durations (blue bars indicate high power) produces a more efficient tissue effect with less collateral tissue heating compared to a continuous beam (continuous green bar at lower power) emitting the same average power (fluence). Modified unpublished Lumenis, Inc. illustration.

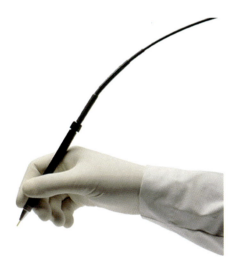

Figure 15.6. A semi-flexible waveguide delivers the carbon dioxide laser to the handpiece, where a variable aperture determines the power density. Power density is also affected by distance of the tip from the tissue. Modified unpublished Lumenis, Inc. illustration.

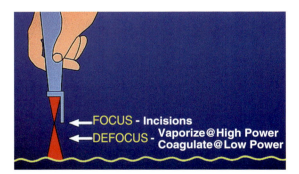

Figure 15.7. The carbon dioxide laser delivered through a focusing handpiece. When the stylus touches the tissue, maximum power density is delivered. The handpiece can be moved away from the tissue to defocus (diminish) the power density. Modified unpublished Lumenis, Inc. illustration.

Laser Delivery

CO_2 Lasers

CO_2 laser energy is delivered entirely in a noncontact fashion; only the laser beam contacts the tissue. Delivery options include a hollow flexible reflective waveguide (Figure 15.6) that channels the energy to a tip of variable diameter (the tip controls power density) or an articulated arm containing finely tuned mirrors that reflect the laser beam to a handpiece containing a lens to focus the energy (Figures 15.7, 15.8). A computerized pattern scanner is a very useful accessory for CO_2 lasers. The scanner moves a focused beam continuously around the target area so fast that tissue is vaporized without producing char (Figure 15.9).[9,10] The net effect of using the scanner is that the superficial tissue is removed very efficiently with almost no effect on deeper

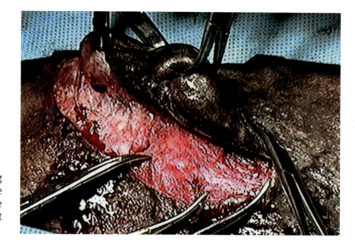

Figure 15.8. A fusiform incision has been created surrounding this cutaneous tumor using a CO_2 laser. The hemostats indicate the only hemorrhage that occurred. The towel clamps provide the necessary tension to accomplish a physiologic incision that will heal primarily when sutured.

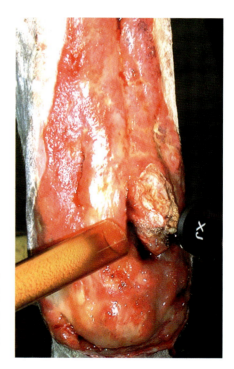

Figure 15.9. A carbon dioxide laser with a scanner attached is used to vaporize granulation tissue. This wound approximates $25 \text{ cm} \times 10 \text{ cm}$, encompassing the entire carpal canal on the palmar/caudal surface of a carpus. The pale area ahead of the laser handpiece and to the right of the smoke evacuator and a cleft into the wound is the crater remaining from removing a mass of granulation tissue elevated 2 cm from the surface. The granulation tissue mass was removed in less than 1 minute; note that there is neither hemorrhage nor charring of the tissue.

tissues,[10,11] making it very effective for superficial debridement or removal of skin tumors (Figures. 15.10a and 15.10b).

Nd:YAG and GAA Diode Lasers

Near-infrared Nd:YAG lasers and GAA diode lasers are minimally absorbed by water but are profoundly absorbed by darker pigments and some protein (Figure 15.4). These wavelengths can be delivered under water or through transparent body fluids. The GAA laser is somewhat more absorbed by water than the Nd:YAG, which makes it a bit more efficient for use in lighter pigmented tissues such as mucous membranes. These wavelengths are transmitted through a flexible quartz fiber (making endoscopic surgery possible) and delivered to the tissue either by free transmission of the light beam from the fiber, similar to a CO_2 laser, or by causing

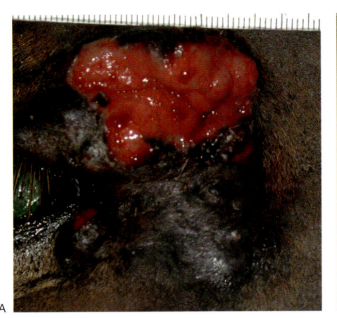
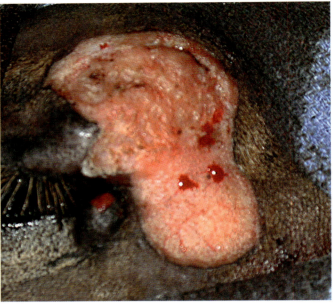

A   B

Figure 15.10. (A) This elevated periocular sarcoid that is partly verrucous and partly fibroblastic is shown before surgery. (B) The same site after the mass was vaporized using a CO_2 laser with a scanner. The amount of hemorrhage is real. Note that there is no char on the wound, and the dermis is intact. The author would apply local chemotherapy following surgery.

the energy to heat the tip of the fiber or an accessory sapphire tip which is applied to tissue in a contact fashion. These contact techniques compensate for the wavelengths' inability to inherently interact with lightly pigmented tissues. Because a heated fiber contacts tissue in the contact delivery, there is thermal necrosis of adjacent skin similar to that seen with electrosurgery. If primary healing of a sutured wound is desired, a CO_2 laser is preferred. If a near-infrared fiber must be used, the principles of minimizing collateral heating described previously should be followed and suture placement should be wider than normal. However, successful first-intention healing can be accomplished using a quartz fiber with the near-infrared lasers if the described principles are followed (Figures 15.11a–d). For the near-infrared wavelengths, contact application also minimizes projection of laser energy into the deeper tissues, which increases the safety substantially.

Health Risks

Appropriate eye protection is required for surgical laser wavelengths. Clear glass with protection from all angles is adequate for the CO_2 laser, but optical density recommendations are specific for the near-infrared wavelengths and should be followed for the capacity of the laser.

All smoke generated from tissue should be evacuated using a filtered laser smoke evacuator, available from any supplier of surgical lasers. Despite reports that insignificant concentrations of bacteria become aerosolized[12] and that horses are not adversely affected by routine upper airway laser surgery,[13] there is sufficient evidence that infectious, carcinogenic, and irritant material is present in laser smoke.[14] The vaporized debris and potentially viable cells or pathogens should not be inhaled by humans or the patient. Surgical suction is inadequate for this task because it is less efficient and the suction lines will eventually foul.

Surgical Objectives

Medical lasers transfer light energy to tissue, which is converted to heat to meet various surgical objectives. The three important tissue interactions include incision/excision, vaporization, or coagulation. Incision/excision can be compared to sharp steel surgery or electrosurgery, and coagulation can be compared to electrosurgery

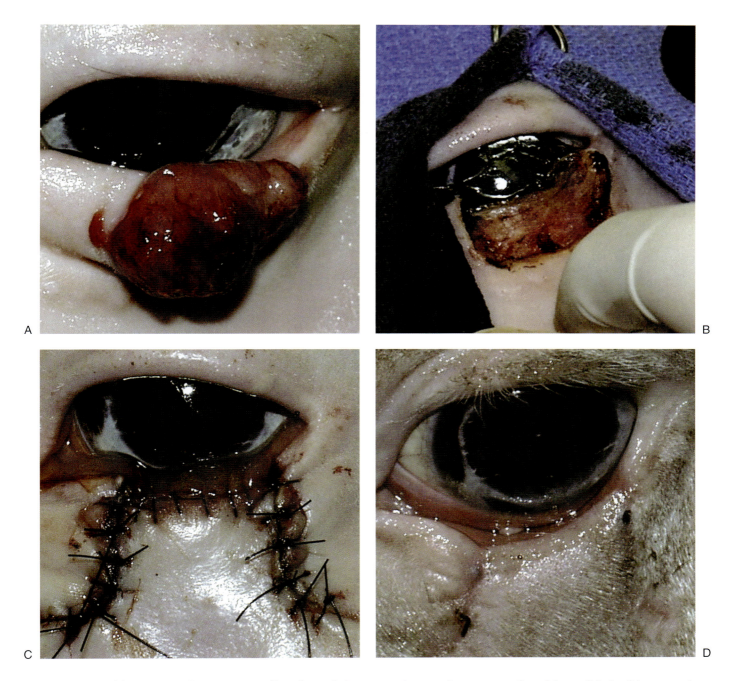

Figure 15.11. (A) This periocular squamous cell carcinoma is large enough to require reconstruction of the eyelid after it is removed. (B) The wound bed, immediately following resection of the mass with a quartz fiber delivering GAA diode laser energy, contains no hemorrhage but there is minimal char. The eye is protected by application of an ophthalmic ointment. Contact laser energy will not be projected across space to the eye. When necessary to protect the globe, the author holds the lids closed and/or covers the area with wet gauze sponges. (C) The wound immediately postoperatively after the half H plasty advancement flap has been apposed with subcutaneous absorbable suture and nylon skin sutures. The conjunctiva has been everted. (D) The wound 2 to 3 weeks postoperatively. Note that there is primary healing of the wound.

to a point, but vaporization has no conventional surgical counterpart. Achieving these effects depends upon power density, wavelength of the laser light, and the properties of the target tissue. In contrast to electrosurgery, laser coagulation can be applied to larger expanses of tissue by "painting" with the defocused CO_2 laser hand-piece, which is a useful procedure to minimize serous transudate in dead spaces that must be closed. The tissue effect is superficial coagulation of protein and mildly visible physical deformation characterized by contraction or blanching of tissue.

Clinical Applications

Wound Debridement

The CO_2 laser is effective for wound debridement.[15] Superficial necrotic tissue and microorganisms will be removed to a large extent;[16–18] however, complete sterilization of the wound is unlikely.[12] Efficient superficial vaporization can be performed without damaging the deeper tissue, but heating of deeper tissue should not be allowed. The thermal effect approximated 85 microns using pulsed CO_2 laser energy for excision debridement of rat burn tissue,[19] meaning that necrotic, contaminated, soft tissue can be vaporized leaving minimal hemorrhage. Importantly, mineral debris or soil may not be vaporized and therefore must be removed by more traditional means (e.g., irrigation and sharp debridement). A CO_2 laser with a pattern scanner can very precisely remove a superficial contaminated layer of tissue from an open wound while sparing the deeper tissue. Freshening skin edges requires a fine touch with the laser to preserve tissue; thus, a scalpel may be more precise in this regard.

Removal of Exuberant Granulation Tissue

Removal of granulation tissue is required when it becomes exuberant or to prepare a wound for skin grafting. The CO_2 laser is absorbed entirely by the surface of the granulating wound and therefore can be used to debulk tissue very effectively (Figure 15.9). The near-infrared wavelengths delivered in a noncontact fashion are not desirable for the vaporization of granulation tissue. However, contact vaporization or excision of granulation tissue with the GAA diode or Nd:YAG laser is safe and effective for areas intended to be left open to heal by second intention (Figure 15.12). The procedure is almost bloodless.

Graft Bed Preparation

Because the purpose of preparing the granulation bed for grafting is to stimulate angiogenesis, we should concern ourselves with the vascularity of the recently lasered surface. The Nd:YAG and GAA diode lasers are

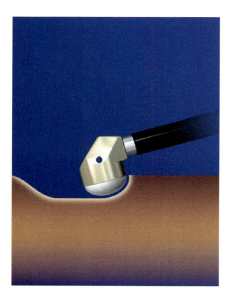

Figure 15.12. Contact vaporization using a sapphire tip on an Nd:YAG laser. The power density is sufficient to vaporize tissue and the laser effect is confined to the surface; however, considerable heating of tissue occurs.

among the most efficient lasers at hemostasis. Whether they are delivered in contact or noncontact fashion, superficial microvascularity is likely to be coagulated, a disadvantage for surface skin grafting. Alternatively, the CO_2 laser equipped with a scanner has been shown to prepare a graft bed with subsequent acceptable graft take.[1,20,21] Excision debridement with a focused CO_2 laser, as with a scalpel, would also work well, but a scanner is much simpler. Blood flow to the most superficial granulation tissue is of less concern when pinch, punch, or tunnel grafts are used.

Cutaneous Masses

Lasers are particularly well-suited for resection of masses because the resulting dead space tends less toward seroma formation and peri-incisional edema is reduced. The procedure itself is more efficient without the typical hemorrhage associated with sharp dissection (Figure 15.8). Combined with tension, a plane of dissection can be developed to effectively remove the necessary tissue (Figure 15.8). The improved visibility facilitates accurate dissection through the marginal tissue, avoiding tumor cells. CO_2 laser dissection particularly reduces the chance of seeding neoplastic cells because nothing touches the tissue with noncontact delivery. When the wound is to be left open, there will be reduced hemorrhage and exudation in the early postoperative period. However, larger vessels should be ligated. Bandaging may remain an advantage to facilitate final healing.

It is an advantage when marginal neoplastic cells absorb laser energy or become vaporized. However, the surgeon should consider the laser delivery device to be the same as a scalpel with regard to attempting complete excision. Collateral heating of tissue is an imprecise factor and should not be counted upon to clean up the margins. This concern should be addressed with local chemotherapy.

Char

Char occurs when "lasered" tissue remains in situ and cools. Intraoperatively, char absorbs and reduces penetration of laser energy, adding to tissue heating, and diminishes surgical precision because it flares and disrupts uniformity of the laser procedure. Accumulated char negatively affects the sutured wound because it is a foreign body. Delivering an adequate power density to efficiently vaporize tissue reduces char.

The CO_2 laser with a scanner will produce no char after superficial vaporization. Ablation of masses with Nd:YAG or GAA diode lasers will leave char because the laser penetrates to depths at which the power density diminishes. Nevertheless, this is a very efficient technique for removing some pigmented masses where deeper penetration is not a danger.

When char occurs and the tissue is accessible, char can be removed by abrasion with a gauze sponge. It should be removed because black char can completely block penetration of near-infrared lasers. These wavelengths are more efficient hemostatic agents than those of the CO_2 laser, but more collateral heating is produced, which can be suited for debulking large vascular masses that will heal by second intention.

Nonsurgical Laser Therapy

Healing Effects

Photomodulation of cellular activity has been widely proposed to produce biological responses. LLLT outputs are in the mW range, which is very low compared to surgical lasers. In contrast to the photothermal effect of surgical lasers, the effect is photochemical. One school of thought is that laser energy stimulates cytochrome production and mitochondrial respiratory activity, leading to increases in ATP and cellular activity.[22] Another is that calcium channels are activated, allowing Ca influx into the cell.[23] More recent work by updated methods may shed favorable light on these theories.[24]

Many earlier reports are difficult to interpret based upon information provided, and many lacked experimental control or refereeing during the publication process. Although still inconsistent, recent reports are more encouraging. One explanation for the variable success of LLLT studies is that the specific laser effect may be dose- (fluence, total laser energy) and tissue-dependent.[25] Where one fluence may produce a desired effect, a slight variation may be detrimental.[25,26] Because up-regulation of cells is a proposed effect which may affect only dormant cells, cells that are already active may not be affected, thus showing no effect.[27]

Wavelength must be considered because any potential laser effect will be limited by the depth of penetration.[27] Wavelengths reported to be useful for LLLT fall in the 500–1,100 nm range ([visible]red or near-infrared wavelengths).[22,27]

At 632 nm, the helium-neon (He-Ne) laser penetrates tissue adequately to exert an effect on appropriate cells. In vitro, 3% of the emitted He-Ne laser energy penetrated through 2 cm skin (including subcutaneous fat) biopsies, and transmission of laser energy through granulation tissue was 2.5 times more than skin.[28] Helium-neon laser irradiation of experimental equine pharyngeal sulfuric acid burns was reported to accelerate healing compared to untreated wounds.[29] However, no benefit of He-Ne or GAA diode laser irradiation of burns on the backs of rats was found,[30] and diode laser energy produced no beneficial effect on wounds on the dorsal surface of fetlocks in horses.[31]

Biostimulation of cells in the wound healing process would directly benefit surgical and trauma patients. One in vitro/in vivo combined study demonstrated that He-Ne irradiation increased conversion of fibroblasts to myofibroblasts in human gingival tissue,[32] which would increase the rate of granulation and contraction of wounds. Fibroblast proliferation was indirectly stimulated in vitro by addition of secretions from He-Ne-irradiated macrophages.[22] For more information regarding the relationship between macrophages to fibroblast and granulation tissue formation, see Chapter 1.

Antimicrobial Effect

The presence of a healthy wound is an inhibitor of bacterial growth in itself,[33] whether it was facilitated by medical treatment or stimulated by LLLT. However, a specific phototherapeutic effect on bacteria has been reported.[34] Interactions between wavelength and bacteria and between wavelength and fluence were observed, showing that there are likely hundreds of permutations of LLLT on various species of bacteria. Specifically from this study, *P. aeruginosa* growth was inhibited by the 810 nm diode laser delivering $5 \, J/cm^2$, whereas *E. coli* growth was accelerated by the same wavelength at $0.015–0.03 \, J/cm^2$. *S. aureus* growth increased 27% following 905 nm irradiation at $50 \, J/cm^2$.[34]

Promotion of Healing

Surgical lasers applied at reduced power densities have been reported to promote healing and relieve pain and inflammation. In controlled studies, increased area of skin flap survival was reported after treating with the 830 nm diode ($600 \, mW/cm^2$ for fluence of $36 \, j/cm^2$) and the defocused CO_2 lasers ($300 \, mW/cm^2$, fluence unavailable).[22] (Note that the power densities are expressed in milliwatts.) Although lacking controls, a therapeutic benefit for fetlock synovitis has been reported in horses with the CO_2 laser applied for 6 minutes, producing a fluence of $60 \, J/cm^2$.[35] The far-infrared CO_2 laser energy dissipates almost entirely in the outer $100 \, \mu m$ of tissue, which implies that heating of tissue is the mechanism of action.[36] Fifty percent more CO_2 laser energy ($91 \, J/cm^2$) caused an approximate 5°C increase in skin temperature and a 2- to 3-fold increase in skin perfusion.[37] Histologic changes consisted of focal subdermal cleft formation, which were believed to be reversible; more energy produced more profound effects.[38] There is insufficient information to make direct comparisons of the two laser techniques, but tissue warming would seem to be responsible for any effect.

Conclusion

In summary, lasers present advantages for removal of tissue with minimal hemorrhage or from sites inaccessible to conventional instruments. Superficial wound debridement of wounds can be facilitated with a focused CO_2 laser or a CO_2 laser with a scanner, and granulating masses can be debulked by vaporization with the CO_2 laser or by excision with either the CO_2 or the near-infrared lasers. Preparation of granulation beds for grafting is expedited by relatively blood-free debulking with the CO_2 laser used by hand[15] or with a scanner.[10] Additionally, the laser is well suited for reconstructive procedures in which wounds are to be excised for primary closure.

Clearly, LLLT holds promise for benefits in wound healing. However, specifications for the patient, tissue, and wavelength must be defined through controlled and prospective studies before a predictable effect can be expected.

Experience with laser procedures is required to ensure effective application. Vaporization of surface tissue using a CO_2 laser is a convenient way to begin, but practice for incising tissue with proper distracting tension and rate of movement is required. The decision to use a laser versus a conventional instrument should reflect the case at hand. In some situations, such as freshening skin margins, conventional surgery no doubt still hold an advantage.

References

1. Graham JS, Schomacker KT, Glatter RD, et al: Efficacy of laser debridement with autologous split-thickness skin grafting in promoting improved healing of deep cutaneous sulfur mustard burns. Burns 2002;28:719
2. Mison MB, Steficek B, Lavagnino M, et al: Comparison of the effects of the CO_2 surgical laser and conventional surgical techniques on healing and wound tensile strength of skin flaps in the dog. Vet Surg 2003;32:153
3. Sanders DL, Reinisch L: Wound healing and collagen thermal damage in 7.5-microsec pulsed CO_2 laser skin incisions. Lasers Surg Med 2000;26:22
4. Demidov VP, Rykov VI, Putyrskii LA, et al: The use of the carbon dioxide laser in the surgical treatment of breast cancer. Vopr Onkol 1992;38:42
5. Savay L, Jori J, Czigner J: Laser lingual tonsillotomy. Acta Chir Hung 1992;33:87
6. Lanzafame RJ: Laser/light applications in general surgery. In: K Nouri, ed. *Lasers in Dermatology and Medicine*. In press: Springer
7. Holmberg DL, Brisson BA: A prospective comparison of postoperative morbidity associated with the use of scalpel blades and lasers for onychectomy in cats. Can Vet J 2006;47:162
8. Fortune DS, Huang S, Soto J, et al: Effect of pulse duration on wound healing using a CO_2 laser. Laryngoscope 1998;108:843
9. Domankevitz Y, Nishioka NS: Effects of a rapidly scanned carbon dioxide laser on porcine dermis. J Burn Care Rehabil 1997;18:206
10. Kauvar AN, Waldorf HA, Geronemus RG: A histopathological comparison of "char-free" carbon dioxide lasers. Dermatol Surg 1996;22:343
11. Grover S, Apfelberg DB, Smoller B: Effects of varying density patterns and passes on depth of penetration in facial skin utilizing the carbon dioxide laser with automated scanner. Plast Reconstr Surg 1999;104:2247
12. Mullarky MB, Norris CW, and Goldberg ID: The efficacy of the CO_2 laser in the sterilization of skin seeded with bacteria: survival at the skin surface and in the plume emissions. Laryngoscope 1985;95:186
13. Engelbert TA, Tate LP Jr, Malone D, et al: Influence of inhaled smoke from upper respiratory laser surgery. Vet Radiol Ultrasound 1994;35:319
14. Alp E, Bijl D, Bleichrodt RP, et al: Surgical smoke and infection control. J Hosp Infect 2006;62:1.
15. Palmer SE: Instrumentation and techniques for carbon dioxide lasers in equine general surgery. Vet Clin North Am Equine Pract 1996;12:397
16. al-Qattan MM, Stranc MF, Jarmuske M, et al: Wound sterilization: CO_2 laser versus iodine. Br J Plast Surg 1989;42:380
17. Lee JS, Tarpley SK, Miller AS, et al: CO_2 laser sterilization in the surgical treatment of infected median sternotomy wounds. South Med J 1999;92:380
18. Reid AB, Stranc MF: Healing of infected wounds following iodine scrub or CO_2 laser treatment. Lasers Surg Med 1991;11:475
19. Green HA, Domankevitz Y, Nishioka NS: Pulsed carbon dioxide laser ablation of burned skin: in vitro and in vivo analysis. Lasers Surg Med 1990;10:476
20. Acikel C, Ulkur E, Celikoz B: Carbon dioxide laser resurfacing and thin skin grafting in the treatment of "stable and recalcitrant" vitiligo. Plast Reconstr Surg 2003;111:1291
21. Acikel C, Ulkur E, Guler MM: Treatment of burn scar depigmentation by carbon dioxide laser-assisted dermabrasion and thin skin grafting. Plast Reconstr Surg 2000;105:1973
22. Schindl A, Schindl M, Pernerstorfer-Schon H, et al: Low-intensity laser therapy: a review. J Invest Med 2000;48:312
23. Smith K: The photobiological basis of low level laser radiation therapy. Laser Ther 1991;3:9
24. Karu T: High-tech helps to estimate cellular mechanisms of low power laser therapy. Lasers Surg Med 2004;34:298
25. van Breugel HH, Bar PR: Power density and exposure time of He-Ne laser irradiation are more important than total energy dose in photo-biomodulation of human fibroblasts in vitro. Lasers Surg Med 1992;12:528
26. Lanzafame RJ, Stadler I, Kurtz AF, et al: Reciprocity of exposure time and irradiance on energy density during photoradiation on wound healing in a murine pressure ulcer model. Lasers Surg Med 2007;39:534
27. Hawkins D, Houreld N, Abrahamse H: Low level laser therapy (LLLT) as an effective therapeutic modality for delayed wound healing. Ann N Y Acad Sci 2005;1056:486
28. Kolarova H, Ditrichova D, Wagner J: Penetration of the laser light into the skin in vitro. Lasers Surg Med 1999;24:231
29. Gomez-Villamandos RJ, Santisteban Valenzuela JM, Ruiz Calatrava I, et al: He-Ne laser therapy by fibroendoscopy in the mucosa of the equine upper airway. Lasers Surg Med 1995;16:184
30. Cambier DC, Vanderstraeten GG, Mussen MJ, et al: Low-power laser and healing of burns: a preliminary assay. Plast Reconstr Surg 1996;97:555

31. Petersen SL, Botes C, Olivier A, et al: The effect of low level laser therapy (LLLT) on wound healing in horses. Equine Vet J 1999;31:228

32. Pourreau-Schneider N, Ahmed A, Soudry M, et al: Helium-neon laser treatment transforms fibroblasts into myofibroblasts. Am J Pathol 1990;137:171

33. Nelson JS: Lasers: state of the art in dermatology. Dermatol Clin 1993;11:15

34. Nussbaum EL, Lilge L, and Mazzulli T: Effects of 630-, 660-, 810-, and 905-nm laser irradiation delivering radiant exposure of 1–50 J/cm^2 on three species of bacteria in vitro. J Clin Laser Med Surg 2002;20:325

35. Lindholm AC, Swensson U, Mitri ND, et al: Clinical effects of betamethasone and hyaluronan, and of defocalized carbon dioxide laser treatment on traumatic arthritis in the fetlock joints of horses. J Vet Med Series A 2002;49:189

36. Alster TS, Kauvar ANB, Geronemus RG: Histology of high-energy pulsed CO_2 laser resurfacing. Semin Cutaneous Med Surg 1996;15:189

37. Bergh A, Nyman G, Lundeberg T, et al: Effect of defocused CO_2 laser on equine tissue perfusion. Acta Vet Scand 2006;47:33.

38. Bergh A, Ridderstrale Y, and Ekman S: Defocused CO_2 laser on equine skin: a histological examination. Equine Vet J 2007;39:114.

16 Bandaging and Casting Techniques for Wound Management

Jorge Gomez, DVM, MS, Diplomate ACVS and Ted S. Stashak, DVM, MS, Diplomate ACVS

Introduction

Bandaging, bandage splinting, and in some cases casting can be very important components of successful wound management. Bandages protect the wound from environmental contamination, including contact with flies, which may reduce the chance of sarcoid transformation of the wound. If properly applied, bandages effectively absorb wound exudate/discharge and at the same time reduce limb edema.[1] Following application, bandages increase limb temperature, which favors angiogenesis and increases tissue metabolism and wound healing. They also reduce CO_2 loss from the wound surface, thus reducing the pH which is detrimental to bacterial growth but favorable to oxygen release from hemoglobin at the wound surface.[2] Bandaged distal limb wounds also heal 30% more rapidly than do similar non-bandaged wounds.[3] A disadvantage to bandaging is that in wounds of the distal extremities it may encourage the development of exuberant granulation tissue.[4-9]

Splints made of polyvinyl chloride (PVC) plastic pipe or cast material affixed to the outside of the bandage can effectively immobilize highly mobile regions (e.g., fetlock, carpus, and hock).

Casts provide the most effective rigid external immobilization. They are often recommended and used for treatment of lacerations involving the coronary band, heel bulbs, and fetlock regions, and for any injury that compromises the integrity of a soft tissue support structure (e.g., tendons and/or ligaments). Casts are also recommended for sutured full-thickness wounds of the distal limb (carpus/tarsus and below) that are perpendicular or oblique to the limb's long axis and for distal extremity wounds that are sutured under tension.[10]

This chapter will focus on the techniques for applications of bandages, bandage splints, and casts to different regions of the body.

Bandage Layers and Materials

Bandages are usually composed of three layers: a primary or contact layer referred to as a "dressing"; a secondary or intermediate layer; and a tertiary or outer layer.[11]

A variety of wound dressings are available, ranging from passive adherent/non-adherent to interactive and bioactive products that contribute to the healing process. Many of the newer dressings are designed to create a moist wound healing environment which allows the wound fluids and growth factors to remain in contact with the wound, thus promoting autolytic debridement and accelerating wound healing.[12] For more information regarding wound dressings, see Chapter 3.

The main purpose of the secondary (intermediate) layer is to absorb fluids (e.g., serum, blood, exudate, etc.), bacteria, and necrotic debris from the wound. This layer should be thick enough to collect and absorb moisture, pad the wound against trauma, and "splint" it to prevent excessive motion. Materials used in the secondary layer are cotton pads (e.g., Gamgee™, CombiRoll™, RediRoll™) and conforming (elastic) gauze (e.g., Kling™, Comform™, Specialist Cast Padding™), which are applied to conform to the shape of the limb (Table 16.1).

The tertiary layer is usually composed of a material which is stiffer than that used for the secondary layer. The purpose of this outer layer is to hold the previous layers in place, prevent contamination and trauma, apply pressure to minimize swelling of the limb, and decrease flexion and extension of the limb. This final layer should be porous yet waterproof. Elastic self-adhesive bandages (e.g., Vetrap™, Powerflex™, Elastikon™, SECUR-Wrap™) are frequently used as the tertiary layer (Table 16.1). The tertiary layer should be applied with constant pressure that is gradually increased as the bandage is wrapped in a distal to proximal direction. The most proximal and distal aspects of the cotton pad (secondary layer) are initially left uncovered to avoid creating pressure points that may affect the cutaneous circulation. As a final step the proximal and distal ends of the

Table 16.1. Bandage materials.

Bandage material	Description	Common use	Source
Gamgee™	Cotton bandage	Secondary layer	3M Animal Care Products, St. Paul, MN
CombiRoll™	Cotton bandage	Secondary layer	The Franklin-Williams Co., Lexington, KY
RediRoll™	Cotton bandage	Secondary layer	The Franklin-Williams Co., Lexington, KY
Kling™	Conforming gauze	Support dressing	Johnson & Johnson, New Brunswick, NJ
Comform™	Conforming gauze	Support dressing	Covidien Animal Health/Kendall, Dublin, OH
Specialist Cast Padding™	Cast padding	Hock and carpal wounds	BSN Medical, Brierfield, UK
Vetrap™	Elastic self-adhesive	Hold secondary layer in place	3M Animal Care Products, St. Paul, MN
Powerflex™	Elastic self-adhesive	Hold secondary layer in place	Andover Coated Products Inc., Salisbury, MA
Elastiant™	Elastic adhesive	Hold secondary layer in place	Vet-One, Hampshire, UK
SECURWrap™	Elastic adhesive	Hold secondary layer in place	Securos, Charlton, MA
Elastikon™	Elastic adhesive	Hold secondary layer in place	Johnson & Johnson, Skillman, NJ

cotton pad are covered with an adhesive bandage tape (e.g., Elastikon™, Elastiant™) that adheres to both the outer bandage layer and the skin. This is done to keep the bandage in place and to prevent foreign material (e.g., wood shavings, dirt, etc.) from entering between the skin and the bandage, which may cause skin sores and wound contamination.

Bandaging Techniques

Wounds involving the hoof and pastern regions, the superficial (SDFT) and deep (DDFT) digital flexor tendons, carpus, hock, head, and trunk require special techniques to hold the bandages in place and avoid complications associated with bandaging.

Hoof and Pastern Regions

The foot can be bandaged for protection after treatment of penetrating wounds and complete avulsion injuries of the hoof wall and coronary band, and following hoof wall and sole resection.[10] Generally, the open wound is debrided (if applicable), irrigated with a dilute antiseptic solution, and then dressed with either a topical antibiotic or antiseptic ointment (e.g., povidone-iodine), an antimicrobial dressing (Kerlix AMD™ Covidien Animal Health/Kendall, Dublin, OH) or a debridement dressing (e.g., Wet-to-Dry or Cursalt™ Covidien Animal Health/Kendall, Dublin, OH) before the bandage is applied (Figure 16.1). (See Chapter 2 for more information regarding preparation of a wound and Chapter 3 for more information regarding selection of a wound dressing). Cotton bulk, sheet, or pad, folded on itself, is placed over the dressing for padding and further protection (Figures 16.2a and 16.2b), after which the foot is wrapped with elastic self-adherent tape (Figure 16.2c) and a multipurpose polycoated (duct) tape is used to cover the bottom of the foot (Figure 16.2d). Duct tape is preferred because it is more waterproof than other self-adhesive bandage materials. As an alternative, a rubber boot can be applied to the foot to protect and waterproof it (Figure 16.3).

If duct tape is used, a square patch can be made slightly larger than the surface area of the bottom of the foot by placing (sticking) the adhesive side of the tape onto a non-adherent surface (e.g., wall, table top, stainless steel surface). Each strip of tape is torn at the appropriate length, after which it is adhered to another strip by overlapping the edges. To provide a double thickness, a second layer of tape is placed over the first at a 90° angle, giving a cross-hatched appearance (Figure 16.4). The tape patch is then applied to the bottom of the foot, after which the redundant edges are folded up over the hoof wall. Duct tape is then used to hold the foot protection in place (Figures 16.2c and 16.2d).

Pastern wounds involving the coronary band or heel bulb regions are bandaged in a manner similar to the hoof except the bandage extends proximad to cover the wound in the pastern region. Most of these wounds are best managed with a phalangeal (foot/pastern) cast, which will be discussed later. Lacerations of the mid and proximal pastern region may be managed by bandaging the region without including the bottom of the foot. Elastic tape is used to attach the distal end of the bandage to the hoof wall.

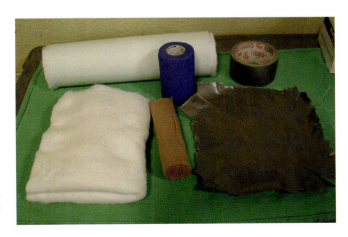

Figure 16.1. Material needed for a foot bandage. Left, cotton padding; middle, brown conforming gauze and elastic self-adhesive bandage (e.g., Vetrap™); and right: duct tape roll and patch.

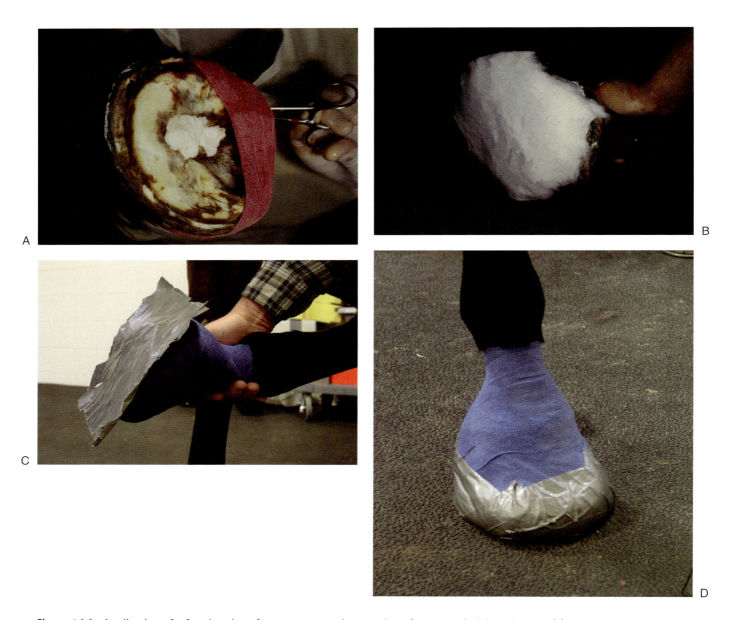

Figure 16.2. Application of a foot bandage for treatment and protection of an open draining abscess. (A) The wound in the sole is packed with an antimicrobial dressing. (B) Bulk cotton padding is applied to the bottom of the foot and then held in place with brown gauze. (C) Elastic self-adhesive tape (blue) is used to secure the cotton padding to the bottom of the foot and the patch of duct tape is applied to the bottom of the foot. (D) The bandage is complete.

Flexor Tendon Lacerations

Lacerations of the SDFT and the DDFT require special bandaging, splinting, and casting techniques to decrease tension on the wound edges and permit adequate healing.

Following proper preparation, the wound site is explored to determine the extent of the injury to the flexor tendons. Lacerations affecting >50% of the diameter of the SDFT and/or DDFT should be immobilized with the fetlock fixed in partial flexion. Following the application of an appropriate dressing (primary layer) that is held in place with sterile conforming gauze (e.g., Kling™), a laminated cotton roll bandage (e.g., CombiRoll™) is applied to the distal aspect of the limb from the coronary band to the proximal aspect of the metacarpus/metatarsus and secured with conforming gauze. Finally, the bandage is secured with self-adhesive tape (e.g., Vetrap™, SECURWrap™).

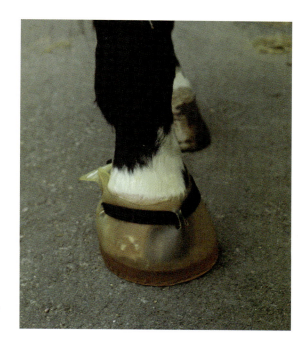

Figure 16.3. One of many types of plastic boots used to keep the hoof dry and clean.

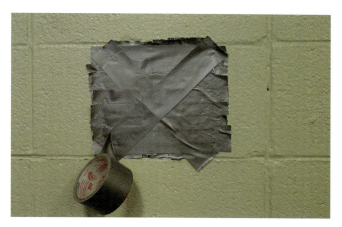

Figure 16.4. A patch of duct tape formed for use on the bottom of the foot.

If the horse is to be transported to a facility for further treatment, a PVC pipe bandage splint or a commercially available distal limb splint (Kimzey™, Woodland, CA) should be applied prior to transport. Although the Kimzey™ splint is one of the most effective in immobilizing the distal limb (Figure 10.11), an effective splint can be constructed using PVC material. The PVC pipe splint is affixed to the dorsal surface of the fore limb or the plantar surface of the pelvic limb using 5 cm white adhesive tape (Figures 10.12a 10.12b). To be most effective, the splint should extend down to the ground level in both cases. In the case of a fore limb laceration, the fetlock is pulled dorsally into the splint, placing the joint in flexion; in the case of a hind limb laceration, the foot is pulled in a plantar direction into the splint, which places the fetlock joint in partial flexion.

In most cases, a lower limb fiberglass cast or a Kimzey™ splint can be used for treatment. If a cast is selected it is applied from the bottom of the hoof to the proximal region of the metacarpus or metatarsus. An exception to this would be a flexor tendon transected at the proximal limits of the metacarpus/metatarsus; in this case the cast would extend proximad to include the carpus and tarsus. A wedge of wood or a folded roll of fiberglass casting tape, placed on the bottom of the hoof at the heel, elevates the heel and improves weight bearing (see lower limb casting, discussed later in this chapter, for more details). A Kimzey™ splint keeps the fetlock in partial flexion and prevents complications associated with the prolonged use of a cast, while enabling open wound management (see splints, discussed later in this chapter, and Chapter 10 for more information regarding treatment of tendon lacerations).

Carpus

Wounds on the dorsal surface of the carpus heal better when the carpus is immobilized in extension. Bandaging the carpus requires special care to avoid placing excessive pressure over the medial and lateral tuberosities of the distal radius and over the accessory carpal bone. These prominent and superficial structures are predisposed to the development of cutaneous sores from pressure and, in some cases, movement. An adhesive primary dressing is preferred (e.g., Covaderm Plus™, Powell, TN; Stery Strip™, St. Paul, MN). Alternatively a non-adherent dressing can be held in place with conforming gauze, which is secured to the skin using an elastic adhesive bandage (e.g., Elasticon™) placed at the distal or proximal extent of the primary layer or for greater security at both ends (Figures 16.5a and 16.5b). This will prevent the primary layer from slipping distad on the limb.

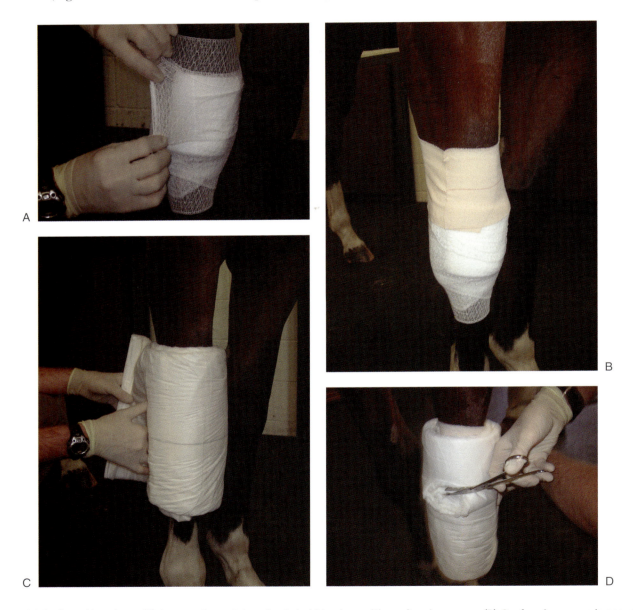

Figure 16.5. Carpal bandage. (A) A non-adherent dressing is held in place with conforming gauze. (B) Conforming gauze is secured to the skin at the proximal extent of the bandage with an elastic adhesive bandage. (C) A cotton pad is used as a secondary layer. (D) A plug of cotton is removed from the cotton pad overlying the accessory carpal bone on the palmar surface of the carpus. (E) (next page) A self-adhesive bandage has been applied over the cotton bandage and elastic adhesive tape is used to secure the bandage at its proximal and distal limits. (F) (next page) A circle of self-adhesive bandage was removed, overlying the accessory carpal bone in this case.

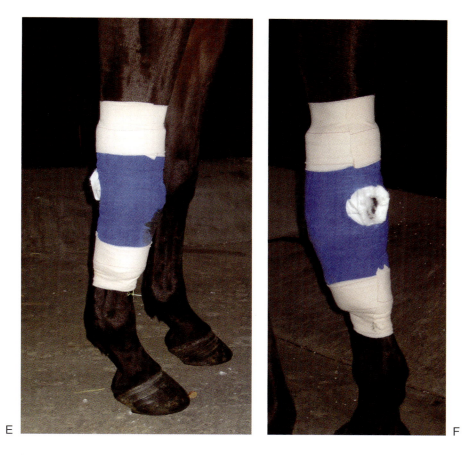

E

F

Figure 16.5. *Continued*

A cotton pad (e.g., CombiRoll™) may be used as a secondary layer, from which a plug of cotton is removed to minimize pressure over the bony prominences (Figures 16.5c and 16.5d). The secondary layer (cotton pad) can be secured with conforming gauze placed in a figure-8 pattern, after which an elastic self-adhesive bandage is applied, starting from proximal to distal. Elastic adhesive tape is used to secure the bandage at its proximal and distal limits (Figure 16.5e). A circle of the elastic self-adhesive bandage can be cut over the accessory carpal bone (Figure 16.5f).

Hock

The conformation of the hock and the combination of forces generated by the reciprocal apparatus impose some important considerations when applying a bandage to this region. Horses are reluctant to accept restricted movement of this region and frequently disrupt the bandage by hyper-flexing their hocks. The primary and secondary layers should be applied so as to avoid excessive circumferential pressure over the point of the hock (calcaneal tuberosity).

Using the same techniques as described for the carpus, a figure-8 bandage is applied, starting with complete loops of conforming gauze on the distal region of the crus and continuing with figure-8 loops below and above the point of the hock, thus leaving this prominence uncovered (Figures 16.6a and 16.6b). As a tertiary layer, a self-adhesive bandage (e.g., Vetrap™) is applied circumferentially over the cotton padding, from the most distal to the most proximal extent of the bandage (Figure 16.6c). Finally, elastic adhesive tape is used to secure the bandage at its proximal and distal limits to the hair (Figure 16.6d).

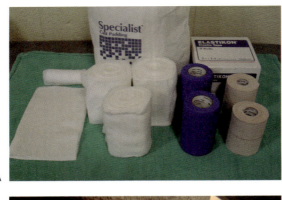

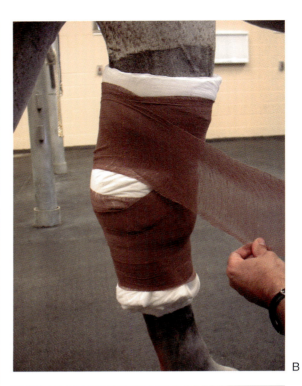

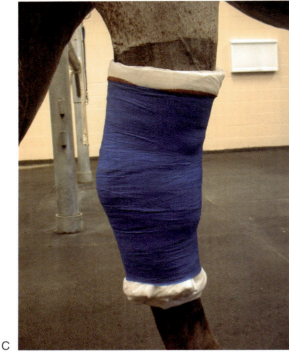

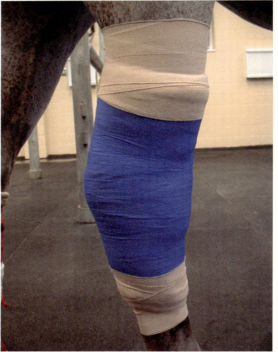

Figure 16.6. Hock bandage. (A) Materials needed for bandaging the hock. Left, dressing and conforming gauze; middle, specialist cast padding; and right, elastic adhesive bandage. (B) Brown conforming gauze is applied over the cotton bandage, leaving the point of the hock uncovered. (C) A self-adhesive bandage is applied over the cotton bandage from the most proximal to distal limits of the bandage. (D) Elastic adhesive tape is used to secure the bandage at its proximal and distal limits.

As an alternative, an adhesive or non-adhesive dressing can be used as a contact layer, which is held in place with conforming gauze. As a secondary layer, two or more rolls—according to the desired thickness—of a thin cotton bandage (Specialist Cast Padding™) can be applied circumferentially, from the distal third of the gaskin to the proximal third of the metatarsus. As a tertiary layer, a self-adhesive bandage (e.g., Vetrap™) is applied circumferentially over the cotton padding from the most distal to the most proximal extent of the bandage (Figure 16.6c). Finally, a length of elastic adhesive bandage (e.g., Elastikon™) is applied longitudinally to the plantar aspect of the limb over the tertiary layer from the most proximal to the most distal extent of the bandage (Figure 16.7a). Two or three loops of the same elastic adhesive bandage material are applied at the gaskin and metatarsal regions to secure the bandage in place (Figure 16.7b). The elastic adhesive bandage, placed longitudinally on the plantar surface of the bandaged limb, helps prevent disruption of the bandage when the hock is flexed (Figure 16.7c).

For large wounds on the dorsal and/or plantar aspect of the hock, applying a rigid bandage and/or splint to the distal limb with the fetlock in partial flexion can significantly decrease the range of motion of the hock, thereby increasing survival time of the bandage and allowing optimal wound healing.

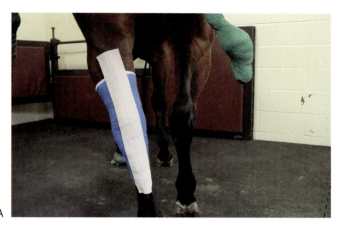

A

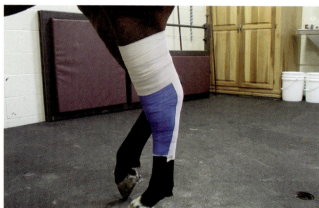

B

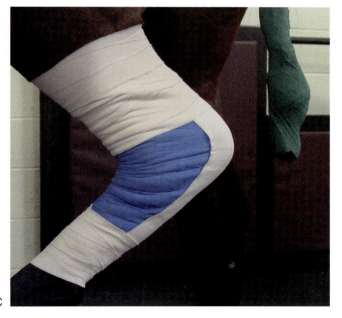

C

Figure 16.7. Alternative hock bandage. (A) A strip of elastic adhesive tape (e.g., Elastikon™) is placed longitudinally over the plantar surface of the hock region. (B) The strip of Elastikon™ is held in place at its proximal limit by circumferential rolls of the same tape. (C) Bandage complete; both the proximal and distal limits of the strip of Elastikon™ are secured with the same tape. The strip of Elastikon™ prevents disruption of the bandage during hock flexion. Courtesy of Dr. D. Peters.

Full Limb Bandage

A full limb bandage can also be used to cover wounds on the dorsal surface of the carpus or hock to decrease limb flexion and prevent bandage slippage. A laminated cotton roll bandage (e.g., CombiRoll™) is applied to the distal region of the limb from the coronary band to the proximal region of the metacarpus/metatarsus and secured with brown conforming gauze bandage (Figures 16.8a and 16.8b). A second roll of laminated cotton is applied immediately proximal to the distal roll from the most proximal region of the metacarpus/metatarsus to the most proximal region of the antebrachium or the mid-gaskin for the front and the hind limbs, respectively (Figure 16.8c). Two more rolls of laminated cotton are applied over the first rolls and in the same fashion from the coronary band to the most proximal region of the antebrachium/mid-gaskin, and then secured with elastic self-adhesive bandage. A fifth laminated cotton roll is placed over the carpus/hock and held in place with elastic self-adhesive bandage. Finally, an elastic self-adhesive bandage (e.g., Vetrap™) is applied from the coronary band to the most proximal limit of the bandage (Figure 16.8d). To increase stiffness of the bandage, a PVC half pipe splint can be customized and applied on the palmar surface of the forelimb. See the section on splinting for more details.

Head

A head bandage may be used to cover and protect a sutured laceration or a wound left open to heal by second intention, or it can be used to apply pressure. Elastic adhesive tape (e.g., Elastikon™) can be used to hold a sterile dressing in place, after which a 15 cm orthopedic stockinet is used to cover the head and the sterile dressing for further protection.

The application of the stockinet is as follows: the length of the stockinet required to cover the site is measured from the pole rostrally (Figure 16.9a) and the stockinet is cut if a single layer is to be used or folded back on itself (doubled) for more protection (Figure 16.9b) prior to cutting. The stockinet is rolled outward (Figure 16.9c) and then pulled over the face to the poll region and unrolled rostrally to cover the head (Figure 16.9d). Holes for the eyes and ears are cut in the stockinet. The rostral and caudal limits of the stockinet are secured with elastic adherent tape (e.g., Elastikon™) (Figure 16.9e).

To cover wounds that require some pressure (e.g., enucleation or a sinus flap), a figure-8 self-adhesive bandage is wrapped above and below the eyes and around the circumference of the throat latch, nasal bones, and the mandible (Figure 16.10). Horses are usually very tolerant of this type of bandage. Skin Bond® (Smith & Nephew, Hull, UK) can be used to increase the adhesion (stickiness) of the elastic bandage, thus reducing the amount of material required (Figures 16.11a–d).[13] Additionally, a 15 cm orthopedic stockinet may be applied over the head for further protection.

If further protection of a wound site is needed (e.g., following repair of an unstable facial fracture), a cast helmet can be made by forming moistened fiberglass cast tape over a mound of cotton padding that is covering the site. The moistened cast tape is unrolled and arranged in an accordion-like manner so that it completely covers the entire circumference of the cotton mound. Each strip of cast tape should overlap the next strip by at least half its width. Once the cast material has cured, it is secured in place with an elastic adhesive bandage (Figure 16.12).[13] An advantage to the cast helmet is that it can be removed and replaced as needed. In most cases it is used only during recovery from anesthesia and for transporting the horse in a trailer. However, it can be used in the post-operative period as needed.

Trunk, Neck, and Upper Limb Regions

Stent or tie-over bandages are suitable to cover sutured wounds or those left open to heal by second intention on the trunk, neck, and upper limb regions. A tie-over is achieved by placing loops of a heavy, non-absorbable suture (#1 or #2) through the skin, 3 cm apart and parallel to the wound edges (Figure 16.13a). The bandage that is applied to cover the wound is held in place by lacing umbilical tape through the previously created suture loops (Figure 16.13b). The bandage can be changed as needed. This type of bandage prevents retraction of the wound edges, keeps the wound free of contaminants, applies pressure to the wound, and provides a moist environment that is conducive to epithelialization. To place a stent bandage, sutures inserted at a variable distance from the wound margins are used to tie over a sterile dressing (Figure

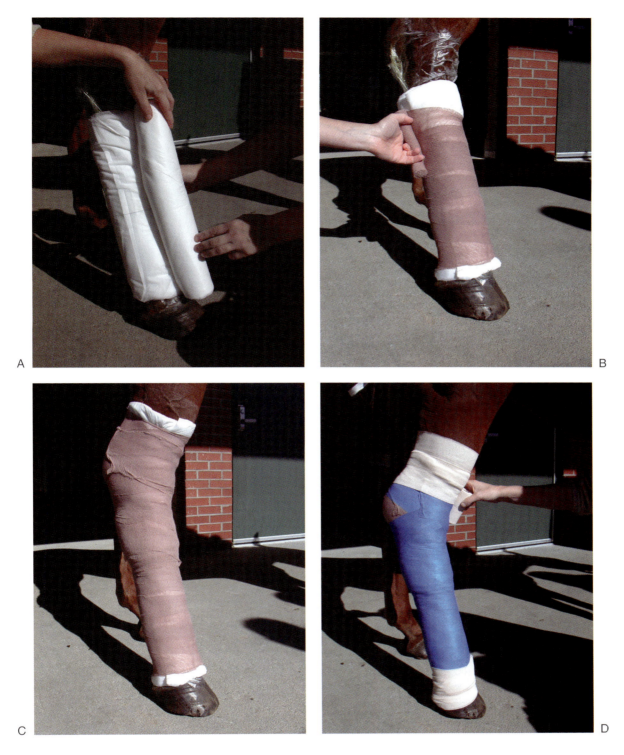

Figure 16.8. Full hind limb bandage. (A) A laminated rolled cotton bandage is applied from the coronary band to the proximal metatarsus. (B) Brown conforming gauze is used to secure the rolled cotton bandage. (C) A second rolled cotton bandage has been applied from the proximal metatarsus to the mid-gaskin region. Brown conforming gauze is used to secure the second cotton bandage. (D) Vetrap™ is used to secure the secondary layer and Elastikon™ is used to secure the proximal and distal limits of the bandage.

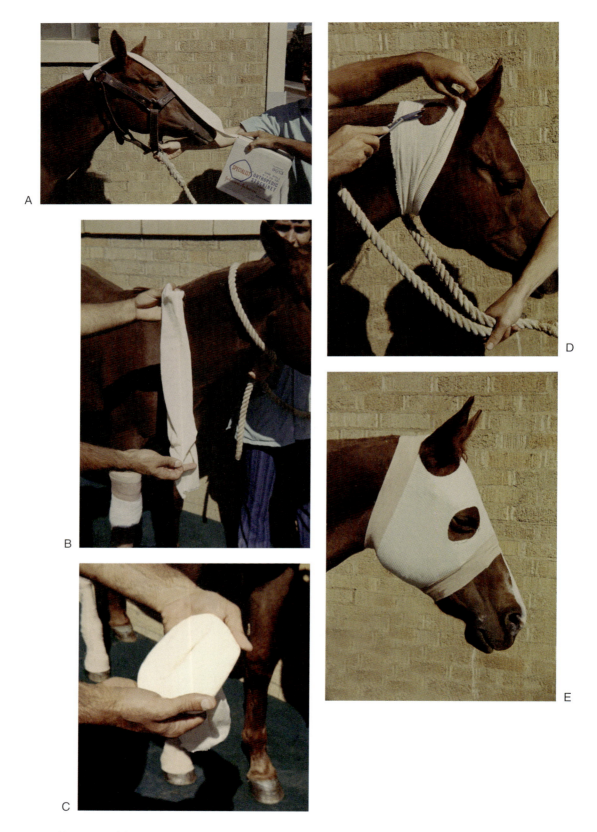

Figure 16.9. Head bandage. (A) Stockinet is measured from the poll rostral to the mid-nasal region. The stockinet is cut if a single layer is used. (B) The stockinet is doubled for greater protection. (C) The stockinet is rolled. (D) The stockinet is unrolled rostral from the poll. (E) Ear and eye holes have been cut and Elastikon™ is used to secure the caudal and rostral extents of the stockinet to the skin.

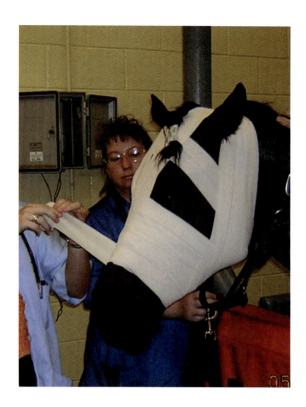

Figure 16.10. A figure-8 self-adhesive bandage is wrapped above and below the eyes and around the circumference of the throat latch, nasal bones, and mandible.

16.14). Stent bandages provide covering and pressure on the incision and decrease tension on the primary incision line.

Bandage Splinting

Bandage splinting is useful to manage wounds that need long-term immobilization yet frequent monitoring. Splints made of PVC pipe can be affixed to the outside of a bandage to reduce carpal and/or fetlock flexion. Thus, they are most effective when used to immobilize wounds involving extensor tendons as well as those involving the dorsal fetlock and dorsal carpal regions. Splints made from fiberglass casting tape are more effective in reducing hock flexion. They can be made either from cast material formed to the caudal aspect of the bandaged limb only, or from cast material that is wrapped circumferentially around the bandage, after which the cast is bivalved. Either approach is effective in the treatment of large wounds involving the dorsal hock region that may or may not be treated with skin grafting (Figure 16.15).

Polyvinyl Chloride Pipe

A half- (for the fetlock) or full limb (for the carpus) bandage is applied to the affected limb. Because it is often difficult to keep the splint in the proper position, it is most beneficial to apply conforming gauze, which is secured to the limb with an elastic adhesive tape (e.g., Elastikon™) before the secondary layer of cotton padding is applied. Otherwise, the cotton often shifts around the limb, causing the splint to become displaced. The cotton padding is secured to the limb with conforming gauze and elastic self-adhesive bandage. Additional cotton padding is usually applied to protect the limb from the PVC pipe splint before it is affixed to the bandage.

Generally 8 cm diameter PVC pipe is cut in thirds or halves, longitudinally, and the sharp ends are rounded. The PVC pipe can be made from a single piece or the components can be taped together, which is stronger than a single piece (Figures 16.16a and 16.6b). The PVC pipe is affixed to the palmar/caudal surface of the limb and

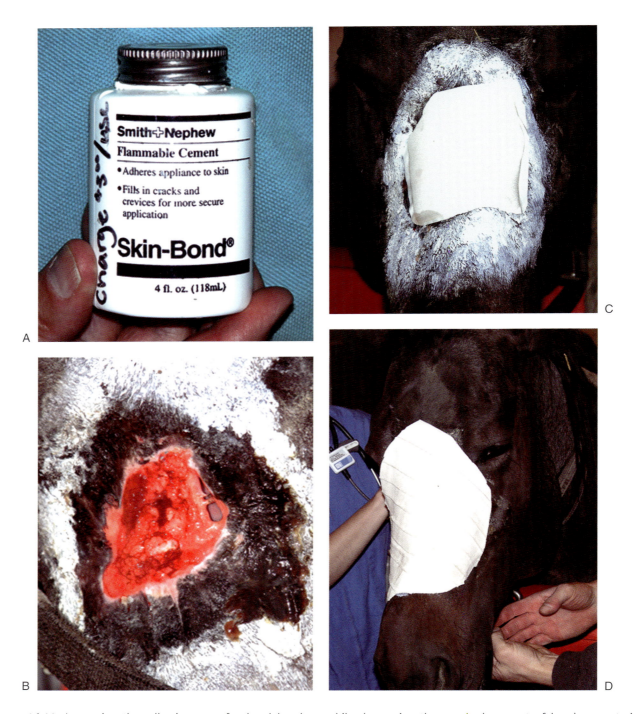

Figure 16.11. Increasing the adhesiveness of a head bandage while decreasing the required amount of bandage material. (A) Skin Bond® can be used to increase the adhesiveness of the elastic adherent tape. (B) Skin Bond® is applied around the perimeter of this healing nasocutaneous fistula. (C) A dressing is applied over the nasocutaneous fistula. (D) Elastikon™ is cut and adhered to the area where the Skin Bond® was applied.

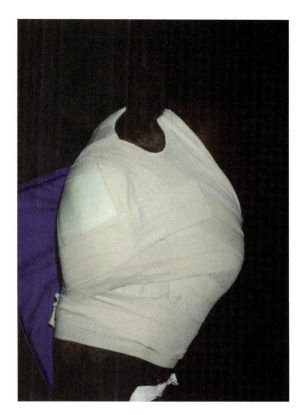

Figure 16.12. A cast helmet was used to cover/protect the repair site following surgical repair of a fracture of the supraorbital process.

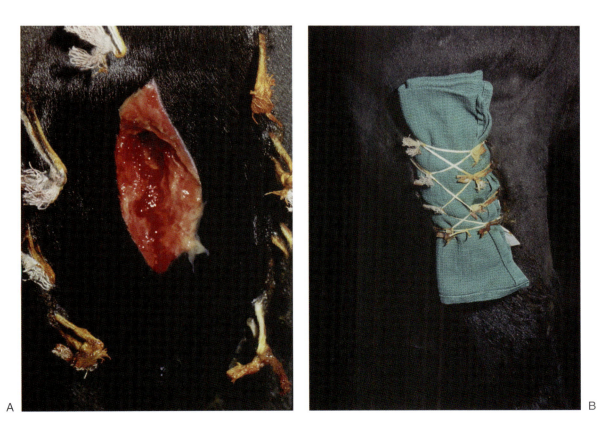

A

B

Figure 16.13. Tie-over bandage. (A) Loops of heavy, non-absorbable suture are placed in the skin parallel to the wound edges. This full-thickness wound entered the elbow joint. (B) A sterile towel is held in place by lacing umbilical tape through the previously created suture loops.

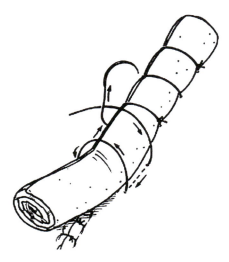

Figure 16.14. Illustration of a stent bandage being applied, over a sutured wound, with interrupted sutures.

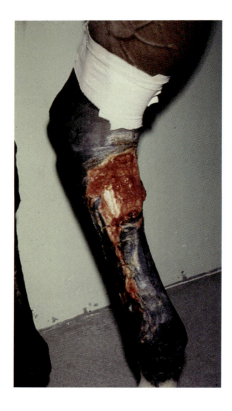

Figure 16.15. Large degloving wound involving the dorsal hock region that would benefit from a cast splint.

secured with self-adhesive bandage tape (Vetrap™) and 5 cm white non-elastic adhesive tape (Figure 16.16c). The non-elastic tape reduces the tendency for the splint to rotate independently from the bandage. To prevent the splint from slipping down the limb, elastic adhesive bandage tape (e.g., Elastikon™) should be wrapped around the distal extent of the splint to secure it to the bandage.

For the carpus, the PVC splint should extend from the distal metacarpus to the proximal radius (Figure 16.16c). For the fetlock, the PVC pipe should extend from the heel bulbs to the proximal metacarpus or metatarsus. To prevent fetlock flexion, as in the case of transected extensor tendons, extra cotton can be added to fill in the space between the phalanges and the full limb pipe splint (Figure 16.17). Alternatively, a full limb plastic splint can be heated and bent to fit the pastern region (Figure 16.18).

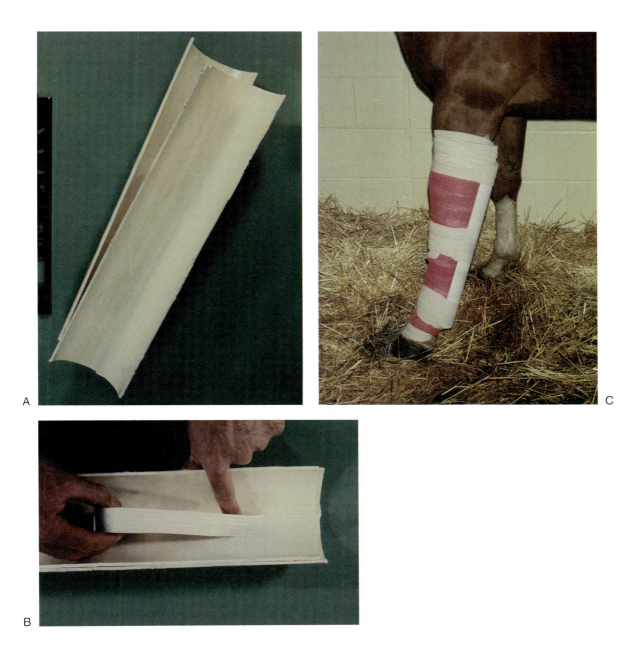

Figure 16.16. PVC pipe splint application. (A) 8 cm diameter PVC pipe has been cut in half, longitudinally. (B) The two components of the PVC pipe are taped together. (C) The splint has been affixed to the caudal/palmar surface of the bandage to prevent carpal flexion. The splint extends from the mid antebrachium to the distal metacarpus.

Cast Material

Even though a cast splint is most effective for preventing hock flexion, it can also be used for the same purpose at the carpus and fetlock. PVC pipe is usually selected for these other regions, due to the cost of materials and the convenience. However, on an angled hock the application of PVC tubing is impractical. The cast splint is made from four to five rolls of 12 cm–15 cm fiberglass cast tape that is affixed to the back of the limb over a bandage. Alternatively, a commercial splint (OrthoSplint™) made from nine layers of fiberglass tape impregnated with polyurethane resin can be used (Figure 16.19). The splint should extend from the distal metatarsus to the mid- or proximal crus.

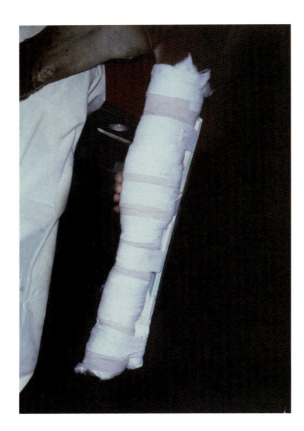

Figure 16.17. Extra cotton padding has been added to fill in the space between the phalanges and a full limb pipe splint. The extra padding will prevent fetlock flexion.

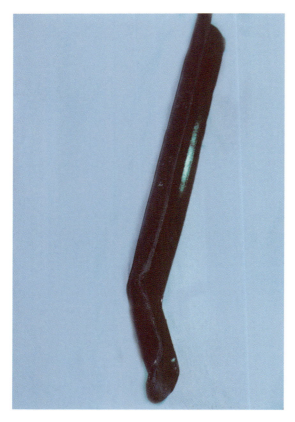

Figure 16.18. The plastic splint was heated and bent to fit the contour of the pastern region, thus preventing flexion of the fetlock.

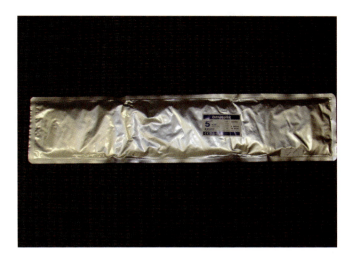

Figure 16.19. OrthoSplint™.

The technique for making the splint from fiberglass casting tape is as follows: First, a full hind limb bandage is applied (described previously). Once complete, the bandage area where the splint is to be affixed is covered with a water-impervious material (e.g., disposable plastic OB sleeve or plastic food wrapping sheets). The first cast tape is unrolled on the plantar/caudal surface of the hind limb to the proper length, then folded back on itself repeatedly in a slight overlapping manner (from side to side). Additional rolls of cast tape are unrolled (rapidly to circumvent curing) in a similar fashion and attached to the first roll to make a splint. The splint is dipped in water, stripped of excess moisture, and placed on the caudal surface of the limb. It is manually molded to the limb, after which the splint is held in place with conforming gauze.

The cast material is allowed to set for 2 to 3 minutes and then removed by cutting the plastic wrapping as well as the conforming gauze with scissors. Rubbing the cast with a gloved hand, lubricated with water or cream, helps laminate the cast tape layers. The splint should be allowed to cure for at least 20–30 minutes before affixing it to the bandage Figure 16.20a.

As an alternative (the second author's preference), the first roll of casting tape is dipped in water and applied to the caudal limb as described. It is conformed to the bandage by hand rubbing, after which it is held in place with conforming gauze. Once the cast splint has set (firm enough to act as a mold), it is removed and more cast tape is added to it to form the splint. Once cured, the splint cast is affixed to the bandage with either non-elastic 5 cm white tape or self adhesive elastic bandage (e.g., Vetrap™) (Figure 16.20b). Adhesive tape can be used to secure the splint at its proximal and distal limits.

To construct a bi-valved cast splint, a half-limb or full limb bandage is applied, depending on the need, as previously described. Several rolls (four to five) of fiberglass cast tape are applied over the bandage to increase its strength and ensure immobilization (Figure 16.21a). Once the cast cures, usually within 20–30 minutes, it is cut laterally and medially into two longitudinal halves (bi-valved) to allow removal for dressing changes and wound treatment (Figure 16.21b). After re-bandaging the wound, the two half-casts are re-applied and secured with elastic self-adhesive tape (Figures 16.21c, 16.21d, and 16.21e).

Casting

Casts are frequently used to immobilize wounds involving the distal limb, including those involving the flexor tendons, the fetlock and pastern, coronary band, and heel bulbs regions. These injuries typically heal more quickly and with less scarring when the limb is immobilized.

Selected Products

Various fiberglass casting tapes are commercially available (Table 16.2). Fiberglass is preferred over plaster of paris because of its shorter curing time[14] and greater strength and durability.[15–20] Curing refers to the irrevers-

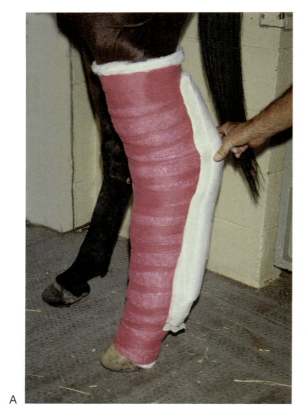
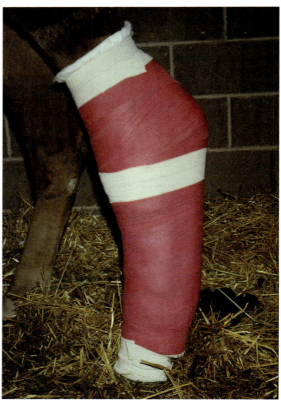

A   B

Figure 16.20. Cast splint for the hind limb. (A) The cast splint has cured and is ready to apply to the hind limb. (B) Vetrap™ is used to affix the cast splint to the bandage. Elasticon™ is used to prevent the end of the self-adherent tape from unraveling (center) and to further secure the splint proximally and distally.

ible transformation of the soft, flexible, resin-impregnated casting tape into a firm, rigid material; curing time refers to the time it takes for the material to achieve full strength. Following submersion in warm water, most fiberglass cast tape products cure within 20–30 minutes,[14] compared to plaster, which takes 24–72 hours to completely cure.[19]

Because a significant proportion of the strength in the fiberglass cast is derived from bonding between layers, correct application of the tape is important. Most fiberglass tape companies recommend that the strips of material be overlapped by 30%–50%[19] and for the tape to be further conformed and laminated by rubbing it with the gloved hand. It is important that the cast be rubbed with the open hand while avoiding finger pressure, which may create a depression in the material, leading to the formation of a pressure point on the soft tissues underlying the cast.

A variety of padding materials are used to protect the soft tissues of the limb against abrasion by the cast material (Table 16.2). Stockinet applied in a double layer is often used for this purpose. While cotton stockinet may retain moisture, polyester or polypropylene stockinets allow passage of moisture and exudate, and therefore are considered more appropriate for use under a fiberglass cast.[18] Stockinet should conform to the limb and be wrinkle-free following its application.

Orthopedic casting felt customarily has been applied over stockinet at sites where there is an increased risk of pressure developing. It is still commonly applied as a ring surrounding the circumference of the limb at the top of the cast and occasionally it is placed over anatomic prominences with little soft tissue covering (e.g., accessory carpal bone, calcaneal tuberosity, etc). Problems may arise if the felt either slips distad, creating a pressure point, or compresses, leaving a space for movement to occur between the soft tissue and cast. Both can lead to the development of skin sores (see Cast Complications discussed later). A resin-impregnated water curable cast foam (e.g., Custom Support Foam™, Procel Cast Liner™) applied over the stockinet was shown in

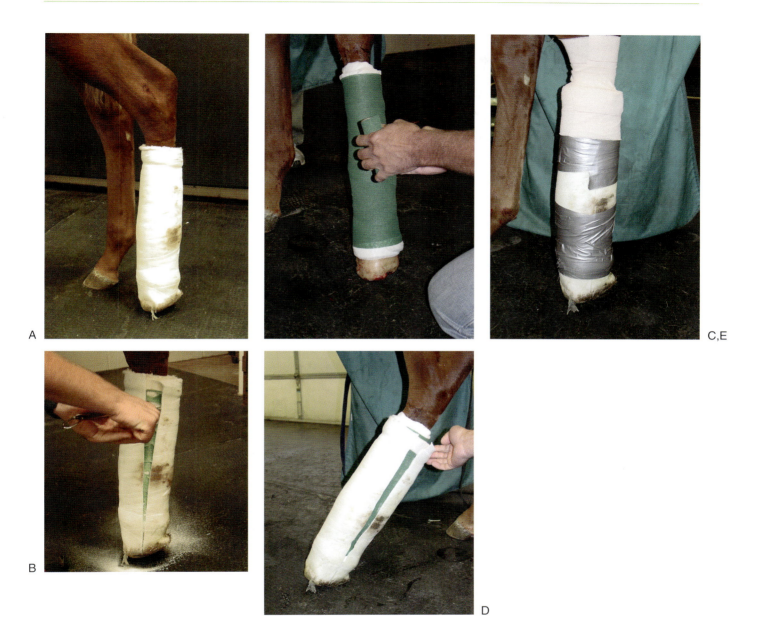

Figure 16.21. Half-limb (lower) bandage cast. (A) Fiberglass cast material has been applied over the lower limb bandage. (B) The cast has been cut and is being split, laterally and medially, into longitudinal halves (bivalved) so the bandage can be changed. (C) Following bandage change. (D) The cast is re-applied to the limb. (E) The body of the cast is secured with duct tape while Elasticon™ is used to cover the opening at the proximal extent of the cast.

early clinical evaluations to reduce the incidence of skin sores without increasing the weight of the cast or decreasing its permeability.[21]

Techniques

Casts of various lengths are used according to the location of the injury. A phalangeal cast that covers the hoof and pastern is recommended for wounds involving the hoof wall, coronary band, heel bulbs, or distal pastern region. For wounds involving the fetlock and/or the flexor tendons, application of a lower limb cast,

Table 16.2. Casting materials and splints.

Material	Common use and estimated set and weight-bearing times	Source
Stockinet™	First layer between skin with or without a bandage and cast padding	3M Animal Care Products, St. Paul, MN
Custom Support Foam™	Padding layer between cast and stockinet	3M Animal Care Products, St. Paul, MN
Procel Cast Liner™	Padding layer between cast and stockinet	W.L. Gore & Associates, Flagstaff, AZ
Orthopedic Felt	Extra padding proximal end of the cast and over bony prominences	Hartman-Conco Inc., Rock Hill, SC
Delta-Lite™	Fiberglass fabric, polyurethane resin casting tape Set: 7 minutes Weight bearing: 20 minutes	Johnson & Johnson Products Inc., New Brunswick, NJ
Dynacast Extra™	Fiberglass fabric, polyurethane resin casting tape Set: 10 minutes Weight bearing: 30 minutes	Smith & Nephew, Hull, UK
Vet Cast™	Fiberglass casting tape Set: 3–5 minutes Weight bearing: 20 minutes	3M Animal Care Products, St. Paul, MN
Scotch Cast™ and Vet Cast Plus™	Fiberglass casting tape Set: 3–5 minutes Weight bearing: 10 minutes	3M Animal Care Products, St. Paul, MN
Orthocast Plus™	Fiberglass casting tape Set: 5 minutes Weight bearing: 20 minutes	Securos, Charlton, MA
PVC splint	Immobilize limb Frequent removal to monitor a wound	Custom made
OrthoSplint™	Fiberglass cast splint Immobilization	Securos, Charlton, MA

which extends from the bottom of the hoof to the most proximal extent of the metacarpus or metatarsus, is recommended. Tube (sleeve) casts, extending from the most distal region of the metacarpus/metatarsus to the proximal region of the antebrachium/crus (gaskin), are suitable to manage some wounds over the carpal and tarsal joints. To ensure efficiency, the equipment and materials needed for preparation of the patient/wound and cast application should be acquired in advance of the planned procedure (Box 16.1).

Phalangeal (Foot Pattern or Slipper) Cast

Wounds of the coronary band and the pastern are subjected to significant motion that favors wound dehiscence, proliferation of granulation tissue, and delayed healing.[22–24] A phalangeal cast applied with the horse sedated (this method is preferred by the authors) or under general anesthesia is the recommended approach to manage wounds of these regions. Before applying the cast, the shoe should be removed and the sole and frog cleaned and trimmed. A non-adherent synthetic dressing is applied over the wound and is secured with one-third to one-half of a roll of sterile conforming gauze (Box 16.1). A double layer of stockinet is applied from the bottom of the hoof to 4 cm–5 cm past the planned proximal extent of the cast. At the proximal extent of the pastern a 2.5 cm–3 cm wide band of orthopedic felt is applied to the circumference of the pastern, over the stockinet, and secured with 2.5 cm white adhesive non-elastic tape. One layer of resin-impregnated cast liner (e.g., Custom Support Foam™, Procel Cast Liner™) is then applied (Figure 16.22a).

In the standing, sedated horse, 1 roll of 12.5 cm fiberglass cast tape can be used to cover the bottom of the foot. The cast material is unrolled and repeatedly folded back and forth on itself accordion-style; it is then

Box 16.1.

Preparation of the Patient, Materials, and Equipment Needed for Cast Application

Preparation of the Foot and Limb

- **Foot**
  1. Remove shoe, trim and clean foot.
  2. Treat/pack sulcus with gauze soaked in povidone-iodine (Betadine™ Solution, Purdue Frederick Co., Norwalk, CT) if thrush is a problem.
- **Limb**
  1. Clip hair around wound.
  2. Irrigate and debride wound.
  3. Suture wound if indicated.
  4. Apply appropriate dressing and secure it with a half roll of sterile conforming gauze.

Equipment and Materials Needed for Cast Application

- Scissors to clip excessively long hair (e.g., palmar/plantar pastern region)
- Stockinet of 5–10 cm diameter, depending on the size of the limb, rolled to form two layers
- Cast padding
  A. Orthopedic felt: ½ cm thick, cut to fit the region
  B. White non-elastic self-adhesive tape 2.5 cm to secure the felt in place
  C. Resin-impregnated cast foam
  D. Gloves and a bucket of warm water
- Cast
  A. Rubber gloves to apply the cast
  B. Fiberglass cast material needed
     a. Mature horses: In general, the number of rolls depends on the size of the horse
        - Phalangeal cast: One roll of 12.5 cm cast tape (bottom of the foot), two to three rolls (hoof and pastern region) of 10 cm cast tape
        - Lower limb cast: Six to seven rolls, including material for heel wedge
        - Full limb cast: Seven to nine rolls of 10–12.5 cm cast tape, including the heel wedge
        - Sleeve cast: Four to five rolls of 10 cm or 12.5 cm cast tape
     b. Immature horses
        I. Foals
           - Lower limb and sleeve casts: two to three rolls of 7.5–10 cm cast tape.
           - Full limb casts: Uncommon application for wound management; four rolls of 7.5–10 cm cast tape.
        II. Weanlings and yearlings
           - Lower limb and sleeve casts: Three to four rolls of 7.5–10 cm cast tape.
           - Full limb: Uncommon; five to six rolls of 7.5–10 cm cast tape
  C. Cast protection
     a. Hoof acrylic (e.g., Technovit™)
     b. Tongue depressor
     c. Elastic self-adhesive tape
        I. To cover the opening at the top of the cast.
        II. To cover the bottom of foot (Technovit™) to help prevent the horse from slipping during recovery from anesthesia and while walking on a slippery surface.

applied to the bottom of the foot which is subsequently placed on the ground in the normal standing position. A plastic bag can be placed under the bottom of the foot to protect the flooring. The remainder of the cast is applied up to the mid-portion of the orthopedic felt (Figure 16.22b); usually two to three rolls of 10 cm fiberglass tape are used. Once complete, the stockinet is cut to within 7.5 cm above the upper limits of the

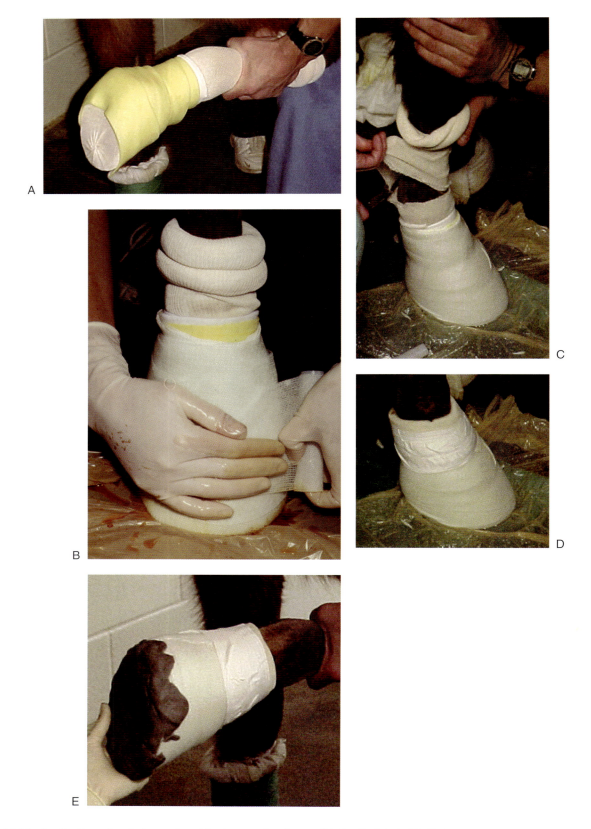

Figure 16.22. Application of a phalangeal cast in the standing horse. (A) The limb is held off the ground to apply a single layer of cast padding (Custom Support Foam™) to the pastern and hoof regions and a fiberglass cast tape to the bottom of the foot (not shown). A ring of orthopedic felt, underlying the foam, was placed at the proximal pastern. (B) A roll of 12.5 cm fiberglass cast tape has been applied to the bottom of the foot. The remainder of the cast is being applied to the pastern up to the mid-portion of the orthopedic felt in the standing horse. (C) Excess stockinet is cut in preparation of rolling it distad over the cast. (D) The rolled stockinet is being secured to the cast with 5 cm white non-elastic tape. (E) Technovit™ has been applied to the bottom of the cast.

cast (Figure 16.22c). The stockinet is then rolled distad and attached to the cast with 5 cm white inelastic adhesive tape (Figure 16.22d). After the cast hardens (about 5 to 7 minutes), an acrylic protector (Technovit™, Jorgensen Laboratories, Loveland, CO) is applied to the bottom of the cast to improve resistance and impermeability (Figure 16.22e).[13] Elastic adherent bandage is applied to the top of the cast to prevent contaminants (e.g., dirt, bedding, etc.) from migrating between the cast and skin.

Alternatively, the upper part of the cast can be applied first. Two to three rolls of 10 cm fiberglass cast tape are applied, beginning 1 cm below the proximal edge of the orthopedic felt and rolled distad to the bottom of the foot, without covering the sole. After 5 to 7 minutes (enough time for the cast to harden), the hoof is picked up and two rolls of 4 in (10 cm) fiberglass cast tape are applied to the bottom of the hoof to cover the sole and the hoof wall. Technovit™ is applied to the bottom of the cast to minimize wear upon weight bearing.[11]

Another approach to applying a hind limb phalangeal cast is to have the horse stand with both hind feet on a block of wood (5 cm × 15 cm × 20 cm); the toe of the affected limb rests on the board. It is important that the sole of the affected limb remain parallel to the ground and that the toe does not become elevated.[25] Positioning the foot in this manner allows the majority of the cast to be applied with the limb fully weight bearing. Once the cast dries, cast material is applied to the toe region while the limb is extended craniad. Technovit™ is applied to the bottom of the hoof for protection.[25] Whenever a phalangeal cast is applied while the horse is standing, the patient must not walk until the cast has cured (20–30 minutes).

When the cast is applied to a horse under general anesthesia, two wires placed through holes made in the white line, 2 cm medial and lateral to the dorsal midline of the hoof, are used to pull the phalanges into extension while the cast material is being applied (Figure 16.23).[22]

The phalangeal cast is usually removed in 10–14 days, at which time the wound is re-examined. A new cast can be applied at this time if necessary.

Distal (Lower, Short-, or Half-) Limb Cast

It is usually best to apply a distal limb cast while the horse is under general anesthesia; however, there are circumstances in which it should be applied in the standing animal (e.g., a horse at risk for general anesthesia). The limb must be clean. The stockinet is measured, cut, and rolled in such a fashion that it becomes a double layer that will cover the limb (Figures 16.24a–c). The foot should be prepared as described in Box 16.1. These steps are particularly important if the cast is to remain on the limb for a prolonged period (4 to 6 weeks). If the hair on the palmar or plantar pastern and fetlock regions is long, it should be trimmed. If a bandage is required to protect/cover a wound, a sterile non-adherent dressing is secured using $< \frac{1}{2}$ roll of sterile conforming gauze. One layer (outward rolled) of the stockinet is unrolled, beginning at the sole, to above the carpus/tarsus. The other roll is twisted at the bottom of the foot to hold it in place and unrolled in a similar manner as described for the first layer, such that two layers cover the limb (Figure 16.25a and 16.25b). The stockinet should fit snugly, conform to the limb, and be free of wrinkles (Figure 16.25b). Generally, a ring of orthopedic felt is applied to the proximal limit of the metacarpus/metatarsus and secured with 2.5 cm

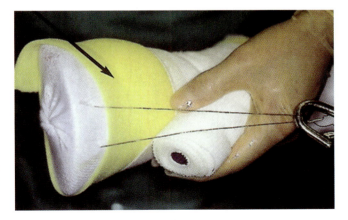

Figure 16.23. Application of a phalangeal cast in the anesthetized horse. Two wires placed through holes made in the white line 2 cm medial and lateral to the dorsal midline of the hoof are being used to pull the phalanges into extension. Courtesy of Dr. D. Knottenbelt.

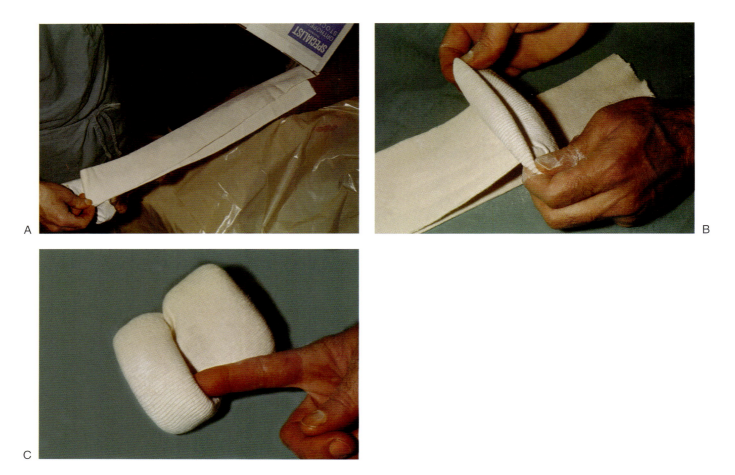

Figure 16.24. Preparation of the stockinet for application. (A) The length of stockinet is measured against the limb. Twice this length will be required to make a double layer to cover the limb. (B) The stockinet is folded in half. One end is rolled outward, the other end inward, and both rolled ends will meet in the center. (C) The rolled stockinet is ready for application.

non-elastic white tape (Figure 16.25b). A layer of cast padding (e.g., Custom Support Foam™, Procel Cast Liner™) is applied over the stockinet prior to application of the cast material (Figure 16.25c). Excessive padding should be avoided because, when compressed, it can increase limb movement within the cast and consequently the chances of developing skin sores. There are specific instructions on how to handle each type of padding material. Some materials will start to set as soon as they are exposed to air; therefore, they are kept packaged until needed.

The limb should be positioned according to the injury. When treating a flexor tendon laceration or a severe heel bulb laceration generating considerable tension upon suture apposition, it is best to cast the limb with the fetlock relaxed in a slightly flexed position. For most other problems the limb can be cast in extension by applying pressure to the toe region and dorsal surface of the carpus in the forelimb, and plantar hock and cranial stifle regions of the hind limb.

The cast tape should be submerged in warm water. Generally the hotter the water the more rapidly the cast material will cure. The drier the cast, the less one layer will laminate to another. Usually two to three rolls of 10 cm cast tape are used first because it is easier to conform to the limb than the 12.5 cm or 15 cm tape. To apply the cast one can start at the bottom or the top; the top is preferred by the authors. The cast is best applied by unraveling the material in close apposition to the limb. The cast material should be overlapped by at least one-third to one-half (the authors' preference) its width, and the first layers applied with minimal circumferential tension (Figure 16.26a). The cast should be applied from the top to just above the sole

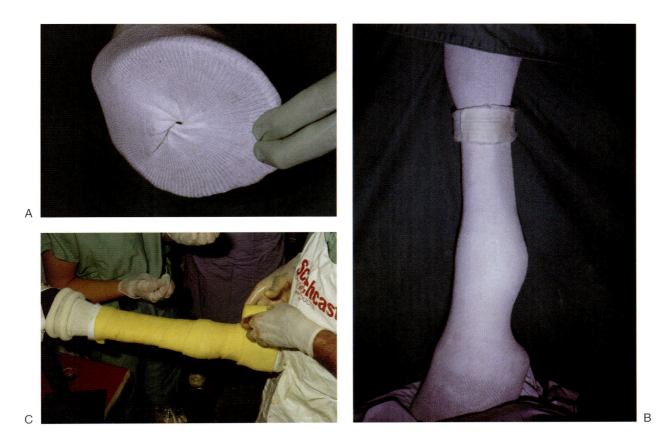

Figure 16.25. Application of the stockinet. (A) The outward and inward rolls of stockinet have been twisted at the bottom of the foot. The twist should be located at the palmar/plantar third of the sole to avoid adding length to the toe region. (B) The two rolls of stockinet have been applied to the limb; note that there are no wrinkles and they conform to the limb. A layer of orthopedic felt has been applied over the stockinet at the proximal metacarpus. Phalanges are fixed and maintained in an extended position by the pressure being applied to the toe region. (C) A layer of Custom Support Foam™ has been applied over the stockinet.

of the foot; the foot will be incorporated in the cast after the upper part hardens (sets). When it is necessary to change directions of the cast tape to conform it to the limb, it is better to make one large fold rather than multiple small ones.

Application of the second roll should start where the first roll ended. It is good practice to make several wraps at the proximal extremity of the cast in an effort to ensure an equivalent thickness to the rest of the cast. The stockinet at the top of the cast should be folded down over the first layers of cast and incorporated into the subsequent layers, leaving a nice rounded edge around the top circumference of the cast.

After each roll of cast tape has been applied it should be rubbed with the open gloved hand, moistened with water or cream, to better conform and laminate the material. Once the upper part of the cast hardens, the limb is supported with the open hand (not the fingertips, which could create pressure points in the cast material) at the level of the fetlock. The bottom of the foot is cast by unrolling the casting tape and applying it circumferentially around the foot so that one-third of the cast tape width covers the outer hoof wall and the remaining two thirds cover the sole. Applying the cast tape in this fashion will usually ensure coverage of the entire bottom of the foot. When one-third of the roll of casting tape remains it can be used to wrap the dorsal and solar surfaces of the hoof to create a smooth covering to the ground surface.

A heel wedge is applied at this time; its height is adjusted to allow the horse to walk more easily by decreasing the break over force generated during walking. This technique is also very effective in decreasing the pressure exerted by the cast at its dorsal proximal extent on the metacarpus or metatarsus. The heel wedge is formed

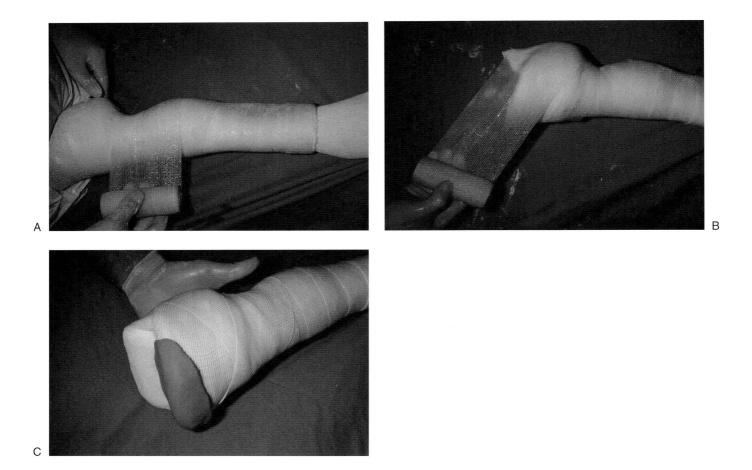

Figure 16.26. Cast application. (A) Casting tape is being applied to the limb. Enough room is available on the underside of the limb to allow circumferential application without lifting the limb. (B) A partial roll of cast tape (heel wedge) has been secured to the heel region with cast tape. (C) Hoof acrylic has been applied to the toe region.

from one-third to one-half of a roll of 10 cm cast material. It is rolled up, dipped in water, shaped to fit the heel, and attached with the remaining cast material (Figure 16.26b). The bottom of the cast is best protected with Technovit™ (Figure 16.26c). Elastic adhesive tape (e.g., Elastikon™) is applied to the top of the cast and the hair just proximal to it. Once the horse recovers from general anesthesia a rubber boot with a wooden block attached to the bottom can be applied to the hoof of the unaffected limb in an attempt to equalize the length of the fore-limbs (Figure 16.27).[26]

Full Limb Cast

The principles for applying a full limb cast are identical to those for a half-limb cast except that orthopedic felt may be applied as a strip over the accessory carpal bone and the medial tuberosity of the radius (fore limb) or the calcaneal tuberosity and the dorsal surface of the hock (hind limb). The strips of orthopedic felt are held in place with 2.5 cm white non-elastic adhesive tape. However, since the advent of cast foam padding, the authors have discontinued using the orthopedic felt over these prominences. A full fore limb and hind limb cast should encase the foot and extend to the proximal third of the antebrachium and crus respectively.

If the horse is under general anesthesia and in lateral recumbency the limb should be cast while it is in the uppermost position; this will avoid the abnormal limb position that occurs with pressure applied to the muscles on the downside limb. While this is not so important for the fore limb, it is still recommended in most cases even if the horse must be rolled over to cast the limb. The limb to be cast should also be positioned so that it is

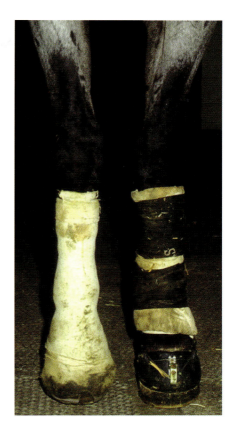

Figure 16.27. A rubber boot to which a block of wood is attached to the bottom has been applied to the foot of the unaffected limb. Note that the limb lengths appear equivalent.

parallel to the ground. If the limb is uppermost it maybe positioned and stabilized using a limb support (e.g., leg brace) placed under the proximal antebrachium for the fore limb or under the proximal crus for the hind limb.

During recovery it is best to place the horse so the cast limb is uppermost. This allows the down limb to flex and extend so the horse can stand. In all cases horses should be observed closely when recovering from general anesthesia after a full limb cast has been applied. Assistance during recovery is recommended.

Cast Applied in the Standing Horse

Distal or full limb casts can be applied to well mannered, sedated, standing horses. Although the principles for applying standing casts are the same as those for casts applied under general anesthesia, applying the cast to the foot can be awkward. It is easiest to cast the foot first, followed by the limb. The limb is elevated to expose the sole, the distance from the toe to the heel is measured, and three-fourths to a full roll of 12.5 cm cast tape is applied first to the solar surface (accordion-style), and then it is held in place by wrapping the cast tape over the dorsal and solar surfaces of the hoof wall. Once complete, the foot is placed on the ground and the remaining rolls of cast tape are applied with the horse weight-bearing. A plastic disposable garbage bag placed under the foot will keep the floor clean. At least 20–30 minutes should pass after the cast is applied before the horse is allowed to move.

Tube (Sleeve) Cast

A tube cast can be applied to either the fore or hind limb to immobilize the carpus or tarsus. It is usually applied from the proximal antebrachium in the fore limb or proximal crus in the hind limb to the proximal extent of the proximal sesamoid bones. Following application of the stockinet, a ring of orthopedic felt is placed at the level of the proximal limits of the proximal sesamoid bones. Another ring of orthopedic felt is applied at the proposed upper limits of the cast (Figure 16.28a). Cast foam or a bandage is often used as cast padding. The cast is usually made using four to five rolls of 10 cm–12.5 cm fiberglass casting tape (Figure 16.28b). The advantages of a sleeve cast over a full limb cast are ease of application, economy of cast material, and comfort (the foot is exposed and the fetlock can flex).

Cast Complications

Horses are not ideal candidates for cast immobilization because most return to weight bearing and ambulation shortly following application, which continually stresses the cast and may lead to complications.[19] Complications associated with casts include skin sores and cracking or breaking of the cast. Full limb cast complications include fracture of the radius or tibia, rupture of the peroneus tertius, coxofemoral luxation, and effects associated with prolonged immobilization.

Skin Sores

Skin sores more commonly result from movement of soft tissues underlying or at the top of the cast than from static pressure (Figure 16.29). Compression of the cast padding, reduced limb swelling, or an ill-fitting cast

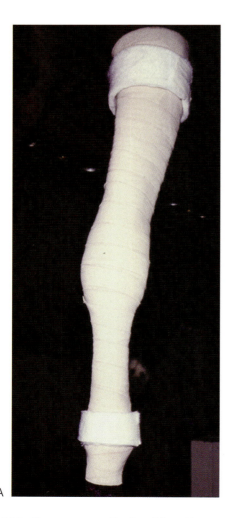
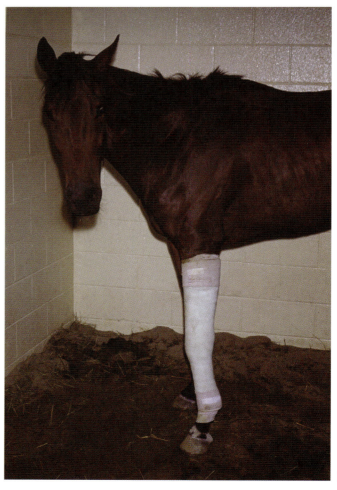

A   B

Figure 16.28. Sleeve cast application. (A) In this case Elasticon™ applied over Kling gauze™ was used instead of orthopedic stockinet to pad the limb. A ring of orthopedic felt has been placed at the proposed proximal and distal limits of the cast. Custom Support Foam™ can be applied at this point. (B) Four rolls of fiberglass casting tape were used to make this forelimb sleeve cast.

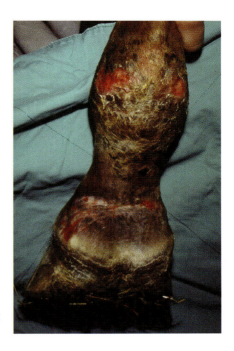

Figure 16.29. Movement-related skin sore over the proximal sesamoid bones following casting for 2 weeks.

can create space between the cast and soft tissue, thus providing the opportunity for movement-related skin sores. If the limb was markedly swollen at the time of cast application, it may be necessary to remove the cast within 48 hours and apply a new one. Breakage of the cast at the sole or phalangeal regions can also cause increased movement of the soft tissues within the cast. Other causes include foreign materials (e.g., shavings or dirt) becoming entrapped between the cast and the skin or poorly applied casts which may cause excessive pressure at bony prominences.

Signs indicating the presence of a skin sore include visual evidence of a sore at the top of the cast, excessive swelling proximal to the cast, and/or drainage. Drainage can occur at the top of the cast or seep through the cast. Increased lameness, exudate oozing through the cast, increased body temperature, and an elevated white blood cell count are all signs that indicate the presence of a full-thickness skin sore (Figure 16.30). Limiting exercise will reduce movement of the soft tissues underlying the cast and therefore decrease the risk of skin sores. The sole of the cast should be monitored daily for excess wear and disruption because protrusion of the foot through the bottom of the cast will allow motion of the phalanges, which increases the risk of developing cast sores.

The most common sites for skin sores are the top of the cast on the proximal aspect of the metacarpus and metatarsus, the plantar surface of the mid-metatarsus, the palmar and plantar surfaces of the sesamoid bones (Figure 16.29), as well as the heel bulbs and bony prominences (e.g., accessory carpal bone, calcaneal tuberosity, and distal medial aspect of the radius).[27]

Cast sores can be serious, particularly if the sore extends to involve a synovial cavity or tendon. The cast should be removed or replaced at the earliest signs of skin sores or increasing lameness.

Long Bone Fractures, Rupture of the Peroneus Tertius, and Coxofemoral Luxation

Long bone fractures have been associated with casts that terminate in the middle instead of the proximal region of the radius, tibia, metacarpal, and metatarsal regions. Terminating the cast in the middle of these long bones causes stress to concentrate at the top of the cast, making the bones susceptible to fracture.[19]

Rupture of the peroneus tertius has been seen with full hind limb casts following recovery from anesthesia and after the horse has struggled with the cast. The peroneus tertius, a component of the reciprocal apparatus, passively flexes the tarsocrural joint when the femorotibial joint is flexed. The excessive tension exerted upon the peroneus tertius when the stifle is flexed and the hock is fixed in extension within the cast is thought to be the cause of the rupture.

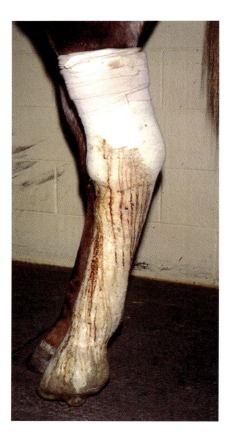

Figure 16.30. Example of a cast that is well overdue for removal and replacement if needed. The cast was applied 2 weeks earlier while at another hospital to treat a severe hock laceration. The horse was subsequently referred for evaluation.

Coxofemoral luxation has been reported in two foals following the application of either a full limb cast or a tube cast (sleeve cast) to the hind limb.[28] The coxofemoral luxation in the foal with the full limb cast was believed to occur while it was struggling to stand from being in lateral recumbency, with the cast limb up. Tube casts had been applied to all four limbs in another foal to counteract localized compressive forces occurring during ambulation. The luxation probably occurred when the foal either fell or while it was trying to stand from a recumbent position.

Long-term Complications

Long term complications related to casting include muscle atrophy, tendon laxity (particularly flexor tendons in immature horses),[29] reduced range of joint motion, bone demineralization (osteopenia), and lameness.[30] Recovery from the long-term complications associated with casting is generally proportional to the time of immobilization. While 30 days of immobilization of a joint has been shown to exert minimal effect on the biochemical content of articular cartilage,[30] 8 weeks of immobilization following 7 weeks of rehabilitation of the metacarpophalangeal joint were insufficient to restore bone density[31] or joint function or values for joint measurements (e.g., range of motion, circumference)[32] in the cast limb.

Another complication of long-term casting is contraction of the cast foot, as a consequence of the lack of weight bearing on the affected limb. In general, once the cast is removed, the foot has been properly trimmed, and the animal returns to normal weight bearing, the foot contraction resolves within a short period of time without further complications.

Cast Care

Cast complications, to a large degree, can be obviated by proper application and appropriate post-application care. This section will focus on the latter. Elastic adhesive tape (Elasticon™) should be applied to the top of the cast and to the hair proximal to the cast to prevent bedding material from entering the cast. The tape should be removed to examine the top of the cast for a rub sore; therefore it is usually changed every 3 to 4 days.

The horse should be confined to a clean, dry box stall that is protected from inclement weather. A soft pliable floor (e.g., rubber mat) that provides good footing with suitable bedding that will not accumulate around the cast is ideal. Wood shavings, sawdust, paper products, and short length straw are satisfactory bedding materials. If support limb laminitis is of concern, sand 15 cm deep can be added to the floor with bedding placed on top. The stall should be bedded with enough material to make recumbency comfortable for the horse. If uneven limb length is a problem, a piece of wood can be affixed to the bottom of a rubber boot, after which the boot is applied to the noncast foot to equalize the length of the limbs (Figure 16.27). In all cases, soiling of the cast should be avoided.

The horse should be monitored (twice daily is ideal) for rectal temperature, respiration and peripheral pulse (vital signs), appetite, fecal output, and any reluctance to use the cast limb or increased duration of recumbency.[11] Any change in vital signs and decrease in appetite may indicate pain, inflammation, or infection associated with the soft tissues underlying the cast. Palpation of the cast for evidence of looseness or local heat should be performed, particularly in areas commonly affected by movement-related skin sores. Special attention should be given to the top of the cast because this is one of the most common sites for a skin sore to develop. The cast should also be checked for cracks and excessive wear at the bottom. The support limb digital vasculature should be palpated twice daily for signs of increasing pulse pressure, which may indicate an impending laminitis.

To evaluate limb use, the horse should be walked 3 to 5 step in a straight line, then turned to the right and to the left so the cast limb is on the inside of the turn and then the outside of the turn. This will allow for observation of subtle changes in willingness to bear weight on the cast limb; a shortened stance phase of the stride, compared to that observed at the previous exam, is an indication that the horse is bearing less weight on the cast limb. Nonsteroidal anti-inflammatory agents should be used judiciously to avoid masking the signs of impending cutaneous sores.

Casting Periods

Casts are left in place for variable periods depending on their purpose and whether complications develop. For the clean, sutured, uncomplicated wound they are usually left in place for 10–14 days. If used for the treatment of tendon laceration or rupture or a joint luxation casts are usually required for 4 to 6 weeks or even longer, according to the specific situation. In general, long-term casts should be replaced and the soft tissues evaluated every 4 to 6 weeks. The growth rate of foals precludes prolonged use of a single cast and the cast should be changed in 12–14 days.[19]

The decision to remove the cast is an important one. The criteria used are: the way the horse is wearing it, the reason for its use, and whether healing has progressed to the point that the horse can bear weight on the limb without re-injury. Horses wearing casts should be observed daily as described under Cast Care.

One of the earliest signs that a cast is not being worn well is a change in the horse's weight-bearing pattern. (See Cast Complications for more details.) Later signs include pointing the foot, pawing the ground repeatedly, rubbing the outer surface of the cast on fixed objects, or biting it. Swelling of the limb above the cast usually indicates significant inflammation of the underlying soft tissues. Moisture at the top can be expected when a cast is applied over open wounds but it indicates skin sores, infection, or possible wound dehiscence when the cast was applied over a sutured wound. Specifically, a bad odor emanating from the top of the cast, moisture, and an elevated rectal temperature usually indicate infection. Ideally, the cast should be removed at the earliest signs of improper wear or use. It is better to risk premature removal of the cast than to allow a skin sore or wound dehiscence to progress to the point that the damage created by the cast is worse than the damage that initially led to its application.[10]

Cast Removal

Cast removal is performed either with the horse under general anesthesia or while it is standing. General anesthesia is preferred if the cast is being changed. On the other hand, the cast is best removed in the standing, sedated horse if this is to be the end of the cast period, since there is less chance of re-injury to the treated limb compared to that which may occur during recovery from general anesthesia. In those cases in which it is impossible to remove the cast in the standing horse, the cast should be cut evenly down the lateral and medial sides, to bisect it, so that it can be reapplied temporarily during recovery from general anesthesia if deemed necessary. Alternatively, distal limb immobilization to protect a laceration of the extensor and or flexor tendons during recovery can be provided with custom-made PVC splints or a commercially available metal splint (Kimzey™).

Prior to cast removal, the equipment needed for the procedure should be obtained (see Box 16.2). When an oscillating cast cutter (saw) is used, grooves should be cut into the surface of the cast down its medial and lateral sides, then joined by a groove made across the bottom (solar surface) of the cast. The grooves serve as markers for the ensuing full thickness cut through the cast. The cast saw should be embedded using gentle pressure until the full thickness of the cast has been penetrated. This will be perceived as a lack of resistance to the oscillation of the saw blade. Generally, this is best done at the top of the cast under which orthopedic felt has been applied. This full thickness cut is continued distad to include the proximal lateral surface of the hoof wall. The same full-thickness cut is then performed on the medial side. Finally, a full-thickness cut is made in the cast overlying the hoof and sole regions. Great care should be taken to avoid traumatizing the skin. In the standing horse, skin injury is usually accompanied by an adverse reaction (e.g., pulling the limb away or kicking). In the deeply sedated or anesthetized horse, serious injury to soft tissue, including a synovial structure, can occur. In the case of synovial involvement, the prognosis may be guarded and prompt repair is recommended.[18]

Box 16.2.

Equipment and Materials Needed for Cast Removal

Equipment for Cast Removal

- Electric extension cord
- Cast cutter (oscillating saw)
- Cast spreader
- Heavy duty scissors to cut cast padding and stockinet
- Screwdriver to help pop the acrylic off the bottom of the foot

Material to Clean and Treat the Limb

- Bucket of warm water and soap to clean the limb, plus a dry clean towel
- Sterile saline and antiseptic soap (should not have contact with open wound) to clean the wound site, plus a clean sterile towel to dry the wound site
- Suture removal scissors, if indicated
- Topical wound ointment (antiseptic or antibiotic), if indicated
- Wound dressing
- Bandage material
- Splint, if indicated

Once the full thickness of the cast has been cut, cast spreaders are used to expand the width of the saw cut to permit cast removal. As the halves of the cast are separated, heavy duty scissors can be used to cut the orthopedic felt and the stockinet. Once the cast has been removed the site of injury and the rest of the soft tissues underlying the cast should be evaluated and appropriate treatment applied. In most cases this involves washing and drying the limb, cleansing the wound, applying an appropriate dressing followed by bandaging, and in some cases splinting the limb. If another cast is to be applied, any skin sore must be cleansed and then treated with an antiseptic ointment followed by the application of wound dressing, conforming gauze, and Elasticon™ bandage. This approach protects the skin sore from further trauma and usually allows it to heal uneventfully.

Conclusion

The appropriate use of bandages and casts constitutes a very important part of successful management of wounds in horses. Bandaging not only protects the wound from further contamination, but it also limits edema and creates an environment conducive to more rapid healing.[3] The main disadvantage of bandaging wounds of the distal extremities is that it may encourage the development of exuberant granulation tissue; this problem can largely be avoided with proper wound care.

Bandage splints, and in some cases casts, can be very important components of wound management, particularly when they are used to immobilize injured tissue in a region subject to high motion (e.g., carpus and tarsus) and high tension (e.g., wound sutured under tension). In most cases, casts are preferred for the management of an injury compromising the integrity of a soft tissue support structure (e.g., flexor tendon and/or ligament).

The materials and techniques required to bandage and immobilize the most commonly affected anatomical regions in the horse have been reviewed. Information in this chapter should enable the practitioner to protect a wound from the external environment and effectively immobilize an injured site to facilitate wound healing.

References

1. Stashak TS: Selected factors that affect wound healing. In TS Stashak. ed. *Equine wound management (1st edition)*. Philadelphia: Lea and Febiger, 1991, p.19
2. Knighton DR, Silver IA, Hunt TK: Regulation of wound-healing angiogenesis. Effect of oxygen gradients and inspired oxygen concentration. Surg 1981;90:262
3. Wollen N, DeBowes RM, Liepold HW, et al: A comparison of four types of therapy for the treatment of full thickness wounds of the horse. Proc Am Assoc Equine Pract 1987;33:569
4. Fretz PB, Martin GS, Jacobs KA, et al: Treatment of exuberant granulation tissue in the horse: evaluation of four methods. Vet Surg 1983;12:137
5. Berry DB, Sullins KE: Effects of topical application of antimicrobials and bandaging on healing and granulation tissue formation in wounds of the distal aspect of the limbs in horses. Am J Vet Res 2003;64:88
6. Bertone AL: Management of exuberant granulation tissue. Vet Clin North Am Equine Pract 1989;5:551
7. Barber SM: Second intention wound healing in the horse: the effect of bandages and topical corticosteroids. Proc Am Assoc Equine Pract 1990;35:107
8. Wilmink JM, Stolk PWT, van Weeren PR, et al: Differences in second-intention wound healing between horses and ponies: macroscopical aspects. Equine Vet J 1999;31:53
9. Theoret CL, Barber SM, Moyana TN, et al: Preliminary observations on expression of transforming growth factor β1, β3, and basic fibroblast growth factor in equine limb wounds healing normally or with proud flesh. Vet Surg 2002;31:266
10. Stashak TS: Bandaging and casting techniques. In TS Stashak, ed. *Equine wound management (1st edition)*. Philadelphia: Lea and Febiger, 1991, p.258
11. Gomez JH, Hanson RR: Use of dressings and bandages in equine wound management. Vet Clin North Am Equine Pract 2005;21:91
12. Stashak TS, Farstvedt E, Othic A: Update on wound dressings: indication and best use. Clin Tech Equine Pract 2004;3:148
13. Stashak TS: Selected bandaging and casting techniques. Proc North Am Vet Conf 2007;21:212
14. Berman AT, Parks BG: A comparison of the mechanical properties of fiberglass cast materials and their clinical relevance. J Orthop Trauma 1990;4:85
15. Houlton JEF, Brearley MJ: A comparison of some casting materials. Vet Rec 1985;117:55
16. Mihalko WM, Beaudoin AJ, Krause WR: Mechanical properties and material characteristics of orthopedic casting materials. J Orthop Trauma 1989;3:57
17. Rowley DI, Pratt D, Powell ES: The comparative properties of plaster of Paris and plaster of Paris substitutes. Arch Orthop Trauma Surg 1985;103:402
18. Lindsay WA: Casting materials and techniques. In N White and J Moore, eds. *Current practice of equine surgery (1st edition)*. Philadelphia: Lippincott, 1990, p.151
19. Murray RC, DeBowes RM: Casting techniques. In AJ Nixon, ed. *Equine fracture repair (1st edition)*. Philadelphia: W.B. Saunders, 1996, p.104
20. Bartels KE, Penwick RC, Freeman LJ, et al: Mechanical testing and evaluation of eight synthetic casting materials. Vet Surg 1985;14:310

21. Bramlage LR, Embertson RM, Libbey CJ: Resin impregnated foam as a cast liner on the distal equine limb. Proc Am Assoc Equine Pract 1991;37:481
22. Booth TM, Knottenbelt DC: Distal limb casts in equine wound management. Equine Vet Edu 1999;11:273
23. Blackford JT, Latimer FG, Wan PY, et al: Treating pastern and foot lacerations with a phalangeal cast. Proc Am Assoc Equine Pract 1994;40:97
24. Janicek JC, Dabareiner RM, Honnas CM: Heel bulb lacerations in horses: 101 cases (1988–1994). J Am Vet Med Assoc 2005;226:418
25. Fitzgerald BW, Honnas CM, Plummer AE, et al: How to apply a hindlimb phalangeal cast in the standing patient and minimize complications. Proc Am Assoc Equine Pract 2006;52:631
26. Stokes M, Hendrickson DA, Wittern C: Use of an elevated boot to reduce contralateral support limb complications secondary to cast application in the horse. Equine Pract 1998;20:14
27. Stashak TS: Methods of therapy. In TS Stashak, ed. *Adams' lameness in horses (4th edition)*. Philadelphia: Lea and Febiger 1987, p.840
28. Trotter GW, Auer JA, Warwick A, et al: Coxofemoral luxation in two foals wearing hindlimb casts. J Am Vet Med Assoc 1986;189:560
29. Kelly NJ, Watrous BJ, Wagner PC: Comparison of splinting and casting on the degree of laxity induced in the thoracic limbs in young horses. Equine Pract 1987;9:10
30. Richardson DW, Clark CC: Effects of short-term cast immobilization on equine articular cartilage. Am J Vet Res 1993;54:449
31. van Harreveld PD, Lillich JD, Kawcak CE, et al: Effects of immobilization followed by remobilization on mineral density, histomorphometric features, and formation of the bones of the metacarpophalangeal joint in horses. Am J Vet Res 2002;63:276
32. van Harreveld PD, Lillich JD, Kawcak CE, et al: Clinical evaluation of the effects of immobilization followed by remobilization and exercise on the metacarpophalangeal joint in horses. Am J Vet Res 2002;63:282

Index

Page references followed by f stand for figures; page references followed by t stand for tables.